HEALTH CARE AND COST CONTAINMENT
IN THE EUROPEAN UNION

Health Care and Cost Containment in the European Union

Edited by

ELIAS MOSSIALOS and JULIAN LE GRAND

The London School of Economics and Political Science

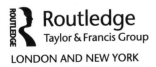

LONDON AND NEW YORK

First published 1999 by Ashgate Publishing

Reissued 2018 by Routledge
2 Park Square, Milton Park, Abingdon, Oxon, OX14 4RN
52 Vanderbilt Avenue, New York, NY 10017

Routledge is an imprint of the Taylor & Francis Group, an informa business

Copyright © Elias Mossialos, Julian Le Grand 1999

All rights reserved. No part of this book may be reprinted or reproduced or utilised in any form or by any electronic, mechanical, or other means, now known or hereafter invented, including photocopying and recording, or in any information storage or retrieval system, without permission in writing from the publishers.

Notice:
Product or corporate names may be trademarks or registered trademarks, and are used only for identification and explanation without intent to infringe.

Publisher's Note
The publisher has gone to great lengths to ensure the quality of this reprint but points out that some imperfections in the original copies may be apparent.

Disclaimer
The publisher has made every effort to trace copyright holders and welcomes correspondence from those they have been unable to contact.

A Library of Congress record exists under LC control number:

ISBN 13: 978-1-138-38591-7 (hbk)
ISBN 13: 978-0-429-42697-1 (ebk)

Contents

About the authors	*viii*
Acknowledgements	*xii*

PART ONE

1 Cost containment in the EU: an overview

Introduction	1
Section I: Health care systems	3
Section II: Health care spending	42
Section III: Cost containment measures	62
Section IV: Cost containment measures in practice	71

Elias Mossialos and Julian Le Grand

2 Cost containment and health expenditure in the EU: a macroeconomic perspective — 155
Panos Kanavos and John Yfantopoulos

3 Is there convergence in the health expenditures of the EU Member States? — 197
Adelina Comas-Herrera

PART TWO

4 Cost containment and health care reform in Belgium — 219
David Crainich and Marie-Christine Closon

5 Health care and cost containment in Denmark — 267
Terkel Christiansen, Ulrika Enemark, Jørgen Clausen and Peter Bo Poulsen

vi *Health Care and Cost Containment in the European Union*

6   Cost containment in Germany: twenty years experience   303
Reinhard Busse and Chris Howorth

7   Health care and cost containment in Greece   341
Aris Sissouras, Anthony Karokis and Elias Mossialos

8   Health care and cost containment in Spain   401
Guillem Lopez i Casasnovas

9   Twenty years of cures for the French health care system   443
Pierre-Jean Lancry and Simone Sandier

10   Health expenditure and cost containment in Ireland   471
Jenny Hughes

11   Cost containment and reforms in the Italian
National Health Service   513
Giovanni Fattore

12   Health care and cost containment in Luxembourg   547
Elias Mossialos

13   Developments in health care cost containment in
the Netherlands   573
Mirjam van het Loo, James P Kahan and Kieke G H Okma

14   Health expenditure and cost control in Austria   605
Engelbert Theurl

15   Health care reform and cost containment in Portugal   635
*João Pereira, António Correia de Campos, Francisco Ramos,
Jorge Simões and Vasco Reis*

16   Cost containment in Finnish health care   661
Unto Häkkinen

17   Health care reforms and cost containment in Sweden   701
Anders Anell and Patrick Svarvar

Contents vii

18 Cost containment and health care reforms in the British NHS 733
Giovanni Fattore

Index *783*

About the Authors

Anders Anell
Director, Swedish Institute for Health Economics, Lund, Sweden.
Associate Researcher, Centre for Business and Policy Studies, Stockholm, Sweden.

Reinhard Busse
Director, Health Care Services and Health Services Unit, Department of Epidemiology and Social Medicine, Medizinische Hochschule Hannover, Germany. Visiting Fellow, LSE Health, London School of Economics and Political Science, UK.

Guillem Lopez i Casasnovas
Professor of Economics, University Pompeu Fabra, Barcelona, Spain.

Terkel Christiansen
Professor of Economics, Centre for Health and Social Policy, Odense University, Denmark.

Jørgen Clausen
Research Assistant, Centre for Health and Social Policy, Odense University, Denmark.

Marie-Christine Closon
Professor of Economics, Centre d'Etudes Interdisciplinaires en Economie de la Santé, Université Catholique de Louvain, Belgium.

Adelina Comas-Herrera
Research Assistant, Personal Social Services Research Unit, London School of Economics and Political Science, UK.

António Correia de Campos
President, National Institute of Public Administration (INA), Portugal.

About the Authors   ix

David Crainich
Teaching Assistant in Economics, Facultés Universitaires Saint-Louis, Brussels, Belgium.

Ulrika Enemark
Assistant Professor in Economics, Centre for Health and Social Policy, Odense University, Denmark.

Giovanni Fattore
Lecturer in Public Management, Istituto di Economia Aziendale "G Zappa", Università "Luigi Bocconi", Milan, Italy. Research Associate, LSE Health, London School of Economics and Political Science, UK.

Unto Häkkinen
Research Director, Health Services Research Unit, National Research and Development Centre for Welfare and Health, Helsinki, Finland.

Chris Howorth
Research Assistant, LSE Health, London School of Economics and Political Science, UK. Research Associate, Royal Holloway School of Management, University of London, UK.

Jenny Hughes
Health Economist, Glaxo Wellcome Ireland. Former Newman Scholar in Health Economics, Centre for Health Economics, University College Dublin, Ireland.

James Paul Kahan
Senior Scientist, RAND Europe, The Netherlands.

Panos Kanavos
Lecturer in Health Policy, Department of Social Policy and Administration and LSE Health, London School of Economics and Political Science, UK.

Anthony Karokis
Research Associate, Department of Operational Research, University of Patras, Greece.

Pierre-Jean Lancry
Director, Department of Information, Research, Evaluation and Quality, l'Assistance-Publique Hôpitaux de Paris. Former Director, CREDES (Centre de Recherche, d'Etude et de Documentation en Economie de la Santé), France.

Julian Le Grand
Richard Titmuss Professor of Social Policy, Department of Social Policy and Administration, London School of Economics and Political Science. Chairman, LSE Health, UK.

Mirjam van het Loo
Research Assistant, RAND Europe, The Netherlands.

Elias Mossialos
Director, LSE Health, London School of Economics and Political Science, UK.

Kieke G H Okma
Senior Policy Advisor, Netherlands Ministry of Health, Welfare and Sport, The Netherlands.

João Pereira
Assistant Professor of Health Economics and Head of the Health and Social Sciences Department, National School of Public Health, New University of Lisbon, Portugal.

Peter Bo Poulsen
Fellow in Health Economics, Centre for Health and Social Policy, Odense University, Denmark.

Francisco Ramos
Secretary of State for Health, Portugal.

Vasco Reis
Adviser at the General Directorate of Health (Ministry of Health). Assistant Professor of Health Administration, National School of Public Health, New University of Lisbon, Portugal.

Simone Sandier
Research Director, ARGSES (Arguments Socio-Economiques pour la Santé). Former Research Director, CREDES (Centre de Recherche, d'Etude et de Documentation en Economie de la Santé), France.

Jorge Simões
Hospital Administrator, Coimbra University Hospital. Adviser to the President of the Republic, Portugal.

Aris Sissouras
Professor of Operational Research, University of Patras, Greece. Director, Institute of Social Policy, National Centre for Social Research, Athens, Greece.

Patrick Svarvar
Senior Project Manager, The Swedish Institute for Health Economics, Lund, Sweden.

Engelbert Theurl
Professor of Economics, Institut für Finanzwissenschaft der Leopold-Franzens-Universität Innsbruck, Austria..

John Yfantopoulos
Associate Professor of Social Policy, Department of Political Science and Public Administration, Athens National University, Greece.

Acknowledgements

The editors would like to acknowledge the support of the European Commission through grant SOC 95 201552 05F01 and the research assistance of Govin Permanand and Kristen Goliber. They are also grateful to the European Commission for a Human Capital and Mobility Grant ERBCHRXCT 940673, which brought together a number of European scholars to discuss issues concerned with health care and cost containment in the EU. The editors are in debt to Sarah Moncrieff for her expert help with the preparation of the manuscript.

1 Cost containment in the EU: an overview

ELIAS MOSSIALOS AND JULIAN LE GRAND

Introduction

Throughout Europe in the 1980s and early 1990s, health care was both a personal and a political priority. More and more Europeans were demanding quality health care: care that was delivered efficiently, equitably and with a due regard for the needs and wants of the patient. All Member States of the European Union have health care systems that are largely publicly funded; hence their governments faced enormous pressures to provide extra funds to meet these demands. Political debates were dominated by health issues; other government departments watched – and resented – scarce government resources being diverted to the Ministry of Health; employers and employees protested bitterly as taxes or social insurance contributions rose to meet health needs.

Moreover, government itself seemed partly to blame. More and more government officials and academic analysts subscribed to Aaron Wildavsky's Law of Medical Money: 'medical costs rise to equal the sum of all private insurance and government subsidy'. There seemed to be no mechanism by which health systems were self-stabilizing.[1] So, inevitably and unsurprisingly, most governments began to look at methods of containing their own health expenditures. Budgets for health sectors and health providers were set; restrictions on publicly funded treatment were introduced; and direct and indirect controls over health service providers were imposed. Perhaps in consequence, the growth in health spending in many countries began to slow.

However, as we approach the twenty-first century, the problem has not gone away. The growth in health care spending in most countries has indeed been reduced; but it has not stopped. Indeed in some Member States it continues to grow as fast as ever. And many of the pressures that contributed to

2 Health Care and Cost Containment in the European Union

expansion are still there; in fact some, such as the rise in public expectations, are more intense than before. It may be that the early years of the new millennium will see a resumption of uncontrolled growth in health spending. It is therefore crucial that the experience of cost containment in Europe over the last fifteen years be described and analysed, so as to understand that experience, and to determine, as best we can, which methods were successful and which were not. That is the aim of this book.

The book is divided into two parts. In Part I we provide an overview of health policies and cost containment measures in the EU Member States during the last fifteen years. This begins with two background sections: a review of some aspects of the current systems of health care in the European Union, and a review of recent expenditure trends. The next section provides a new method of classifying cost containment measures. The following section uses this classification scheme to summarise the measures adopted by the different Member States and discusses such evidence as exists concerning their impact. It endeavours to draw some conclusions about the effectiveness of different measures: inevitably, given the methodological and data difficulties involved, these are rather tentative. Additional chapters examine the determinants of health expenditure trends in the EU, and whether there is convergence in these trends.

Part II complements the first, examining in detail cost containment policies in each EU Member State. The authors of the country-based chapters were given a specific framework and guidelines to produce their chapters. The aim was to address similar questions and issues and have a standardised structure. However, inevitably there has been some divergence in the way different authors decided to analyse and examine some of the policies and issues. Their analyses reflect particular priorities in different countries and the authors' own preferences and style. The country-based chapters refer to developments up to mid-1997.

I : Health care systems

Health care systems within the European Union have fundamental similarities; on the other hand, they also differ in a bewildering variety of ways. By way of background to the rest of this book, in this chapter we summarize some of the principal differences and similarities. We concentrate on eight key areas: finance, provision, payment systems for hospitals and doctors, the supply of doctors, the extent of patient choice and three areas where there previously has been little comparative information: dental care, out of hospital care and the regulation of pharmaceuticals.

1.1 Finance

This section begins with a general discussion of sources of finance for health care expenditure. It is followed by sub-sections looking in more detail at the three principal sources of funding: taxation and social insurance, voluntary health insurance and direct payments or charges.

1.1.1 Sources of finance

The principal sources of health care finance in the EU Member States are presented in Tables 1.1 and 1.2. Table 1.1 (overleaf) shows the sources of funding in selected Member States in the 1980s and Table 1.2 (page 6) the sources of funding in the 1990s. The data presented in the tables are those provided by the authors of the country chapters in this volume, unless otherwise stated. There are two limitations to the tables: it was not always possible to report data for the same year, and data for three countries (Austria, Ireland and Italy) were not available for the 1980s.

Most countries rely primarily on taxation or social insurance contributions. But it is worth noting that private expenditure in the form of direct payments is high in Greece (40 per cent of total funding), Italy (31 per cent), Portugal (37 per cent) and Finland (21 per cent). It is also relatively high in Belgium (17 per cent), Denmark (17 per cent), France (17 per cent), Sweden (17 per cent) and Spain (16 per cent). The systems of charging vary signif-

4   *Health Care and Cost Containment in the European Union*

Table 1.1 Sources of health care finance in the EU in the 1980s (percentages)

EU Member State	Taxation	Social insurance	Voluntary health insurance (VHI)	User charges*	Other
Belgium (1987)	39.0	36.0	–	12	13
Denmark (1987)	84.5	–	–	15.5 (including VHI)	–
West Germany (1986)	10.8	64.8	6.6	7.4	10.5
Greece (1987)	33.7	25.4	–	40.9	–
Spain (1986)	19.0	59.3	4.8	15.3	1.6
France** (1985)	5.2	73.2	5.4 (*Mutuelles*)	14.8 ***	–
Luxembourg (1985)	29.1	59.2	–	8.9	2.7
Netherlands (1990)	10.0	65.0	16.0	9.0	–
Portugal (1980)	66.0	5.2	0.6	28.2	–
Finland (1990)	73.0	10.8	3.6	12.6	–
Sweden (1985)	81.4 ****	8.7	negligible	10.0	–
UK (1987/8)	78.8	12.9	5.4	2.9	–

Notes:
* including direct payments
** research, training, administrative and preventive care costs not included.
*** includes VHI.
**** includes 63.8 per cent local taxes and 17.6 per cent general taxes.

Sources: Authors' research based on data provided by the authors of the country chapters of this book and Hills,1995[2] for the UK.

The European Union: Health Care Systems   5

icantly from country to country and this is discussed in more detail below.

The picture becomes slightly different if premiums to voluntary health insurance (VHI) are added to direct payments. For instance, private expenditure expressed in these terms accounts for 19 per cent of total expenditure in Denmark, 23 per cent in Spain, 24 per cent in France, 22 per cent in Ireland, 22 per cent in the Netherlands, 22 per cent in Austria and 9 per cent in the UK.

Table 1.3 (page 8) summarizes the main methods of financing health care, illustrates their main variants and gives examples from the EU Member States.

1.1.2 Taxation and social insurance

In eight countries the principal source of funding is taxation. This takes the form of mainly central taxation (Spain, Portugal, Ireland and the UK), mainly local taxation (Denmark and Sweden), a combination of central and local taxation (Finland), and of general taxation with payroll taxes (Italy). Even where rights to health care are not based on the payment of employee and employer insurance contributions, payroll contributions may still be collected and used for health services as in Italy, Sweden, Finland and the UK.

The taxes in this group are mainly general in form. Hypothecated taxation is not very important in most EU Member States with the exception of Italy, where payroll and other earmarked taxes accounted for 36.7 per cent of total funding in 1995. Hypothecated taxes based on income also exist in the UK, Sweden and Finland, but they do not exceed more than 15 per cent of total funding. In Belgium hypothecated taxes – including so-called 'sin' taxes: taxes on alcohol and tobacco products – account for about 5 per cent of the total funding of health care. Austria is currently planning to introduce hypothecated sin taxes on a small scale.

Other member states rely more heavily on insurance of one kind or another. In the Netherlands the system is mainly financed by a mixture of social and private insurance. Those (about 40 per cent of the population) exceeding an income ceiling have to leave the statutory sickness funds and are encouraged to join a voluntary health insurance scheme. Only 1 per cent choose not to join a scheme – mainly the very wealthy. In Belgium and Greece finance is by a mixture of taxation and social insurance, with the proportion of public expenditure financed by social insurance being about half in Belgium and slightly under half in Greece. The majority of health

6   *Health Care and Cost Containment in the European Union*

Table 1.2 Sources of health care finance in the EU in the 1990s (percentages)

EU Member State	Taxation	Social insurance	Voluntary health insurance	User charges (including direct payments)	Other
Belgium (1994)	38	36	–	17	9 (a)
Denmark (1996)	80.7	–	1.9	17.4	–
Germany (1995)	11.0	64.8	7.1 (b)	7.3	9.8 (c)
Greece (1992)	33.3	24.1	2.1	40.4	–
Spain (1995)	59.3	15.3	7.0	16.3	1.7
France (d) (1994)	3.6	71.6	7.0 (*Mutuelles*)	16.5 (e)	1.3
Ireland (1993)	68.1	7.3	8.6 (f)	13.9	2.1 (g)
Italy (1995)	64.6 (h)	-	2.6	31.2	2.4 (h)
Luxembourg (1992)	30.0	49.8	2.0	7.9	2.8
Netherlands (1996)	10.0	68.0 (i)	15.0	7.1 (includes other sources)	–
Austria (1992)	24.0	54.0	7.5	14.0	–
Portugal (1995)	55.2	6.0	1.4	37.4	–
Finland (1994)	62.2 (j)	13.0	2.2	20.8	1.8 (k)
Sweden (1993)	69.7 (l)	13.4 (m)	negligible	16.9	–
UK (1993/4)	78.8	12.3 (n)	5.6 (o)	3.2 (p)	–

Notes and *Sources* – see facing page.

The European Union: Health Care Systems 7

Notes:

(a) Includes premiums for voluntary insurance, VAT and hypothecated taxes.
(b) This percentage includes premiums of those who have joined private health insurance funds.
(c) Includes accident insurance, retirement funds expenditure, direct expenditure by employers.
(d) Research, training, administrative and preventive care costs not included.
(e) Includes VHI.
(f) Includes VHI expenditure, other non-household expenditure and private capital expenditure.
(g) Includes receipts under EU regulations, i.e. European Social Fund, European Regional Fund.
(h) General taxation accounts for 27.9 per cent and payroll and earmarked taxes for 36.7 per cent. 'Other' are regional revenues.
(i) Includes the compulsory exceptional medical expenses scheme (AWBZ), which covers the entire population for long-term care.
(j) National government: 29.2 per cent, municipalities: 33 per cent.
(k) Includes private insurance, direct expenditure by employers and relief funds expenditure.
(l) Includes 64.2 per cent local taxes and 5.5 per cent general taxes.
(m) Social insurance (payroll earmarked tax).
(n) Earmarked tax (National Insurance).
(o) Private health insurance premiums and other private medical payments (grossed up from Family Expenditure Survey data).
(p) Mainly prescription charges.

Sources: Authors' research based on data provided by the authors of the country chapters of this book and Hills, 1995[2] for the UK.

---

care for the compulsorily insured is financed by social insurance contributions in Germany, France, Luxembourg and Austria. The German health system is financed through a social insurance system separated from the government in terms of revenue collection and micro charging levels. The role of the state in social provision and financing of health care services is largely restricted to providing a regulatory framework within which this provision takes place.[3] There are nearly 800 social sickness funds (*Gesetzlichen Krankenversicherung* – GKV) all of which are independent, non-profit-making organizations. Eighty-eight per cent of the population have membership in the sickness funds; 75 per cent are compulsory members of these organizations and 13 per cent voluntary members.[3] The provision of health care is on a 'payment in kind' or third party payer principle,

8   *Health Care and Cost Containment in the European Union*

Table 1.3 Financing health care: sources of funding, main versions and examples in the EU Member States

Sources of funding	Main versions	Examples in the EU Member States
Taxation	Central, local, both	Mainly central: UK, Ireland, Portugal, Spain Mainly local: Denmark, Sweden Mixed (local and central): Finland
Hypothecated taxes	Income related taxes, Sin taxes, other taxes	Income-related taxes: Italy, Finland, Sweden, UK (National Insurance) 'Sin' taxes: Belgium, Austria
Social insurance	Single fund, multiple funds	There are a Union of Sickness Funds and 9 other funds in Luxembourg, about 800 separate funds in Germany and 5 federations of funds in Belgium. In Greece, 84% of the population is covered by 2 funds and in France 75% of the population is in one fund. In Austria there are 15 nationwide funds organized on occupational lines
Top-up voluntary health insurance provided by sickness funds/social insurance	Covers co-payments, upgraded hospital facilities and better access to services	Insurance funds in the Netherlands and Belgium
User charges	Flat rate, deductible, percentage of price/fee	Deductibles in Sweden and the Netherlands, flat rates in the UK Percentage of price/fee in most other countries
Voluntary health insurance	Supplementary to statutory health insurance	Several countries
	Substitutes for statutory health insurance	Germany (~10% of the population) Netherlands (40% of the population)

Source: Authors' research.

The European Union: Health Care Systems   9

and most specialist out patient care is carried out through ambulatory physicians. The 13 per cent of the population who are voluntary members of the GKV are persons who are entitled to choose to be insured in the GKV, with private health insurers or not at all (only 0.3 per cent of the population elect to have no insurance). Sixty per cent of the privately insured persons (that is, 6 per cent of the population) are effectively ineligible to take GKV cover.* A further 2 per cent of the population is covered under free governmental health care. From these figures it may be seen that the Social Health Insurance scheme in Germany enjoys a high degree of acceptance within the population.[3] This support for the social scheme is often seen as a sign of the high quality of the German sickness funds but it is argued by Busse *et al.*[3] that the possibility of steep rises in premium level** and the fact that each additional family member must be paid for under private insurance (unlike the social sickness insurance) are additional factors which must be considered.

In some countries there have been significant changes during the last 15 years. In Spain general taxation replaced social insurance as the predominant source of funding. In most countries the role of voluntary health insurance increased moderately and direct payments as revenue generating mechanisms increased significantly in many countries. We discuss each of these in more detail below.

1.1.3 Voluntary health insurance

Voluntary health insurance, although not yet significant in many EU Member States, is a growing sector in most of them. The coverage of the population ranges from under 0.5 per cent in Sweden to more than 85 per cent in France. However, these figures are misleading since both the concept and the coverage of VHI differ significantly from country to country.

There are two main types of VHI in the European Union. First, there is VHI that substitutes for, and is mutually exclusive from, the statutory health insurance scheme (Germany and the Netherlands). Second, there is VHI that

---

* These are *Beamte*, roughly translated as civil (public) servants, and include police officers, university professors and other public officials with decision-making powers.[3]

** Persons who leave the social health insurance scheme are ineligible to return to it unless their income falls below the statutory minimum.

10   *Health Care and Cost Containment in the European Union*

is supplementary to public entitlement (most other countries). The insurers may be both non-profit and for-profit. This is the case in France where the *Mutuelles* (supplementary insurance funds) coexist with private for-profit insurers, although they cover different benefits. In Belgium and the Netherlands additional VHI is offered by both the sickness funds and private insurers.

Most VHI companies or organizations contract with providers and pay them directly. Others reimburse patients' expenses or co-payments (as in France). In a number of cases VHI companies own networks of doctors and hospitals. This is the case of *Seguro de Assistencia Sanitaria* companies in Spain which could be considered as US-style Health Maintenance Organizations. The British United Provident Association (BUPA) and Private Patients Plan (PPP) Healthcare in the UK are hospital owners. PPP Healthcare recently formed a joint venture with Columbia/HCA Healthcare, the largest provider of health care in the US, to take a 50 per cent stake in four major London private hospitals.

VHI companies provide cash benefits, benefits in kind, accident insurance, critical illness coverage and coverage for long-term care. But the mixture and the weight of different kinds of insurance products differ considerably from one country to another, and their analysis is beyond the scope of this overview. However, it is worth noting that many insurance companies have recently changed their products in a number of EU countries, usually replacing the provision of luxurious private hospital care with budget plans that are fixed cash payments. The role of VHI in each EU Member State is further analysed and examined in section IV of this chapter.

1.1.4 Co-payments

Two main forms of co-payment have been implemented in the Member States: a percentage of payment, and deductibles. In the latter case the insured bears a fixed amount and any amount in excess is borne by government or the insurer. Deductibles can apply to specific cases or for a certain period of time (usually a financial year or a year since the first payment by the insured).

Two countries apply deductibles as a form of co-payment. In Sweden the deductible applies to the whole population and for all services, though people suffering from diabetes mellitus are exempted. This raises serious

The European Union: Health Care Systems   11

equity issues especially for the young, the unemployed, the elderly and single parent families. In the Netherlands, as of 1997, all ZWF (sickness funds) insured as well as privately insured face a co-insurance of 20 per cent of medical costs up to a maximum of NLG 200/ECU 93.47; or NLG 100/ECU 46.73 for people dependent on social security income. This co-payment is waived for GP visits, dental care (when covered) and hospital costs of pregnancy. The government is planning to abandon deductibles and introduce income-related co-payments in the near future.

In 1995, 10 per cent of the French population received completely free health care because they had no means to pay the usual co-payments.[4] In Spain there is a co-payment ceiling per prescription for chronically ill patients. In 1996, this was set at PTE 439 /ECU 2.24. In Sweden the ceiling for total patient co-payments in most county councils (except for in-patient and dental care) is SEK 2,400/ECU 282 per year. There are plans to exclude all those over 20 years old from free dental care, although pregnant women and the mentally ill are exempted. Since 1992 the county councils have no responsibility for chronically ill patients. Instead, the communities charge patients for long-term care. The charge differs according to the income of the patient, rising to a maximum of SEK 1,000 per day (on average SEK 600/ECU 70.50). Very poor elderly people are excluded from paying for long-term care.

Irish health care policy follows the principle of giving full eligibility for all necessary services free of charge to the lowest income group, and of providing necessary services to those outside this group at a cost they can afford.[5] On the basis of this principle two groups of people have been defined; those with full eligibility (Category I) and those with limited eligibility (Category II).[6] Full eligibility entitles patients to a full range of publicly financed health services as well as to all prescribed drugs and medicines listed in the General Medical Services (GMS) code book. The decision on which individuals are classified as Category I is means tested and depends mainly on a person's financial and family circumstances, though chronic illnesses may also be taken into account. 35.8 per cent of the population was classified as Category I in 1995. Category II patients are liable to user charges for general practitioner services and prescribed drugs. However, Category II patients are entitled to a refund from the health board in excess of IEP 90/ECU 113.42 in co-payments for pharmaceutical care in 1996. Those without medical cards but certified as having need for regular ongoing medical treatment can apply to the health board to receive autho-

12 *Health Care and Cost Containment in the European Union*

rization to pay only up to IEP 32/ECU 40.33 per month.

In Germany there is a ceiling for total patient co-payments (except for in-patient and dental care). This is equal to 2 per cent of income for mandatory members of sickness funds and 4 per cent of income for voluntary members of sickness funds. In general, children and low income people are exempted from co-payments. Such an exemption structure makes cost sharing in Germany socially tolerable. In Portugal patients suffering from chronic diseases (diabetes, cancer, asthma and so on) and pensioners whose pension is below the national minimum wage enjoy a 15 per cent reduction in the co-payment rate for pharmaceutical care (the rates are 15/45 per cent). However, their prescriptions have to be authorized and dispensed in a hospital. For GP and specialist consultations, the flat rate co-payment does not apply to pensioners with pensions lower than the minimum wage, persons with low family income (unemployed and those receiving supplementary income benefits), pregnant women, children under 12 years, the disabled, patients suffering from a number of chronic diseases and drug addicts on recovery programmes. In Greece only some pharmaceuticals, especially those for long-term illnesses, are excluded from co-payments.

In Belgium preferential treatment is given to several groups, including the disabled, pensioners, widows/widowers and orphans (VIPOs), unemployed and low income families. There is also an income protection scheme. Co-payment levels for the above groups are much lower compared with other categories. In addition, if cost-sharing expenditure exceeds an annual ceiling then insurance picks up the full cost of treatment above this ceiling. This ceiling is linked to the household income. Cost sharing for pharmaceuticals is not included in the ceiling. In Denmark pensioners, low income families and the disabled are either exempted from co-payments or pay reduced co-payment rates. Catagories of people exempted from co-payments vary between municipalities. Individuals can apply directly to the National Board of Health to ask for exemption from charges for pharmaceutical care. In Austria low income people are exempt from co-payments and in Luxembourg the social assistance scheme or the local social services offices cover the co-payment of those with insufficient income. A 1986 law established a minimum income level for each household depending on the age and number of its members. Medical examinations of pregnant women are also fully covered.

In Finland there is no cost sharing for a number of services including hospital treatment for those under 18, dental care for those under 19, pre-

The European Union: Health Care Systems   13

ventive care and immunizations, treatment of some communicable diseases and psychiatric ambulatory care. Registered individuals suffering from certain specified diseases qualify for 75 to 100 per cent reimbursement of pharmaceutical costs in excess of a fixed charge of FIM 25/ECU 4.29. In Italy those under 6 years and those over 65 are exempted from user charges for pharmaceuticals if household income is under ITL 70 million/ECU 3,573. People under 10 years and those over 60 are exempted from user charges for specialist care if household income is under ITL 70 million. In 1994 a co-payment applied to only 11.9 per cent of the drugs included in the positive list, which amounted to 14.1 per cent of pharmaceutical expenditure for the products included in the list. Approximately 40 per cent of the marketed drugs in Italy are not reimbursed. Co-payments for specialist care accounted for 42.2 per cent of total expenditure in 1994. In the same year, 34.5 per cent of the population was exempted from co-payment for specialist care.[7]

Finally, in the UK exemptions from prescription charges include those under 16 or full-time students under 19, those aged 60 or over, those receiving income support or on low incomes, pregnant women or those who had a baby during the previous 12 months, those receiving a war or Ministry of Defence disablement pension and those suffering from a specified medical condition. NHS dental treatment is provided free of charge if treatment starts when the recipient is under 18 or is a full-time student under 19. In addition, those on Disability Working Allowance, Income Support, Income-based Job Seekers Allowance or Family Credit schemes, and pregnant women or women who had a baby during the previous 12 months, are entitled to free dental care. Low income people and war pensioners may get help with the cost of dental treatment. Several population groups are also exempted from user charges for NHS sight tests, the cost of eye-glasses or contact lenses, NHS wigs and fabric supports, and NHS hospital travel costs.

1.2 Provision

Many EU health care systems are based on a combination of state finance and state provision. That is, the state not only finances much health care but also owns and operates the principal agents of health care delivery, such as hospitals, primary care centres, ambulance services and so on. For instance,

14 *Health Care and Cost Containment in the European Union*

hospital beds are over 90 per cent publicly owned in Denmark, Sweden, Finland and the United Kingdom, between 80 and 90 per cent publicly owned in Italy and Portugal, and over 50 per cent publicly owned in Spain, France, Greece and Ireland.

Elsewhere there is greater variety. Only about half of hospital beds are publicly owned in Germany and most of the remainder are owned by non-profit hospitals. In Belgium, Luxembourg and the Netherlands most of the acute hospitals are private. In Belgium and Luxembourg, and in private hospitals in France, the doctor is normally separately paid on a fee-for-service basis for services supplied to in-patients. Elsewhere, the hospital pays its doctors on a salary basis.

Some of the tax-financed, state-provided systems are experimenting with independence for their own providers coupled with a greater use of private or non-profit providers operating in market or quasi-market systems of delivery. The most comprehensive reform of this kind was the internal market introduced in the United Kingdom in 1991; however, Sweden, Italy and Finland are also encouraging local purchasers (counties, local health units or municipalities) to experiment with new provider patterns. Also, payers in some insurance based systems are being transformed into purchasers of services and imposing budgets on each contracted health sector. In Greece and Portugal, private services are contracted to supplement those owned by insurers. Portugal is also planning a more general separation of purchasers from providers. This will be done through the enhancement of the role of regional agencies which currently have an advisory role on resource allocation, quality assurance and planning. The current position with respect to integrated and contracted systems is summarized in Table 1.4.

As the product of perhaps some of the most radical changes in recent years, the UK's system is worth describing in more detail. Under the Conservative Government reforms of 1991, most secondary care providers remained publicly owned, but were constituted as independent 'trusts' with their own budgets and decision-making powers. They contracted with two kinds of purchasers: a health authority, commissioning services for the population of a fixed geographical area; and GP fundholders, primary care practitioners who were given a budget to purchase certain kinds of secondary care (mostly elective surgery) for the patients on their practice lists. In theory both kinds of purchasers could shift contracts from provider to provider in order to obtain better services. In practice it tended to be the GP fundholders who were more flexible in this regard;[9] and when the Labour

The European Union: Health Care Systems   15

Table 1.4 Principal methods of providing services in the EU Member States in 1997

EU Member State	Integrated services	Contracted services
Belgium		All services
Denmark	Hospitals in a small number of counties	Hospitals in most counties, GPs, specialists outside hospitals, most dentists and physiotherapists, pharmacies
Germany		All services
Greece	Doctors, hospitals	Pharmacies, few private hospitals, most dentists, many private doctors
Spain	Specialists, hospitals, 60% of GPs	Pharmacies, dentists and private hospitals
France		All services
Ireland	Public hospitals, specialists	Private non-profit hospitals, GPs, pharmacies
Italy	Public hospitals, specialists	Private hospitals, GPs and private specialists, pharmacies
Luxembourg		All services
Netherlands		All services (since 1994, sickness funds may selectively contract with doctors)
Austria		All services
Portugal	GPs, some specialists, public hospitals	Private hospitals, some doctors in rural areas, pharmacies, labs for X-ray and pathology, most dentists
Finland	Health centres	Hospitals, pharmacies, private out-patient care services
Sweden	Health centres, pharmacies, 60% of dentists	Hospitals, private doctors (8% of doctors), private hospitals (approximately 1% of beds), 50% of dentists
UK	Community services	Public hospitals, GPs, private hospitals, most dentists, pharmacies

Sources: Authors' research, Abel-Smith and Mossialos, 1994.[8]

16   *Health Care and Cost Containment in the European Union*

Government was elected in 1997, it was not surprising that (despite some rhetoric to the contrary) they decided to build on this aspect of the previous government's reforms. Under Labour's proposals, the purchaser/provider split and independent trusts are to be retained.[10] Purchasers will now be so-called Primary Care Groups, groups that, like health authorities, will cater for specific geographical areas (although much smaller ones) but, like GP fundholding, will be GP-led. The process of implementation is due to begin in April 1999.

1.3 Payment systems: hospitals

The methods of financing hospitals in the EU Member States have changed significantly over the last 15 years. There is a clear move from open-ended retrospective funding of hospital activities to the establishment of prospective budgets. In some countries hospital activities or functions are taken into account in setting the budget. Other countries use case-mix payments. These are either based on Diagnosis Related Groups (DRGs) or on purchaser-provider contractual agreements.

There are four main types of hospital financing in the EU Member States. They are:

- prospective budgets mainly based on historical spending (Denmark, Greece and France);

- prospective budgets based on hospital activities or functions (Germany, Ireland, Luxembourg, the Netherlands and Portugal);

- prospective budgets combined with activity-related payments. In this case part of the hospital expenditure is fixed and another part is not budgeted (Belgium, Spain and Austria); and

- activity-related payments, which may be case-mix-based payments (Sweden and Italy) or purchasing packages of hospital services (the UK and Finland).

This is summarized in Table 1.5. However, this mostly reflects the current situation and does not deal with any planned changes. These are discussed in more detail below.

Table 1.5 Payment systems for health care providers in the European Union

EU Member State	Hospitals: prospective budgets	Activity or service-related payments	Payment of first contact doctor and access to specialist services
Belgium	Prospective budget for hotel costs and clinical biology. No budget for medical acts	All Patients DRGs for nursing activities	Fee-for-service
Denmark	Prospective global budgets	Experiments with DRGs – but probable use for measuring and comparing productivity	Mixed: capitation and fee-for-service. Extra billing for Group 2 patients (2.5% of the population) Group 1 (97.5% of the population) – R – no referral is required for ear, nose and throat specialists and ophthalmologists Group 2 (2.5% of the population)
Germany	3 types of prospective budgets		Fee-for-service
Greece	Prospective budgets	Plans to introduce activity-related payments	Salary (NHS doctors), fee-for-service (private doctors)
Spain	10 regions: prospective global budgets combined with activity-related payments	Catalonia: case-mix adjustments, Andalucía: experiment with DRGs, Basque Country: activity-related payments	60% GPs salary and capitation, 40% GPs capitation, R

Note: R: Access to specialist services by referral.

Table 1.5 (continued) Payment systems for health care providers in the European Union

EU Member State	Hospitals: prospective budgets	Activity or service-related payments	Payment of first contact doctor and access to specialist services
France	Prospective global budgets to be gradually combined with activity-related payments		Fee-for-service. Extra billing for Sector 2 doctors (26% of total office-based doctors); 12.5% of doctors joined a new scheme of 'médecin référant'
Ireland	Prospective global budgets; Case-mix (DRG type) measures define part of the budget		Capitation plus fee-for-service for special services (General Medical Services Scheme (GMS) – 1/3 of the population), R, fee-for-service (Category II eligibility)
Italy		Activity-related payments	Capitation plus fee-for-service for special services, R
Luxembourg	Prospective global budgets combined with activity-related payments		Fee-for-service
Netherlands	Prospective functional budgets taking into account hospital activities		Capitation (low income), fee-for-service (high income), R
Austria	Prospective fixed budget for part of hospital activities	case-mix (DRG type)-based payments	Fee-for-service combined with capitation

The European Union: Health Care Systems 19

EU Member State	Hospitals: prospective budgets	Activity or service-related payments	Payment of first contact doctor and access to specialist services
Portugal	Prospective global budgets taking into account hospital activities	Case-mix (DRG type) activity-related payments to be introduced	Salary, R. No referral is required for civil servants, personnel of the military forces and bank employees
Finland		Purchasing of packages of hospital services. DRG-based prices are being developed	Salary, some capitation, R. No referral is required for private specialist care covered by National Sickness Insurance
Sweden	Case-mix systems and prospective per case payments (mostly based on DRGs) complemented by price, volume and quality controls		Salary, private doctors on a regulated fee-for-service basis. Mixed capitation and regulated fee-for-service payment for the family doctor system in some counties. Referral is not mandatory. There is direct access to specialists in many counties at a higher fee
UK		Activity-related annual purchaser/provider contracts	Capitation, some expenses (staff and premises costs) are reimbursed directly. GPs receive target payments for achieving particular levels of coverage for childhood immunization and cervical cytology screening, R

Note: R: Access to specialist services by referral.
Source: Authors' research.

20   *Health Care and Cost Containment in the European Union*

1.3.1 Prospective budgets based on historical spending

In two of the three countries which fall under this category, Greece and France, activity or function-related payments are being gradually introduced or are planned.

In Greece prospective budgets for each hospital are set on a historical basis but they are always overshot. There are plans to introduce activity-related payments for major diseases and interventions. These plans may not be implemented in the near future because of the lack of appropriate information systems and patient records.

In France prospective global hospital budgets were established in 1984. Since 1996, regional hospital agencies are responsible for allocating funds to individual hospitals on the basis of the overall regional budget. The agencies negotiate contracts with individual hospitals. Negotiated contracts take into account the relative hospital costs and activity levels and last for three to five years. They also outline development programmes on the basis of the General Regional Health Organization Plans (SROS). Although there is no fixed budget for private hospitals, regional agencies sign contracts with them. These contracts outline activity levels and specify agreed spending targets.

In Denmark since 1993, contracts have been gradually introduced between counties and individual hospitals. Tenders for the treatment of patient groups have also been introduced. From the early 1980s, global prospective hospital budgets at the county level replaced the former highly specified budget for each hospital. Small investments are made out of the current budget. More significant investments require specific allocation at the county level. The budget reflects historical trends and its annual setting involves a highly political negotiation process. DRGs have been tried on an experimental basis; however, if their use is extended, this will probably be more for measuring and comparing hospital productivity than for paying hospitals.

1.3.2 Prospective budgets based on hospital activities or functions

In Germany there were three types of prospective budgets until 1997. Type I budgets included 70 case-related fees (25 per cent of all cases) covering full costs of combinations of specific diagnosis and interventions. Type II included 150 procedure fees covering specific interventions. Type III included all other cases, which were reimbursed on a per diem basis covering non-medical costs and a clinical department charge covering medical costs. There were also combinations of Type II and Type III budgets.

There were spending targets with different adjustment factors. For case-related fees the hospital received 50 per cent of the fee when it delivered less or more than the agreed volume. For per diem payments, if the hospital delivered more than the agreed patient days, it could keep 25 per cent and refund 75 per cent of the fixed daily rate. If it delivered less then the hospital still received 75 per cent of the agreed daily rate for the non-delivered days. This 75 per cent reflects the fixed production costs. Finally, for each case and procedure a number of points were allocated by the Ministry of Health. The monetary conversion factor was negotiated at the state level. The per diems were negotiated between the sickness funds and each hospital.

The growth rate of these budgets was linked to the growth rate of contributions to health insurance. Early in 1997, the fixed hospital budgets were replaced by individually negotiated target budgets. Joint committees of doctors and sickness funds, and not the Ministry of Health, are responsible for determining the list of prospective case and procedure fees.

In Ireland, there are three different types of hospital payments. Voluntary Public Hospitals receive annual funding directly from the Department of Health. Voluntary health insurance has introduced ceilings for private hospitals' budgets. If the ceiling is exceeded then the hospital is paid on a system based on variant marginal cost pricing (25 to 40 per cent of actual cost). Budgets for Health Board hospitals are determined by Health Boards on a historical expenditure basis adjusted for inflation, pay awards and projected changes in service provision. Since 1993, case-mix measures (DRGs) are taken into account in setting part of the hospital budget.

In Luxembourg prospective budgets take into account activity-related payments (not linked with specific diagnosis), non-activity-related payments for hospital maintenance and lump-sum payments for specific treatments. In the Netherlands historical budgets were replaced in 1988 by functional budgets. The functions on which the budgets are defined include medical function (diagnosis and treatment), hotel function, specialized services (such as cardiac surgery) which also provide care to those living outside the hospitals' catchment area, and a 'settlement' function related to infrastructure (energy, maintenance and so on). Medical and hotel functions are part

22 *Health Care and Cost Containment in the European Union*

of the budget negotiated with the health insurance agencies, whereas the compensation for special services and the settlement function are determined by the Central Agency for Health Care Tariffs (GOTG). In 1992 the rate for day care visits was raised and weighted rates for admissions and first out-patient visits were introduced.

In Portugal in 1996, prospective budgets for individual hospitals were introduced taking into account hospital activities and planning priorities. DRGs have been developed and are to be implemented. In 1998, 20 per cent of the hospital budget was based on DRGs. A Hospital Monitoring Agency has been established in Lisbon and similar organizations have been created in all other regional authorities. Their role is to monitor hospital activities on behalf of consumers and help hospitals plan their activities, including budgets. From the early 1990s, insurance companies were billed by hospitals on a DRG based system. However, most of them failed to fulfil their obligations and as a result hospital deficits increased.

1.3.3 Prospective budgets combined with activity-related payments

In Belgium there are two different types of prospective global budgets for costs of patient days: for accommodation costs and for nursing activities based on APDRGs (All Patients Diagnosis Related Groups). There is no budget for medical activities (including surgical operations) which are paid on a fee-for-service basis.

In Spain, in the ten regions which are centrally managed, there are agreements that link global hospital budgets with activity-related payments on the basis of resource-weighted health care units (UPAs). In Catalonia payments are based on case-mix adjustments (mostly based on DRGs) but their real impact is still marginal. In Andalucía there are experiments with DRGs. In the Basque Country there are activity-related payments (patient management categories). Nonetheless, in all regions, although the financing system is supposed to be prospective, in practice it is still retrospective.

Since 1997 in Austria, a case-mix system based on DRGs has been utilized. From 1991 the cost of hospital treatment per case was collected in 20 hospitals, and on the basis of this information homogeneous groups of patients were derived. A regression tree algorithm was used to construct cost-homogeneous groups. There are additional elements taken into account to calculate hospital payments, which include specific allocations for day surgery, long-term care and use of intensive care units. At federal level the Hospital Co-ordination Fund (HCF) allocates funds to different provinces according to the number of inhabitants, the number of hospital days, training needs and hospital deficits. The health insurance funds allocate resources as block transfers to different provinces based on the number of days of care in their hospitals. This system is expected to change in 1998. The part of the hospital budget allocated by the HCF and health insurance can be considered as a prospective fixed budget. An additional part, which is not fixed, is funded by the provinces and local communities. Provincial hospital committees allocate budgets to individual hospitals.

1.3.4 Activity-related payments

In Italy until 1992, hospitals were managed by local health authorities and were funded on the basis of historical spending. After the 1992 reforms hospitals should have been funded on a per case basis. However, in practice the actual impact of the new method of funding is marginal.

In Finland since 1993, municipalities have purchased packages of hospital services and have been gradually moving into a DRG-based pricing system. Prices differ between municipalities and there are no national guidelines. In theory there may be competition between providers, but in practice this does not happen.

In Sweden there are significant variations between county councils. In about 50 per cent of the county councils there are case-mix systems and prospective per case payments (predominantly based on DRGs) complemented by price, volume and quality controls. In some cases per diem payments complement per case payments. Psychiatric, primary and geriatric care are reimbursed through a combination of global budgets and fee-for-service payments. There are significant variations in payment systems between county councils and hospitals.

In the UK, since the 1991 internal market reforms, hospitals have been funded by Health Authorities on the basis of annual block contracts, and by GP fundholders usually on cost-per-case contracts. In theory, both kinds of purchaser are free to choose providers from the NHS hospitals and the private sector. In practice, with some exemptions, actual hospital funding by Health Authorities (who provide the bulk of such funding) is mainly based on historical spending which is taken into account in the annual negotia-

24 *Health Care and Cost Containment in the European Union*

tions. Private hospital contracting is negligible. Both kinds of purchaser are to be replaced in 1999 by Primary Care Groups: GP-led purchasing groups covering up to 100,000 people.

1.4 Payment systems: doctors

Table 1.5 also indicates the method of paying office-based or point of first contact doctors. In three countries (Ireland, Italy and the UK) they are paid on a capitation basis, in four by salary (Greece, Portugal, Finland and Sweden), in four by fee-for-service (Belgium, Germany, France and Luxembourg), though France also has about 2000 health centres with salaried doctors. Portugal is planning to introduce a capitation scheme in 1998. In France, the office based doctors convention introduced a voluntary scheme in 1987 which offered the possibility to doctors of becoming 'médecin référants'. Patients who join this scheme have a moral commitment not to visit a specialist directly. Doctors must keep a detailed record of their patients' treatment regimes and 10 per cent of their prescriptions must be for generic drugs. Doctors who join this scheme receive an additional annual fee of FRF 150 per registered patient. Up to the end of 1997, only 12.5 per cent of doctors had joined this scheme. Most were reluctant because of the fear that they may be more controlled by the health insurance system because of the detailed patient records they are obliged to keep.

Denmark has a mixture of capitation and fee-for-service payment for all general practitioners; in Spain 60 per cent of general practitioners are paid by capitation and 40 per cent by salary. In Austria, since January 1995, doctors' fees are partially based on a capitation scheme. Doctors receive a quarterly lump sum based on the number of patients who have been consulted. In the Netherlands, for low income patients, doctors are paid on a capitation basis, whereas a fee-for-service system applies for high income patients. For specialists, on average, private fees are about twice as high as the fees for sickness funds (public insurance scheme) patients. Most specialists are paid on a fee-for-service basis regardless of the type of insurance fund that reimburses them. Based on the Health Care Prices Act (WTG) of 1980 a specially appointed autonomous body, the Central Office on Health Care Prices (COTG) sets out guidelines for the composition and calculation of prices. After approval by the government these guidelines are used by representative organizations of providers and insurers to negotiate the

The European Union: Health Care Systems 25

actual charges which in turn have to be approved by COTG. The associations of GPs and specialists, on the one hand, and those of sickness funds and private insurers, on the other, are designated by law as negotiators.

Doctors have to accept the negotiated rate of payment in all Member States except France, where 26 per cent of office-based doctors have opted to be able to levy higher fees. Their patients are only reimbursed a fixed percentage of the negotiated fee and the doctors have to pay for their own pensions and observe other conditions. In Denmark there is extra billing for Group 2 patients (2.5 per cent of the population).

Doctors can be faced with changed incentives by altering the relative value scale under fee-for-service systems of payment, as in Germany. Doctors have been paid relatively less for diagnostic tests in France and Germany with the aim of reducing supplier-induced demand. Table 1.6 gives examples of services included in the Relative (or Unified) Value Scale in Germany and the number of points per service to be reimbursed.

Table 1.6 The German Relative Value Scale In 1996

Service	Number of points
Basic fee per patient per 3 months	60–575 depending on specialty of doctor and status of patient (working/retired)
Surcharge for regular care per 3 months by nephrologists for patients needing dialysis, oncologists for cancer patients or rheumatologists for patients with rheumatoid arthritis	900
Consultation fee	50
Consultation fee (home visit)	400 (non-urgent), 600 (urgent)
Antenatal care per 3 months	1,850
Health check-up	780
ECG	250
Osteodensitometry	459

Source: Busse and Schwartz, in press.[11]

26   *Health Care and Cost Containment in the European Union*

One of the weaknesses of the Relative Value Scale is that it only lists services and not the indications that justify these services. This mechanism has protected the high level of clinical freedom of German doctors which is only limited by internal control mechanisms within the doctors' associations. Doctors who prescribe more services compared with their colleagues have to justify their decisions to escape financial penalties.[12] This scheme operated until early 1997 in combination with fixed budgets for ambulatory care for regional associations of doctors. Since early 1997 fixed budgets have been replaced by volume targets. Since there are no effective sanction mechanisms to prevent supplier-induced demand it is probable that volume targets will not be respected.

Specialists serving compulsorily insured out-patients are salaried in Spain, Greece, Portugal, UK, Finland and Sweden and under the GMS scheme in Ireland. In the other Member States, some or all are paid on a fee-for-service basis.

1.5 Doctor supply

Most Member States have specific restrictions on the number of doctors entering publicly financed systems. In Germany the number allowed to enter insurance practice is controlled by the Regional Physicians' Associations which issue licences for insurance practice in particular specialities.[8] Since 1993, the number treating sickness funds members has been regulated by law. A ceiling was set for main specialities and comparable cities and regions at 110 per cent of the average number of doctors in 1990. There were no adjustments for population age, sex, morbidity or supply of hospitals. In Ireland, the Health Boards limit entry of general practitioners to the GMS service for lower income patients. The number and type of hospital consultants is regulated by the Hospital Council. Since 1991, consultants have been able to commit themselves to different categories of hospital appointment. These vary in salary levels and the facility to work in private practice, in association with the service commitment in public hospitals. The number of consultants working in public hospitals declined from 1,085 in 1984 to 1,064 in 1995. In contrast, the number of other hospital doctors increased from 1,824 in 1984 to 2,430 in 1993. In Italy the central government has imposed strict limitations on regions and local health units mainly by freezing staff hiring. Despite these efforts the number of doctors

The European Union: Health Care Systems   27

and dentists employed by the NHS increased from 79,820 in 1987 to 100,372 in 1994. In Spain, Finland, Sweden and Portugal the number of posts for doctors is controlled by the central government. In Sweden the number of practising doctors has stabilized in recent years. In Portugal no new posts for doctors were authorized between 1986 and 1989.[8] In Austria sickness funds limit the number of doctors they contract; also some doctors have decided not to sign contracts with insurance funds. In the Netherlands there is state control over the number of consultants working in hospitals. However, entry to practice under health insurance is open to all doctors. In Denmark it is the responsibility of each county to indicate which parts of the system are open or closed to the entry of further specialists and general practitioners. Nonetheless, there are no explicit manpower controls. Manpower supply is mainly influenced by the limited number of training posts for medical doctors.

In the UK, since the start of the National Health Service, entry to general practice in overdoctored areas has been heavily restricted, but there has been no attempt to place an overall limit on general practitioners entering the NHS. In December 1997 the Medical Workforce Standing Committee recommended that the number of medical students increase by 20 per cent above the current number of 4,894 intakes per year. This was in order to cope with an over-reliance on doctors from overseas (who make up 25 per cent of the doctor workforce)[13] and additional demands as the population ages and employment patterns change, partly because of the increase in the number of women working part-time (who currently account for 54 per cent of admissions to medical schools). Entry to practice under health insurance or the health service is open to all doctors in Belgium, France and Luxembourg. NHS posts are strictly controlled in Greece but entry to practice under health insurance is open to most doctors.

1.6 Patient choice

Patients have free choice of general practitioner, family doctor or office-based doctor in Belgium, Luxembourg and France. In Germany and Austria patients have free choice among sickness funds doctors. In the Netherlands free choice of doctors is restricted to twice a year among doctors who are contracted by a health insurance fund. In Sweden there is free choice of NHS and contracted private doctors, and in the UK there is free choice for

28   *Health Care and Cost Containment in the European Union*

those aged 16 or over, while parents or guardians choose for children under 16. In Italy there is free choice of GP from a list of doctors approved by the region. This is also the case of Category 1 patients (full eligibility) in Ireland. In Denmark Group 1 patients (97.5 per cent of the population) can change their doctor once in a period of six months, whereas for Group 2 there is free choice. In Finland choice is limited. In Greece patients cannot choose insurance funds or doctors working in hospital out-patient departments. Some patients have free choice of office-based doctors contracted out by health insurance. In Spain patients choose their GP, paediatrician and gynaecologist from a list of local doctors, and in Portugal they also choose their NHS GP or specialist or contracted out doctors from a list.

Patients have free choice of public or private hospitals in Germany, France, Luxembourg and Austria. In Belgium, the Netherlands and Italy patients have free choice among those hospitals approved by health insurance or government. In Denmark, since October 1992, patients have been given a degree of freedom to choose their hospital. The precondition remains that a referral from a general practitioner should be made. However, patients who need basic hospital treatment cannot choose to be treated in one of the specialized hospital departments located in university hospitals. In Sweden there is free choice between regional public hospitals and approved private ones. In Portugal patients can choose among public hospitals and, in practice, this is also the case in Greece. There is free choice of hospital in Finland, Ireland and Spain.

In the UK fundholding GPs determine the hospitals for their patients, in theory in consultation with the patient. For the patients of GPs who are not fundholders, the choice depends on the contracts made by the Health Authority; any referrals made to hospitals with whom the Health Authority does not have a contract (so-called extra-contractual referrals) may have to be approved by the Health Authority. This system is due to be abolished under the new Labour Government, but at the time of writing it is not clear with what it will be replaced.

1.7 Dental care

It has been estimated that capitation payment schemes result in higher utilization of dental services but also in greater emphasis on preventive care.[14] However, the most common method of payment for dental treatment is fee-for-service. This can lead to excess provision of services and induced demand. Birch[15] conducted an analysis of individual courses of treatment and suggested that supplier-induced demand was present within dental provision of the British NHS. A study in Finland examined ulitization of dental care as measured by dental expenditure. The data came from a sample of 1,779 employees, whose dental expenditure was refunded up to a maximum of 99.75 per cent. Money price elasticity was small, but significant (-0.069). General and personal inducement appeared to have a considerable effect on utilization, but did not have any systematic connection with the dentist/population ratio.[16] However, another study in Norway found that dentists in areas of excess supply were able to maintain their workload by increasing the demand for and the utilization of their services.[17] Elderton and Nuttal[18] examined the agreement between 15 dentists when they planned treatment for the same group of 18 young adults and found that there was a fivefold difference among the dentists in the cost of the planned treatment, much of which was restorative. Wide variation was found among the dentists as to which tooth surfaces required restoration.

Despite this evidence, the only countries in the EU where a universal capitation payment scheme exists are the UK for the NHS dental services (but this is eroding – see below) and Ireland for dentists employed by the Health Board. In the Netherlands the 'cluster charge' links preventive dental care with a fee-for-service system. Patients covered by statutory health insurance are entitled to preventive treatments, check-up, plaque removal and oral hygiene instruction. For each patient who attends this session of preventive care at least once a year, the dentist can claim a standard fee (the 'cluster charge').[19] In several countries there is limited provision of dental care to the elderly and young (usually under 18 year olds) in public health care settings. In this case dentists are paid on a salary basis (Greece) or capitation (Spain, Italy). In Germany dentists are paid on a fee-for-service basis which takes into account a Relative Value Scale. Within the fixed budget system, Relative Value Scales are relative values for allocating proportional payments out of the budget. However, fixed budgets were lifted in early 1997 and it is possible that total dental expenditure will increase, despite the lifting of budgets being combined with further exclusion of some dental services from reimbursement (surgical services and dentures for those born after 1978). For all others these services have to be provided privately, as the sickness funds contribute only a flat amount. Since 1990 in the UK, dentists have been paid on a capitation basis for providing continuing care to chil-

30   *Health Care and Cost Containment in the European Union*

dren up to age 18 and for patients over 18 on the basis of a two-year rolling contract for which monthly payments are made. Dentists receive fee-for-service payments for fillings of deciduous teeth, difficult extractions, orthodontics and so on. However, many dentists have refused to take on new NHS patients and have preferred to expand private practice by charging the full cost of care to their patients.

Table 1.7 shows the relative domination of private practitioners in each country. The countries with the lowest percentage in private practice (Denmark, Finland, Ireland and Sweden) are, not surprisingly, those with a large publicly funded dental service. Overall, the number of inhabitants per practising dentist in the EU was 1,700 in 1996, with the lowest in Greece (908) and the highest in Spain (2,688). In those countries with fewer dentists the number is increasing annually.[19]

The availability of data on dental health care expenditure and utilization of services is scarce. The OECD data bank does not include detailed data on dental expenditure. These data are also lacking from most of the national statistics on health expenditure. Part of the problem is that dental care is provided by the private sector in most countries. Also most dental services are excluded from reimbursement, hence the indifference of public authorities to collecting data. Where there is coverage of dental care by the public entitlement system or publicly financed and privately provided care, high co-payment rates apply. The only exception to the rule is Luxembourg.

In 1995, the Netherlands excluded from reimbursement dental care for adults (apart from preventive care and specialist surgical care). Sweden increased significantly co-payments in 1997. In Spain the NHS only covers extractions, treatment of medical complaints (oral pathology) and surgery. Private dental expenditure accounted for 25 per cent of private health expenditure or 5 per cent of total expenditure on health. Murillo and Gonzalez[20] estimated that private expenditure on dental services increased significantly between 1980 and 1989, from PTE 3,470 per household (real expenditure) to PTE 6,459.

In Belgium public expenditure on dental care remained stable in the early 1990s and accounted for 2.4 per cent of total public expenditure on health. However, during the same period a number of services were excluded from reimbursement and co-payments were significantly increased. In Finland dental expenditure accounted for 5.9 per cent of total health expenditure in 1994 and this percentage has remained relatively stable over the last 15 years. In 1994, 56 per cent of dental expenditure was private. Those

The European Union: Health Care Systems 31

Table 1.7 Total number of practising dentists and percentage in 'private practice', hospitals and public dental services in 1996

EU Member State	Total number practising	Number of inhabitants per practising dentist	% in 'private practice'*	% in hospitals	% in public dental service
Belgium	7,410	1,363	97	3	0
Denmark	5,466	951	64	5	29
Germany	59,900	1,358	95	4	1
Greece	11,460	908	92	n.a.	n.a.
Spain	14,550	2,688	93	5	2
France	39,457	1,041	94	n.a.	n.a.
Ireland	1,400	2,549	65	3	26
Italy	36,600	1,561	97	3	5
Luxembourg	269	1,491	100	0	0
Netherlands	6,900	2,223	100	n.a.	n.a.
Austria	3,648	2,197	80	8	5
Portugal	4,000	2,472	100	5	0
Finland	4,880	1,041	53	6	39
Sweden	8,650	1,011	44	4	52
UK**	22,034	2,645	82	12	8
EU15	226,624	1,700	90	–	–

Notes:
n.a. not applicable or data not available.

Percentages may add up to more than 100% because some dentists work part-time in more than one setting.

* 'Private practice' is defined as non-salaried, in premises privately owned by the dentist(s). The precise term for this type of practice varies across Europe: for example, 'liberal practice' in France and 'general practice' in the UK. The proportion of 'private practioners' who work full-time varies between countries and some will also work part-time in hospitals or a public dental service.

** In the UK a small proportion of dentists in general practice are salaried employees of the NHS.

Source: Anderson *et al.*, 1997.[19]

who were born before 1956 bear the full cost of dental care. Others are subsidized either by municipalities (free care for those under 18, subsidized for those aged between 19 and 40) or the National Health Insurance (for those aged between 19 and 40).

In 1995, private expenditure on dental care in France accounted for 54.8 per cent of total expenditure; 40.1 per cent was through direct payment and the remainder through private insurance payments. The *Mutuelles* covered 13.6 per cent and compulsory health insurance only 31.5 per cent. The relevant figure for 1980 was 48.5 per cent. It is expected that in the future private expenditure will increase further.

In Germany there were regional fixed budgets for dental care until 1997. Cost sharing is high (up to 50 per cent) and a number of services are not reimbursed. Expenditure rose significantly between 1993 and 1995 when the fixed budgets were abolished and this led to their reinstatement in 1996. In 1996, expenditure on dental care (including dentures) accounted for 9.6 per cent of total sickness funds expenditure. In 1995, total dental expenditure accounted for about 14 per cent of total health expenditure. Most of this was for restorative and prosthetic care.

1.8 Out-of-hospital care

In nearly all countries provision of nursing homes and homes for the aged is budeted separately by local government or social security, or is largely left to the private sector. The elderly person often has to pay more for care in an old people's home than in a hospital, and it can be very expensive if the private sector is used without any subsidy. In the Netherlands care in nursing homes is financed under a separate national insurance scheme and care in old people's homes is financed out of the national budget. Only in Ireland does the same budget which pays for health care also pay for old people's homes, but provision is poorly coordinated with the hospitals.

Nursing home care appears to be most fully developed in the Netherlands, where there are more occupied beds in nursing homes than in hospitals. Many countries are recognizing the need to make more provision for the elderly by the allocation of small hospitals for their care. It has been estimated in Germany that 17 per cent of hospital patients do not need hospital care; as a result, insurance for long-term care has been introduced.[8] Following an experiment in one county in Denmark, municipalities now have to pay the county (which provides the hospitals) for each day any patient stays in hospital while waiting for a place in an old people's home. This had the immediate effect of forcing the municipalities to make further provision.[8] In addition, since 1996, patients who are older than 80 years are entitled to two home visits by social services per year with the aim of preventing unnecessary hospitalization or institutionalization and of clarifying whether senior citizens are in need of social services.[21] In 1998, this scheme was extended to those over 75 years.

Home nursing is poorly developed in Belgium, France, Germany and Luxembourg (where there are plans to develop it). It is virtually non-existent in Greece, very low but growing in Portugal and Italy, and only being developed in one region of Spain. It is provided in the Netherlands by not-for-profit organizations with government subsidy. It is provided by the Health Boards in Ireland but on a limited scale. It is more extensive in the United Kingdom. The most comprehensive and dynamic service appears to be provided in Denmark where home nurses with cars are available to visit patients, even during the night in most municipalities, to provide medical services and supervision.[8]

In Denmark, Ireland, Italy, Portugal, Spain and Sweden nursing home organizations receive a fixed budget from central or local governments, based on the number of inhabitants or the elderly in their catchment area or on the number of staff. Patients need no referral. Nursing care in these countries is financed by general or local taxation.[22]

In Denmark home care and home nursing are financed by local municipalities in cases of permanent need. Municipalities can charge non-terminally ill users for home care services. The charge per hour is means tested and cannot exceed DKK 82 or the cost of the service provided. There are significant differences in the provision of home care in terms of hours allocated per recipient per week among different municipalities; for instance, Skaerbaek provides 5.2 hours per week per recipient whereas Copenhagen provides only 3.8 hours.[23]

In the UK it is important to distinguish what is meant by home care, as the type of care involved determines the mechanism for financing care. Medical home nursing care provided by community/district nurses or community psychiatric nurses is provided and funded entirely from local health authority budgets and users of these services do not make a contribution towards these costs. An allowance of specialist equipment such as incontinence pads would be available to all individuals and again these would be

34   *Health Care and Cost Containment in the European Union*

free of charge. Other equipment used in home care would be provided on loan.

If, however, home care refers to assistance with activities of daily living or the instrumental activities of daily living such as help with getting dressed, toileting or shopping, a different model applies. Any public help with these activities is at the discretion of local authority social services, based on an assessment of the needs of individuals. Local authority social services are not obliged to provide or enable any services of this type at all. However, if they do provide such help directly or through a contract with a private or voluntary organization they may require a contribution from individuals based on their level of income. Many local authorities simply do not have the resources to fund home care and thus individuals are left to make their own arrangements with the private or voluntary sectors.

In Austria, Belgium, Luxembourg, Germany and France, home nursing care is mainly financed through a health insurance scheme. Nursing home institutions are financed on a fee-for-service basis. Patients need a referral to gain access to home nursing services. In Luxembourg only technical nursing activities are reimbursed and more basic nursing care, such as bathing or help with getting out of bed, has to be partly paid for by patients.[22] In Austria a preventive nursing home scheme was introduced in 1993 with the objective of granting people in need of care a statutory claim to nursing benefits. The prerequisites to claim flat cash nursing benefits include a permanent need of nursing and help owing to a physical or mental handicap; a nursing need of more than 50 hours per month; and need for care and help is required for at least six months.[24] In 1996, 264,596 Austrians (3.3 per cent of the population) received home nursing benefits.

A long-term care insurance pay-as-you-go scheme was introduced in Germany in 1995, after a long process of political negotiation and compromise. The scheme provides benefits in cash or kind for both community and institutional care and is based on compulsory contributions evenly split between employees and their employers. The rate is 1.7 per cent, up to a ceiling of DEM 6,000 per month.[25] Patients undergo a medical check by a special service of long-term care insurance (LTCI) and are placed in one of the following categories: Grade I, needing considerable care, Grade II, needing extensive care, and Grade III, needing very extensive 24 hours a day care. Entitlements differ according to the grade.[26] The home nursing institution receives a fixed monthly amount per patient according to the patient's dependency level. It is also possible to provide patients with budgets to buy their own nursing care. In Sweden there are plans to introduce a similar scheme to finance long-term care.

The new care insurance scheme in Germany has encountered problems. Employers were strongly opposed to the additional social insurance and suggested that a private scheme financed solely by employees be established. They feared that an insurance based model would lead to an increase in non-wage labour cost, although they could not deny the need for reform.[26] Critics also doubted whether the revenues provided by the present contribution rates would be sufficient if more professional services entered the market. The rates reflect the current availability of services and it is unclear what will happen if expenditure exceeds revenues.[27]

In Denmark care provided in nursing homes is mainly financed by municipalities (90-95 per cent) and user charges (mainly for rent) cover about 5-10 per cent. In Finland home nursing care is financed out of general taxation but patients need a referral, whereas in the Netherlands nursing care is financed by a compulsory health insurance scheme and nursing home organizations receive a fixed budget based on the number of personnel. No referral is needed. There are currently plans to change the method of allocating budgets to take into account the number of hours of care provided.[22] In southern EU Member States families still play an important role in the provision of home care. In Spain in 1995, 72 per cent of home care was provided by family members.[28]

In six EU Member States (Denmark, Germany, Ireland, Portugal, Spain and the UK) there is no co-payment for home nursing care.[22] In Belgium and the Netherlands there is a small membership fee that has to paid to the nursing home institution. In 1996, this was NLG 50 and between BEF 500–1,000 per family per year in the Netherlands and Belgium, respectively. In France and Belgium most families have additional supplementary insurance which covers co-payments to nursing home institutions. In Italy there is no co-payment for home nursing services provided by the NHS, although there are different levels of co-payments for services provided by private organizations and by social services of the communities. Co-payment levels are income-related. In Finland patients have to pay part of the expenditure. This share (between 11 and 35 per cent of care cost in 1994) varies according to the size and income of the family. For occasional nursing care the co-payment is FIM 30 per visit by a nurse. In Greece the co-payment is 20 per cent and in Sweden it depends on the institution providing care (county councils/health care or municipalities/social services). In

36   *Health Care and Cost Containment in the European Union*

the case of county councils the co-payment varies and in 1995 was about SEK 50 per nursing home visit. Co-payments are not income-related and are part of the overall ceiling of co-payments. Since the 1992 reforms the responsibility for the long-term medical care of elderly people has shifted from the health services/county councils to the municipalities. Care for the elderly, apart from long-term medical care, was always the responsibility of the municipalities.[29] Some municipalities include co-payments in the total home care charges (which also include home help). It is estimated that on average people pay about SEK 600 per month for home care services. Most municipalities use an income-related charge system and the individual's co-payment is also dependent on hours of care provided.[22]

Kerkstra and Hutten[30] found that that there seems to be a relation between the way of funding and the organizational structure of home nursing in the EU Member States. In Member States where the organizations receive a fixed budget, based on the number of inhabitants or the demography of the catchment area, home nursing is mainly provided by one type of organization and is freely accessible to the patients. In this situation there is little competition among the organizations, and the catchment areas of the regional organizations do not tend to overlap. On the other hand, in countries where organizations are reimbursed according to a fee-for-service principle and a referral of a doctor is required, home nursing is provided by different types of organizations and also by independent nurses. It seems that fee-for-service reimbursement stimulates competition between providers and a market-oriented home care. The consequence of a fee-for-service method of funding is that mainly costs of technical nursing procedures and some basic care are reimbursed; this leaves little room for nurses to perform preventive and psychosocial activities or to provide more integrated care.[30]

1.9 The regulation of pharmaceuticals

Government strategies for cost containment in the pharmaceutical sector include measures to influence the supply and demand sides of the market and interventions designed to counter market failure in health care and the monopoly character of the industry (Table 1.8).

Demand-side strategies operate on patients (for example, cost sharing and development of a market for OTC products). The aim is to make

The European Union: Health Care Systems   37

Table 1.8 Recent cost containment strategies in the pharmaceutical sector

---

Demand-side strategies

---

1   Operating on patients

Cost sharing (all countries)

Developing a market for over-the-counter (OTC) products

Health education programmes (the Netherlands, UK)

2   Operating on principal agents (doctors and pharmacists)

(a) *Payment systems*

Capitation or salary payment for first-contact doctors (several countries, including Spain, Ireland, Italy, the Netherlands, Finland, Sweden, the UK)

Paying pharmacists on a flat rate, not a percentage basis (the Netherlands and the UK)

(b) *Budgets for pharmaceutical expenditure*

Fixed budgets for doctors (fundholding GPs in the UK)

Indicative budgets for doctors (non-fundholding GPs in the UK, Germany, Ireland)

Fixed budgets for pharmaceutical expenditure (Spain, Italy)

Target budgets for pharmaceutical expenditure (Belgium, Denmark)

(c) *Policies encouraging cost-effective prescribing and delivery of pharmaceuticals*

Practice guidelines (France)

Use of cost-effectiveness studies (mainly in France, Finland, Sweden, the UK, but not in a systematic way)

Information and feedback to physicians (Denmark, Germany, the Netherlands, Finland, Sweden, the UK)

Prescription auditing (several countries, but not in a systematic way except in the Netherlands and the UK)

Encouraging generic substitution (several countries, but mainly contingent upon doctor's agreement)

Promoting the use of generics (mainly Denmark, Germany, the Netherlands, the UK)

38   *Health Care and Cost Containment in the European Union*

Table 1.8 (continued) Recent cost containment strategies in the pharmaceutical sector

---

Supply-side strategies operating on the industry

Price controls (all countries except Germany for most patented products)

Reference prices (Denmark, Germany, Italy, the Netherlands, Sweden)

Profit control (UK)

Industry contributions when budgets are exceeded (Germany in 1993)

Revenue targets for the industry (France)

Positive and/or negative lists (all countries)

Controlling the number of products (mainly Denmark, the Netherlands)

Ceilings on promotion expenditure (Spain, UK)

Taxes on promotion expenditure (France, Sweden)

Development of a market for parallel imports (Denmark, Germany, the Netherlands, UK)

Source: Authors' research.

patients price-sensitive and price-conscious and to address the problem of moral hazard in the health care markets. Demand-side strategies also operate on health care providers (doctors and pharmacists who act as patients' agents). These strategies aim to control induced demand and to make the provision of pharmaceutical care more cost-effective. The objective is to change the behaviour of providers through financial incentives or penalties or other regulatory measures.

One way of attempting to influence providers' behaviour is by changing the method by which doctors are paid. Doctors paid a salary or on a capitation basis have less incentive to overprescribe. Another way is to introduce budgets for family doctors or office-based doctors. The main supply-side strategy operating on the industry is price control.

All Member States control either the prices or the profits of the pharmaceutical industry, the exceptions being Germany and Denmark, with partial indirect control in Luxembourg. Germany, Denmark, Italy, Sweden and the Netherlands have introduced a reference price system for non-patented medicines. The UK controls prices indirectly through the Pharmaceutical

The European Union: Health Care Systems 39

Price Regulation Scheme (PPRS) which is a profit control system. The PPRS regulates the profits that companies make from their sales to the NHS. The scheme does not cover branded generic products. While the general agreement is negotiated between the Department of Health and the Association of British Pharmaceutical Industries, details are negotiated between the DoH and the individual companies. It operates at the level of a company's total business with the NHS, rather than in relation to individual products. The scheme measures profitability in terms of the return on capital employed: the regulator's objective is to prevent pharmaceutical companies from making excessive profits from the NHS. For companies which do not have any significant capital in the UK, profitability is assessed on the basis of return on sales.

Table 1.9 (overleaf) shows the methods of regulating or influencing pricing. The underlying mechanisms are shown in the right-hand column, though some have recently been superseded by budgets (as in France). What is noticeable is the widespread introduction of multiple systems of control over the past few years. Other controls have been superimposed on the basic systems of influencing or controlling prices, such as price control, profit control or a reference price system.

With respect to price controls, there is no objective way of establishing the 'real' price of a product. Products share the capital equipment of the company, its overheads, its research and development costs, and its sales promotion costs because several of the company's products may be promoted together. The cost of production and, to some extent, the costs of packaging depend on the level of sales, as the earlier French system of price control explicitly recognized. The French system, before company revenue budgets were introduced, stopped trying to determine the costs of production and allowed higher prices to be charged for products that contributed to the national economy.

Two of the EU member states that use price controls (France and Belgium) attempt to assess the innovativeness of the product or its advantage over existing treatments or at least how its price compares with those of existing treatments. But the price advantage to be conceded cannot be determined objectively. For many years, because higher prices were paid for new products, there was an incentive for companies in France and Belgium to develop a stream of products that were similar to existing ones. This prompted the Belgian authorities to set specific criteria for the reimbursement of new products. A new product is reimbursed provided that its price

40 *Health Care and Cost Containment in the European Union*

Table 1.9 Main means of regulating or influencing the price of drugs in 1997

EU Member State	Underlying mechanism to regulate or influence prices
Belgium	Prices based on improvement on existing therapy*
Germany	Free pricing, plus a reference price system excluding most patented drugs
Denmark	Across-the-board price freezes until March 2000, plus a reference price system**
Spain	Prices based on 'cost'
Finland	Prices are regulated
France	Priced according to medical effectiveness and by negotiation with each company
Greece	Prices fixed based on cost, transfer price and lowest price in the EU
Ireland	Prices in Denmark, France, Germany, the Netherlands and the UK
Italy	Average prices of Germany, Spain, France and UK, plus a reference price system
Luxembourg	Prices of Belgium, free pricing if no price in Belgium
Netherlands	Maximum prices are the average of those in Belgium, France, Germany and the UK, plus a reference price system including most patented drugs
Austria	Prices based on 'cost' (based on production costs in locally based pharmaceutical company)
Portugal	Lowest price among Spain, France and Italy
Sweden	Negotiated price and a reference price system excluding patented drugs
UK	Profit regulation

Notes:
* The cost of a product is reimbursed if its price does not exceed the price of any patent medicine containing the same active substance or 110 to 150 per cent of the price of a patent medicine with an equal therapeutic effect.
** In 1998, the members of the pharmaceutical industry association agreed with government that health insurance expenditure should be limited to a 0.8% increase over that of the previous year. The limit for 1999 was set at 3% over the 1998 ceiling. If expenditure exceeds the limit, and a company has a sales growth (for similar products in the same period the previous year) of more than the limit, it should contribute to eliminating the overrun during the next 3 months through price reductions.
Source: Authors' research.

does not exceed the price of any patent medicine containing the same active substances or 110 to 150 per cent of the price of a patent medicine with an equal therapeutic effect.

Greece, Portugal and Ireland broadly compare their prices with those in other European countries; and Italy and the Netherlands use prices based on the average prices of other countries. Italy introduced an average price system based on the prices of the four largest markets in the European Union: those of Germany, France, the UK and Spain. The Italian authorities use Purchasing Power Parities (PPPs) for the calculation of the 'average price'. The 'average' recommended Italian price is the arithmetic mean of the 'standardized' national prices in the four markets. In 1996, the Dutch government also introduced an average European price based on prices in Belgium, France, Germany and the UK.

Other measures that may influence price levels and stimulate price competition include the development of markets for generics and parallel imports and the imposition of revenue or fixed budgets for the industry. Controls on the number of products and promotion expenditure also aim to mitigate the industry's influence on providers. Negative lists are designed to shift to the consumer the full cost of pharmaceutical care for several treatments or treatment options. Another aim of negative lists is to reduce consumption of drugs with questionable effectiveness. However, they may have the undesired effect of switching prescribing to more expensive products included in the positive list.

Cost sharing is the most common measure employed by countries to influence consumer demand. The development of a market for OTC products also aims to shift part of the cost of pharmaceutical care to consumers. Demand-side measures acting on health care providers (mainly doctors and pharmacists) include introducing expenditure ceilings through prospective budgets for doctors, exercising influence on authorizing behaviour and encouraging generic substitution. Much depends on the incentive to the pharmacist. A pharmacist has no incentive to substitute generics if he or she is paid on the basis of a percentage of the price, even if this is a regressive proportion. One reason why generic penetration has been high in the Netherlands and UK is the payment of a fixed fee per drug item to the pharmacist. By allowing pharmacists to retain a third of the savings the Netherlands encourages them to use generics and provides incentives for pharmacists to seek these lower prices. In most countries current systems of remunerating pharmacists do not provide any incentives for generic substi-

42 *Health Care and Cost Containment in the European Union*

tution even where substitution is encouraged. Table 1.10 shows the differences in the methods of remunerating the pharmacist.

Table 1.10 Method of remunerating the pharmacist

EU Member State	Method of remuneration
Greece, Italy, Spain, Portugal	Percentage margin
Belgium, Luxembourg	Percentage margin up to a maximum
Finland	Percentage margin for acquisition costs plus regressive margin
France, Germany, Austria	Regressive margin according to price
Denmark, Sweden	Fixed fee plus regressive margin
Ireland, Netherlands, UK	Fixed fee per prescription

Source: Authors' research.

Supply-side measures focus on regulating prices, reimbursement and promotion expenditure. They include price or profit control schemes; the introduction of positive and negative lists for pharmaceutical products; developing a market for parallel imports, with the aim of stimulating price competition; and limiting promotion expenditure.

The structure of the health care system and the extent of the monopsony power of buyers of health and pharmaceutical care are also expected to influence the decision-making process and the type of measures adopted by different purchasers or payers of care. However, industrial policy also affects decisions in several countries. Countries with a strong pharmaceutical industry that is a major exporter are reluctant to implement strict price control schemes.

II : Health care spending

In this section we examine and compare some of the trends in health care spending among the Member States of the European Union. This raises some difficult methodological issues. International comparisons are only as

The European Union: Health Care Spending   43

good as the data on which they are based. The administrative and statistical systems in the Member States differ, and the data collected are designed to serve the more specific needs of individual health care systems rather than comparative purposes. Each Member State has its own way of classifying health expenditure which often arises out of its organizational pattern, and in consequence what is classified as health care expenditure may differ in different countries. There are also problems in ensuring that expenditure data, expressed as they normally are in national currency units, are comparable in value terms across countries. The section begins with a discussion of some of these problems. It continues with an examination of the relevant trends, and concludes with a discussion of some of the upward pressures on health spending.

1.10 Methodological issues

The principal methodological difficulties that arise in making international comparisons of expenditure trends can be grouped under two headings: classification problems and value comparisons.

1.10.1 Classification problems

There are substantial differences between definitions of variables, terminology employed and methods of collection. Data inaccuracies may affect the reliability of the information. Expenditure comparisons face difficulties in drawing the boundaries of health expenditure. For instance, health expenditure statistics in different Member States vary in the extent to which they include programmes financed by agencies or ministries other than the Ministry of Health, such as those for military personnel, school health services and occupational health. There are varying practices in the financing of medical and dental education, and nurse education and training. In addition any changes in definition over time have to be examined and taken into account.

Of particular concern is the classification of services for the elderly and chronically ill. In some countries care for the elderly in nursing homes or home care is part of the social services budget. Even whether an institution

44 Health Care and Cost Containment in the European Union

is called a long-stay hospital or a nursing home varies internationally, although the institutions concerned may be performing the same function. If patients have to pay for anything not called a hospital, they will try and stay in a free hospital if possible. These problems are most pronounced in the case of the chronically disabled, the elderly, the mentally ill and mentally handicapped. In France nursing home patients and the elderly and frail are often found in the same institution. Some homes for the elderly in several countries provide skilled nursing and are thus treating cases similar to those in nursing homes or hospitals elsewhere.

Friers et al.[31] analysed comparative statistics representing institutionalized residents in seven countries and found significant differences in age, length of stay, in summary measures of physical and cognitive functioning and case mix. Additionally, within countries there was little homogeneity in nursing home service. Friers et al. argue that these differences strengthen the position that the term 'nursing home' does not provide a sound basis for cross-national comparisons and that these comparisons need to adjust at the level of the individual resident for differences in resident populations.

Detailed bilateral comparisons illustrate some of the problems. The purpose of bilateral comparisons is to define comparable sets of activities and to exclude services provided under different headings (for instance, as health care in one country and as social care in another) with a view to explaining differences in the levels of spending. The statistical service of the Netherlands has attempted to produce common comparable baskets for health services and draw bilateral comparisons between different countries. For instance, in the case of the comparison between the Netherlands and Denmark, it was established that the common comparable basket comprised 79 per cent of the measured total costs of health care in the former and 90 per cent in the latter.[32] The disparity mainly reflected differences in the classification of social services and long-term care expenditures.

The case of Sweden provides another illustration of the point. In 1985, care for the mentally handicapped was shifted from the health care budget to the education and social services budget. This resulted in a 5 to 6 per cent fall in total health expenditure in 1986. Further, in 1992, the responsibility for the care of the elderly in nursing homes was transferred to municipalities and hence the associated expenditure came off the health budget. The result was an apparent 'one-off' 16 per cent fall in public health care expenditure (in 1991 prices) and a fall in the percentage of Gross Domestic Product (GDP) taken by that expenditure from 9.3 per cent to 7.4 per cent.

Similarly, Austria recalculated its health care basket in 1993, thereby reducing health spending as a proportion of GDP from 9.4 per cent to 8.0 per cent. The recalculation involved new measures of private consumption, a shift of some expenditure to the social services budget, the exclusion of veterinary services and of subsidies to employers for loss of working days due to sickness of their employees, and a re-estimation of pharmaceutical expenditure.[33]

When attempts are made to break down health expenditure by category, the problem of comparability becomes even more important. The most crucial problems are the boundaries between in-patient and out-patient care and between hospitals and other types of institution. In Greece, for example, out-patient health centres were, until very recently, financed via hospital budgets and thus were classified as in-patient expenditure. There are also problems in comparing health service inputs and activity indicators between countries; for instance, the definition of a qualified nurse differs between Member States. Definitions of hospital beds are even more variable. Measures of activity are often dictated by payment methods and these vary both between countries and within a single country over time. Generally, hospital statistics present problems of validity in almost every Member State.

1.10.2 Value comparisons

There are several problems in making comparisons of the value of health expenditures across countries. Exchange rates and Purchasing Power Parities (PPPs) are the two principal methodologies that have been used to convert values of different currencies into a common denominator, thus allowing comparative research. However, the use of either presents important conceptual and practical problems. Exchange rates do not adequately reflect relative purchasing power across countries, because the equilibrium set of exchange rates only reflects the prices of internationally traded goods, rather than the prices of non-tradeables, such as health care. Thus they attach little weight to non-marketed commodities, and they are also not commodity-specific. In addition, different exchange rate policies have a considerable impact on the values of the relevant variables, even if there is no underlying change in the position of the health sector. So exchange rate depreciation or appreciation alters the ratio of domestic to international

46 Health Care and Cost Containment in the European Union

prices, and thereby changes the relationship between depreciating and appreciating countries. Consequently, international comparisons of commodities and analyses based on exchange rates are, at best, approximations.[34]

PPPs are calculated on the basis of a basket of goods theoretically common to all countries and are used as a benchmark. As international price deflators, PPPs have none of the problems of the exchange rates so international comparisons based upon them have significant conceptual advantages. However, they present a number of measurement-related problems, especially when applied to the health sector. First, PPPs are estimated only every five years and much can change within the health care sector over that length of time. In particular, medical care technology changes in ways that make techniques of only a decade ago seem archaic, providing some particularly striking illustrations of the difficulties involved in measuring quality-adjusted prices. Second, medical services are generally measured on the basis of a very small sample of prices and on weakly comparable volume indices. Third, there is a bias towards pharmaceutical prices (228 prices out of a total of 294 calculated in the PPPs), this despite the fact that hospital services and practising medical personnel account for over two-thirds of the total spending on health care.[34]

Fourth, there is a more general issue concerning public and semi-public sector services which do not carry a market price. The health sector is characterized to a large degree by the absence of markets to determine prices, especially on the public health side, since public health cannot, by definition, be individualized.[34,35] But even where markets do exist they are incomplete because of important market failures and government intervention. Consequently, many prices used for PPP comparisons will be artificial.[36]

Overall, making international comparisons of expenditure trends is a hazardous business; a fact that needs to be borne in mind when, as in the next section, we try to examine these trends.

1.11 Trends in health care expenditure

There are major differences in per capita expenditure on health care among the Member States. Table 1.11, based on the OECD data bank[37] shows that the highest spending countries in 1996 in terms of purchasing power parities (PPPs) are Germany (USD 2,222), Luxembourg (USD 2,206) and

Table 1.11 Per capita spending in USD PPPs (Purchasing Power Parities) in 1990 and 1996

EU Member State	1990	1996
Belgium	1,247	1,683
Denmark	1,069	1,430
Germany	1,642	2,222
Greece	389	748
Spain	813	1,131
France	1,539	1,978
Ireland	748	923
Italy	1,322	1,520
Luxembourg	1,499	2,206*
Netherlands	1,325	1,756
Austria	1,180	1,681
Portugal	616	1,077
Finland	1,292	1,389
Sweden	1,492	1,405
UK	957	1,304
EU average (unweighted)	1,142	1,472

Notes: * 1995 for Luxembourg.

Source: OECD Health Data, 1997.[37]

France (USD 1,978) which spend about three times that of the lowest (Greece). Belgium, Italy, the Netherlands and Austria are above the unweighted EU average (USD 1,497). Spain, Ireland, Portugal and Greece are the lowest spending countries in the EU. However, as discussed above, the use of PPPs presents several problems and data based on them should be treated with some caution.

Even when expenditure is expressed as a percentage of Gross Domestic Product (GDP), large disparities remain (see Table 1.12 overleaf). Germany is the highest with 10.5 per cent of GDP devoted to health care in 1996, followed by France, the Netherlands, Portugal, Austria and Belgium all with shares of GDP expenditure above the (unweighted) EU average of 7.8 per

Table 1.12 Total expenditure (TE) and public expenditure (PE) on health as a percenatge of GDP (1971–96)

EU Member State	1971		1981		1986		1991		1996	
	TE	PE	TE	PE	TE	PE	TE	PE	TE	PE
Belgium	4.2	3.6	7.2	5.8	7.6	6.0	8.0	7.0	7.9	6.9
Denmark	6.4	5.5	6.8	5.8	6.0	5.1	6.5	5.5	6.4	5.1
Germany	6.3	4.5	8.7	6.5	8.6	6.3	9.6	7.5	10.5	8.2
Greece	3.4	1.9	3.7	3.2	4.5	3.6	4.2	3.4	5.9	4.9
Spain	4.1	2.7	5.8	4.6	5.6	4.5	7.1	5.6	7.7	5.9
France	6.0	4.5	7.9	6.3	8.5	6.5	9.1	6.8	9.7	7.8
Ireland	6.3	4.5	8.4	6.9	7.7	5.9	6.8	5.3	7.6 (a)	6.1
Italy	5.5	4.9	6.8	5.3	6.9	5.3	8.4	6.6	7.6	5.3
Luxembourg	4.2	n/a	6.4	6.0	5.9	5.3	6.5	6.0	7.0 (b)	6.5
Netherlands	6.3	4.8	8.1	6.1	8.0	5.8	8.6	6.4	8.6	6.8
Austria	5.4	3.5	8.2 (c)	5.7	6.9	5.6	7.2	5.4	7.9	5.9
Portugal	2.9	1.7	6.2	4.0	7.0	3.7	7.2	4.5	8.2	4.9
Finland	5.9	4.3	6.7	5.3	7.4	5.9	9.1	7.4	7.5	5.6
Sweden	7.5	6.5	9.5	8.7	8.6	7.7	8.7	7.6	7.3	5.9
UK	4.6	4.0	5.9	5.3	5.9	5.0	6.5	5.4	6.9	5.8
EU average (unweighted)	5.3	3.5	7.1	5.7	7.0	5.5	7.6	6.0	7.8	6.1

Notes:
(a) 1994 for Ireland.
(b) 1995 for Luxembourg.
(c) According to the previous system of measuring health care expenditure.
Source: OECD Health Data, 1997.[37]

The European Union: Health Care Spending 49

cent. At the other end of the spectrum, Greece spends 5.9 per cent of its GDP. Despite the well known association between national income and health care expenditure (total and as a percentage of GDP), the pattern does not wholly reflect the wealth of the countries concerned. Relatively wealthy countries, such as Denmark and the UK, spend less as a proportion of GDP than poorer countries such as Ireland and Portugal.

Table 1.12 also indicates trends in total and public health care expenditure as a proportion of GDP in the Member States from 1971 to 1996. After rapid increases in the first decade, the proportion grew much more slowly between 1981 and 1991 and between 1991 and 1995 in all countries. In Belgium, Denmark, Italy, Finland and Sweden, health care expenditure as a proportion of GDP actually fell between 1991 and 1996; however, the Swedish figures are in large part a consequence of the reclassification change noted in section 1.10.1. Over the same period, health care expenditure remained stable in the Netherlands. Since 1981, the figures have increased steadily in Spain, coinciding with a period of economic growth and of health service development. In the UK, expenditure as a proportion of GDP increased after 1990 by 0.4 per cent, coinciding with the introduction of the reforms of the National Health Service. Between 1991 and 1996, the percentages of GDP devoted to health expenditure increased in Portugal (1.0 per cent), Germany (0.9 per cent), Ireland (0.8 per cent), Austria (0.7 per cent) and France (0.6 per cent).

Ireland is an interesting case. It managed to reduce significantly the percentage of GDP devoted to health expenditure between 1981 and 1991 (from 8.4 per cent to 6.8 per cent). The most remarkable savings were achieved in the hospital sector: while total health expenditure at constant 1980 prices declined by 8 per cent between 1980 and 1988, expenditure on hospital services declined by almost 15 per cent over the same period. The savings in the hospital sector were accomplished by the closure of some hospitals, a 20 per cent decline in the number of acute hospital beds, a 19 per cent decline in average length of stay and a 25 per cent decline in hospital bed-days, with just a 5 per cent decline in discharges from the acute hospital system.[6]

Some problems with the data should be noted. The classification issues concerning Sweden and Austria were discussed in the previous section. With respect to Austria it should be noted that the 1997 version of the OECD Health Data included these changes which are backdated to 1983. Before this year data are not comparable, so an apparent reduction of health

Table 1.13 Annual growth rate of total per capita health expenditure in the EU Member States (at constant 1990 prices)

EU Member State	1976–80		1981–85		1986–90		1991–96	
	Volume (a)	Real (b)	Volume (a)	Real (b)	Volume (a)	Real (b)	Volume (c)	Real (b)
Belgium	3.83	4.33	1.38	2.17	3.41	3.48	1.24	0.62
Denmark	3.00	1.23	1.58	1.43	1.66	2.69	1.91	1.44
Germany	2.97	3.11	0.59	2.23	1.14	1.62	2.65	2.74
Greece	4.05	4.34	4.55	3.19	2.07	0.35	7.82	7.95
Spain	1.94	1.90	0.71	0.75	11.51	10.15	0.85	2.60
France	5.32	4.21	4.66	2.91	4.46	3.79	2.74	1.92
Ireland	6.37	7.79	-2.15	-0.21	-1.21	2.05	4.03	-0.56
Italy	5.63	7.26	2.81	2.45	4.20	6.90	0.83	-1.20
Luxembourg	8.04	6.86	2.14	1.91	5.55	7.73	3.79	5.974 (e)
Netherlands	1.51	3.12	0.87	0.58	2.84	3.64	1.98	1.46
Austria	2.26	4.28	-5.23 (d)	-3.55 (d)	2.19	3.81	0.66	2.89
Portugal	n.a.	3.98	-0.38	1.03	3.98	3.77	3.19	4.21
Finland	2.54	2.42	2.43	4.85	3.53	5.17	-6.22	-2.93
Sweden	3.05	4.55	1.37	0.70	1.33	1.81	-9.136 (f)	-2.967 (f)
UK	1.70	2.33	1.63	2.41	1.47	3.39	1.32	3.20

Notes:

n.a. not available.

(a) Current national total per capita expenditure on health deflated by a weighted health specific deflator.

(b) Current national total per capita expenditure on health deflated by GDP deflator.

(c) 1991–93 for Belgium, Denmark, Greece, Italy, Luxembourg, Portugal and Sweden, 1991–94 for all other Member States.

(d) This decline mainly reflects changes in the system measuring health expenditure.

(e) 1991–95.

(f) In Sweden the decline is mainly due to significant cost shifting to the social services budget.

Source: Authors' estimates based on OECD Health Data, 1997.[37]

The European Union: Health Care Spending 51

spending between 1981 and 1991 was not significant. According to the re-calculation in 1983, the percentage of GDP spent on health was 6.5 per cent.

The German data are not comparable after 1990 (the year of the unification of the Federal Republic of Germany with the former German Democratic Republic). The OECD data bank includes data for West Germany only before the unification and for both West and East Germany after the unification. The figures for Greece and Portugal are also questionable. Greece is almost certainly heavily underreporting its health spending, as national accounts do not capture the size of the private or the parallel economy sector. Portugal may be underestimating its public expenditure on health in recent years. An indicator of this is the fact that the public debt to suppliers (not included in the reported health expenditures) was equal to about one-quarter of the health budget in 1993. However, these are only estimates since the government has not published any official data concerning the size of the debt.[38] Finland had a significant fall in Gross Domestic Product between 1990 and 1991, mainly owing to the loss of exports to the Soviet Union; the subsequent revival of GDP, rather than a dramatic fall in health spending, explains the reduction in that spending as a percentage of GDP from 9.1 per cent in 1991 to 7.5 per cent in 1996.

Finally in this section, for completeness, Table 1.13 shows the annual growth rate of total per capita health expenditure in the EU Member States at constant 1990 prices in 'volume' terms (current national total per capita expenditure on health deflated by a weighted health-specific deflator) and in 'real' terms (current national total per capita expenditure on health deflated by the GDP deflator). The first is an indication of changes in the actual volume of resources used; the second is an indication of changes in the opportunity cost of those resources.

1.12 Health expenditure by category

1.12.1 Public/private

In the EU public expenditure accounts on average for three-quarters of total expenditure (see Table 1.14 overleaf). The proportion is highest in Luxembourg (98.8 per cent) followed by Belgium, the UK, Sweden and Denmark with more than 80 per cent of total expenditure. Portugal has the

52   *Health Care and Cost Containment in the European Union*

Table 1.14 Public expenditure on health as a percentage of total health expenditure (1971–95)

EU Member State	1971	1981	1991	1995*
Belgium	86.0	81.5	88.1	87.8
Denmark	85.6	85.0	83.3	83.0
Germany	72.0	75.0	73.1	73.5
Greece	56.8	84.4	75.7	75.8
Spain	64.6	78.7	78.9	78.2
France	74.8	79.5	74.7	78.4
Ireland	72.5	82.8	77.2	76.0
Italy	89.1	78.4	78.3	70.0
Luxembourg	n.a.	92.9	97.3	98.8
Netherlands	76.5	75.2	73.8	77.5
Austria	63.8	69.5	65.5	63.4
Portugal	59.7	64.3	55.5	56.0
Finland	72.7	79.7	81.1	75.2
Sweden	86.8	91.9	88.3	83.4
UK	87.0	88.9	83.7	84.1
EU average (unweighted)	74.9	80.5	78.3	77.4

Notes:
n.a. not available.
* 1994 for Denmark, Greece, Ireland, Luxembourg, Austria, Finland, Sweden, UK.
Source: OECD Health Data, 1997.[37]

lowest share of public expenditure with 56 per cent; the share is also low in Austria (63.4 per cent) while, in the remaining Member States, public expenditure ranges between 70 and 80 per cent.

During the 1980s and early 1990s, the public share of total health expenditure decreased in all Member States except in Belgium, Luxembourg and the Netherlands. The reduction was most marked in Greece, Ireland, Italy and Portugal. These trends were based on OECD data which only provide data for total and public expenditure on health. A somewhat different picture was given in the previous section, where we discussed sources of funding for health care in the Member States. The data there, based on sources provided by the authors of the country-based chapters of this book, give higher percentages for private expenditure on health (includ-

The European Union: Health Care Spending 53

ing user charges and voluntary health insurance) compared with the OECD data. The differences may reflect problems of definition. The OECD does not provide any explanation on what constitutes the difference between total and public expenditure on health. It may be well the case that part of the private expenditure (user charges) is publicly administered and thus it may be classified as public expenditure.

1.12.2 Sector

In most countries for which data are available, the majority of health resources are devoted to in-patient care (Table 1.15, overleaf). Denmark, Greece and Ireland are shown in the OECD data as allocating over 55 per cent of resources to in-patient care while Austria, Italy, the Netherlands, Spain and Sweden allocate between 45 and 55 per cent. But Germany, Belgium, Luxembourg and Portugal only devote about a third of their health resources to in-patient care.

Ambulatory care provided by doctors outside hospitals consumed almost half of total expenditure in Luxembourg and Finland, over 30 per cent in Belgium and Italy, while in Spain it was less than 15 per cent. Expenditure on pharmaceuticals varied widely among Member States, from over 25 per cent of the total in Portugal to under 11 per cent in the Netherlands and Austria; again these data should be treated with some caution in view of definitional problems.

In several EU countries the share of in-patient care increased during the 1980s. This was particularly the case in Greece and Portugal; but Spain, Germany, France, Finland, Italy, Sweden and the Netherlands reduced the share of resources on in-patient care during the same period.

1.13 Upward pressures on expenditure

During the last two decades several factors have combined to exert upward pressure on health expenditure in the European Union. One is demography: all European countries have ageing populations, with higher levels of chronic diseases and disability. Another is expansion of coverage by public health systems. Costs have also increased because of improvements in technology. In addition, other cost-increasing factors include higher real income,

Health Care and Cost Containment in the European Union

Table 1.15 Expenditure by sector as a percentage of total health care expenditure (latest available year and 1980)

EU Member State	Latest available year (LAY)	Hospital care (a)		Ambulatory care (b)		Pharmaceuticals (c)	
		LAY	1980	LAY	1980	LAY	1980
Belgium	1994	36.0	33.1	36.5	39.2	17.5	17.4
Denmark	1994	60.9	65.1	21.1	21.1	11.1	9.1
Germany	1993	31.3	32.6	26.9	33.4	18.9	13.1
Greece	1992	59.2	48.9	n.a.	n.a.	23.5	34.8
Spain	1993	48.7	54.1	11.4	12.6	18.2	21.0
France	1994	44.8	48.1	27.0	24.8	16.5	15.9
Ireland	1994	56.9	n.a.	n.a.	n.a.	11.5	11.2
Italy	1995	47.7	46.7	30.1	27.5	18.1	13.7
Luxembourg	1994	32.1	31.3	52.1	49.5	15.6	14.5
Netherlands	1994	52.3	57.3	28.8	27.7	10.7	7.9
Austria	1995	45.6	n.a.	24.0	20.2	10.9	12.0
Portugal	1993	31.5	28.7	n.a.	n.a.	25.6	19.9
Finland	1994	40.9	48.4	49.4	39.9	12.8	10.7
Sweden	1993	52.8	n.a.	n.a.	n.a.	12.5	6.5
UK	1993	42.9	53.5	n.a.	n.a.	15.3	12.8
EU (d)		45.6	45.7	30.7	29.6	15.9	14.7

Notes:

n.a. not available.

(a) Total expenditure on in-patient care: current spending only. Public expenditure for Ireland, Portugal and Sweden.

(b) Total expenditure for all out-patient medical and paramedical services.

(c) Total expenditure for the purchase of medical and paramedical services.

(d) Unweighted average of available data.

Source: Authors' estimates based on OECD Health Data, 1997.[37]

The European Union: Health Care Spending   55

increasing number of doctors (mainly specialists), medical inflation in excess of the general consumer price index, tax concessions for private health insurance, increasing administrative costs and fee-for-service payment systems. All these are discussed in subsequent chapters in more detail; here we simply outline some of the principal arguments concerning the first three factors mentioned: ageing, coverage and technology.

1.13.1 Ageing

The overall impact of ageing on health care expenditure is not entirely clear. It has long been recognized that people need to use more health care as they get older. However, Fuchs[39] claimed that the relationship between health care utilization (and thus costs) and age is biased by the fact that the percentage of people in their last year of life is increasing rapidly with age. He hypothesized that, if mortality in all age groups above 65 were assumed to be constant, then the relationship between health care costs with age would also be constant. An analysis of US Medicare data has shown that the payments associated with an additional year of life and the average annual payments over an enrollee's lifetime both decreased as the age of death increased.[40] A recent study in Germany showed that the most costly patients are those who die young. Lifelong hospital utilization for persons who die at 50 or later is directly proportional to the number of years lived.[41] Evidence from the US also suggests that, contrary to common belief, the costs of those who die aged 80 or over are about 80 per cent of the costs of those who die aged 65 to 79.[42] Moreover, these costs are heavily concentrated in nursing home and home care costs. It seems therefore that it is the 'younger old' rather than the very old who get expensive high-technology care. Harrison et al.,[43] on the basis of a number of assumptions, estimated that demographic change in the UK will require an extra 8.25 per cent growth in real expenditure between 1994 and 2014, which is slightly less than the estimated growth of 10.3 per cent from 1974 to 1994. They therefore concluded that pressures arising from demography and morbidity are likely to have a modest impact in the future.

However, Meerding et al.[44] reached a different conclusion. They estimated the demands on health care resources caused by different types of illnesses and variation with age and sex and they reported the proportion of the health care budget spent on each category of disease and cost of health care per person at various ages. After the first year of life, costs per person for children were lowest. Costs rose slowly throughout adult life and increased exponentially from age 50 onwards until the oldest age group (95 or above). The top five areas of health care costs were mental retardation, musculoskeletal disease (predominantly joint disease and dorsopathy), dementia, a heterogeneous group of other mental disorders, and ill-defined conditions. Stroke, all cancers combined and coronary heart disease ranked 7th, 8th and 10th, respectively. Meerding *et al.* concluded that the main determinants of health care use in the Netherlands are old age and disabling conditions, particularly mental disability. They also argued that their study is more comprehensive than previous ones in including data on all health care costs[45] and that this explains why the Dutch results seem at variance with the Medicare study that shows decreasing costs with the oldest ages. The US study did not include long-term care for elderly people or care in nursing and old people's homes.

Of course the cost of health care for any age group depends on the forms of care that are considered appropriate to that group. In the case of the elderly, these can differ dramatically within the EU countries. Typical in this respect is the North–South division, whereby institutional care for the elderly in the North is paralleled by family care in the South.

1.13.2 Coverage

The extension of coverage of the population by compulsory health insurance has contributed to rising health care costs in several countries. In all Member States except the Netherlands, compulsory health insurance as defined by the International Labour Office covers over 90 per cent of the population.[8] Universal rights to health care were extended over a period of 36 years, as Table 1.16 illustrates. Universal coverage was extended to the whole population with the establishment of national health systems in Italy, Portugal, Spain and Greece in the late 1970s and early 1980s (although for Greece only with respect to access to public hospitals). In Ireland only those on low incomes are covered for primary care (the General Medical Services scheme). Those not covered have to make considerable co-payments for specialist and in-patient care. In the Netherlands virtually all those not compulsorily covered are members of voluntary insurance schemes. Only 1 per cent of the population is uninsured (most often the very wealthy). On the

Table 1.16 Percentage of population covered by compulsory health insurance in 1960 and 1996

EU Member State	1960	1996
Belgium	58.0	99.0
Denmark	95.0	100.0
Germany	84.0	92.2
Greece	30.0	100.0
Spain	50.0	99.3
France	80.0	99.5
Ireland	85.0	100.0
Italy	87.0	100.0
Luxembourg	100.0	100.0
Netherlands	71.0	74.1
Austria	78.0	99.0
Portugal	18.0	100.0
Finland	100.0	100.0
Sweden	100.0	100.0
UK	100.0	100.0

Source: OECD Health Data, 1997.[37]

other hand, provision for serious and prolonged disability and sickness has long been universal. Only about 60 per cent of the population is compulsorily covered for hospital and specialist services. Very nearly universal rights (about 99 per cent coverage) are now found in Belgium, France and Luxembourg and about 90 per cent are covered by the statutory insurers in Germany. In Germany all those not covered by sickness funds are members of a compulsory private insurance scheme. In Belgium the self-employed and employers are only covered for the heavy risks – in-patient care and certain diseases such as cancer and tuberculosis. Those not covered are the very poor, immigrants and the wealthy.

1.13.3 Technology

Health care technology[46,47] is perceived to encompass all of the instruments, equipment, drugs and procedures used in health care delivery, as well

58 *Health Care and Cost Containment in the European Union*

as the organizations supporting delivery of such care.* Technological innovation has brought profound changes in the delivery of health care services over the last 50 years, and has led to a reduction in mortality, a limitation of the incidence and duration of many diseases, and a significant improvement in both the quality and quantity of life across all population groups. There are a growing number of previously untreatable conditions for which treatments or cure have become available, such as chemotherapy for childhood leukaemia and certain solid tumours; there are new treatments that have replaced or supplemented existing treatments, such as thrombolytic drugs for myocardial infarction; and there are new techniques for diagnosis and treatment, such as minimally invasive surgery. Furthermore, the diffusion of drugs and technology from tertiary centres has greatly increased their availability, and thus their utilization.[48]

However, expansion in the utilization of medical technologies is deemed partly responsible for the rapid escalation of health care costs in the developed world.[49-53] Apart from increased prices, patient complexity and the intensity of services have been found to be the main factors underlying hospital cost increases in the US.[54] Strictly speaking, improvements in technology could be cost reducing, contributing, for instance, to a reduction of length of stay in hospitals and hence to saving in hospital costs. However, reductions in the average cost of treatment of a given quality (reductions in the cost per unit) can coexist with increases in total costs if there is a big enough increase in the number of treatments carried out. In fact the perceived improvements in quality brought about by medical technology are such that any reductions in average costs are generally swamped by the irresistible pressure for more to be done.

But does technology always bring about actual improvements in quality? New technologies can be used to replace older and much less expensive technologies for routine use when, for many conditions, the outcome using the old technology may be just as good as with the new.[55] The impact of technology on health care costs has at best been estimated in a rather indirect way, treating technology as a residual,[56] or at the micro level, looking at the impact on growth in hospital costs.[57] Also the vast majority of these studies cover only a fraction of in-patient care: not surprisingly since aggregate data on technology are scarce.

---

*The World Health Organisation and the US Office of Technology Assessment used almost the same definition.

The European Union: Health Care Spending   59

There is some evidence on the existing stock of technology in different countries in the EU. From this evidence it emerges that there are considerable differences within the EU regarding capital investment in medical technologies. Table 1.17 shows how intensity in standard technologies differs not only among countries with dissimilar income levels, but also among these with similar standards of living (for instance, the number of magnetic resonance imagers (MRIs) in the UK versus the same number in France, Germany and the US).

Table 1.17. Frequency of selected technologies in different countries in 1990 (per million population)

Country	Scanners	MRIs	Lithotripters
Australia	13.7	0.6	0.4
Canada	7.0	0.7	0.4
China	0.3	0.02	0.18
France	7.2	1.2	0.7
Germany	12.2	2.3	1.7
India	0.2	0.02	0.02
Japan	55.4	6.5	2.5
Mexico	2.2	0.2	0.17
Netherlands	7.3	0.9	0.8
Sweden	10.5	1.5	1.2
UK	4.3	0.9	0.3
US	26.8	8.4	1.4

Source: Banta, 1995.[58]

It is possible, however, that such figures underestimate the impact of technology on the increase in health spending because in many countries technological innovation is funded by revenue, rather than capital expenditure, or because alternative ways of financing the purchase of medical equipment, for instance long-term leasing or, even, donation make it undetectable in national statistics.[58] Even less is known about the utilization rates of different 'big ticket' medical technologies* across countries (although there is –

---

* 'Big-ticket' applies to large-scale, costly technologies, such as scanners, whereas 'small-ticket' applies to small-scale technologies, such as laboratory equipment.

60 Health Care and Cost Containment in the European Union

conflicting – evidence about its effectiveness when compared with 'small ticket' technology*).[52,53,59,60] Thus, despite technological innovation in medical treatment being undoubtedly responsible for some part of the escalation of health care costs, little is known about its aggregate impact on health spending or about its impact relative to that of other factors.

A partial exception is pharmaceuticals. Three studies have suggested that new expensive drugs are the most significant factor affecting pharmaceutical expenditure. Jönsson and Gerdtham estimated that real drug expenditure in Sweden increased by 95 per cent between 1974 and 1993.[61] During the same period, the relative price of drugs fell by 35 per cent. The number of prescribed drugs increased by 22 per cent but most of the increase in real drug expenditure can be attributed to a residual which increased by 146 per cent during the period 1974–93. The authors identified five factors affecting the residual:

- the introduction of new drugs into areas where there were no other drugs available;

- the switch from inexpensive to expensive drugs;

- the introduction of new and cheaper generic drugs;

- the sale of old drugs in larger packages;

- the sale of old drugs in smaller packages.

Of these, Jönsson and Gerdtham argued that the switch to more expensive drugs was the most important factor.

Lopez-Bastida and Mossialos estimated that in Spain, while real drug expenditure increased by 264 per cent between 1980 and 1996, the relative price of drugs fell by 39 per cent and the number of prescribed items increased by 10 per cent.[62] Most of the increase can be attributed to new products, whose impact on health expenditure trends increased by 442 per cent between 1980 and 1996. They analysed pharmaceutical consumption data within different therapeutic categories and concluded that the switch to more expensive drugs was the most important factor which led to a significant increase in pharmaceutical expenditure.

In the UK it was estimated by the Department of Health that demo-

---

* For an overview of the attempts by the EU Member States to assess technological developments, see Cranovsky R, Matillon Y, Banta D, 1997.[63]

The European Union: Health Care Spending   61

graphic factors accounted for 0.3 per cent of the annual growth of the UK drugs bill between 1982 and 1992. Other more important factors included product mix (new products), which accounted for 5.5 per cent of the annual growth in the same period. Prescriptions per capita accounted for 2.7 per cent growth, quantity per prescription 1.1 per cent, and the price of the basket of existing products 1.4 per cent.[64]

However, most of the new, highly priced products are not significant innovations. Table 1.18 shows the market shares of new products on the market of six EU Member States between 1991 and 1993. Market shares of novel products are low in all the countries examined and this may reflect the small number of innovative products introduced on the relevant markets. However, market shares of new products which do not offer real improvements are very high in Spain, Italy and Germany where strict price control systems or reference prices are in force.

Table 1.18 Impact of new products on total pharmaceutical spending on products introduced in 1991, 1992 and 1993 (percentage of market share)

EU Member State	1991			1992			1993		
	A (%)	B (%)	C (%)	A (%)	B (%)	C (%)	A (%)	B (%)	C (%)
Germany	10.7	4.3	1.9	9.5	3.4	0.8	7.4	1.9	0.5
Spain	13.4	5.5	2.2	13.0	5.4	1.1	12.7	5.7	0.4
France	8.5	5.4	1.8	6.5	3.2	0.1	7.2	2.3	0.3
Italy	15.8	8.3	0.9	14.4	7.9	0.9	1.3	5.9	1.2
Netherlands	10.3	6.4	1.3	7.5	5.1	2.4	9.1	5.3	1.8
UK	5.1	3.8	1.9	5.5	3.2	0.5	6.3	2.7	1.0

A = all new products, B = new chemical entities, C = novel products.
Source: Cueni, 1995.[65]

1.14 Conclusion

After rapid increases in the 1970s, the proportion of health care expenditure in GDP grew much more slowly between 1981 and 1991 and between 1991

62 *Health Care and Cost Containment in the European Union*

and 1995 in all countries. In some (Belgium, Denmark, Italy and Finland) health care expenditure as a proportion of GDP actually fell between 1991 and 1996. This is despite pressures for increased spending arising from the ageing of the population, increases in coverage and improvements in technology. It is at least probable, therefore, that this was due to some of the cost containment measures that most Member States introduced over that period; these are discussed in the next two sections.

III : Cost containment measures

As is illustrated in Part II of this book, almost all the member states of the European Union have introduced an enormous number of measures over the last 15 years aimed directly or indirectly at containing public health care costs. It will greatly simplify our subsequent discussion if these can grouped together in a form that is useful for analytic purposes. Cost containment measures can be classified in a number of ways. The most common is to divide them into those designed to affect the demand for publicly funded health care and those designed to reduce its supply.[48,66] However, this is not quite refined enough for our purposes here, and we adopt a slightly different, threefold classification: budget shifting, budget setting and direct and indirect controls. In this section we explain these in more detail.

1.15 Budget shifting

Possibly the most common method of reducing public health expenditure is to try to shift health care expenditure on to some other budget: either that of the patients themselves or that of other, non-health-related, parts of the government's budget. Expenditure can be shifted onto patients either directly through introducing charges or co-payments for the use of medical services or indirectly through reducing the range of services covered by the public health systems. Both of these can lead to a greater take-up of privately funded voluntary health insurance, which can also be encouraged by other means, such as tax incentives. Expenditure can be shifted onto the other parts of the government budget by the simple expedient of reclassifying

The European Union: Cost Containment Measures   63

health spending as another form of public spending, by measures to encourage potential users of health services to use other parts of the government service instead, or by subsidizing private expenditure in health care through the tax system.

1.15.1 Co-payments

It is well known that one of the major factors leading to upward pressures on public health expenditures is the phenomenon of 'moral hazard'. Under most public health systems, patients are not required to pay the costs of medical treatment they receive and therefore neither they nor their doctors have any incentive to economize on that treatment. The moral hazard problems can be reduced by requiring the individual patients to pay a charge, or make a co-payment, for the use of public health services, one that reflects part of the costs of medical care received. In theory, this should have two effects. First, it should discourage the so-called 'frivolous' use of health services: consultations and treatment that are unwarranted by the severity (or rather lack of it) of the condition concerned. This should reduce the utilization of medical services overall, hence reducing the share of national resources devoted to health care, and also reduce the pressures on the public budget. Related to this, charges can be used as an incentive device to encourage cheaper forms of medical service utilization. For instance, charges can be levied on patients who go straight to hospital without being referred by primary care practitioners, but not on those who are referred, thus encouraging the gatekeeping role of primary care and perhaps a greater use of primary care services themselves.

Second, the use of co-payment systems can relieve pressure on the public budget through raising revenue that can be used to contribute to the government expenditure on health care. This is in partial conflict with their role in discouraging the use of services; for the more effective charges are in discouraging service use, the less revenue they will raise.* Their revenue-gen-

---

* Strictly, the relationship between an increase in charges, its impact on use and on the revenues raised will depend on the price-elasticity of the service concerned. If the elasticity is greater than one, then a 1 per cent increase in charges will bring about a greater than 1 per cent fall in the use of the service concerned and a fall in overall revenue; if it is less than one, then the fall in service use will be less than 1 per cent and revenue will rise.

erating capacity will depend crucially on any exemptions that are part of the system, with the more people exempted the lower the revenue raised.

Most of the authors who have studied the operations of co-payment systems in practice are sceptical about their supposed benefits ever being achieved to any significant extent.[67] The co-payments are usually set too low to discourage use sufficiently; alternatively, if they are raised to a level high enough to affect use (as in France), the individuals concerned often take out private health insurance to cover the charges, with the consequence that the charges have little impact on use. Moreover, in so far as they do discourage use, they appear to discourage that which is 'worthwhile' as much as that which is frivolous.[67] Further, their revenue-raising capacity is usually severely affected by extensive exemption systems that are administratively expensive to operate and that exempt very large proportions of users.

Also it may not be equitable to increase cost sharing. The poor generally have worse health and need more services than the better-off. Under a co-payment scheme their health care bill could suddenly become very substantial when an expensive illness strikes. Moreover, some patients with chronic illnesses need expensive drugs for a long time.

Means-tested charges are often proposed as a way of making cost sharing more equitable. However, it is difficult to devise systems that are not abused and in which people pay according to their means. Who is to determine capacity to pay – the doctor, the pharmacist, some social welfare agency or patients themselves? Operating an effective means test for occasional expenditure is bound to be expensive administratively and can be divisive socially.[67]

1.15.2 Treatment restrictions

Reducing the number and type of treatments that are publicly funded can lead to a 'one-off' reduction in public health care costs. The reduction could be based on an examination of evidence concerning effectiveness, cost-effectiveness, and/or other considerations such as whether the treatment is largely cosmetic. Restrictions can take the form of positive or negative lists. A positive list details the treatments that will be funded publicly; a negative list details those that will not. Both kinds have been introduced within EU Member States, most notably for pharmaceutical care.

The way the restrictions are implemented depends on the type of health

The European Union: Cost Containment Measures   65

system. In national health systems with purchaser/provider splits, the purchasers may be instructed not to purchase treatments on a negative list, or only to purchase those treatments on a positive one. In national health systems, without purchaser/provider splits the instructions go straight down to the providers themselves. In social insurance systems with reimbursement, the insurers simply refuse to reimburse patients for any expenses in relation to treatments on a negative list, or confine themselves to reimbursement of treatments on a positive list.

In a sense, treatment restrictions can be viewed as the ultimate form of co-payment, in that the payment for the restricted treatment is shifted entirely onto the patient. That is, patients are not actually forbidden to have the treatment concerned; rather, if they do wish to have the treatment, it will have to be paid for entirely out of their own resources.

1.15.3 Public budget shifting

Public health care spending can be reduced by simply reclassifying certain kinds of spending so that they come out under other parts of the government budget (such as social services). Of course this is simply an accounting change, and does nothing to address the fundamental problems of cost containment. More substantive changes can be achieved through tax incentive systems that encourage individuals to take out private health insurance, the cost of which will appear as reduced revenue to the government, instead of increased spending.

1.16 Budget setting

Traditionally, many health services, public or private, operated with what we might call national budgets or indeed with no budget at all. That is, all the relevant agents, from the government down to local health centres, operated on what was effectively an ex post system of reimbursement. Thus, in such systems, hospitals and doctors operated on a fee-for-service basis, providing treatment to patients and then sending on bills for the treatments concerned to the relevant payments agency (such as the social insurance fund or private insurance company). If the payments agency had not enough

66 Health Care and Cost Containment in the European Union

funds to meet these bills, then, provided it had the power to do so, it raised levies on the population it covered, either through raising premiums, as in the case of private insurance companies, or through raising contribution rates in the case of social insurance funds. If the agency did not have that power, as some social insurance funds, for instance, did not, it asked for money from the government. And if the government could not pay the extra out of allocated funds it made an appropriation, diverting spending from elsewhere, increasing government borrowing or raising taxes in one form or another.

Such systems have an obvious problem: no-one has any incentive to economize, since overspending can always be passed on to someone else. Hence they are extremely vulnerable to upward cost pressures. However, they also have an obvious solution: the introduction of fixed or hard budgets as crucial points in the system. If budgets are allocated to the relevant agents, and those agents have a strong incentive to spend within their budget (either through penalties for overspending, through rewards for underspending, or both) then cost pressures can be contained.

The budgets can be set at any (or all) levels. There could be an overall budget cap at government level, with the government committing itself to a fixed allocation for public health spending. Different sectors could be given a fixed budget (in-patient care, ambulatory care, pharmaceuticals). In systems with a split between purchasers and providers, the purchasers could be given fixed budgets; in systems with no such split, the providers could be allocated budgets directly. Finally, patients themselves could be given a budget to spend on their own care, as they chose.

The budgets themselves can take different forms. They can be 'hard' in the sense described above, that is, with penalties for overspending and perhaps also rewards for underspending. The penalties can take the form of requiring the agent concerned to repay any overspending out of subsequent years' allocation, or only partial reimbursement of overspending or, ultimately, of a complete withdrawal of budgetary power. In systems where the budget is used to reimburse fee-for-service providers, the fees can be automatically adjusted retrospectively to make sure that total expenditure remains within budget. The rewards can involve retention by the agent of some or all of any surplus made.

An alternative to hard budgets is target or 'shadow' budgets, where a record is kept of the costs of the transactions undertaken by the agent concerned, who is made aware of any overspending or underspending, but

The European Union: Cost Containment Measures   67

where no immediate penalties are applied and overspending is automatically met. Such budgets are less likely to be effective instruments of cost containment than hard budgets. However, they might not be totally ineffective; most agents would prefer to be known as running the kind of operation that keeps within a budget. 'Naming and shaming' agents who habitually overspend can have a salutary effect on behaviour.

Budgets can be set in a variety of ways. For agents serving a fixed population they can be set on a capitation basis: that is, the agent receives a fixed amount per person covered, regardless of the actual use made of the system. To take account of variations in need between different populations, the amount per person may be adjusted according to various risk factors such as age or health record: however, the more risk adjustments made, the more complex the system. Alternatively, budgets can be set according to historical spending or activity levels; however, unless those levels are an accurate reflection of needs, both now and in the future, this may simply perpetuate past inefficiencies in resource allocation.

Budgets do have their problems as instruments of cost containment. First, hard budgets with penalties for overspending but no rewards for underspending encourage agents to spend up to their limit.[68] Second, most types of budget offer incentives for cream skimming and budget shifting; that is, for agents to select the people covered by their budget so as to favour those who will make the least demands on the budget and to shift other, more expensive patients onto other budgets (their own or those of other government agencies). Third, if budgets are successful in containing costs, then they are likely to create a need for rationing and waiting lists may develop, which can create political problems. Faced with these difficulties, governments may be tempted to relax budgetary constraints; if this happens too frequently and if agents begin to suspect that, if they overspend, there will be little or no penalty, then incentives for cost containment will quickly evaporate.

The main advantage of hospital budgets is that the cost is fixed for both the insurer/purchaser and the hospital, and the latter can plan in advance the most efficient use of the limited resources. However, efficiency gains depend on how budgets are set and the extent to which managers are held accountable.[69] It is also possible to adapt budgets to productivity by using case-mix weightings or DRGs as indicators of hospital activity and performance.[70] Systems without provision for budget adjustment for higher productivity may create incentives to minimize costs but can affect the quality

68   *Health Care and Cost Containment in the European Union*

of services negatively if budgets are inadequate. In addition, budgets can play an important role in health reforms that include decentralization of the decision-making process in the health system and devolution of responsibilities on resource allocation to local hospital managers.[71]

The main disadvantages of hospital budgets, in addition to the problems discussed above, are that the hospital has no incentive to increase its productivity by shorter lengths of stay, because the more patients are admitted to a fixed number of beds, the larger the number of expensive early days of care which have to be financed out of the fixed budget, with the associated treatment and diagnostic costs. Therefore reduction in lengths of stay or even the introduction of day surgery may be impeded.[67,72] There is also a risk of undertreatment of admitted patients to keep within budget limits. In addition, budgets allocated on the basis of historical practice create institutional inertia that tends to lock in existing patterns of resource use.[72]

Nevertheless, global budgeting can be a useful initial phase between the use of traditional line-item budgeting and the adoption of capitation or activity-related payments. The further development of management capacity, accounting and information systems may lead to mixed hospital payment systems that include both budgeting and activity-related payments. These may be a better way of paying the hospital, taking into account productivity gains and quality improvements.

1.17 Direct and indirect controls

Governments can try to affect health care costs through direct and indirect controls on the way in which providers supply health care. Fees or payments made to providers can be controlled, and the prices of pharmaceuticals and other medical supplies can be regulated, as can the profits of pharmaceutical companies or other medical suppliers. The adoption of new, expensive technologies can be controlled and, conversely, the introduction of new, cheaper technologies (such as day surgery) required or encouraged. Also the 'inputs' into the system can be regulated, with governments imposing restrictions on capital investments or the supply of medical personnel.

As with other methods of cost containment, direct or indirect controls have their difficulties. The imposition of any kind of restriction or control is likely to encourage costly efforts to evade them. Even if they are not evad-

The European Union: Cost Containment Measures 69

ed, there is likely to be a 'balloon' effect, with the compression in one part of the system leading to expansion elsewhere. This is especially the case where one element of expenditure is controlled, but others are not. So if, for instance, the prices of pharmaceuticals are kept low, the demand for drugs expands, the quantity purchased increases and total expenditure on pharmaceuticals may increase. If the supply of doctors is restricted, their wages may increase, and again the overall wage bill for doctors may increase. Switching to cheaper technologies may simply expand the total volume of procedures undertaken and lead to no overall reduction in expenditure. Only if several elements are controlled simultaneously (price and quantity, wages and employment, technology and volume) are direct controls reasonably certain to have an influence in the right direction, but extending controls in this way inevitably complicates the system.

Some of these problems can be illustrated by the Diagnosis Related Group (DRG) methodology, a method of price control which some governments have introduced or encouraged purchasers or providers to adopt. DRGs are groups of diagnoses, each of which has a prospectively set fixed rate (fee) attached to it; a provider paid according to DRG procedures simply receives the fixed rate (fee) per patient regardless of the cost of the treatment.

The experience with DRGs has shown that there are several advantages and disadvantages to their use. Hospital payments are based on the kind of admissions and the (marginal) revenue of the provider is linearly related to the number of admissions. However, this is not linked to the volume of services provided or the length of stay. The rationale is that, within each DRG category, there is a homogeneous and observable product. Therefore a fixed fee for all admissions classified under a DRG category is established. Accordingly, a prospective fixed fee per admission per DRG category denotes a fair distribution of risks and provides a sufficient incentive scheme.

Nonetheless, efficiency incentives are related, on the output side, to the number of hospital admissions, and, on the input side, to the intensity in the use of resources per admission. Output efficiency is only associated with the number of hospital admissions and with health status. Losses in the hospital revenues resulting from the DRG payment system could be offset if doctors modified their admission policies to produce more profit. If this occurred, the net effect of a DRG programme would be to exacerbate hospital cost inflation.[73] Wennberg *et al.*[73] classified all non-obstetrical medical and surgical hospitalizations in Maine, US for the years 1980 to 1982 into DRGs and measured variations in admission rates among 30 hospital market areas. Hysterectomy rates varied by a factor of 3.5, but 90 per cent of medical and surgical admissions fell into DRGs for which admission rates were even more variable, suggesting that professional discretion plays an important part in determining hospitalization for most DRGs.

The fixed payment encourages hospitals to eliminate unnecessary services, to specialize in the types of care they do best and to reduce complications (such as hospital acquired infections) as these add to costs without generating revenue. However, low payment rates may lead hospitals to slow the adoption of new, useful technologies,[74] increase hospital admissions, decrease the volume of services to some individuals and shift services outside the hospital.[75]

DRG payment systems may also lead to cost shifting. Hospital costs can be reduced by shifting patients to other sectors of the health care system.[76] These other sectors may include out-patient departments and long-term care facilities.[77] In addition, the incentive to discharge may be too strong, so that very frail and elderly patients are prematurely discharged.[78] A study in the US showed that some of the cost reductions (or slowing down of the rise in costs) attributed to the prospective payment system are merely phantom savings. Hospitals may simply be shifting costs from Medicare to the Veterans Affairs system.[79] Furthermore, there is the problem of 'DRG creep', where hospitals classify as many cases as possible as severe.[80] The hospital has the incentive to manipulate the system to its advantage in two ways. First, when the diagnosis is not clear-cut the more lucrative of the possible diagnoses may be claimed – 'diagnostic escalation'.[81] Second, patients may be discharged and re-admitted soon afterwards so that two stays can be claimed for the same diagnosis. Hsia *et al.*[82] studied the accuracy of the coding for DRGs in hospitals receiving Medicare reimbursement. The study revealed an error rate of 20.8 per cent in DRG coding. Errors were distributed equally between physicians and hospitals. Small hospitals had significantly higher error rates. A statistically significant 61.7 per cent of coding errors favoured the hospital. These errors caused the average hospital's case-mix index – a measure of the complexity of illness of the hospital's patients – to increase by 1.9 per cent. As a result, hospitals received higher net reimbursement from Medicare than was supportable by the medical records.

Prospective payment by DRG requires some extra administration, and administrative costs are known to increase, but hospital management obtains improved information.[83]

Several classification systems have been proposed as replacements for, or refinements of, the DRG system. However, all of them, including DRGs face a common problem. As Russell[80] points out:

> "Both in principle and in practice, it is difficult to devise a way of measuring severity that reflects only the patient's condition and not what is done for the patient. Measuring what is done for the patient comes back to measuring costs, and the whole purpose of prospective payment is to get away from reimbursing costs."

1.18 Conclusion

Any of these three methods for containing the costs of public health care – budget setting, budget shifting or direct and indirect controls – has its advantages and disadvantages. Their relative effectiveness can only be judged by experience; and to that experience, as demonstrated in the countries of the European Union, we now turn.

IV : Cost containment measures in practice

Measures corresponding to each of the three kinds of cost containment measure discussed in the previous section – budget shifting, budget setting and direct and indirect controls – were implemented by our countries during the period with which we are concerned. In fact, the period can be broadly divided into three distinct phases, each corresponding to one of the three kinds of cost containment: controls during the late 1970s and early 1980s; budget setting in the mid- and late 1980s, and budget shifting during the 1990s. However, each kind continued to exist and to be implemented in the next period.

Boxes 1.1a, 1.1b and 1.1c illustrate the emphasis on the kind of cost containment and describe the main measures introduced in the three periods. They also examine the model of purchasing and provision of services in different health systems.

72 *Health Care and Cost Containment in the European Union*

Box 1.1a Cost containment measures in EU Member States, 1970s–2000s: mid-1970s/mid-1980s

Emphasis: Direct and indirect controls

Purchasing/provision of services: Public integrated model dominant in systems mainly financed by taxation (Beveridge type); public contract model dominant in systems financed by statutory insurance (Bismarck type). Payers gradually transformed into purchasers in some social insurance-based systems.

Budget shifting
- Role of cost-sharing still small
- Voluntary health insurance negligible except in the Netherlands, Germany, Austria and France
- Exclusion of services from reimbursement limited but spa treatment excluded in Italy. Elsewhere, negative lists for drugs introduced and parts of dental care no longer covered in several countries

Budget setting
- Budget ceilings for hospitals (prospective global budgets in France, historical budgets in Denmark)
- Target budgets for each contracted sector (Germany and the Netherlands)
- Relative value scales for payment of doctors (Germany) or hospital services (diagnostic tests in Belgium)
- Changing doctor payment systems (capitation payments in Italy, salaried GPs in Portugal, salaried specialists in Irish hospitals)

Direct and indirect controls
- Controls of hospital staff numbers (Ireland, Spain)
- Controls on prices (pharmaceutical products, per day payments in hospitals)
- Controls on volume (e.g. maximum number of items per prescription)
- Controls on hospital beds (most countries)
- Controls on capital investment and new technology
- Incentives to develop alternatives to hospital care (Northern European countries)
- Manpower controls (numerus clausus in medical and dental schools, controls over entry to specialist training)
- Doctors' profiles with or without sanctions for excess prescribing

The European Union: Cost Containment Measures in Practice   73

Box 1.1b Cost containment measures in EU Member States, 1970s–2000s: mid-1980s/mid-1990s

Emphasis: Budget setting

Purchasing/provision of services: Public contract model replaces the public integrated model in Denmark, Sweden and the UK. Also the predominant model for the hospital sector in Finland and in Italy. Purchasers in some insurance-based systems set budgets for each of the contracted sectors, negotiate doctors' fees, prices and volume of services.

Budget shifting
- Significant increases in co-payments
- Increasing role of voluntary health insurance
- More drugs included in negative lists and even more switched to OTC status
- More services excluded from reimbursement (mainly dental care, cosmetic surgery, ophthalmic care)

Budget setting
- Introduction of fixed or target budgets for overall or public expenditure on health
- Sectoral budgets for health services, mainly for hospitals and pharmaceutical care
- Individual fixed or target budgets for doctors (UK, Ireland)
- Relative value scales for payment of doctors (Luxembourg and the fee–volume trade-off payment system in France)
- More countries introduce capitation for payment of first contact doctors
- Fee-for-service payments are introduced in capitation-based systems to encourage preventive medicine (immunizations, screening) and day surgery
- Performance-related payment systems for hospitals are introduced in several countries (DRG type or activity-related)

Direct and indirect controls
- Price control systems for pharmaceuticals in all countries except in Germany and the UK
- Reference price systems for non-patented pharmaceuticals in Germany, Sweden and Denmark and for all pharmaceuticals in the Netherlands and Italy
- More incentives to develop alternatives to hospital care (mainly in Belgium and Denmark)
- Further reduction in hospital beds
- Practice guidelines for office-based doctors with financial penalties (France and Austria)
- Technology Assessment Institutions were established in several countries

74 *Health Care and Cost Containment in the European Union*

Box 1.1c Cost containment measures in EU Member States, 1970s–2000s: late 1990s/early twenty-first century

Emphasis: Budget shifting, rationing and evidence-based purchasing decisions

Purchasing/provision of services: Public contract model dominant in most countries. The role of private finance, but not necessarily private provision, increases.

Budget shifting
- Increases in user charges
- More pharmaceuticals switched to OTC status
- Reduction in the number of those exempted from paying co-payments (e.g., wealthy pensioners)
- Reduction in the number of diseases exempted from co-payment
- Explicit rationing decisions
- A greater role for voluntary health insurance
- Alternatives to hospital care and long-term care coverage schemes are further developed, but mainly financed by private sources

Budget setting
- Fixed budgets replace target budgets
- Budgets are combined with activity-related payments
- Sectoral budgets are replaced by budgets for individual providers

Direct and indirect controls
- A greater role for Health Technology Assessment in coverage and purchasing decisions
- Further controls on capital investment and new technology
- Further reduction in hospital beds
- Development and use of sophisticated information systems
- Further manpower controls (mainly doctors)
- More investment in developing management competence

Source: Abel-Smith, 1992[66] and authors' research.

Let us examine the different cost control approaches in more detail.

1.19 Budget shifting

The principal types of budget shifting measures undertaken by our countries in the 1980s and 1990s involved an increased use of co-payments. Treatment restrictions on the whole were confined to pharmaceuticals and dental care; public budget shifting was relatively rare.

1.19.1 Co-payments

Virtually all the countries in our study used co-payment systems to control pharmaceutical expenditures and expenditures on dental care. Most of them also used co-payment systems as a means of cost containment for ambulatory and hospital services, either raising existing charges or introducing charges on services previously provided free, especially during the late 1980s and the 1990s (see Table 1.19 overleaf). Exceptions include Spain and Greece. Denmark has co-payments for dental care, auxiliary services and treatments by physiotherapists and chiropractors, but has not changed these very significantly in recent years. Luxembourg has various co-payments but again has not changed them much during our period.

Austria introduced a small index-linked charge for consultations in 1988, a cost-sharing scheme for spa services in 1996 and a small charge for consultations in 1997. Between 1992 and 1995, Belgium increased co-payments for in-patient care and ambulatory consultations, in some cases by 60 per cent or more. Between 1990 and 1995, Finland increased its hospital in-patient, out-patient and health centre charges by 20 percentage points more than the consumer price index. In 1993 and 1995, France increased patients' financial contributions to hospital care expenses, with the hospital co-payment nearly doubling in absolute terms. Co-payments in Germany were extended during the 1990s to cover hospital in-patient days, rehabilitation facilities and ambulance transport, and were extended further following the 1997 Second Statutory Health Insurance Restructuring Act. In 1987, Ireland introduced charges for out-patient and in-patient care for two-thirds of the population. In 1994 in Italy, co-payments for out-patient care were introduced, whereby patients were required to pay the full cost up to a limit. In 1996, the Netherlands extended its cost-sharing measures (until then largely confined to home care and nursing homes) to co-payments for regular medical services up to a limit in any one year. In 1992, Portugal introduced

76   *Health Care and Cost Containment in the European Union*

Table 1.19 Cost sharing for GP and specialist visits, pharmaceuticals, in-patient care and dental care in 1996

Belgium (1995)	
GP	7.6% for VIPOs (disabled, pensioners, widows/widowers and orphans whose income is less than a predefined ceiling). 30% for other categories. For GP home visits: 7.9% for VIPOs and 34.9% for other categories.
Specialist	8.45% for VIPOs and 40% for others.
Pharmaceuticals	0, 20, 40, 50, 75 or 85% (for VIPOs). Flat rate for generic products.
In-patient care	For VIPOs: 1st to 8th day: BEF 156/ECU 4; 9th to 90th day: BEF 103/ECU 2.7; >90 days: BEF 226/ECU 5.9. Other categories: 1st day: BEF 1,366/ECU 35.46; 2nd to 8th day: BEF 366/ECU 9.5, 9th to 90th day: BEF 259/ECU 6.7; >90 days: BEF 490/ECU 12.7.
Dental care	Mostly private, limited services are free for those under 18, high co-payments or full charge for others.
Denmark	
GP	Extra billing for Group 2 patients (2.5% of the population).
Specialist	Extra billing for Group 2 patients.
Pharmaceuticals	0, 25, 50 or 100%.
In-patient care	Nil.
Dental care	Free for those under 18. Flat rate for operations and some other services, 35% or 55% (age differentiated co-payment)/ 60/100% for other services.
Germany	
GP	Nil.
Specialist	Nil.
Pharmaceuticals	DEM 9, 11 or 13/ECU 4.6, 5.6 or 6.6 depending on pack size plus the difference from the fixed reimbursed level (1997).
In-patient care	DEM 12/ECU 6.3 per day up to 14 days per calendar year.
Dental care	Those under 18 are exempted. Others: for regular check-ups and regular fillings: nil; for dentures and crowns 50%. There is a 40% rate for those with at least five years' regular check ups.

Greece

GP	**Nil.**
Specialist	Nil for office-based doctors. GRD 1,000/ECU 3.3 for hospital specialists.
Pharmaceuticals	10, 25 or 100%.
In-patient care	Nil.
Dental care	No co-payment for those under 18 for NHS-provided services. 25% for dental prostheses. Extra billing is the usual practice in the private sector (>95% of dentists).

Spain

GP	Nil.
Specialist	Nil.
Pharmaceuticals	0,10 or 40%. Patients who are chronically sick have to pay 10% of the cost up to a maximum of PTE 439/ECU 2.24.
In-patient care	Nil.
Dental care	Free regular check ups for those under 18; free extractions for the whole population. No coverage for all other dental services.

France

GP	30%.
Specialist	30% (25% for visits to public hospitals).
Pharmaceuticals	0, 35 or 65%.
In-patient care	20% plus small co-payment for lodging expenses (FRF 70/ECU 10.8), no co-payment from day 31 on for acute care. No co-payment for long-term care beds.
Dental care	30% for prevention, X-rays and surgical operations. up to 80% for dentures and orthodontic treatment.

Ireland

GP	Category One eligibility: nil. Category Two eligibility: IEP 15–20/ECU 18.9–25.2 depending on the area and doctor.
Specialist	Category One and Two patients: nil for consultant services. Category Two patients: IEP 12/ECU 15.12 for hospital accident and emergency department without referral.
Pharmaceuticals	Category One eligibility: nil. Category Two eligibility: up to IEP 90/ECU 113.42 per quarter. No co-payment for certain long-term illnesses and disabilities.

78   *Health Care and Cost Containment in the European Union*

Table 1.19 (continued) Cost sharing for GP and specialist visits, pharmaceuticals, in-patient care and dental care in 1996

In-patient care	Category Two patients: daily charge of IEP 20/ECU 25.2 (up to a maximum of IEP 200/ECU 252 per any consecutive 12 month period) for stays in public wards.
Dental care	Category One, pre-school and national school children: nil. Others (paying the full rate of Pay Related Social Insurance): nil for dental examinations, diagnosis and scaling. Subsidized treatment for fillings, extractions, dentures and root canal therapy. For the remainder of the population, the full cost of treatment is charged.

Italy

GP	Nil.
Specialist	ITL 70,000/ECU 35.7.
Pharmaceuticals	Flat rate (ITL 3,000/ECU 1.53) for class A products (for severe and chronic illness). ITL 3,000/ECU 1.53 plus 50% of price for class B products (drugs of therapeutic importance). 100% of charge for class C products (drugs for minor ailments).
In-patient care	Nil.
Dental care	Mostly private. Free treatment to low income people is available in the health centres of the NHS.

Luxembourg

GP	35% plus extra co-payment of 20% for the first home visit within a period of four weeks.
Specialist	Same as GPs.
Pharmaceuticals	0, 20 or 40%.
In-patient care	LUF 214/ECU 5.45 per day for second-class hospital beds. Additional charges for first-class beds. Also additional charges for doctors' fees in first-class beds (66% on top of the fixed fee).
Dental care	Expenditure for dental services included in the list of medical and dental services covered by health insurance exceeding the amount of LUF 1,200/ECU 30.5 is reimbursed at 80% rate. There are different co-payments for other dental services.

The Netherlands (a)

GP	Nil.
Specialist	Nil.
Pharmaceuticals	Nil.

In-patient care	NLG 8/ECU 3.74 per day.
Dental care	Dental care for those under 17 is free. For adults, preventive care and specialist surgical care are also free. For all other treatments there is 100% charge.

Austria

GP	20% of the population (farmers, civil servants, employers) pay 20%.
Specialist	20% of the population (farmers, civil servants, employers) pay 20%.
Pharmaceuticals	ATS 42/ECU 3.13 per prescription.
In-patient care	ATS 50–60/ECU 3.72–4.47 per day (depending on the province and hospital) for up to 28 days.
Dental care	20% of the population (farmers, civil servants, employers) pay 20%. Up to 50% of costs for crowns and bridges.

Portugal

GP	ESP 300/ECU 1.87–ESP 600/ECU 3.73 for a home visit.
Specialist	ESP 400/ECU 2.48 for district hospitals, ESP 600/ECU 3.73 for tertiary hospitals.
Pharmaceuticals	0,30 or 60%.
In-patient care	Nil.
Dental care	Mostly private.

Finland

GP	Municipally provided services: either an annual payment of FIM 100/ECU 17.16 or a charge per consultation for the first three consultations (maximum FIM 50/ECU 8.58). NHI scheme: 60% of the basic tariff established for private physicians plus extra billing.
Specialist	Municipally provided services: a maximum of FIM 100/ECU 17.16 per consultation. NHI scheme: 60% of the basic tariff established for private physicians plus extra billing.
Pharmaceuticals	Flat rate (FIM 50/ECU 8.58 per prescription) and 50% co-payment.
In-patient care	Municipally provided services: FIM 125/ECU 21.45 per day for short-term care. For long-term in-patient care charges are linked to the patient's income.

80 *Health Care and Cost Containment in the European Union*

Table 1.19 (continued) Cost sharing for GP and specialist visits, pharmaceuticals, in-patient care and dental care in 1996

Dental care	Dental care for those under 18 is free. 10% for oral or dental examinations or preventive treatment; 40% for other treatments. Orthodontic and prostheses treatments are not covered.

Sweden

GP	SEK 60–140/ECU 7.00–16.40 depending on county council (average SEK 107).
Specialist	SEK 100–260/ECU 11.75–30.55 for hospital-based specialist (average SEK 193). (b)
Pharmaceuticals	SEK 160/ECU 18.80 for first drug prescribed and SEK 60/ECU 7.00 for each additional. (c)
In-patient care	Maximum SEK 80/ECU 9.40 per day.
Dental care	No co-payment for those under 20 years. High co-payments with ceilings for all others. (d)

The United Kingdom

GP	Nil.
Specialist	Nil.
Pharmaceuticals	Flat rate of GBP 5.80/ECU 7.12 in 1998. (e)
In-patient care	Nil.
Dental care	80 per cent of treatment cost up to GBP 325/ECU 400. (f) Basic NHS check-up: GBP 4.24/ECU 5.21. Full care assessment GBP 13.68/ECU 16.81.

Notes:

(a) As of 1997 all ZWF (sickness funds) insured as well as privately insured face a co-insurance of 20% of medical costs up to a maximum of NLG 200/ECU 93.47, or NLG 100/ECU 46.73 for people dependent on social security income. This co-payment is waved for GP visits, dental care (when covered) and hospital costs of pregnancy.

(b) Depending on county council and whether the patient had a referral or not.

(c) Since 1997 the patient pays the full cost of pharmaceutical care up to a ceiling of SEK 400/ECU 47, and a fixed percentage of drug prices up to a ceiling of SEK 1,300/ECU 153. Only diabetic drugs will be free to chronically ill.

(d) As from March 1997, adult patients pay the full cost of dental care up to SEK 700/ECU 82, 65 per cent of the cost up to SEK 13,500/ECU 1,586 and thereafter 30 per cent of the cost.

(e) 83 per cent of prescriptions are excluded from co-payment.

(f) In 1997.

Source: Authors' research.

The European Union: Cost Containment Measures in Practice   81

co-payments for almost all forms of care. Fees for visiting hospital physicians relative to primary care physicians were raised by the county councils in Sweden during the 1990s, with the aim of steering patients towards primary care. Although the UK has not introduced co-payments for medical services other than for dental care and pharmaceuticals, both it and Belgium have increased the use of charges by shifting long-term patients out of acute and chronic hospital beds (where care is provided largely free), into nursing and residential homes (where the charges are higher).

However, despite increases in the use of co-payments, these have never been the most important mechanism for cost containment. Nor has the extent of co-payments increased continuously. In all countries the issue is a matter of heated controversy between the political parties, probably because of its visibility. Co-payments can be increased when the economic position deteriorates and then reduced when economic prospects improve. In addition its extent may depend on which political party is in power. In fact, except for Portugal and France, the magnitude of cost-sharing has been modest. In France there has always been a greater role for the 'ticket modérateur' (cost-sharing) throughout the history of the French health insurance scheme. However, 83 per cent of the population have private insurance that pays all or part of patients' share of the costs, thus lessening its impact.[84] More recently cost sharing has played a more significant role, mainly as a revenue-generating measure, in Sweden, Finland and Denmark. In the first two countries, out-of-pocket expenditure increased significantly in the 1990s, but the exclusion of services from reimbursement might have contributed more to this trend than co-payment increases.

Concerning pharmaceutical care, the proportion of the cost paid by the patient varies by type of drug in Denmark, France, Greece, Italy and Portugal and for certain classes of drug in Belgium. In Germany, it now varies according to pack size. It is a flat rate in the UK and for some drugs in Belgium. In Spain the patient pays a standard proportion of the cost. There are extensive exemptions in Belgium, Germany, Denmark, Spain, Italy, and the UK. In addition, in several countries the percentage of items exempted from co-payment is high.

Most of the evidence concerning the effectiveness of co-payments as a means of cost containment comes from studies of their use with respect to cost sharing for pharmaceuticals. Evidence from the only randomized control trial available – the RAND Health Insurance Experiment (HIE) – suggests that lower levels of cost sharing were associated with higher pharma-

82 *Health Care and Cost Containment in the European Union*

ceutical expenditure overall.[85] In this study cost sharing was not combined with increased use of generic products.[86] However, there may have been a health impact. Brook *et al.*,[87] using the RAND HIE data, found that low income patients exempted from cost sharing had significant improvements in visual acuity and significant reductions in blood pressure compared with non-exempt patients. Other studies showed that demand for prescription drugs was reduced by a direct contribution from the patient. However, the price elasticities which measure the scope of the decrease in drug consumption are low (-0.1 to -0.6).[88] Fattore, in this volume, reviewed several studies conducted in the UK and showed that higher charges are associated with a decrease in pharmaceutical consumption.[89] These studies also suggest that the demand for drugs is relatively inelastic.

Several studies have suggested that user charges have a significant effect on the demand for dental care.[90] Yule *et al.*[91] estimated that in the UK the main effect has been on the volume of treatment provided, rather than the number of patient consultations. The introduction of a proportional system for the non-exempt patients in 1988 (75 per cent of treatment cost up to a maximum including dentures) had a significant impact on overall treatment volumes.

Yule *et al.*[91] also compared the impact of the UK policies with the results of the RAND Health Insurance Experiment in the US. In the RAND HIE the transition to lower charges at the beginning of the experiment resulted in a large, temporary surge in utilization in the first year, which was also the case after the introduction of the NHS dental care in the UK. In the middle years of the study demand stabilized, allowing the long-term effects of dental insurance to be assessed. Those facing zero charges had 34 per cent more dental visits and 46 per cent higher dental expenses than those paying 95 per cent of dental costs.[92] The utilization of low income groups was more sensitive to charges than that of high income groups.

According to Yule *et al*,[91] the fact that prosthetic treatments were most affected by patient charging was consistent with the UK findings. In terms of dental health status, it was estimated that the population with poorest dental care was found to benefit most from subsidized care. However, it is debatable to what extent high user charges influence utilization trends compared with the dentist's decision to treat and recall patients.[93] It is also debatable to what extent higher dental expenditure and access to dental services improves dental health. What is clear, however, is the evidence that the utilization of low income groups is more responsive to cost sharing than is

The European Union: Cost Containment Measures in Practice   83

that of more wealthy groups.[94]

The country chapters in this book report little evidence concerning the impact of the introduction or extension of charging on utilization, revenues and costs. However, such as there is tends to support the view of the sceptics. In Portugal, where empirical studies were reported, the impact of cost sharing on utilization was found to be negligible. In Finland the decline in expenditures was associated more with decrease in supply than with demand-side factors. In Germany some of the areas where co-payments were extended were those where expenditure increased the fastest.

What is also clear is that co-payment systems tended to be complex and expensive to implement. Despite some evidence of its effectiveness as a device for encouraging greater use of the general practitioner as a gate-keeper, Austria may abolish its system of consultation charges because of the expense. Hospital patient charges in Greece have had a minimal effect, since for administrative reasons most hospitals simply do not levy the charge. In Portugal there are many examples of service providers forgoing charges because of the bureaucracy involved.

In addition there are significant population groups exempted from co-payment charges which further limits the impact of cost sharing both as a cost containment and as a revenue-generating measure. Reduced charges or exemptions for those on low incomes and for other categories (for example, pregnant women or the chronically sick) vary between EU member states (see section 1.1.4). Several Member States, including Sweden, Germany, Belgium, Finland, Ireland and the Netherlands, have introduced income protection schemes by setting a ceiling for all co-payments. Overall, the scope for increases in charging for basic medical care services as a cost containment measure in Europe seems to be extremely limited.

1.19.2 Rationing and treatment restrictions

Outside the pharmaceutical and dental care areas, most of our countries have not used treatment restrictions as a way of shifting spending onto patients. However, there have been some moves in most countries towards establishing priority-setting frameworks or guidelines for decision making to help explicit rationing decisions in other areas. We will now examine all these areas in some detail, beginning with the role of positive and negative lists for pharmaceuticals, and then examining payment decisions for new

84 *Health Care and Cost Containment in the European Union*

expensive (bio)pharmaceutical products in a number of countries, trends in dental care provision, and the attempts of different EU Member States to establish rationing guidelines.

1.19.2.1 Positive and negative lists for pharmaceuticals All EU member states have introduced positive or negative lists for pharmaceuticals. It is worth noting that in its judgment in the Duphar Case,* the Court of Justice of the European Communities ruled that under a compulsory national health care scheme Member States are entitled to exclude certain medicinal products from reimbursement or to allow reimbursement only for certain products, on condition that the choice of the excluded products (in the case of a negative list) or of the included products (in the case of a positive list) involves no discrimination regarding the origin of the products and is carried out on the basis of objective and verifiable criteria.

Some countries with positive lists also have negative lists, and a positive list subsumes a negative one. Ireland extended its negative list of drugs for General Medical Service patients in 1982. Germany removed health insurance cover from some minor drugs in 1983 and more of these drugs in 1991. In 1984, the UK removed a range of drugs from the National Health Service – mainly those obtainable without prescription – and the list was extended in 1992. In 1993, Spain removed 800 drugs from its list and extended the list in 1998. From 1993, the cost of non-allopathic drugs was no longer reimbursed in the Netherlands. Belgium, Austria, Denmark, Finland, France, Italy, the Netherlands, Sweden and Portugal have positive lists of what can be paid for, as does Greece (which does not enforce the list effectively).

How effective are restrictions of this kind? In 1984, the UK Department of Health estimated that limiting prescriptions in seven selected groups could save the NHS up to GBP 100 million a year. Later the estimate was reduced to GBP 75 million a year. The Department was criticized for not disclosing how these figures were calculated. Critics also pointed out that it is almost impossible to assess the impact of changing patients to products that could still be prescribed within the NHS.[95]

In 1986, Reilly *et al.*[96] reported that orders for H2-histamine antagonists increased after prescriptions for antacids were restricted. Such 'switching up' could significantly limit the savings from a limited list. This is not

---

* See judgment at the European Court of Justice of 7 August 1984 in Case 238/82.

a good example, however, because at the time the growth rate of prescriptions for H2-histamine antagonists was high and it continued to be high for many years.

Two studies have shown that the introduction of the UK limited list resulted in a reduction in the rate of prescribing. Ryan and Birch[97] used a time series regression model and estimated that the list reduced the rate of prescribing by 300,000 items per month. O'Brien[98] estimated that the impact of the policy was to reduce the rate of prescribing by some 260,000 scripts a month. The first study used data for the period January 1979 to December 1985 and the second study data for the period January 1969 to December 1986. The limited list was introduced in April 1985. We do not know, therefore, to what extent this measure had a lasting effect or resulted in a once-and-for-all reduction of the rate of prescribing.

In Spain a negative list of 892 products was introduced in 1993. The expected savings were estimated to be PTE 23,000 million (about 4.7 per cent of the pharmaceutical budget). It was subsequently estimated that there was a 'one-off' saving of PTE 2,000 to 3,000 million, because most of the medicines excluded from reimbursement were replaced by others that were still reimbursed. A recent study concluded that there were no real savings but that there were important changes in the prescribing patterns. Garcia-Alonso[99] estimated that the consumption of antitussives combined with other preparations declined dramatically after the cost of these products stopped being reimbursed. However, the cost of antitussives that were not combined with other preparations continued to be reimbursed and their consumption doubled in 1994. In addition, in 1994, prescriptions for several vitamin products (mainly combinations of different vitamins) declined significantly, whereas sales of calcium not in combination increased by 1 million, as did iron preparations not in combination; both preparations were reimbursed.

In Ireland, in October 1982, 150 items were removed from the list of drugs available free of charge in the GMS. There was a significant reduction in prescribing rates in the final quarter of 1982 and by 1983 it was 20 per cent less than the 1981 figure. It was seven years before the actual prescribing rate returned to its previous high level, though by 1984 the annual rate of increase was back to its earlier level.[100]

There were, however, additional effects which diminished the extent to which financial savings were achieved. It was estimated that deletion of cough and cold preparations was associated with a threefold increase in the

86   Health Care and Cost Containment in the European Union

prescription of carbocisteine (a mucolytic agent of doubtful efficacy) which was retained on the list. Similarly the exclusion of antacids from the list resulted in a major rise in prescriptions for H2-histamine antagonists.[101]

In Italy the drug reclassification and extension of the negative list resulted in significant changes concerning the consumption in values of a number of products. There are no detailed studies available to evaluate the long-term effects of the change, but the impact in 1994 was significant.[102] The consumption of the delisted products was reduced by 28 to 80 per cent, whereas the consumption of those included in the positive list increased by 10 to 47 per cent. This is evidence of 'swapping up' policies.

1.19.2.2 Paying for new expensive (bio)pharmaceutical products   The financing of new expensive pharmaceutical products and especially biotechnology products has caused significant controversy in several countries. The issue of reimbursement of new protease inhibitors in France early in 1996 generated a hot debate, which was triggered by the National AIDS Council proposal that the choice of recipient be made by national lottery. The National Advisory Ethics Committee stated that a lottery scheme should be the last resort and held only at local hospital level when the choice could not be made on medical criteria. It is believed that the outcry of AIDS groups led the prime minister openly to oppose the lottery idea. A committee of experts has now been given the job of defining eligibility criteria.[103]

The case of beta-interferon, one of the first drugs that was authorized by the European Medicines Evaluation Agency, is also worth examining. The policy responses of EU Member States towards beta interferon differed extensively. Although in all countries hospital use of the product is either recommended or restricted, some countries have centrally established eligibility criteria for the use of the product and Finland has left it to the responsibility of local hospitals. In Spain treatment is limited to 16 neurological centres and there is a centralized registration system of all patients receiving treatment. Italy went a step further to produce a special Ministerial Decree[104] for the use of the product and named in the Decree the doctors responsible for its use in each designated provincial centre.

Denmark was the only country where the Ministry of Health produced an evaluation report of the product, in cooperation with a number of experts.[105] According to the report a number of criteria should be established concerning the use of beta-interferon. These include the severity of the disease, side effects, patients' compliance, the pharmacological administration of the product and the impact on the health system in terms of changes in the organization and personnel. The Ministry also launched a Reference Programme for beta-interferon. This programme is limited to this specific drug, but it may set a precedent for the future. The programme includes the guidelines for eligibility, criteria for treatment with beta-interferon, practice guidelines for doctors prescribing the drug and the establishment of a national clinical database of those who are eligible to receive treatment but do not necessarily do so.

In the UK the NHS Executive issued Circular EL(95)97 on 15 November 1995.[106] The Circular asked purchasing authorities and providers to develop and implement local arrangements to manage the entry of such drugs into the NHS, in consultation with other key interests, especially GPs and patient interest groups; and, in particular, to initiate continued prescribing of beta-interferon through hospitals. The NHS Executive also suggested that they take into account a number of issues raised in a Clinical Advice Report on beta-interferon. The report was produced by the Standing Medical Advisory Committee in consultation with the Association of British Neurologists, the Joint Consultants Committee, the Royal College of General Practitioners and the General Medical Services Committee, and following discussions with the Multiple Sclerosis Society.[107] The Circular strongly emphasized that GPs should be encouraged not to prescribe beta-interferon drugs themselves and instead to refer patients who apparently fulfil the indications for this form of treatment to a local hospital neurologist for special assessment or reassessment. Where treatment is appropriate it is suggested that the drug be prescribed by the specialist.

Finally, it is worth noting that representatives from the Ministries of Health of Italy, Germany and France met in December 1995 with the aim of preparing guidelines for the use of beta-interferon. It is not known what was the result of this meeting, but it is the first time that government officials have met to discuss policy developments for a specific product and this may set a precedent for the future.

1.19.3 Priority setting in health care: the EU experience

In the 1990s, several governments (Denmark, Germany, Spain, France, the Netherlands, Finland and Sweden) established committees to set priorities in health care. This section reviews their approaches.

88 *Health Care and Cost Containment in the European Union*

1.19.3.1 The Danish County Councils and the Danish Council on Ethics*
Since 1992, in the county of Funen the authorities signed with hospitals have defined how many patients are to be treated within a specified framework. There are also specific resource allocation mechanisms within the hospitals regarding allocation of resources to different wards. The contracts include guidelines that define how priorities are to be set in case the framework fails to provide optimum treatment to all patients. It is recommended that patients with the most serious conditions and for whom the lack of treatment would be catastrophic if they were not treated should be treated first.

The order of priority is presented in Box 1.2.[108]

Box 1.2 Treatment priorities in the Danish county of Funen in 1996

1. Treatment of possibly fatal illnesses and illnesses in acute need of treatment.

2. Treatment of illnesses that may have serious consequences later if not treated.

3. Treatment of diseases for which the applicability of the treatment is documented and which may have serious consequences later if not treated.

4. Treatment of diseases whenever this implies an improvement in the quality of life and health, but where the consequences of not treating them are less grave than for treatments that are given higher priority.

In the case of a hospital ward exceeding its planned provision of services specified in the contractual agreement with the county, services will continue to be provided, taking into account the treatment priorities. The guidelines for treatment priorities apply to individual hospital wards and there are no criteria on how priorities should be set between different wards.

In addition, since 1993, a contracts system has been operating between the county of Storstrøm and hospitals. In 1995 and in 1996, the county initiated consultations mainly with hospital managers as to how priorities should be established for hospital treatment. Two criteria were established to define the priority-setting framework. These are the severity of illness or disease and the documented applicability of the treatment.

---

* This section is based on a report published by the Danish Council on Ethics in 1996.[109]

The European Union: Cost Containment Measures in Practice   89

Based on the above criteria a list of seven priorities was established. It was decided that this list would be a guide in the decision-making process and would not include specific diagnoses because of the recognition that there may be significant differences in the need for treatment between individual diagnoses.[110] The seven priority categories are listed in Box 1.3.

Box 1.3 Treatment priority categories in the Danish county of Storstrøm

1. Acute patients.
2. Sub-acute patients.
3. The patient's life and mobility are in danger.
4. Patients whose quality of life has been impaired considerably.
5. Patients with a reduced quality of life.
6. Patients whose quality of life has been reduced to some extent.
7. Non-efficacious treatment.

The Danish Council on Ethics published a report on priority setting in the health service in 1996.[109] The Council emphasized that the establishment of general and partial goals for the health service does not help taking specific decisions in everyday practice in health service. These goals are often general and they are mainly concerned with principles. However, they are helpful when considering health care reforms or evaluating existing patterns of financing and delivering care. In this case the following questions should be asked. Are we doing the right thing? And could we do it differently?

The Council suggested three broad guidelines which may be appropriate in priority-setting situations:

- All people are to have equal access to the services of the health system across geographical and social boundaries. The basic rule must be that of equal treatment for equal cases.

- The people who have the greatest need of the health system services are to be treated first. The Council emphasized that the question of need does not only depend on the gravity of the condition, but also on how acute the condition is, and the possibility of doing something about it.

- No patient groups should be excluded from coverage; in the priority-setting framework the needs of the weaker groups should be taken into account.

90 Health Care and Cost Containment in the European Union

Finally, the Council emphasized that cost-efficiency and effectiveness are crucial issues in taking value for money decisions. However, cost-effectiveness should be only taken into account in conjunction with the three broad guidelines that the Committee recommended. To some extent this final recommendation is self-contradictory.

1.19.3.2 Germany In Germany, in January 1993, the Federal Minister of Health requested the Advisory Council for Concerted Action in Health Care to prepare an expert opinion on the development of social health insurance beyond the year 2000. Among the questions asked were "Which benefits should remain an essential part of social health insurance after the year 2000? Are some statutory benefits no longer justified for reasons of health and social policy based on the principle of solidarity and subsidiarity? Should new benefits be provided by health insurance schemes?"

The Council reported in 1994 that in its opinion the cutting of legally anchored aspects of health care could only be carried out under the slogan "rationalizing before rationing". Whenever improvements in effectiveness and efficiency of medical care within the framework can be achieved, this should have priority over the limitation of benefits. It suggested medical, economic and sociopolitical criteria for categorizing benefits. Medical criteria could include the degree of life saving and improvement in the quality of life involved in a particular treatment. Economic factors of importance were cost-effectiveness, insurability and price-elasticity of a particular treatment. Other economic criteria could be whether the need for a particular treatment could be avoided by responsible personal behaviour and whether such behaviour represents a major financial risk. Sociopolitical criteria could include cases of hardship and economic stress.

In its 1994 interim report,[111] the Council also identified areas for health targets as a precondition for an outcome-oriented health care policy and grouped them into three dimensions, namely medical targets, strategies and areas of support. In the 1995 report,[112] two examples were elaborated in some detail: antenatal screening and care, and diabetes care for both children and 'young' seniors.

1.19.3.3 Spain In February 1994, a working group of the Interterritorial Committee, which coordinates the regional health services of Spain, proposed a basic package of care to be provided under the National Health Service. It developed criteria for excluding services: lack of sufficient evidence of clinical effectiveness, no proven impact on life expectancy, no increase in patient self-reliance or diminution of patient distress. On this basis it recommended the exclusion of in vitro fertilization, sex change interventions, aesthetic surgery, psychoanalysis, hypnosis and spa treatment. In the case of new treatments, the criteria proposed for inclusion were clinical effectiveness, the absence of cost-effective alternatives and the availability of technology and health professionals to provide the treatment.

In 1995, the parliament issued a Decree on a Guaranteed Health Care Entitlement (GHCE – *Catalogo de Prestaciones*). Five types of care are considered in the GHCE: primary care, specialized care, pharmaceuticals, complementary services (such as ambulance services) and health care information and documentation. All currently provided health services were to be included in the basic package.[113] The exclusion criteria – which refer to future reimbursement decisions – include activities or procedures for which there is no sufficient scientific evidence of clinical safety and efficacy, or those which are clearly outdated in relation to others available; those which have not sufficiently proved their effective contribution to prevention, treatment, cure or improvement in life expectancy; and activities which relate merely to leisure, rest, comfort, sport and aesthetic or cosmetic improvement. Six types of service are specifically excluded: health reports and certificates not legally required, voluntary health checks, aesthetic surgery not required by accident or illness, spa and rest care, sex change, and psychoanalysis and hypnosis.

1.19.3.4 France In 1994, in France the Ministry of Health defined priorities on the basis of three criteria: severity, frequency and socioeconomic impact of diseases. The method employed was the Delphi technique and it involved the use of a questionnaire survey.[114] The questionnaires were sent to 125 experts, including health care administrators, members of the High Level Committee on Public Health, Ministry of Health civil servants specializing in information systems, representatives from regional health observatories, representatives from insurance funds and complementary insurance funds (*Mutuelles*) and researchers.

Three sets of questions were developed and disseminated. The emphasis in the first set was on defining the most important health problems. Respondents were asked to define the eight most important problems in France and the four major determinants of health, apart from age and sex, and to list the criteria they have used to define the problems and their deter-

92 Health Care and Cost Containment in the European Union

minants. The second set of questions asked respondents to rank the eight problems and the four determinants according to their importance. It also included questions concerning problems in the organization of the health system.

Finally, the third set of questions asked the respondents to rank again the health problems and suggest specific proposals for the improvement of the four most important problems of organization. The outcome was that the highest priority problems were considered to be accidents, major types of cancer, AIDS and other sexually transmitted diseases, mental illness, senility and dependence, perinatal issues, iatrogenic and nosocomial disorders and infections, child abuse and neglect, pain and backaches.

1.19.3.5 The Netherlands The 'Dunning Committee' was established in 1990 by the Secretary of State responsible for health in the Netherlands. The main task of the Committee was 'to examine how to put limits on new medical technologies and how to deal with the problems caused by scarcity of care, rationing of care, and the necessity of selection of patients for care'. This was at a time when publicly financed health care was to be extended to the whole population.

Three main questions appeared on the Committee's agenda:[115]

- Why make choices?

- Between what do we have to choose?

- How should we make choices?

The Committee published its report in November 1991 and emphasized that, even if more resources were to be available for health care, explicit choices would still be necessary.[116] The Committee used the community approach to define health. It defined health as the ability to participate in society. Thus inability to participate determined need and care made participation possible. According to the Committee equal access to health should be determined by needs not demands. The Committee discussed the proposition that preference should be given to the young on the grounds that those who have reached the age of about 70 have had 'a fair innings' and rejected it. The Committee claimed that it would conflict with the universal right to self-determination. There was no reason to assume that old people appreciated their lives less than young people, which would be ignored if one were to consider years of life instead of lives. Every individual patient is to decide

The European Union: Cost Containment Measures in Practice 93

for him/herself at what moment his/her life can be considered complete. On this issue, the Committee clings to a liberal perspective in health care rather than a communitarian one.[117] Implicitly the Committee rejected the counting of quality adjusted life years (QALYs) as a criterion for establishing priorities.

They recommended that each health care intervention should go through four different sieves: was the care necessary, was it effective, was it efficient and should it be left to individual responsibility? Figure 1.1 (overleaf) illustrates the Committee's approach of priority setting. The Committee decided that necessary services fell into three groups. First, there were those services which could benefit every member of the community and which guaranteed normal functioning as a member of the community or protected existence as a member of the community. From a community point of view, these had the highest priority. These included facilities which guaranteed care for those members of the society who could not care for themselves – nursing homes, psychogeriatric units and homes for the mentally handicapped. The second were facilities and services which again benefited all members of the society but were principally aimed at restoring ability to participate in social activities; these included emergency medical services, care of premature babies, prevention of infectious diseases and centres for acute psychiatric patients. They also included services to prevent serious injury to health in the long run, such as care for people with serious chronic disorders, such as cancer, heart disease, sensory disorders and chronic psychiatric disease, but also preventive maternity care, care for children and newborns, vaccinations and identification of risks to health. In the third and last group were services the necessity of which is determined by the severity of the disease and the number of persons with that disease.

Effectiveness was confined to confirmed and documented effectiveness. Efficiency would eliminate services of low effectiveness and high cost. Finally, the Committee thought that limits could be set on solidarity when the costs were high and the chance of an effect was very slight. These could be left for individual payment.

The Committee gave four examples. Excluded from basic care would be:

- in vitro fertilization, on the grounds that one does not have a right to the ability to have children and that it is not more than 30 per cent effective;

- homeopathic medicines, on the grounds that their effectiveness had not been sufficiently demonstrated;

94 *Health Care and Cost Containment in the European Union*

Figure 1.1 The 'Dunning Committee' criteria to develop a basic health care package

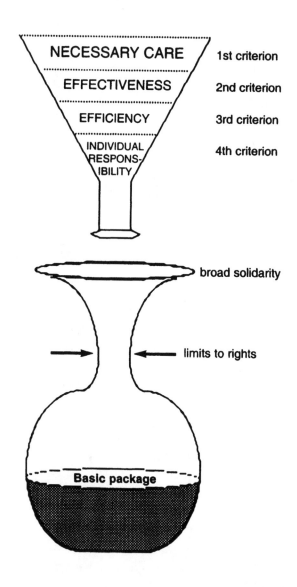

Source: Government Committee on Choices in Health Care, 1992.[116]

The European Union: Cost Containment Measures in Practice   95

- dental care for adults, on the grounds that this could be left to individual responsibility, given good dental care and prevention for the young; and

- homes for the elderly on the grounds that nursing care of residents was essential care: housing costs and living costs should be an individual responsibility unless nursing assistance was needed and the individual was unable to meet the costs.

In addition, the Committee suggested that two other issues should be further examined:

- reducing people's demand for health services through campaigns about not putting too much pressure on the health care system;

- reducing the doctor's readiness to prescribe medicines and offer examinations in cases where it is not strictly necessary, for instance through performing a careful reduction of the doctor's right of professional self-determination and through changing the payment system so that doctors are no longer paid on a fee-for-service basis.

1.19.3.6 Finland The economic recession and international initiatives on priority setting led to the appointment by the Finnish National Research and Development Centre for Welfare and Health (STAKES) of a working group to recommend health policy priorities for Finland.[118] The report focuses on the process of establishing priorities and the underlying values. The report deals with ethical, economic and administrative issues surrounding the choices process but does not offer specific guidelines for prioritizing services or interventions for individuals or groups. The purpose of the report was to promote the debate about choices not only among health professionals and decision makers but also among the public.

The report emphasized that priority should be given to cases where intervention is needed to preserve or rehabilitate the age-specific functional capacity. Decisions should take into account the expected individual health benefit and the expected quality and length of life, and it was underlined that the prolongation of life by all possible means is not the only or most important goal. In addition, the working group recommended that the state and local authorities organize health care in a manner that guarantees the same level of publicly funded health services for everyone. Finally, the working group recommended that the government and local authorities ensure that

96 *Health Care and Cost Containment in the European Union*

the quality, effectiveness and efficiency of new health care interventions be evaluated.

1.19.3.7 Sweden A Commission was set up by the government in 1992. Its 1995 report emphasized the distinctions between effective and ineffective care and between justified and unjustified care.[119] Ineffective care included:

- routine taking of specimens;

- mammography outside the age groups 50-70;

- tests for the exclusion of hypothetical risks;

- treatment of gastritis with antacid preparations;

- preventive treatment of high cholesterol blood levels with drugs, except in hereditary forms or severe situations;

- continued treatment for an incurable disease after the treatment had proved to be inappropriate;

- terminal care which prolonged the process of dying without palliative effect;

- surgery for minor prostate disorders; and

- several treatments for low back pain.

The Commission rejected the idea of priorities being based on age, low birth weight or lifestyle, social or economic status. It defined three principles which should form the basis for the decision-making process:

(a) the principle of human worth,

(b) the principle of need and solidarity,

(c) the principle of cost-effectiveness.

These principles are listed in hierarchical order (that is, the principle of human worth should be the first to be taken into account).

On the basis of this framework the Commission listed priority groups for the clinical activity/level and for priority setting at the political/administrative level. These are presented in Box 1.4.

In considering administrative priorities, the Commission inserted a further category in II – population-based prevention and health screenings of

The European Union: Cost Containment Measures in Practice   97

Box 1.4 Swedish priority-setting framework

Priority groups for political/administrative prioritization

Priority groups in clinical activity

I. Treatment of life-threatening acute diseases and diseases which, if left untreated, will lead to disability or premature death. Treatment of severe chronic diseases. Palliative terminal care. Care of diseases which have led to a reduction of autonomy.

Ia. Treatment of life-threatening acute diseases and diseases which, if left untreated, will lead to disability or premature death.

Ib. Treatment of severe chronic diseases. Palliative terminal care. Care of diseases which have led to a reduction of autonomy.

II. Habilitation/rehabilitation, together with provision of aids and prevention having a documented benefit.

II. Habilitation/rehabilitation, together with provision of aids and individualized prevention which are not integral parts of care.

III. Treatment of less severe acute and chronic diseases.

III. Treatment of less severe acute and chronic diseases.

IV. Borderline cases.

IV. Borderline cases.

V. Care for reasons other than disease or injury.

V. Care for reasons other than disease or injury.

---

documented cost-efficiency. The Commission stressed that too little attention was given to the Ib group of clinical activities compared to groups II and III. In addition, the Commission suggested that where involuntary childlessness is concerned it seems reasonable to limit the number of attempted treatments, to tighten up the indications so that only childless couples are treated, or to raise user charges. In terms of clinical priority setting, the doctor responsible should decide, on the basis of his/her knowledge concerning the suffering of the persons concerned and the specific prospects of treatment succeeding, which cases are to be offered in vitro fertilization. The Commission also recommended that, with the exception of extreme cases, treatment of shortness of stature not due to hormonal or other abnormalities should not be publicly funded. On the same basis, resources for psychotherapy should primarily be devoted to the treatment of cases satisfying current criteria of mental disorder. Furthermore, it was recommended that

98   *Health Care and Cost Containment in the European Union*

care for reasons other than disease or injury (group V) should not be publicly funded. The Commission also suggested that public funding should be available to pay for priority groups I to III at the political/administrative level. It also stated that, since the overwhelming share of health care is publicly funded, there is no objection, within this context, to introducing such concepts as basic security or minimum levels.

1.19.3.8 The impact of the proposals for priority setting in different EU Member States The reports produced by different committees in several EU Member States have been widely discussed and debated internationally. The way they were presented created the impression that in fact their proposals were to be implemented or that at least they would have a significant impact on national policy making. Was this the case or were they simply academic exercises?

To comprehend how policy evolves in different countries it is important to analyse the decision-making framework which, especially in insurance-based systems such as those of Germany and the Netherlands, involves several stakeholders which can veto decisions. The role of the central government is also crucial, as is the weight of organized interest groups. In Finland the report on priorities was not commissioned by government. In Spain the proposals had legislative authority; however, they mainly referred to future reimbursement decisions and left currently provided services intact; indeed, it is worth noting that the Guaranteed Health Care Entitlement actually implied a slight increase in the range of services that are publicly funded. It is also doubtful to what extent the criteria for the exclusion of services from a basic package will be actually employed. France adopted a disease-based approach to define broad priority areas. Further work in this field will elaborate the initial methodological framework and suggest more specific proposals. Currently, the public debate is focusing more on specific programmes than on rationing.[120]

In Germany it is expected that the Advisory Council will recommend a reform of the reimbursement system to take into account outcomes of health interventions[121] to modify existing input and process-oriented remunerations (for example, budgets and fee-for-service, respectively) by the degree to which a provider (or all providers in a region) meet defined goals. To what extent these recommendations will be taken on board will depend on the role of powerful stakeholders, including the regional associations of hospital and doctors. In Denmark the categories for priority treatment in the

The European Union: Cost Containment Measures in Practice   99

county of Storstrøm triggered heated debates. In addition, it has proved difficult to place all patients on a seven-point list and the two criteria for priority setting (severity of illness and disease and possibility of effective treatment) were in some cases contradictory. It was also very difficult to convey the information on cost-effectiveness of different treatments and to take it into account in the decision-making process.

In two EU Member States the impact of the rationing proposals was more significant. In the Netherlands the Ministry of Health commissioned several projects to analyse and examine the proposals of the 'Dunning Committee' and discuss them with health professionals and the public. These projects in many cases confirmed support for the criteria employed by the Committee. This further strengthened the technology assessment programmes funded by the Sickness Fund Council and the development of clinical guidelines and GP standards for care based on scientific evidence. The Cabinet response (in June 1992) to the Committee's suggestions focused primarily on promoting appropriate care, giving a major role to health care professionals in defining standards of care and treatment protocols.[115] The Cabinet did not refer to explicit choices in health care. In addition, the application of criteria to reimbursement decisions was difficult. It was not easy to define what necessary care is and decide when it should be left to individual responsibility.[122] This was clearly the case concerning the government's proposal to exclude oral contraceptives from reimbursement for women over 21. The decision did not materialize as legislation because of strong opposition from women's organizations. But the task of applying the Committee's criteria has been effective in other cases and the government has withdrawn homeopathic drugs and dental care for adults from the scope of health insurance.

The priority-setting framework in Sweden was criticized for being vague and lacking specific recommendations regarding real priority-setting situations. Others have pointed out that unreasonably low priority was given to infertility treatment.[123] However, elsewhere there have been positive reactions to some of the Commission's recommendations. Some county councils excluded infertility treatment from reimbursement or reduced resources allocated to this type of treatment. Several hospitals have attempted to operationalize the Commission's recommendations and produce specific operational plans.

The debate about priority setting may also affect policies related to the waiting time guarantee introduced in 1991–92 for ten diagnoses: hip replacements, cataract surgery, coronary artery bypass, coronary angioplasty, cholecystectomy, prosthetic hyperplasia, prolapse of uterus, incontinence, inguinal hernia and hearing aid fitting. The guarantee is an agreement between the government and the federation of county councils and is not regulated by law. According to the agreement the patient has the right to be treated/operated on within three months from the time a specialist has assessed the medical need for an operation. If that is not possible in the hospital the patient was referred to, then the patient can have access to hospital services in another hospital with full coverage of the costs by the county council.

The first two years after the implementation of this policy the waiting time was less than three months in all hospitals in Stockholm; but by 1995 four out of eight hospitals no longer met the guarantee.[124] There is currently some discussion about changing the idea of waiting time guarantee from elective surgery to chronic diseases according to the recommendations of the Swedish Parliamentary Priorities Commission.

In December 1996, the government forwarded to parliament for consideration a report on general principles for decision making in the health sector. The report was based on the proposals of the Commission and suggested four levels of priority groups instead of the proposed five. The government strongly underlined the need for research, follow-up and public discussion on how priorities are made in a more constrained health care situation. It proposed a special national committee for this task. A decision on the proposal was approved by parliament in Spring 1997.[125]

Overall, pessimism over the effectiveness of these priority-setting proposals may not be fully justified, but their implementation does require their 'ownership' by all the relevant stakeholders; and this is far from easy to obtain.

1.19.3.9 Voluntary health insurance We will now examine in some detail the development of voluntary health insurance (VHI) in the EU and the impact of the EU regulatory framework.

In Germany and the Netherlands those exceeding a certain income ceiling are entitled (Germany) or obliged (the Netherlands) to leave the social insurance scheme. In both countries VHI offers similar but improved benefits compared with the statutory insurance scheme. The benefits provided by public and private insurers are mutually exclusive. In Germany VHI covers 10 per cent of the population. The benefits provided by private insurers are similar but more generous because private insurers provide better hotel

The European Union: Cost Containment Measures in Practice 101

facilities at hospitals and coverage for dental care (up to 80 per cent and in some cases up to 100 per cent). However, the insured have to pay additional contributions for their dependents.

In the Netherlands those earning more than an income threshold and the self-employed are entitled to join VHI. VHI companies offer different levels of care with different premiums. Generally, the benefits they cover are similar to those provided by the sickness funds. VHI companies also cover the rest of the population mainly for dental care, maternity care, medical aids and other services excluded from reimbursement. The difference with the German system is that, in Germany, VHI covers only those exceeding the income ceiling and cannot be extended to the rest of the population to cover for benefits not covered by statutory health insurance. In addition, in the Netherlands the sickness funds are now entitled to provide top up private insurance and merge with commercial insurance companies.

Unlike the case of Germany, in Austria the public and VHI schemes are not mutually exclusive but in fact private health insurers only offer limited services. The number of policies has recently declined but the number of policies taken out for health insurance is very high (34 per cent of the Austrian population holds a private insurance contract, with 13 per cent holding a standard supplementary cost/ambulatory doctor contract and 21 per cent holding a special variant that offers a daily cash allowance in the case of hospitalization).[126] VHI mainly covers for hospital expenses (upgraded accommodation) and cash benefits during hospitalization.

In France complementary insurance covers 85 per cent of the population. The mutual benefit societies (*Mutuelles*) which are mutual not-for-profit companies cover two-thirds of the number of insurance policies and almost all the market for individual policies. Private for-profit insurance companies (*Societés d'assurance*) specialize in group policies. Private insurers mainly cover co-payments at primary health care level, co-payments for pharmaceutical care and dental care.

In Belgium the sickness funds (*Mutualités*) offer to their members complementary insurance which mainly covers co-payments and non-reimbursed medicines. The private for-profit insurance market is very small, mainly covering co-payments or upgraded hospital accommodation. Owing to the gradual reduction of state reimbursement many private insurers reduced their level of coverage and, in addition, as in the case of *Royale Belge*, increased their premiums by 100 per cent. 70 per cent of the self-employed are covered by voluntary health insurance for minor risks. In

102 *Health Care and Cost Containment in the European Union*

Denmark mainly Group 2 members (2.5 per cent of the population) are subscribers of VHI, which accounted for 1.7 per cent of total financing of health care in 1995. The number of economically and socially well established persons in Group 2 is markedly higher than in Group 1. The majority of them live in the Copenhagen region.[127] There are no private beds in public hospitals and only six private hospitals in the country (0.5 per cent of total beds). VHI mainly covers part of hospital expenses in the private sector, home care, medical aids, eye care and co-payments for pharmaceuticals. In 1995, 27 per cent of the population was covered by VHI. VHI covers only 12 per cent of co-payments because most of those covered do not suffer from chronic diseases and are members of a scheme which covers only 50 per cent of medicines' co-payment.

In Finland VHI currently accounts for only 2 per cent of financing of health care. VHI mainly covers children because of the significant waiting time and queues in public health services. It also covers hospital expenses in private settings. One-third of children under 15 years old and 10 per cent of adults are covered by VHI.

Less than 0.5 per cent of the population in Sweden purchase VHI, which mainly covers care in private hospitals. In Greece, however, 10 per cent of the population is covered by VHI. The annual growth rate between 1985 and 1995 was higher than 40 per cent. VHI mainly covers upgraded hospital accommodation in public hospitals, cash benefits and the full cost of hospital care in private hospitals. It also covers diagnostic care in the private sector.

In Italy VHI covers about 5 per cent of population. VHI currently accounts for about 2.5 per cent of the financing of health care. It is not yet well developed but is rapidly growing. The premiums are adjusted annually with increases in health care expenditure. Also insurance companies pay the providers directly and do not reimburse patients.

In Portugal VHI covers 8 per cent of the population. Most of the insured are covered indirectly through employment schemes or the purchase of financial services products. Only 1.15 per cent have individual contracts. VHI provides cash benefits for hospital care and total coverage for all other treatments.

In Spain public sector employees can choose the NHS coverage or VHI company; 85 per cent of public employees have opted for private insurance. Paradoxically, the figure for Ministry of Health employees is equal; 6.7 million people have supplementary private insurance (about 17 per cent of the population). Policy holders increased from 5.8 million to 6.7 million between 1990 and 1995. *Seguro de Assistencia Sanitaria* (insurance companies arranging for provision of health services via a network of office-based doctors and hospitals) accounts for 91 per cent of premiums and provides access to a network of office-based doctors and hospitals. Doctors are paid by VHI on a fee-for-service basis or capitation and patients pay a PTE 100 co-payment for visits to GPs and specialists. *Seguro de Reembolso* (insurance companies reimbursing, fully or partially, out-of-pocket expenses by the insuree) accounts for 9 per cent of premiums and reimburses patients' expenses (including dental care). Although the former provides more comprehensive care, the latter covers services not reimbursed by government.

VHI in Ireland is supplementary to public entitlement. Approximately 34 per cent of the population is covered by the Voluntary Health Insurance Board which was established in 1957. This is because it offers better access to certain medical procedures as well as a higher standard of non-medical facilities. Community rating premiums apply (same level of premiums for all, irrespective of sex, age, health status). In addition, VHI is open to enrolment and covers for life. Since the enactment of the 1994 Health Insurance Act the Voluntary Health Insurance Board has lost its monopoly in providing private insurance in Ireland.

VHI in the UK grew steadily until 1990, the year the NHS reforms started to be implemented. In 1995, 10.6 per cent of the population was covered by VHI. The growth rate was significant from 1985 to 1990, but since 1990, despite the good economic climate in 1994 and 1995, there has been a decline in total subscribers and total persons covered. The cost of subscriptions per subscriber increased considerably, by 53.4 per cent, between 1990 and 1995 in current prices and by 25.5 per cent at constant 1995 prices. This reflects a significant upward adjustment of the cost of plans in the 1990s. In 1994, penetration by socioeconomic group ranged from 1 per cent for unskilled manual to 27 per cent for professionals. Private medical insurance penetration by region also differs significantly, with the percentage of population covered ranging between 4 per cent in the North and 20 per cent in Outer London.[128]

Buck *et al.*[129] argue that the much-publicised reforms of the NHS in 1989 unsettled the public and thus the slowdown of the growth in the VHI market at this time was not solely due to the recession in the economy. One of the implications of the reforms was that the new NHS Trusts charged

104 *Health Care and Cost Containment in the European Union*

commercial rates for private beds and this created significant problems for VHI companies. As a result, BUPA now excludes use of NHS pay beds from cover in its new insurance policies. Subscribers' claims peaked in 1990 at 89 per cent of this year's subscription income. The relevant figure was 88 per cent in 1991, 82 per cent in 1992 and only 79 per cent in 1993 and 1994. The decline may reflect changes in packages offered, most notably the replacement of full hospital coverage with fixed cash benefits or BUPA's exclusion from coverage of NHS pay beds.

Private health insurers have preferred to encourage the growth of critical illness plans which, because of their lump sum, non-reviewable nature, provide insurers with a relatively predictable claims experience arising from the negligible impact on incentives to return to work.[130] Critical illness plans, which provide a lump sum to pay for various additional costs incurred by an individual during a prolonged period of ill health, topped 250,000 subscribers in 1994.[129]

1.19.3.10 The impact of the single European market on the development of VHI Developments concerning harmonization of the rules governing VHI in the EU were triggered by the Third Non-Life Insurance Directive,[131] which introduced important changes in the insurance market.

In the past there have been two main models for the supervision of insurance operations in EU Member States: material regulation and financial regulation.[132] The first model applied to Germany where regulation is based on the idea that, if insurers are sufficiently controlled in the type of business they write and the level of premiums at which they write, then there can be no question of insolvency. The supervisory body considers the policies before they are offered for sale. In addition, in Germany only insurers who have specialised in health care can operate in the field of private health insurance to protect policyholders from insolvency arising from other business. Price competition is restricted or prohibited by the use of compulsory tariffs. The second model was implemented in the UK. According to this model the regulator is concerned with establishing that the insurance firm is solvent by means of detailed financial returns on business. The regulator is not concerned with consumer protection issues including policy wording or defining prices.

The transposition into national law of the Third Non-life Insurance Directive [131] has had a significant effect on the so-called 'common insurance' area. There is now the possibility of providing accident and health

The European Union: Cost Containment Measures in Practice   105

cover conjointly with a life insurance contract, and the possibility for accident and health insurers of offering life insurance contracts provided that different classes are administered separately. However, this may have the effect whereby governments insist on life assurance rules and solvency standards also applying to health insurance operations. In addition, there will be a single licence for insurers incorporated in a Member State to conduct operations anywhere within the EU, whether through branches or under the freedom to provide services, subject only to home state regulation. This raises the question of the regulatory ability of the Member State where the company is incorporated to police and monitor activities of the insurance firm in other Member States. It also removes the right of the Member States to operate material supervision. Insurers will be able to fix freely the rates they wish to charge and this may lead to price competition. But insurers may also increase premiums and overcharge. Competition might also be triggered by implementation of uniform rules on the choice of law and harmonization of a number of important elements of contract law to eliminate choice of law as an element of competition. Furthermore, the movement of currency between any of the parties involved in transactions will be unrestricted. However, as long as private health insurance is a substitute for social insurance, Member States can enforce their binding legal conditions and retain their right to prior notification of policy conditions. Germany managed to retain this right. In addition, Germany forbids age-related premiums, to permit the requirement that premiums for health insurance be calculated on a technical basis similar to life insurance.

It is expected that the principle of home country control will bring into competition not only national undertakings but also national regulatory regimes. Strict regulatory regimes may discourage companies from investing in a specific Member State and the risk of reserve discrimination will induce the strictly regulated Member States to reduce their regulatory constraints. Harmonization towards the lowest common denominator may thus take place.

There are still significant barriers to the free movement of insurance services. These include the harmonization of tax regimes in the EU and the definition of a 'common good'. According to the Third Non-Life Insurance Directive, Member States can adopt or maintain such legal provisions to protect a 'common good' in so far as they do not unduly restrict the right of establishment or the freedom to provide services. This may, however, lead to the establishment of 15 different regulatory regimes in the EU.

106 *Health Care and Cost Containment in the European Union*

Tax decisions require unanimity in the Council. The Single Market Programme introduced directives covering tax issues involving parent companies and their subsidiaries and also mergers. There is, however, no uniform treatment of interest and royalty payments and other related matters.

It is not easy to estimate to what extent these developments will affect the provision of VHI in the EU and the cross border implications. Will competition lead to lower premiums or will the deregulated market create incentives to overprice? Will further regulatory developments be necessary? These questions have so far defied resolution and further research is needed to establish what the appropriate regulatory framework in VHI should be in Europe.

Member States find it difficult to live with these new developments. One of the reasons is that the health ministries were not involved in the discussions concerning the harmonization of private non-life insurance in Europe. Private health insurance was, at the stage of the legislative process, a small part of the insurance market which did not attract specific attention. The fact that the Third Non-Life Insurance Directive also covers health insurance may also have escaped the attention of the relevant authorities. An example which illustrates the tensions between a Member State and an insurance firm is that of the Irish government and BUPA International.[133]

BUPA launched its operations in Ireland in November 1996 by announcing its intention to differentiate from voluntary health insurance by offering two ranges of products: the Essential Scheme and the Cash Plans. The first scheme provides cover for essential medical care, while the latter offers the possibility of upgrading hospital accommodation by four extra-payment grades. This has become a highly political issue and BUPA was accused of contravening the principle of community rating since, unlike the prices of the Essential Scheme, the premiums for the Cash Plans vary according to the age of the insured. After lengthy negotiations with the Department of Health and public battles with the VHI, BUPA withdrew the Cash Plans but it is planning to launch a new Cash Plan scheme.

1.19.4 Public budget shifting

As discussed in the section analysing health expenditure trends, the most obvious example of reducing health care expenditure by shifting them onto other parts of the government budget is Sweden. Greece includes GRD 150

The European Union: Cost Containment Measures in Practice 107

billion of health service spending in the general public debt requirements; and treatment abroad is not fully accounted for. Tax relief for elderly people taking out private health insurance was introduced in the UK in 1991, but was abolished in 1997. There is no tax on insurance premiums in Germany, the Netherlands and Greece. Premiums are also deductible from taxable income up to certain maximum sums. In Finland the premiums are not taxed. In France income for premiums paid to private for profit companies is taxed at a level of 7 per cent. The tax rate in Portugal is 5 per cent. In Ireland tax relief is equal to the standard rate of tax (27 per cent). In Belgium hospitalization cost insurance is taxed at the level of 9.25 per cent. An additional premium (parafiscal tax) of 10 per cent is paid to INAMI (Institut National d'Assurance Maladie Invalidité) which is responsible for administering the health insurance system. There is a very small tax on premiums in Italy (2.5 per cent), Austria (1 per cent) and Spain (0.5 per cent), but premiums also receive favourable income tax treatment.[134] In Austria premium payments were, until 1997, 50 per cent tax deductible but this has now been reduced to 25 per cent.

1.20 Budget setting

Countries with national health systems such as the UK and Denmark have always operated with budgets at some (usually most) levels of the system.* In the UK there is a national budgeting process which was first introduced 20 months after the establishment of the NHS in 1948. Hospital and community services are budgeted at national level. Family services, including expenditure on pharmaceuticals and GP practices, are indirectly regulated without an explicit reference to a national ceiling. In Denmark the overall health care budget is negotiated annually between the government and the local governments. In Ireland public expenditure is cash limited and determined by the Department of Health and the Department of Finance.

Table 1.20 (overleaf) shows to what extent overall public health care expenditure is cash-limited in the EU Member States.

In theory it may seem that separate health insurers cannot be bound by this sort of restriction, but in practice, governments have used their power to

---

* An exception is the UK family practitioner service.

108   *Health Care and Cost Containment in the European Union*

Table 1.20 Budget control of public health care expenditure in the EU Member States in 1997

EU Member State	Budgets
Belgium	Health insurance budget is fixed annually by government. Growth rate fixed at 1.5 per cent (excluding inflation) for 1994–98.
Denmark	Overall health budget is negotiated annually and fixed by government and local governments (counties). Local governments cannot increase local taxes.
Germany	There is no overall fixed health care budget.
Greece	A national budget is established annually but never respected.
Spain	A national budget is established annually but never respected.
France	A target budget was voted by parliament for 1997 (1.7 per cent increase on the 1996 budget).
Ireland	Public expenditure is cash-limited and determined by the Department of Finance and the Department of Health.
Italy	A national budget is established annually but never respected.
Luxembourg	Since 1994, prospective fixed budget for health insurance expenditure.
Netherlands	A target budget was decided by government for 1994-98 (1.3 per cent annual increase). This has been increased to 2.4 per cent for 1998.
Austria	There is no overall fixed health care budget.
Portugal	A national budget is established annually on a historical basis but never respected.
Finland	There is no overall fixed health care budget. Government subsidies to municipalities are fixed annually as are contributions to National Health Insurance.
Sweden	There is no overall fixed health care budget. The rate of local taxes is fixed by government. County councils can increase local taxes but there are disincentives (i.e. reduction of government subsidies).
UK	Public expenditure is cash-limited.

The European Union: Cost Containment Measures in Practice 109

restrict or veto any increases in compulsory health insurance contributions and approve any charges levied on patients or impose reductions in the scope of the insurance offered.[8]

In addition, in countries where local taxes represent the main source of health care funding, central governments control directly or indirectly the level of local taxation. Since the early 1990s, in Sweden, county councils and municipalities can raise local taxes to increase funding for health care, but if they do so they will experience a decline in government subsidies equal to 50 per cent of the tax increase. In Denmark the level of local taxes is defined annually by central government as well as the size of the state subsidies to the health budget of local governments. Health expenditure accounts for about 60 per cent of local government expenditure and it is difficult to shift expenditure from other budget lines. In Sweden health expenditure is more than 80 per cent of most county councils' budgets, except for Stockholm, where it is less than 50 per cent. As a result health care is a top priority for local politicians who are directly accountable to local populations by means of elections.

At government level, Spain has an agreement under the Commission for Financial and Fiscal Policy (*Consejo de Politica Fiscal y Financeria*) linking the overall growth in public health care expenditure to the increase in nominal GDP.* However, in practice this agreement has yet to be fulfilled, with health spending being significantly higher than the indicated level. In Italy, Portugal and Greece in principle the overall public health care expenditure is cash-limited. In practice it is always overshot. In the Netherlands the government set a limit of growth of 1.3 per cent for the period 1994-98. The suggestion of the political party D'66 (centre-left reformist party) to increase the target to 1.8 per cent was not accepted by VVD (liberal conservative party) and PvdA (socialists). The growth rate for 1996 was approximately 1.8 per cent according to provisional data.[135] In addition waiting lists for orthopaedic surgery (mainly for hip replacements), ambulatory mental care, heart surgery and ophthalmology increased significantly. As a response the government has decided that in 1998 the target growth rate be 2.4 per cent. The government of Belgium has set a limit on growth of 1.5 per cent (excluding inflation) since 1994. This limit worked in 1994 and 1995, but the budget was exceeded in 1996 and 1997. In France in 1997, parliament decided

---

* Outside the European Union, Costa Rica has gone in the opposite direction, specifying a minimum below which spending as a proportion of GDP must not fall.

110   *Health Care and Cost Containment in the European Union*

that total expenditure should increase by 1.7 per cent. Different expenditure targets were established for hospitals (+1.3 per cent), ambulatory care (+1.4 per cent for specialists and +2.4 per cent for GPs) and different regions. It is unlikely that some of these targets, especially the one regarding specialists, will be met. Health insurance funds negotiate with doctors the target for each practice. The regional branches of the insurance funds are supposed to ensure that targets are met. There are no provisions for individual sanctions for exceeding the target, but the national level for doctors' fees can be reduced.

These kinds of self-imposed budgetary restrictions are more in the nature of the 'target' than 'hard' budgets, since governments in general cannot (or will not) levy penalties on themselves. It is therefore perhaps not surprising that they have not been very effective.

Of those countries with little by way of budget setting at the beginning of our period (mostly those countries with social insurance systems), most introduced budgets at one or more levels during the period. Table 1.21 presents the development of sectoral budgets in the Member States in 1997.

In the 1990s, Germany set sectoral budgets for ambulatory care and for hospitals. There are also negotiated budgets for dental care and negotiable caps for pharmaceutical care at regional level. The budget for ambulatory care worked; the budgets for hospitals did not, partly because budget constraints were effectively soft. A new law making the hospital budgets harder was introduced in 1996; however, sectoral budgets for ambulatory and hospital care were abolished in 1997.

In Ireland prospective annual budgets are allocated to the eight health boards which have the responsibility of allocating funds across the different health programmes as well as ensuring that budgets are respected. Sweden has devolved budgets to county councils, Finland to municipalities, and Italy and Portugal to regions. The Italian changes do not seem to have much effect, perhaps because in practice they are regarded as soft by the relevant agents and therefore not taken too seriously. In Portugal regional authorities have budgets which are divided into sectoral budgets (GPs, pharmaceuticals, materials and so on). These budgets are always overshot. There is no budget for primary health care and primary health care centres have no financial autonomy. In Finland there is no overall budget for public expenditure on health. However, government subsidies to municipality budgets are fixed annually, as are the budgets themselves. The government also fixes levels of health insurance contributions but expenditure by the National Health Insurance is not fixed.

The European Union: Cost Containment Measures in Practice   111

Table 1.21 Sectoral budgets in health care in the EU Member States in 1997

Member State	Sectoral budgets
Belgium	Sectoral target budgets for hospital, pharmaceutical, clinical biology, dental and primary care expenditure.
Denmark	Hospital budgets are fixed annually. Target budgets for primary care and pharmaceuticals.
Germany*	Fixed negotiated budgets for ambulatory and dental care at regional level. Target budgets for hospitals and spending regional negotiable ceilings for pharmaceutical expenditure.
Greece	None.
Spain	Target budgets for primary care, pharmaceuticals, in-patient care, research and training and administrative expenses.
France	Fixed budgets for hospitals, expenditure targets for clinical biology, nursing services, office-based doctors, pharmaceuticals and physiotherapy.
Ireland	Prospective annual fixed budgets for the eight health boards. Sectoral fixed budgets for community care and special and general hospital programmes.
Italy	Fixed budget for pharmaceutical expenditure; in some regions fixed budgets for ambulatory care and private hospital expenditure.
Luxembourg	None.
Netherlands	Expenditure targets for ambulatory, hospital and mental care.
Austria	Part of sectoral hospital budgets is fixed annually. Expenditure limits for some doctors.
Portugal	Sectoral budgets for GPs, pharmaceuticals and materials at regional level.
Finland	Fixed sectoral budgets at municipal level for hospitals and primary care.
Sweden	In many county councils there are fixed budgets at county council level for primary health care centres and individual hospitals. In other county councils budgets are allocated to groups of hosptals. There are no fixed hospital budgets in county councils with separation of purchasers from providers. Pharmaceutical expenditure is controlled indirectly by county councils.
UK	Hospital and community services are budgeted at national level. Family services including pharmaceutical expenditure and GP practices are regulated indirectly.

* During 1997, new systems were introduced: fixed fee-for-service payments and volume targets for ambulatory care; practice-specific soft budgets for pharmaceuticals; individual negotiated target budgets for hospitals were abolished.

112 *Health Care and Cost Containment in the European Union*

In Sweden county council budgets are fixed annually. Budgets are allocated to health centres (group practices). There are no fixed budgets for contracted private doctors who are paid on a fee-for-service basis. However, their contracts specify expected volume levels. There are significant differences between the 26 county councils concerning hospital budgets. In most county councils, activities are organized into geographically based districts. There are two different types of district organization. In the first model each district includes one hospital and several primary health care centres. The district receives a fixed budget from the county council and allocates it to individual hospital departments and to the health centres. Thus the district can be regarded as an HMO (staff model) with a monopoly position in a given geographical area. In the second model, there is a split between purchasers and providers (such as in Stockholm) and each hospital may be individually paid by several purchasers. Finally, in several county councils primary care is organized separately from hospital care. In this case county council hospitals may form a hospital district. Budgets are then allocated to a group of hospitals.

There is no fixed budget for pharmaceutical care but expenditure is indirectly controlled because it is part of the county councils' budget. It is worth noting that a purchaser/provider split exists in less than 50 per cent of the county councils and that in only six of them is this split real. It is expected that in 1999 there will be a significant merger of county councils and of hospitals. This will result in the provision of more than 50 per cent of all services by only three county councils. It is therefore expected that purchaser/provider splits will be further enhanced and implemented.

Some countries with a purchaser/provider split have set budgets for purchasers. In the Netherlands and Belgium the government has devolved budgets to sickness funds. In the Netherlands prospective budgets for sickness funds are based on a capitation formula taking into account age, sex, region and employment status of the insured. Since 1995, in Belgium, part of the prospective budgets for sickness funds (*Mutualités*) is based on a capitation formula taking into account factors such as age, sex, region, mortality rate, income, family structure and unemployment. This is currently 15 per cent and is expected to increase to 30 per cent in 1999. The other part will be based on historical expenditure. In Greece it has been recommended that a unified fund (with a single budget) be introduced, but the recommendation has stalled.[136] In Luxembourg a prospective fixed budget for health insurance expenditure was established in 1994. Policy implementa-

The European Union: Cost Containment Measures in Practice 113

tion is supervised by the Union of Sickness Funds which may activate redressing mechanisms (such as lowering doctors' fees) in the case of budgetary imbalance. In the UK, following the introduction of the internal market reforms in 1991, health authority purchasers and GP fundholders have been given a budget from which to purchase secondary care; the health authorities have to breakeven, but fundholders may keep any surplus from their budget provided that it is spent in a way that benefits patients. Under the new proposals of the Labour Government, Primary Care Groups, which will be replacing both fundholders and health authorities as principal purchasers, will be under the same rules as fundholders. It seems unlikely that this will result in any significant relaxation of budgetary constraints .

At the provider level, in Belgium hospitals have been given a prospective global budget for accommodation costs and nursing costs, but not for medical activities which are still reimbursed on a fee-for-service basis. Similarly, Luxembourg has introduced global budgets for hospitals, excluding payments for doctors who are still paid on a fee-for-service basis. Greece has set hospital budgets, but in practice these are soft and have had little impact on hospital spending. In 1984, global budgets for public hospitals were introduced in France.

In Denmark hospital prospective budgets are fixed annually. There are also expenditure targets for primary health care and pharmaceuticals which are continuously monitored. Since 1983, hospitals in the Netherlands have been given prospective budgets (originally determined on a historical basis but then on a function basis). Expenditure targets exist for ambulatory, hospital and mental care. In 1997, pilot schemes commenced under which one university and nine general hospitals will offer services directly to companies, bypassing the insurers. Ireland switched from a fee-for-service system for paying GPs to a system of capitation budgets in 1989. There has been no systematic study of the effects, but the change is thought to have reduced consultations by 20 per cent. There are also sectoral budgets for community care and special and general hospital programmes. Budgets for public voluntary hospitals (40 per cent of total hospital beds) are negotiated individually with the Department of Health. In Finland there are fixed sectoral budgets for hospital care and primary care. Since the early 1990s, in some Italian regions private hospital expenditure and ambulatory care are explicitly budgeted.

In Belgium the Insurance Committee for Health Care defines annual spending sectoral targets (for hospital, primary care, pharmaceuticals, den-

114 *Health Care and Cost Containment in the European Union*

tal care and clinical biology). In 1987, a quota was introduced for the amount of clinical pathology which can be done per day of hospital care.[137] In addition, the government may activate redressing mechanisms (such as lowering doctors' fees) in the case of budgetary imbalance. In France expenditure targets were first introduced in 1992 for laboratory tests, nursing and private doctors. These were extended in 1994, to cover physiotherapists and pharmaceuticals, and in 1996, to cover office-based doctors. A ceiling has also been placed on surgical theatre costs in private hospitals. Such systems of control are not needed where doctors are paid by salary or some type of capitation system.[8]

In Austria part of the sectoral hospital budget is fixed prospectively. There are budgets for individual hospitals and expenditure limits for a number of doctors. In Spain there are target budgets for primary care, pharmaceuticals, in-patient care, administrative expenditure and research and training.

Finally, there have been some experiments with giving individuals themselves budgets for long-term care in Austria and the Netherlands. It is not known how effective these were. In Austria, according to the preliminary finding of a working group of government representatives, it appears that long-term care institutions raised their charges, in particular for formerly voluntary or largely publicly provided services, as such services were paid directly by households rather than pension insurance funds. Recipients of cash benefits chose to retain most of the payments, or to give them to family members, rather than to spend them on care or market forms of care.[126]

Our countries' experiences with budget setting also reveal some of the problems involved. In Greece hospital budgets were determined by historical costs and hence incorporated past inefficiencies. In France they were again determined on a historical cost basis; in addition, they were thought to discourage the introduction of new technologies and to encourage cream skimming. In Spain, although hospitals are paid on the basis of their activities by using resource-weighted health care units (UPAs), in practice the financing method is still retrospective. In Germany providers allegedly developed escape strategies and waiting lists appeared, both of which contributed to the recent abolition of the relevant budgets. In Portugal supposedly hard budget constraints for hospitals were in fact soft, with expenditures over budget levels being regularly covered, with no penalty for the managers concerned.

On the other hand, where budgets were enforced they did appear to contain costs. In France the introduction of budgets for hospitals in 1984 played a significant role in reducing their share of overall health expenditure.[138] Redmon and Yakoboski[139] examined total in-patient expenditure trends in France between 1960 and 1990 and found that global budgets were successful in slowing expenditure growth. They did so by reducing the volume of services; the relative price of these services remained constant. In Ireland the significant fall in the average length of stay in hospitals (28 per cent from 1980 to 1993) has been attributed not so much to the per-night patient charges as to the efficiency pressures on hospitals resulting from tight budgetary allocations.[140] In Germany the introduction of budgets for sectors and individual providers, although of various forms and efficacy, were generally more successful in containing costs than any other measure. Yakoboski *et al.*[141] found that spending caps reduced nominal expenditures and real resources flowing to the sector, but they found the volume of services unaffected. This implies that, since the volume of services was constant, the relative price of services must have declined. As shown above, the impact of the global hospital budgets in France has been quite the opposite, with a reduction in volume while relative prices remained constant. This may have been why, in Germany, under the previous budget system the fee-for-service Relative Value Scale was floating and prescription of more services meant a lower fee-per-service for the doctor. Busse and Schwartz[142] estimated that prospective payments in the hospital sector have greatly reduced the length of stay, but have not yielded substantial cost savings. They suggested that one of the aims of the 1992 Health Care Structure Act – to increase coordination between the in-patient and out-patient care – has failed because hospitals were reluctant to offer ambulatory surgery because of budgetary constraints and because of the high level of ambulatory surgery by office-based physicians. The future trend in German health care expenditure following the 1997 abolition of these budgets will be an important test of this proposition. There has already been a substantial rise in hospital expenditure in the first quarter of 1997.[143] More generally, countries that have always had some form of budgetary control at key points in their system, such as the UK and Denmark, are among the few countries not to have experienced a cost explosion.

In most countries the largest impact of budget control has been on hospitals. This has led to pressure to reduce lengths of stay, rationalize the stock, transfer hospitals to other uses or sell them and to develop alternatives to care in hospital. However, it is difficult to disentangle the impact of bud-

116 *Health Care and Cost Containment in the European Union*

gets from that of new therapies and technology on hospital utilization. In many Member States, the trend has been for a higher proportion of health expenditure to be devoted to primary health care rather than hospital care. This reverses past trends.[8]

There is some evidence regarding the effectiveness of budgets in the pharmaceutical sector. Four countries have established budgets either agreed with the industry (Denmark, France and Spain) or simply laid down by the government (Italy). In Italy pharmaceutical expenditure is officially budgeted at national level and there are legal provisions for the enforcement of the pharmaceutical budget.

France introduced a system of revenue targets for each company in 1994. This system could establish an inverse relation between price and volume: the more a company sells, the lower the price will have to be. The critical factor is the extent to which the government takes into account the therapeutic value of the company's products. Because this is difficult to do, there may be a tendency to base company targets on earlier sales. The French press has reported that companies have been told that they will be treated more favourably if they invest in France and are willing to develop generic drugs, so that, as a generics market develops, it will be serviced by French and not imported products.

In 1995, the Spanish Pharmaceutical Industry Association (*Farmaindustria*) proposed that the government should establish a drug budget for the next three years, and the industry promised to see that it was observed. An agreement was reached in late July 1995 that limited the growth in social security expenditure on pharmaceuticals to 7 per cent per annum between 1995 and 1997. Companies must repay 56.7 per cent of the gross profit on any sales exceeding the ceiling. The remainder will come from companies whose sales have grown by more than 7 per cent. Of their repayment, 25 per cent will be calculated as a proportion of these companies' volume of sales and 75 per cent from the increase in the value of their sales. The industry has been guaranteed price increases for products costing less that PTE 300 and no regulation of prices for products that are not reimbursable. There is to be a monitoring committee with an equal number of industry and government representatives. However, the growth rate of the market in 1996 was 13.4 per cent, well above the limit of 7 per cent.

The government in Italy has established a fixed budget for pharmaceutical expenditure since 1994. The budget for that year was ITL 10,000 billion – ITL 2,400 billion less than the expenditure in 1993. Ceilings have also

The European Union: Cost Containment Measures in Practice 117

been fixed by law in all subsequent years. Pharmaceutical expenditure fell to ITL 9,772 billion in 1994, and in 1995 the budget was not exceeded. However, it is difficult to disentangle the effect of the budget from that of the massive reduction in the number of products on the positive list.

Some countries seek to change authorizing behaviour by giving doctors responsibility for budgets (as in the UK, where general practitioners could become fundholders) or by offering doctors part of any savings achieved on target, as in Ireland, where 50 per cent of prescribing savings are returned to the practice to be used in its development.[144] Fundholding practices in the UK have an allowance for prescribing within the firm budgets allocated to them by regions, plus the added advantage of being able to allocate funds to drugs, staff and alternative treatments. There is evidence that this has brought about a relative reduction in their prescribing costs.[145] Several comparisons of fundholding practices and non-fundholding suggest that fundholding GPs' prescribing costs increased more slowly than those of non-fundholders. An account of the first five years of the fundholders prescribing costs has shown that fundholding practices reduced the rate of increase in the costs of prescribing initially, though the effects were reduced after the incentives to save were withdrawn when budget setters reduced the budgets of those who were most successful in cutting costs.[146]

In 1993, the government in Germany imposed an overall budget for pharmaceutical costs for each area covered by a Regional Doctors' Association (RDA). Up to DEM 280 million of any expenditure over these budgets had to be paid back by the doctors on a basis each RDA would determine, and any further excess up to DEM 280 million had to be reimbursed by the drug industry. A budget was also fixed for 1994. This time any overspending up to DEM 280 million fell only on the doctors. In line with a stricter monitoring practice introduced the same year, physicians prescribing more than 25 per cent of the average for their speciality were to have their income automatically reduced unless they could prove that their overspending was justified by a particular patient structure. From 1995, an indicative budget was established for each doctor by taking into account the age structure of their patients and the speciality adjusted for geographical variations.

These budgets may have created incentives for office doctors to refer patients to hospitals for in-patient care. The drug budget seems to have been effective in its first year of operation. The drug budget for 1993 was set at DEM 23.9 billion, and spending fell short by DEM 2.2 billion or 9 per cent. These savings were the result of fewer prescriptions (-10.4 per cent) compared with 1992 and a reduction in the value of each prescription (-4.6 per cent). The therapeutic categories most affected by the introduction of the overall budget were peripheral vasodilators, analgesic and anti-rheumatic products. Other categories, such as anti-diabetics, antibiotics and ACE-inhibitors, were not affected. However, referrals to other specialists increased by 9 per cent and referrals to hospitals, where drug budgets do not apply, increased by 10 per cent. Schulenburg *et al*.[147] calculated that these alternative strategies increased the direct costs to the sickness funds by DEM 1.3 billion and incurred indirect costs (loss of productivity) of DEM 1.5 billion.

Where the budgets are firm, as they are for the UK fundholding general practitioners, and any savings can be used to develop the practice, doctors may be tempted to try a cheaper alternative first, and only if this fails to produce results to use a more expensive product such as a broad spectrum antibiotic. Any budget encourages generic prescribing. It is not surprising that, in the UK, fundholding general practitioners prescribe more generic drugs than non-fundholders.[147] Nevertheless, there is still scope for considerable growth in the generics market because the extent to which doctors prescribe them varies widely.[148] Budgets for doctors also discourage doctors from using new and expensive products.[146]

Overall, a cash-limited health service and budgetary controls at different levels restrain cost escalation. A question remains, however, as to what extent this creates an environment to achieve both technical and allocative efficiency gains.[149]

1.21 Direct controls

Most countries have some kind of direct controls over pharmaceutical prices or profits. Some countries with fee-for-service systems for medical care have tried to control fees directly.

1.21.1 Fee control

An example is Belgium, where the government simply reduced doctors' fees by 3 per cent in 1996. In Germany an increase in doctors' services leads to a proportionate drop in the level of the fees paid. This system was also

The European Union: Cost Containment Measures in Practice   119

tried in the Netherlands for specialists but could not be made to work. Austria and Sweden have used DRGs to set hospital fees. In Finland and Portugal DRG-based prices are being developed. There are also experiments in Catalonia and Andalucía in Spain.

Greece sets its reimbursement fees below market rates; this has the consequence that doctors overcharge or transfer patients to private practice. In Luxembourg fees are fixed by negotiation; this is facilitated by Luxembourg's unification of sickness funds, enabling the unified fund to act as a monopsony purchaser.

1.21.2 Input control

Some countries have concentrated on direct controls over the 'inputs' into the health system, either controlling wages and salaries in the health care sector or controlling quantities. In 1997, Spain froze wages in the public health sector. In 1993, doctors in Luxembourg were asked to take a cut in wages, and hospital salaries were controlled. Most countries control the supply of doctors, including Denmark and France (which has tried to reduce the number of doctors). Many countries impose central controls over capital expenditure and have tightened them during our period. These include Belgium, the Netherlands, Finland, Luxembourg, Italy and the UK. Italy tried to limit local health expenditure through freezes or staff hiring and ceilings on the purchases of goods and services. Sweden dramatically reduced the number of support/auxiliary staff in the health sector in the early 1990s.

1.21.3 Doctor supply

A common theme has been controls on entry to medical education (now exercised in all Member States) and to practice under public health insurance. It is increasingly accepted that an excess of doctors in health insurance practice leads to an excess of costs. In some Member States, costs could be saved by increasing the number of general practitioners at the expense of specialists and by establishing a pattern of referral, as specialists are more likely to use expensive specialized services when this is not strictly necessary.

120 *Health Care and Cost Containment in the European Union*

Table 1.22 Practising doctors per capita in the EU Member States

EU Member State	Average growth		Doctors per 1,000 inhabitants		Doctor visits per capita per year		Proportion of specialists	
	1970–80 (a)	1980–94 (b)	1984	1994 (c)	1984	1994 (c)	1984	1994 (c)
Belgium	4.1	3.6	2.7	3.7	7.3 (d)	8.0	40.7	40.5
Denmark	4.5	1.8	2.5	2.9	5.4	4.8	n.a.	n.a.
Germany	3.3	3.1	2.5	3.3	n.a.	12.8	59.7	54.1
Greece	4.1	3.6	2.9	4.0	n.a.	5.3	64.3 (d)	55.7
Spain	5.6	3.0	3.2	4.1	4.4	6.2	n.a.	n.a.
France	1.1	2.4	2.3	2.8	4.5	6.3	42.2	49.6
Ireland	5.6	1.4	1.5	2.0	6.1	6.6	n.a.	n.a.
Italy	4.5	2.7	1.2	1.7	9.5	11.0	n.a.	n.a.
Luxembourg	4.2	2.4	1.7	2.2	n.a.	n.a.	63.8 (d)	62.7
Netherlands	4.3	2.8	2.2	2.5	5.2	5.7	31.5	33.3
Austria	1.9	3.2	1.8	2.6	5.4	6.2	n.a.	52.6
Portugal	7.4	2.2	2.4	2.9	3.0	3.2	29.7	58.0
Finland	6.4	2.9	2.0	2.7	3.4	4.0	48.4	57.0
Sweden	5.3	2.2	2.5	3.0	2.8	3.0	n.a.	68.2
UK	2.6	0.9	1.4	1.5	5.0	5.8	n.a.	n.a.
EU Average (e)	4.3	2.5	2.2	2.8	5.2	6.4	–	–

Notes:

n.a. not available.

(a) Belgium, Ireland, Austria: 1971–80; UK: 1978–80.

(b) Spain: 1980–93; Italy: 1980–92; Luxembourg, UK: 1980–92; Netherlands: 1980–90.

(c) Or nearest available year.

(d) 1985

(e) Unweighted EU average.

Source: Authors' estimates based on OECD, Health Data, 1997.[37]

The European Union: Cost Containment Measures in Practice 121

For example, in Sweden a fundamental problem of the health system is the overutilization of secondary care specialists, resulting in 75 per cent of hospital institutional spending being allocated to hospital consultations. The absence of a gatekeeper scheme has led to escalating costs. In addition, primary care doctors, whose salaries are paid by county councils, are frustrated by a work environment in which they have little control over their work, inconsistent contact with previous patients and low staff morale. As a result, of the 4,000 positions available in the 800 health centres throughout the country, only 2,000 were filled in 1994.[150]

Indicators of the physical volume of inputs in different EU Member States also show a striking diversity. As shown in Table 1.22, the number of doctors per 1,000 inhabitants varies from 4.1 in Spain to 1.5 in the UK. The figure for Italy greatly underestimates the number of doctors in this country. According to the *Federazione Nazionale degli Ordini dei Medici*, in 1990, Italy had 4.5 doctors per 1,000 inhabitants.[48]

The attempts of EU Member States to control the growth rate of the number of doctors were to some extent successful. In most countries the growth rate between 1980 and 1994 was slower than that between 1970 and 1980. The unweighted EU average growth rate was 4.3 for the latter period and 2.5 for the former. The exceptions to the trend have been France and Austria. However, the growth rate continues to be positive in all Member States and this is expected to lead to further controls. At the same time, doctor visits per capita increased in all countries. The only exception was Denmark. The highest rates of visits to doctors are in Germany and Italy (12.8 and 11.0 per head per year, respectively) and the lowest in Sweden (3.0) and Portugal (3.2). Sweden (68.2 per cent) and Luxembourg (62.7 per cent) have the highest proportion of specialists and the Netherlands (33.3 per cent) and Belgium (40.5 per cent) the lowest.

1.21.4 Hospital beds

In several countries there has been firm action to close hospital beds or hospitals or to change them to other uses. Closing beds or hospital wards rather than hospitals has been the focus in most EU Member States. This can be partly explained by the strong political resistance to closing hospitals – although closing hospitals might have been a more logical choice. It has been estimated that at least 30 per cent of hospital costs are associated with

122 *Health Care and Cost Containment in the European Union*

buildings and other fixed facilities. A significant percentage of hospital overhead costs is tied up in 'invisible' assets, and in staff whose numbers are often only indirectly related to bed numbers.[151] Table 1.23 shows that the total number of hospital beds per 1,000 inhabitants has fallen significantly between 1980 and 1995 in most EU Member States. Further analysis of the OECD data shows that in most countries this was mainly done at the expense of chronic or long-stay beds (Table 1.24).

As shown in Table 1.23, the number of hospital beds per thousand inhabitants is highest in the Netherlands (11.3) which has almost three times the ratio of beds in Spain (4.0). In the Netherlands, most hospitals are run by voluntary organizations but, owing to overcapacity, government regulation is heavy. Hospital capacity is strictly regulated by the Hospital Facilities Act (WZV). Before hospital construction may take place a gov-

Table 1.23 Total number of hospital beds per 1,000 inhabitants in the EU Member States in 1980 and 1995(a)

EU Member State	1980	1995	% change between 1980 and 1995
Belgium	9.4	7.6 (b)	-19.1
Denmark	8.1	4.9	-39.5
Germany	11.5	9.7	-15.6
Greece	6.2	5.0 (b)	-19.4
Spain	5.4	4.0	-25.9
France	11.1	8.9	-19.8
Ireland	9.6	5.0	-47.9
Italy	9.7	6.4	-34.0
Luxembourg	12.8	11.1 (b)	-13.3
Netherlands	12.3	11.3	-8.1
Austria	11.2	9.3	-17.0
Portugal	5.2	4.1	-21.2
Finland	15.6	9.3	-40.4
Sweden	15.1	6.3	-58.3
UK	8.1	4.7	-42.0

Notes:
(a) or latest available year.
(b) 1994.

Source: OECD, Health Data, 1997.[37]

The European Union: Cost Containment Measures in Practice 123

ernment licence must be obtained.

Portugal, Spain and the UK have the lowest ratios of in-patient beds to 1,000 inhabitants. In Portugal and Spain the lower level of hospital provision is mainly due to the shortage of chronic or long-stay beds. Germany, Luxembourg, Austria and Italy have the largest percentage of acute beds. By contrast, the Netherlands, with the highest rate of beds per 1,000 inhabitants, has the lowest percentage of acute beds – about 35 per cent of the total. The UK is the country with the lowest ratio of acute in-patient beds to 1,000 inhabitants (2.0).

Hospital restructuring and reorganization is not free from political problems, as the Finish experience shows. In 1991, in Finland the central government abandoned the precise allocation of its subsidies and started

Table 1.24 Acute hospital beds per 1,000 inhabitants in the EU Member States in 1980 and 1995(a)

EU Member State	1980	1995	% change between 1980 and 1995
Belgium	5.5	4.8 (b)	-12.7
Denmark	5.6	4.0 (b)	-28.6
Germany	7.7 (c)	6.9	-10.4
Greece	4.7	–	–
Spain	–	3.2 (b)	-22.6
France	6.2	4.6	-25.8
Ireland	5.6	3.4	-39.3
Italy	7.6	5.5 (b)	-27.6
Luxembourg	–	6.7	–
Netherlands	5.2	3.9	-25.0
Austria	–	6.6	–
Portugal	4.1	3.4	-17.1
Finland	4.9	4.0	-18.4
Sweden	5.1	3.1	-39.2
UK	2.9	2.0	-31.0

Notes:
(a) or latest available year.
(b) 1994.
(c) West Germany only.
Source: OECD, Health Data, 1997.[37]

124   *Health Care and Cost Containment in the European Union*

funding the municipalities with a fixed amount per resident per year. The goals of regional uniformity and central control were abolished and local solutions were encouraged.[152] The system is expected to acquire more local variation and services will reflect the preferences and structures of the local communities. However, tensions over the location of hospital services in the future may arise. The need for further reductions in the number of hospital beds or even hospitals will inevitably lead to conflicts between different local authorities as to where hospital facilities should be located. The threat of hospital closure may also rebound on decision making and cost-effectiveness. Local authorities may well prefer to accept hospital inefficiencies and oppose a rational reorganization because of the threat of diminishing the provision of services within their territory.[152]

1.21.5 Medical guidelines

In 1993, France introduced a system of guidelines – RMOs – (disease management references) for specific diseases, techniques and treatments. These references are used to assess medical practice outside hospitals.[153] They specify when and how to use different procedures, medical examinations, tests or drug prescriptions related to a disease or health condition. Doctors who do not follow these references can be penalized financially or excluded from the social security system. So far 200 references have been developed and accepted by the government. But the guidelines do not apply if the annual contract between government and doctors has not been agreed. In 1996, the government decided to extend the guidelines to all aspects of doctors' activities and to ensure that they are implemented by giving them a legal basis even if there is no contract. Table 1.25 gives examples of the medical references. These are examples of negative guidelines. This may reflect the fact that French doctors overprescribe; certainly, these French guidelines imply some unusual prescription patterns.

EU Member States seldom use cost-effectiveness studies to influence doctors to change their prescribing behaviour. So far such studies have had little impact on pricing and reimbursement decisions.[154]

Examination of profiles of doctors' work and prescriptions thus seems to have only a limited effect; but the extent of the effect may depend on what sanctions are applied and how often they are imposed. In France the scope of practice guidelines is small, but presumably it will expand. It is an

The European Union: Cost Containment Measures in Practice 125

Table 1.25 Medical references in France: examples

Condition	Restriction
Ordinary seasonal respiratory infections in patients without specific risk factors	No use of systemic fluroquinolones
	No use of 2nd and 3rd generation cephalosporins
	No use of Augmentin®
'Ordinary' anxiety symptoms	No use/association of two different types of benzodiazepines
	No use of two different types of hypnotic drugs
Peptic ulcer	No use of two different drugs containing H2-histamine antagonists
	Treatment for acute gastritis should not continue for longer than six weeks
	No use of H2-histamine antagonists in chronic gastritis

attempt to bind doctors into what is judged to be rational prescribing. In so far as some doctors in all countries do not prescribe rationally, practice guidelines are directed at the source of considerable waste, providing the references are well chosen. But how far can the system be extended and where does valid evidence support the chosen therapy? In France the references for particular conditions are agreed with doctors' representatives, so there is a risk that they will be based on a medical consensus rather than evidence. Indeed, some medical references in France have been criticized as being weak recommendations that offer no firm conclusions that could help the physician and therefore unlikely to have any impact on clinical practice.[155]

The guidelines relating to drug prescribing had only a limited effect on spending in 1994, but some of them had a significant impact on prescribing behaviour. Le Fur and Sermet[156] estimated that the 14 pharmaceutical guidelines could have an effect on 14 million prescriptions, equivalent to 1.9 per cent of all prescriptions issued by office doctors in France in 1994. It was argued that one of the main problems was that the guidelines did not address general problems. Where they did, they dealt with the treatment of patients with chronic diseases, where changes in prescribing patterns are not easily influenced in the short term.

126 *Health Care and Cost Containment in the European Union*

1.21.6 Fixed reimbursement levels for pharmaceuticals: reference price systems

A relatively new approach to reducing the cost of pharmaceuticals is the use of a reference price system. In this system a group of similar products is given a specific price that will be fully covered by insurance, subject to co-payment. The use of a reference price as a reimbursement benchmark implies that the government will only pay that particular price. Any excess above the reference price has to be paid by the insured person. The issue of what criteria to use to select of the 'reference' price remains. The objective of the regulators was to make the consumers more fiscally aware and to trigger price competition in the reference-priced part of the market.

The first scheme of this type was introduced by New Zealand. In Europe, Germany was the first to introduce a reference price system. A reference price system was introduced in the Netherlands in 1991, in Denmark and Sweden in 1993 and in Italy in 1996. It has been proposed in Greece, Spain, Italy and Finland, but not implemented.

In the EU member states there are four types of reference price system:

The German piecemeal type: the system was introduced in three stages and it covers the generic market and part of the patented products market.

The Dutch big bang type: the system initially covered 90 per cent of the market, including patented products.

The Danish and Swedish cautious and limited systems which cover only generic products (Sweden) or a limited part of the market (Denmark). In 1997, the Danish reference price system was expanded to cover products with 'equal' therapeutic effect but different chemical structure.

The Italian type which covers all products clustered in groups of identical drugs.

A reference price system was introduced in Germany in 1989. If the price of the drug prescribed exceeds its reference price, the patient has to pay the difference. The reference price system now covers about 80 per cent of drug consumption. There were three stages for the introduction of the reference price system. The first covered identical preparations, the second covered equivalent products or combinations and the third originally covered preparations that were similar pharmaceutically and therapeutically. This has

The European Union: Cost Containment Measures in Practice   127

been changed to therapeutic similarity. Difficulties arise if some products in a group are still under patent and the reference price system cannot be used.

In July 1991, the Netherlands introduced a reference price system for products judged to be interchangeable, taking account of any side-effects, by the criteria of an independent committee of experts who report to the Association of Sickness Funds. Medicines are regarded as interchangeable if:[157]

- they have a similar mechanism of action and similar uses;

- there are no clinically relevant differences between their therapeutic effects and side-effects;

- they are given in the same way; and

- they are used to treat the same age group.

No reference prices were to be established for new, truly innovative drugs that according to the criteria were not interchangeable with other products. However, expenditure continued to rise after the introduction of the system, mainly because of the high prices of new, innovative, fully reimbursed drugs. In 1993, the Ministry of Health decided that new products that were not deemed to be interchangeable would not be covered by the health insurance schemes until the end of 1994.

In Denmark a reference price system was introduced on 1 July 1993. It covers 20 per cent of the drug market in terms of consumption. Groups of products that are identical in both chemical and pharmaceutical terms have been selected. They are grouped on the basis of type of pack. The reference price is fixed as the average of the two cheapest products in the group. Variations of up to 10 per cent are accepted. It is possible to derogate from this general rule and accept differences of up to 50 per cent in case of products used for the treatment of chronic diseases and when packages of generic products differ significantly.

A reference price system was introduced in Sweden in January 1993. As a result, the full cost of a product, less the charge to the patient, will not be reimbursed if a cheaper alternative is available. A maximum discount or reference price is established for each product equivalent to the price of the cheaper alternative plus 10 per cent. If a more expensive product is prescribed, the patient has to pay the difference.

In Italy, the reference price is defined as the cheapest price of a product in a group of identical drugs (same active ingredient, same method of

128 *Health Care and Cost Containment in the European Union*

administration). However, the groups include drugs with different dosages. This imposes a penalty on low dose drugs, because their price, expressed in cost per milligram, will be higher than that of higher dose products. Only the cheapest product in the group of identical drugs is reimbursable. Products with prices above the reference (cheapest) value are delisted (that is, not reimbursed).

The European pharmaceutical industry has consistently argued that reference pricing distorts clinical decision making, deprives patients of a choice of treatment and removes incentives for research into new medicines. Nonetheless, governments argue that these systems have advantages for the industry. First, while the average prices of those products clustered together may be reduced, no firm is denied the market share it can earn by accepting the reference price. Secondly, the system is fully transparent. Thirdly, patented drugs are excluded in Germany, Denmark and Sweden; the company can fix its own prices for these products. Thus these countries are not likely to lose the important position they have secured in world markets.

From the governments' point of view, the weakness of reference price systems, as the experience of the Netherlands and Germany has shown, is that their introduction does not necessarily decrease the drug budget. In 1993, Germany, in addition to the reference price system, cut by 5 per cent prices not covered by the scheme and introduced a firm drug budget for regional associations of doctors, with penalties for exceeding it. The Netherlands also cut prices by 5 per cent. Despite these measures and the introduction of the reference prices for part of the market, pharmaceutical expenditure continued to rise.

But perhaps reference price systems were successful in containing pharmaceutical expenditure by making consumers more cost-conscious and by triggering price competition in the generics market. Certainly, one would expect that the large price reductions would have resulted in significant savings. However, the reference price system stimulated the industry to make a major effort to promote drugs that were not covered. As a result the market share of these expensive products increased, and firms may even have raised the prices of these products to recover losses caused by the reference price system.

The reference price system for pharmaceuticals in Germany illustrates some of these effects. One effect was a switch in prescribing expensive products not covered by the reference price system, for example, new antibiotics. Advertising by the companies has encouraged this trend. In addition,

The European Union: Cost Containment Measures in Practice 129

pharmaceutical companies increased the prices of products not yet affected by the reference price system. Between 1991 and 1992 prices of drugs subject to reference prices decreased by 1.5 per cent whereas the prices of those that were not increased by 4.1 per cent.[158]

Reference prices were set, on average, 30 per cent below the previous price of the brand-name products. The expected boom in the market for generics did not occur. The annual growth of 2 per cent in sales revenue for the generic market before the 1988 Health Care Reform Act has slowed down to about 1 per cent. This may be explained by new, product life-cycle strategies introduced by R&D-based companies – especially the drastic reductions in prices after patent expiry that they implement to create barriers to market entry. Companies also reduced prices of unpatented products because patients were unwilling to pay for the difference above the reference price level.

Reference prices did not prevent increases in volume in all market segments and in some cases physicians prescribed expensive patented products and ignored cheaper alternatives. According to Klauber,[159] another component, the structural component (particularly increasing the package size of prescription drugs), also contributed to increases in pharmaceutical expenditure (Table 1.26). This prompted the government to link co-payments to package sizes.

The year after the new system was implemented in the Netherlands, a total of 308 new products were launched on the market and were classified

Table 1.26 Annual percentage increases in total pharmaceutical expenditure, volume of prescriptions, cost per prescription and 'structural component' between 1988 and 1993 in Germany

Year	Pharmaceutical expenditure	Volume	Cost per prescription	Structural component
1988	8.5	4.1	4.2	2.7
1989	0.4	-3.5	4.1	2.9
1990	6.5	5.3	1.1	1.3
1991	10.8	3.8	6.7	5.1
1992	9.8	3.2	6.3	4.0
1993	-14.5	-10.4	-4.6	-0.8

Source: Klauber, 1994.[159]

130 *Health Care and Cost Containment in the European Union*

according to the criteria for interchangeable products. 176 new products were patented and 82 were classified as interchangeable with existing medicines and therefore the reimbursement for these new products was limited to the previous level. The remaining products were classified as innovative and were therefore fully reimbursed. It was estimated that prescriptions in the non-clustered market rose by 11 per cent, whereas costs rose by 21 per cent. The cost of products clustered as interchangeable rose by 5 per cent.[157]

In Sweden, the year following the introduction of the fixed reimbursement system, the growth of pharmaceutical sales was 1.6 per cent less than the previous year. However, the next year, 1994, the growth was at its highest during the last six years. Zammit-Lucia and Dasgupta[160] found that a fall in sales in the reference price segment of the market was more than outweighed by greater-than-average sales growth in the rest of the market, so that overall sales were largely unaffected. They also found that changes in prescribing structure were the main driver of growth of pharmaceutical expenditure in Sweden and that, following the introduction of the reference pricing, this contributor to growth became even more exaggerated. Trends in Sweden were, therefore, quite similar to the German and Dutch ones.

1.21.7 Developments in length of stay and day surgery

Advances in medical knowledge and technology have created the potential for hospital patients to have a shorter length of stay or to be transferred from an in-patient ward to day surgery. This allows savings to be made in terms of bed provision and nursing care without any loss of quality, at least in terms of patient outcome. There is also a reduced risk of iatrogenic disease and less trauma for children. In addition, there is less disruption and inconvenience caused to the normal day-to-day activities of the patient.

Day surgery, in particular, has been advocated as an efficient means of increasing hospital productivity in the context of cost containment. Many surgical procedures, including a large number for which there are already long waiting lists (for instance, hernia repair, varicose vein surgery, cystoscopy, arthroscopy and cataract removal) can be carried out on patients who enter and leave hospital on the same day. The ten most frequent day-case procedures account for over 50 per cent of the total. Day surgery offers two considerable advantages. First, the service offered to patients can be better organized and suited to their needs, and above all can be provided

The European Union: Cost Containment Measures in Practice   131

sooner as faster throughput allows waiting lists to be reduced. Second, hospital costs are lower and there is no evidence of significant offsetting cost increases for community support or extra care of patients at home. At the same time, outcomes are no different from those of in-patients undergoing the same procedures.

In a study in Canada, one-day tubal ligation and hernia repair were found to be cost-efficient and averaged hospital savings of CAD 86.00 and CAD 115.00 more than in-patient care.[161] However, the precise cost saving achieved through a greater use of day-case surgery depends on the costing assumptions made and the facilities employed.[162, 163]

Some estimates in the UK show that, if all health authorities performed day surgery consistently at readily achievable levels for each of 20 common procedures, an additional 186,000 patients could be treated each year without increasing expenditure, and many other procedures are suitable for day surgery, offering potential for 300,000 additional patients to be treated annually. This is equivalent to about 34 per cent of the day-case and in-patient waiting lists in England and Wales.[164]

Another way of viewing the variations in hospital utilization and efficient resource allocation is to compare the observed lengths of stay with the regional average. In a study in England, the observed length of stay for appendectomy, inguinal hernia and cholecystectomy in the longest stay districts was at least 13 per cent above their regional average. Translation of these differences into number of bed days indicated that about 2,000 more bed days were occupied than expected for the three procedures in the longest stay districts in each region.[165]

Scientific evaluations suggest that the clinical outcomes achieved and levels of patient satisfaction for short-stay and day-case surgery do not differ significantly from more traditional patterns of patient management.[166] Cleary et al.[167] reviewed patients' medical records and surveyed patients between 3 and 12 months after hospital discharge in six teaching hospitals in California and Massachusetts in order to determine the extent to which interinstitutional variations in length of stay are explained by differences in patient characteristics and to determine whether patients in hospitals with shorter lengths of stay had worse outcomes.

They examined a cohort of 2,484 selected patients who had been hospitalized for acute myocardial infarction or to rule out acute myocardial infarction, coronary artery bypass graft surgery, total hip replacement, cholecystectomy or transurethral prostatectomy. They found that significant

132 *Health Care and Cost Containment in the European Union*

interinstitutional differences in length of stay were noted for all conditions except ruling out acute myocardial infarction. Statistical adjustment for case-mix differences accounted for most of the interinstitutional differences in length of stay for total hip replacement but explained few of the differences in the other conditions. When they controlled statistically for other predictors, length of stay did not have a significant impact on deaths, functional status after hospital discharge, the probability of readmission, or patient satisfaction with hospital care.

It is not surprising, therefore, that many European countries have explored the possibility of keeping costs down through encouraging shorter lengths of stay and day surgery. In 1988, day surgery in the UK was 22 per cent of all surgical procedures carried out. By 1992, this figure had increased to 31.3 per cent.[164] Day hospitals and day surgery are well developed in Denmark and Sweden, are rapidly increasing in the Netherlands and are encouraged in Ireland. Germany has amended the payment system of doctors to encourage it.

Elsewhere, however, progress is slow. There is very little day surgery in Greece, Spain or Portugal, though the new hospitals in Portugal are making provision for it. It exists in Belgium, France and Italy, but on a small scale, and is planned for Luxembourg. According to Morgan and Beech[166] barriers to the more widespread adoption of short-stay and day-case surgery include practical and organizational constraints on clinical practice at a hospital level, lack of awareness among clinicians as to how far their practices differ from current norms, and clinical barriers raised by surgeons who do not see short-stay policies as advantageous. Mechanisms to promote changes in clinical practice styles include independent professional audit, peer review and involvement of clinicians in budgeting and resource allocation. The relatively slow rate of adoption of day-case surgery in the European countries can be attributed to a lack of financial incentives and regulatory mechanisms promoting this form of patient management. In addition, day-case surgery carries little intrinsic interest for the majority of surgeons. Failure of day surgery in France is also due to the fact that both hospital surgeons and GPs are reluctant to see post-operative care transferred from an in-patient to an out-patient setting. Barrow *et al.*[168] examined the opinions of general practitioners (GPs) in a North Western Health District in the UK. GPs were asked for their opinions of the relative merits of day and in-patient surgery for patients with similar conditions. GPs gave only a mixed level of support to the idea of further expansion. This related

The European Union: Cost Containment Measures in Practice 133

less to considerations of workload in the primary care team than it did to concerns about readmissions and complications.

The length of in-patient stay has shown a steady decline in most countries. However, again, there are wide variations within countries and between countries. This is illustrated by data from the OECD: [37] the median length of stay in hospitals in Germany, Spain, Finland and the UK for cataract surgery was 11.0 days, 9.3 days, 8.8 days and 6.4 days, respectively in 1986, but had declined to 6.9 days, 4.3 days, 3.6 days and 2.6 days, respectively by 1992.

1.22 Control of medical technology and developments in health technology assessment

In the EU there have been attempts to control expensive medical equipment by, for example, the health maps used in Belgium, France and Luxembourg. Some attempts elsewhere have been unsuccessful because they have excluded the private sector. France has recently extended control to cover expensive medical techniques. In France the health maps were criticized for a lack of rationale in the definition of the heavy equipment list. For instance, a number of conventional X-ray units whose cost was in the same order of magnitude and sometimes higher than the items on the list were not included (for example, conventional angiography units, specialized tables for digestive examinations). In addition, there were no explicit criteria for appreciation of needs or evaluation of individual demands. Whereas in the private sector lack of response from the public authorities within six months resulted in approval of the equipment by default, in the public sector there was no time constraint for approval. Thus the scheme has been used mainly as a cost containment tool rather than as a planning tool as was the original intention.[169]

Several countries have established bodies to assess new technology. Recent developments in the Member States are presented in Table 1.27, overleaf. There are significant developments in France, Spain, Sweden, Finland and the UK and growing activities and interest in other countries. In 1997, Italy decided that pharmaceutical companies should submit cost-effectiveness studies to the Interministerial Committee of Economic Planning (CIPE) for all new pharmaceutical products that are authorized by

134   *Health Care and Cost Containment in the European Union*

Table 1.27 State of health care technology assessment in the EU in 1996–97

EU Member State	Developments
Belgium	Interest, some activity.
Denmark	Substantial activity, mostly funded by Danish Medical Research Council. Danish Institute of Health Technology Assessment established in 1997. Health Technology Assessment Committee within the National Board of Health.
Germany	Growing activity, substantial interest in the Ministry of Health and some insurance funds.
Greece	Interest, some activity. Plans to establish a technology assessment agency.
Spain	Growing activity: 3 technology assessment agencies in communities (Catalonia, Basque Country, Andalucía) and a national one in Madrid.
France	National agency, the Agency for the Development of Evaluation in Medicine (ANDEM), established in 1990. The agency was renamed to ANAES (National Agency for the Evaluation and Accreditation of Health Care) and was given accreditation responsibility for public and private hospitals and advisory role concerning reimbursement decisions for new pharmaceutical products.
Ireland	Growing interest, discussion of establishing a national committee.
Italy	Some activity. Two regional agencies. National law establishing a government office for evaluating technology being implemented.
Luxembourg	Interest.
Netherlands	Substantial activity. Central priority-setting and technology assessment activity funded by the Health Insurance Executive Board. Technology assessment to guide policy making carried out by Health Council.
Austria	Interest. Small technology assessment programme in the National Academy of Sciences with some health-related studies.
Portugal	Interest.
Finland	Substantial activity. National office established in 1995.

The European Union: Cost Containment Measures in Practice   135

| Sweden | **Substantial activity. National agency, the Swedish Council for Technology Assessment in Health Care (SBU), formed in 1987.** |
| UK | Substantial activity focusing on implementation in administration and practice. Research and Development programme of the NHS, emphasizing health technology assessment, formed in 1991. National Coordination Centre for Technology Assessment formed in 1996. A National Institute of Clinical Excellence is to be established to determine what should be used. A Council of Health Improvement will be responsible for dissemination of information. |

Source: Banta, 1996[170] and authors' research.

the centralized process of the European Medicines Evaluation Agency (EMEA). These studies are expected to be taken into account in pricing and reimbursement decisions. Similarly, at present, the Netherlands is also planning to use cost-effectiveness studies for new pharmaceutical products in the decision-making process concerning reimbursement policies.

However, the impact of cost-effectiveness studies and other types of evaluations comparing costs and outcomes on decision making concerning pricing and coverage decisions has still to be felt.[154] A recent study[171] identified the reasons for lack of use of health technology assessment (HTA) information among the countries studied. These included the political nature of the decisions and lack of information on effectiveness, costs and appropriateness. In France cost-effectiveness studies are considered by the committees dealing with pricing and reimbursement of pharmaceuticals, but the real impact on decision making is still insignificant.[172] In Germany there is no use of cost-effectiveness studies in reimbursement decisions.[173] In the Netherlands economic evaluation studies have played a limited role in reimbursement decisions. Elsinga and Rutten[174] have reported and analysed a case study of one drug (simvastatine) for which cost-effectiveness had an impact. Drummond *et al.*[175] reviewed the use of economic evaluation studies in the UK and concluded that the NHS reforms increase the potential for the use of economic evaluation. However, there was no impact on pricing and reimbursement decisions.

Overall, while these experiments are still developing and have had only a moderate impact (outside the field of pharmaceutical care), they are growing and indicate the trend for the future.

In parallel with these developments during the 1980s and early 1990s, a growing body of evidence emerged highlighting variations in the rate at

136 *Health Care and Cost Containment in the European Union*

which health care interventions were used.[176] These variations were observed at all levels, between countries, regions and individual doctors. Subsequent research demonstrated that many of the variations were due to clinical uncertainty, as a result of the lack of good quality evaluative research on which to base decisions.

In the last five years several EU Member States have shown increased interest in the issue of appropriateness of health care interventions, based on the concept that reductions in ineffective treatment may be a valuable strategy in reducing health care costs without reducing health benefits. This strategy included the development of practice and medical purchasing guidelines. These deal with the treatment of specific conditions and are designed to identify appropriate procedures for clinicians to follow. Services or conditions are identified that are of high cost, high medical liability risk and high incidence for the patient population. The purpose of guidelines is to moderate expenditures and improve practice performance. Additional developments include cost-effectiveness guidelines and their potential integration into contractual agreements. Several approaches have been initiated by different Member States.

In the United Kingdom, the Royal Colleges and some specialist associations have been active in developing clinical guidelines.[177–181] Furthermore, partnerships between hospital doctors and general practitioners have been developed and, in some areas, they are being used to inform purchasing decisions. The Cochrane Centre, established in Oxford by the NHS in 1992, provides clinicians with information and support on clinical trials, literature searches, meta-analyses and practice guidelines.

In December 1994, the NHS Executive (NHSE) issued circular EL(94)94 on 'Commercial Approaches to the NHS Regarding Disease Management Packages' in response to approaches to NHS bodies at local level by pharmaceutical companies. The circular suggested that it may be possible to develop pilot projects, but no deals were possible at local level before a number of issues had been discussed nationally.[182] The Department of Health issued a discussion document in June 1996 stating that joint National Health Service/private sector disease management ventures would have to ensure that (a) the agreement is appropriate to a publicly funded service, (b) it is compatible with national agreements for prescribing and dispensing, (c) it represents good value for money, and (d) potential conflicts of interest have been identified and resolved. The second draft of this document, sent out on 30 September 1996, states clearly that

The European Union: Cost Containment Measures in Practice   137

'even where the disease management programmes suggest a preferred form of treatment, the agreement should not override the duty of clinicians to provide a different treatment for the individual patient if this is considered appropriate'.[183] On funding issues, it suggested that mail order pharmacy is inappropriate to the NHS and that purchasers should comply with HM Treasury rules about funding, particularly drug expenditure.

In Germany a number of scientific medical associations have recently produced clinical practice guidelines, but these are rather unsystematic and are influenced by technologies available in tertiary care settings.[184] The increasing interest in producing practice guidelines may reflect the goals of the prospective hospital payment system which is set by the Federal Ministry of Health or the possible introduction of Länder-wide budgets for hospitals.[11] The development of Pharmacy Benefit Managers (PBMs) was not welcomed by the German Pharmaceutical Association, which pointed out that the German system would not be flexible enough to adapt to these new changes compared with the US, where there is a much higher percentage of private health insurers.[185]

In the Netherlands, the Dutch College of General Practitioners had already started its own standard-setting programme in 1987.[186] The programme is independent of both the government and the insurance system, even though it has become fully subsidized. Its progress is being monitored and early results up to 1990 showed that acceptance was high.[187]

Several initiatives have also been introduced in Scandinavian countries. In Denmark, the National Board of Health, in collaboration with scientific societies, has a programme of developing practice guidelines based on systematic reviews of research-based evidence. In Sweden a number of county councils have initiated projects which aim at integrating elements of disease management and clinical guidelines into purchasing organizations' management programmes. The county council in Ostergötland has produced purchasing guidelines for certain diagnoses (for example, for stroke). The Stockholm County Council has also sponsored institutions to develop disease management techniques.

1.22.1 Development of information systems

The extent to which the separation of purchasers from providers can lead to the management of patients' care through aggressive contracting and cost

138 *Health Care and Cost Containment in the European Union*

control will depend on the availability of adequate information systems. A significant flaw in the internal market structure of the UK NHS has been a lack of information on outcome measurements and on cost data. The only information consistently collected by the NHS has been on annual growth in activity, waiting times and the tracking of improvement in health for certain groups.[188] This has created significant problems in resource allocation. There are no uniform accounting rules for the NHS and hospital trusts cannot set prices in line with what the market could afford. Prices of contracts are restrained by a lack of expertise and accounting practices that are oriented towards meeting cash limits rather than reflecting actual cost structures.[189]

One possible approach to reducing unnecessary services would be the further development of medical purchasing guidelines. Aggregate data, analysis and commentary can be useful sources of evidence in clinical decision making. However, it may be inappropriate to require global adherence to guidelines in individual cases as a condition of employment, compensation or evaluation.[190] Practice guidelines would need to be assimilated by providers, incorporated into medical education and promoted through continuing education. Insurers may use them to determine what they are prepared to reimburse as well as in judgments of quality when contracts are placed with providers. Further research is needed on the most effective strategies for changing doctors' behaviour, as simply publishing them has not been found to be effective.[191] However, there is a growing body of literature describing factors associated with success and failure, including the need to ensure that they are developed using explicit methods and are recognized as scientifically valid.[192] As discussed above, initial evidence on the implementation of disease management guidelines (RMOs) in France shows that they have not been very effective in controlling health care costs.

There is also a need to develop patient information systems in health services. These would have two main features. Firstly, they would take detailed note of patient history and the treatments prescribed when the need arose. Such systems are largely unavailable, particularly in primary and in-patient care. Although such systems may exist for the monitoring of pharmaceutical prescribing, dispensing and spending, their impact is still to be felt,[193] while the validity and completeness of the health care data collected in a number of countries are questionable.[194] A survey showed that most information systems related to drug use were used by doctors and less so by administrative and technical staff.[195]

The European Union: Cost Containment Measures in Practice 139

Secondly, information systems would have to deal with the mobility of patients and the need for, in some cases, constant monitoring. Health cards are a way in which a patient's history can be observed. However, their use is still some way off, owing to significant technical problems. France and Germany are the two EU Member States which traditionally have been leading the development of data card technology in a pilot phase.[196] The German card, holding administrative information only, allows access to health care services and to medical and pharmaceutical prescriptions and is an essential element in processing doctors' claims for reimbursement. France passed a law in April 1996 that will introduce an electronic health insurance card and a professional card for doctors and nurses. Other European countries (Belgium, Greece, the Netherlands, Portugal, Spain) have plans to follow a similar direction. However, in all the above cases, the use of the health card is confined to administrative purposes (patient identification, entitlement to care, coverage by social security and health insurance), rather than medical applications (electronic medical file, keeping track of medications and treatment history).

1.23 Conclusion

Sufficient information is lacking on the long-term effects of many of the cost containment measures taken by EU Member States. An obvious difficulty is that one measure is often quickly followed by another – before there is time to see the effects of the first measure. Indeed, often the effective life of different measures to contain expenditure is shorter than the time required to develop and introduce them. Moreover, cost containment measures are seldom introduced singly. Where more than one measure is introduced, it becomes difficult to assess the effect of each measure separately. This confounding is likely to be more pronounced with a major reform.[8]

In addition, what may appear to be the effect of a cost containment measure may in fact be simply a reflection of an international trend. For example, the increase in turnover of hospitals may be due to technological change influencing all or most countries, such as the introduction or spread of keyhole surgery or day surgery. Thus national data need to be compared with international data. But such comparisons need to be carefully chosen and carefully handled in view of the possible lack of comparability of concepts.[8]

140 *Health Care and Cost Containment in the European Union*

However, from the experience of the countries in our study as summarized above, it is difficult to resist the conclusion of previous commentators that budget setting is one of the most effective ways of controlling public health care costs.[66,197] Denmark, Ireland, Italy and the UK all set budgets at a large number of points in their public health systems: all spend a low share of their GDP on health (less than the unweighted EU average) and all have a relatively low rate of growth. Germany succeeded in restraining the growth in its already high share of GDP through the introduction of budgets at various levels. As Germany now relaxes those budgets, it will be interesting to observe the future trajectory of health care costs in that country. France introduced prospective budgets for public hospitals, which again seem to have been reasonably successful in controlling costs.

Nor does budget-setting appear to have many of the adverse effects predicted by commentators. Consumer satisfaction or dissatisfaction does not currently appear to be related to the presence or absence of budgets.[198] It may also be the case that, because overall budgets for health services or for part of the health sector were imposed so late in the day (in most countries in the mid-1980s), waiting for appointments with specialists or admission to hospital is not yet as great a problem in Belgium, Germany, France or the Netherlands as it is in the UK. There may be, therefore, a change in the public's views in the future if health care in Europe becomes more managed, and if the pace of demand outstrips the pace of gains from efforts to increase efficiency. Indeed, this may be one of the factors behind the current relaxation of budgetary controls in Germany.

Budget setting at all levels is facilitated in countries with national health systems funded from general taxation; and it is surely no coincidence that countries with a long experience of such systems, such as the UK, Ireland and Denmark, have relatively low public expenditures on health care, but also relatively low rates of growth. The effectiveness of cost control measures reflects to a very large extent the bargaining strength and power of purchasers and providers.[66,199]

As Evans points out:[200]

"Discretionary power is commonly defended by denial of its existence, the allegation of inevitability. Objective external conditions and forces are claimed to dictate policy decisions with tangible distributional effects. In health policy, such forces include the aging of the population, the extension of technology, and the demands of ethical standards.

The European Union: Cost Containment Measures in Practice   141

> Taken together, these forces create relentless upward pressure on costs, to levels which society 'cannot afford, necessitating sacrifice of the interests of the less eligible'. Yet quantitative analysis of these forces does not sustain the argument; in each case the source of cost escalation is not external pressure but the way in which the health care system itself reacts. Less costly and equally effective options are demonstrably available, but would threaten provider interests and broader ideologies. A spurious cloak of inevitability serves to promote and justify political choices."

Tax-financed systems or systems where there is monopsony power through a single purchaser organization seem to be more successful in containing the growth of health care costs. However, this is not to say that all other kinds of measures are ineffective, or that insurance based systems cannot control costs. Some insurance-based systems (as in the Netherlands) have also been successful in controlling costs through heavily regulating providers' fees and by implementing successful direct control measures. It is also obviously not impossible for countries with social insurance systems to introduce effective budgets, as Germany's highly successful regime indicates.

Certain kinds of budget-shifting measures clearly can work to keep public spending down, as is illustrated by the experience of several EU Member States with respect to treatment restrictions on dental care and pharmaceuticals. Others are of more dubious value, including large-scale extensions of co-payments for basic medical services. To overcome the obvious equity problems associated with these kinds of co-payments, they are often coupled with elaborate exemption systems that are bureaucratic and expensive to enforce; this severely limits both their revenue-raising capability and their deterrent effect on use. In addition, if set sufficiently high, they encourage affected individuals to take out private health insurance to cover them, which further negates any deterrent effect on use.

Given the theoretical objections to the use of direct and indirect controls, and the absence of much positive evidence concerning their effectiveness, it is hard to recommend some of them. However, alternatives to hospital care, technology assessment and control, day surgery and manpower controls do seem to have had an impact.

Purchasing decisions and resource allocation based on evidence-based medicine and cost-effectiveness studies may be more effective in controlling health expenditure in the future. But this will require a long consultation

142   *Health Care and Cost Containment in the European Union*

process and significant investment to document the cost and clinical effectiveness of different treatments and interventions. That presupposes the development of adequate information systems. Although such systems may exist for the monitoring of pharmaceutical prescribing, dispensing and spending, their impact is still to be felt,[193] while the validity and completeness of the health care data collected in a number of countries are questionable.[194] There is also an urgent need for information systems in primary and hospital care. The choice about how much care to buy is complicated by the fact that the information about what services produce what outcomes is not good enough to show what the trade-off is.[80] As Lohr *et al.* point out:[201]

> "If we cannot know with certainty when additional expenditures will bring no further benefits, then we also cannot know with certainty when cost controls will begin to threaten patient well-being or harm quality of care."

In addition, to implement policies and run health care systems in the late 1990s and early in the twenty-first century will require a far higher level of management competence. It is argued that, if public health services are to survive, then managers in these services will need to be highly skilled and knowledgeable and that they will need some of the competencies of modern commercial managers as well as public health knowledge and skills.[202] A recent survey in Italy examined the problems in implementing the latest reforms which aimed at transforming Local Health Care Units into purchasing organizations. Among the most significant issues raised were the lack of mechanisms to evaluate and control the activities performed, the lack of new management tools for economic and human resources, rigid human resources management patterns and difficulties in convincing personnel to adjust to organizational changes.[203]

So what of the future? Although prediction is always a dangerous business, some issues and trends are emerging that could shape cost control policies in the early twenty-first century. Regarding the model of purchasing/provision of services, the public contract model will be dominant in most countries. The role of private finance, but not necessarily private provision, is also expected to increase. Specific measures may include the replacement of target budgets with fixed budgets, combination of budgets with activity-related payments and the replacement of sectoral budgets by budgets for individual providers. Alternatives to hospital care and long-

The European Union: Cost Containment Measures in Practice 143

term care coverage schemes will be further developed, but they will be mainly financed by private sources. In addition, health technology assessment will play a greater role in coverage and purchasing decisions, and further reduction in hospital beds and manpower controls will be part of the cost control portfolio.

Cost containment has been the dominant theme of health policy in most developed countries for two decades. Some successes in controlling costs in some Member States of the European Union should not mask the fact that many of the underlying cost pressures are still active, and indeed are likely to become more so in the coming years. Yet several countries have managed to control health care expenditure or slow down its growth rate. It is therefore important that we learn the lessons from the recent experience of cost containment measures in action over the last 15 years. This book is part of that process.

References

INTRODUCTION

1 Wildavsky A. Doing better and feeling worse: the political pathology of health policy. *Daedalus: Journal of the American Academy of Arts and Sciences* 1977;106:105–23.

SECTION I

2 Hills J. Funding the Welfare State. *Oxford Review of Economic Policy* 1995;11(3): 27–43.

3 Busse R, Howorth C, Schwartz FW. The future development of a rights based approach to health care in Germany: more rights or fewer? In: Lenaghan J (ed.). *Hard Choices in Health Care – Rights and Rationing in Europe.* London: BMJ Publishing Group, 1997.

4 British Embassy. *Labour and Social Affairs Report: France.* Paris: British Embassy, October 1995.

5 Commission on Health Funding. *Report of the Commission on Health Funding.* Dublin: Stationery Office, 1989.

6 Kurunmaki L. *The Irish Health Care System: Cost Containment Measures During the 1980s and 1990s.* LSE Health Working Paper, London, 1998.

7 Mapelli V. Cost-containment measures in the Italian healthcare system, *Pharmacoeconomics* 1995;8(2):85-90.

8 Abel-Smith B, Mossialos E. Cost containment and health care reform: A study of the European Union. *Health Policy* 1994;89(2):89–134.

9 Le Grand J, Mays N, Mulligan J. *Learning from the Internal Market.* London: King's Fund, 1998.

144 Health Care and Cost Containment in the European Union

10 UK Department of Health. *The New NHS: Modern, Dependable.* London: HMSO (Cm 3807), 1997.

11 Busse R, Schwartz FW. Decision-Making and Priority-Setting in Public Health and Health Care in Germany. In: Holland W, Mossialos E with Belcher P and Merkel B (eds). *Priority Setting in Public Health in the EU Member States.* Aldershot: Ashgate, in press.

12 Henke K-D, Murray MA, Ade C. Global budgeting in Germany: lessons for the United States. *Health Affairs* 1994:13(4):7–21.

13 Hinde J. Formulae for growth. *Times Higher Education Supplement* 27 March 1998;10.

14 Rosen HM, Sussman RA, Sussman EJ. The inclusion of capitation reimbursement in solo-practice. *Journal of Public Health Dentistry* 1978;38(2)184–92.

15 Birch S. The identification of supplier-inducement in a fixed price system of health care provision: the case of dentistry in the United Kingdom. *Journal of Health Economics* 1987;7:129–50.

16 Sintonen H, Maljanen T. Explaning the utilization of dental care. Experiences from the Finnish dental market. *Health Economics* 1995;4(6):453–66.

17 Grytten J. The effects of supplier involvement on Norwegian dental services. Some empirical findings based on a theoretical model. *Commumity Dental Health* 1991;8(3): 221–31.

18 Elderton RJ, Nuttal NM. Variation among dentists in planning treatment. *British Dental Journal* 1983;154:201–6.

19 Anderson R, Whitehouse NH, Treasure E. *EU Manual of Dental Practice 1997.* Cardiff: Dental Public Health Unit, University of Wales College of Medicine, 1997.

20 Murillo C, Gonzalez B. El sector sanitario en Espana: situation actual y perspectivas de Futuro. *Hacienda Publica Espaniola* 1993;119:49–58.

21 Ministry of Health. *Health Care in Denmark.* Copenhagen: Ministry of Health, 1997.

22 Hutten JBF, Kerkstra A. *Home Care in Europe: A Country-specific Guide to its Organisation and Financing.* Aldershot: Arena, 1996.

23 Intenrigsministeriet. *Intenrigsministeriets Kommunale Nagletal.* Copenhagen: Intenrigsministeriet, 1997.

24 Federal Ministry of Health and Consumer Protection. *Public Health in Austria.* Vienna: Federal Ministry of Health and Consumer Protection, 1996.

25 Clasen J. Social insurance in Germany: dismantling or reconstruction? In: Clasen J. *Social Insurance in Europe.* Bristol: The Policy Press, 1997.

26 Evers A, Liebing J. The new long term care insurance in Germany: characteristics, consequences and perspectives. In: Harding T, Meredith B, Wistow G. *Options for Long Term Care.* London: HMSO, 1996.

27 Lankers CHR. Pflegeversicherung – The insurance of care in Germany. *Eurohealth* 1996;2(2):28–9.

28 Pinto JL, Selmes MA, Creado B. *Transnational Study of the Socio-economic Impact of Alzheimer's Disease in the European Union: The Spanish Case.* Barcelona: Fundacio ACE, Universitat Pompeu Fabra, Alzeimer Espana, 1997.

The European Union: References   145

29 Bergmark Å. From reforms to rationing? Current allocative trends in social services in Sweden. *Scandinavian Journal of Social Welfare* 1997;6:74–81.

30 Kerkstra A, Hutten JB. Organization and financing of home nursing in the European Union. *Journal of Advanced Nursing* 1996;24(5):1023–32.

SECTION II

31 Friers BE, Schroll M, Hawes C *et al*. Approaching cross-national comparisons of nursing home residents. *Age Ageing* 1997;26 (suppl 2):13–18.

32 Mosseveld van CJPM, Son ven P. *International Comparisons on Health Care Data. Phase I: Intramural Health Care.* Voorburg/Heerlen: Statistics Netherlands, 1996.

33 Österreichisches Statistisches Zentralamt. *Gesundheitsausgaben in Österreich 1993–1995.* Vienna: Österreichisches Statistisches Zentralamt, 1997.

34 Kanavos P, Mossialos E. *The Methodology of International Comparisons of Health Care Expenditures: Any Lessons for Health Policy?* London: LSE Health Discussion Paper, 1997.

35 Kanavos P, Mossialos E. International comparisons of health care expenditures: what we know and what we do not. *Journal of Health Services Research and Policy,* in press.

36 Danish Ministry of Health. *Health Resources and Price Statistics. Working Party on Community Health Data and Indicators.* Copenhagen: Danish Ministry of Health, 1994.

37 OECD. *OECD Health Data 1997.* Paris: OECD, 1997.

38 Gouveia Pinto C. *Competition in the Health Care Sector and Welfare.* Lisboa: Associañao Portuguesa de Economia da Saude, Documento de Trabahlo 1/95, 1995.

39 Fuchs VR. Though much is taken: reflections on aging, health, and medical care. *Milbank Memorial Fund Quarterly: Health and Society* 1984;62(2):143–66

40 Lubitz J, Beebe J, Baker C. Longevity and Medicare expenditures. *The New England Journal of Medicine* 1995;332:999–1003.

41 Busse R. *Medical Costs Do Not Rise With Age.* Paper presented at a seminar organised by LSE Health, London, November 1997.

42 Scitovsky AA. Medical care in the last twelve months of life: the relation between age, functional status, and medical care expenditures. *Milbank Memorial Fund Quarterly: Health and Society* 1988;66(4):640–60.

43 Harrison A, Dixon J, New B, Judge K. Funding the NHS: Can the NHS cope in future? *British Medical Journal* 1997;314:139–42.

44 Meerding WJ, Bonneux L, Polder JJ *et al*. Demographic and epidemiological determinants of healthcare costs in Netherlands: cost of illness study. *British Medical Journal* 1998;317(7151):111–15.

45 Koopmanschap MA, van Roijen L, Bonneux L *et al*. Costs of diseases in an international perspective. *European Journal of Public Health* 1994;4:258–64.

46 Office of Technology Assessment. *Assessing the Efficacy and Safety of Medical Technologies.* Washington DC: US Government Printing Office, 1978.

47 Johansen KS. WHO concept of health technology sssessment. *Health Policy* 1988;9: 349–51.

146 Health Care and Cost Containment in the European Union

48 Abel-Smith B, Figueras J, Holland W, McKee M, Mossialos E. *Choices in Health Policy: An Agenda for the European Union.* Aldershot and Luxembourg: Dartmouth and Office for Official Publications of the European Communities, 1995.

49 Evans RW. Health care technology and the inevitability of resource allocation and rationing decisions – part II. *Journal of the American Medical Association* 1983; 249(16):2208–19.

50 Davis K. The role of technology, demand and labour markets in the determination of hospital costs. In: Perlman M. (ed.). *The Economics of Health and Medical Care.* New York: John Wiley and Sons, 1974.

51 Worthington NL. Expenditure for hospital care and physicians' services: factors affecting annual changes. *Social Security Bulletin* 1975;39:3–15.

52 Altman SH, Blendon RJ. (eds). *Medical Technology: The Culprit behind Health Care Costs?* Washington DC: US Government Printing Office, 1979.

53 Moloney TW, Rogers DE. Medical technology: a different view of the contentious debate over costs. *The New England Journal of Medicine* 1979;301:1413–19.

54 Ashby JL, Craig L. Why do hospital costs continue to increase? *Health Affairs* 1992; 11(2):134–47.

55 Abel-Smith B. The escalation of health care costs: how did we get there? In: OECD. *Health Care Reform: The Will to Change.* Paris: OECD, 1996.

56 Klarman HE, Rice D, Cooper BS. Accounting for the rise in selected medical care expenditures: 1929–1969. *American Journal of Public Health* 1970;60:1023–39.

57 Freeland M, Schendler C. National health expenditure growth in the 1980s: an ageing population, new technologies and increasing competition. *Health Care Financing Review* 1983;3:1–58.

58 Banta D. *An Approach to the Social Control of Hospital Technologies.* Geneva: WHO, SHS paper No 10, 1995.

59 Scitovsky A. Changes in the cost of treatment of selected illnesses, 1971–1981. *Medical Care* 1985;23:1345–57.

60 Showstack JA, Schroeder SA. Use of medical technologies 1972–77: a study of 10 inpatient diagnoses. *The New England Journal of Medicine* 1982;306:706–12.

61 Jönsson B, Gerdtham U-G. *Cost Sharing for Pharmaceuticals: The Swedish Reimbursement System.* Basle: The Pharmaceutical Partners for Better Healthcare, 1995.

62 Lopez-Bastida J, Mossialos E. Spanish drug policy at the crossroads. *The Lancet* 1997; 350(9079):679–80.

63 Cranovsky R, Matillon Y, Banta D. EUR-ASSESS project subgroup report on coverage. *International Journal of Technology Assessment in Health Care* 1997;13(2):287–332.

64 Department of Health. *Pharmaceutical Price Regulation Scheme: Report to the Parliament on the PPRS.* London: Department of Health, 1996.

65 Cueni T. An industrial policy for the pharmaceutical industry in Europe: the way forward. In: *Health Care Reforms and the Role of the Pharmaceutical Industry* (proceedings of a European workshop). Basle: The Pharmaceutical Partners for Better Healthcare, 1995.

SECTION III

66 Abel-Smith B. *Cost Containment and New Priorities in Health Care*. Aldeshot: Avebury, 1992.

67 Abel-Smith B. *An Introduction to Health Policy Planning and Financing*. London: Longman,1994.

68 Aas IHM. Incentives and financing methods. *Health Policy* 1995;34:205–20.

69 Glaser WA. *Paying the Hospital*. San Francisco: Jossey-Bass Publishers, 1987.

70 Donaldson C, Gerard K. *Economics of Health Care Financing: The Visible Hand*. London: Macmillan, 1993.

71 Barnum H, Kutzin J, Saxenian H. Incentives and provider payment methods. *International Journal of Health Planning and Management* 1995;10:23–45.

72 Beech R, Morgan M. Constraints on innovatory practice: the case of day surgery in the NHS. *International Journal of Health Planning and Management* 1992;7:128–35.

73 Wennberg JE, McPherson K, Caper P. Will payment based on diagnosis-related groups control hospital costs? *The New England Journal of Medicine* 1984;311(5):295–300.

74 Kane NM, Manoukian PD. The effect of the Medicare prospective payment system on the adoption of new technology. The case of cochlear implants. *The New England Journal of Medicine* 1989;321(20):1378–83.

75 Young DA. DRGs and prospective payment under Medicare. *Medical Decision Making: An International Journal of the Society for Medical Decision Making* 1985;5(1):7–13.

76 Crane TS. Hospital cost control in Norway: a decade's experience with prospective payment. *Public Health Reports* 1985;100(4):406–17.

77 Carrol NV, Erwin WG. Patient shifting as a response to Medicare prospective payment. *Medical Care* 1987;25:1161–7.

78 Lyles YM. Impact of Medicare diagnosis-related groups (DRGs) on nursing homes in the Portland, Oregon metropolitan area. *Journal of The American Geriatrics Society* 1986;34(8):573–8.

79 Hurley J, Linz D, Swint E. Assessing the effects of the Medicare prospective payment system on the demand for VA inpatient services: an examination of transfers and discharges of problem patients. *Health Services Research* 1990;25(1 Pt.2):239–55.

80 Russell LB. *Medicare's New Hospital Payment System: Is it Working?* Washington DC: The Brookings Institution, 1989.

81 Rodrigues J. Hospital utilization and reimbursement methods in Brazil. *International Journal of Health Planning and Management* 1989;4:3–15.

82 Hsia DC, Krushat WM, Fagan AB *et al.* Accuracy of diagnostic coding for Medicare patients under the prospective-payment system. *The New England Journal of Medicine* 1988;318(6):352–5.

83 Schwartz WB, Mendelson DN. Hospital cost containment in the 1980s. Hard lessons learned and prospects for the 1990s. *New England Journal of Medicine* 1991;324:1037–42.

148 *Health Care and Cost Containment in the European Union*

SECTION IV

84 Collin C, Geffroy L. The health system: reform wanted by government and expected by patients. *The Lancet* 1997;349:791-2.

85 Leibovitz A, Manning WG, Newhouse JP. The demand for prescription medicines as a function of cost sharing. *Social Science and Medicine* 1985;21:1063-69.

86 Anderson GM, Spitzer WO, Weinstein MC, Wang E, Blackburn JL, Bergman U. Benefits, risks and costs of prescription drugs: a scientific basis for evaluating policy options. *Clinical Pharmacology and Therapeutics* 1990;48:111-19.

87 Brook H, Ware JE, Rogers WE *et al.* Does free care improve adults' health? *New England Journal of Medicine* 1983;309(23):1426-34.

88 Huttin C. Use of prescription charges. *Health Policy* 1994:27:53-73.

89 Fattore G. Cost containment and health care reforms in the British NHS. (In this volume.)

90 Yule B, Parkin D. The demand for dental care: an assessment. *Social Science and Medicine* 1985;21(7):753-69.

91 Yule B, Ryan M, Parkin D. Patient charges and the use of dental services: some evidence. *British Dental Journal* 1988;19 September:377-79.

92 Manning WG, Bailit HL, Benjamin B, Newhouse JP. The demand for dental care: evidence from a randomised trial in health insurance. *The Journal of the American Dental Association* 1985;110:895-902.

93 6 P, Jupp B, Bently T. *Open Wide: Futures for Dentistry in 2010.* London: Demos, 1996.

94 Yule B, Parkin D. *Financing of Dental Care in Europe.* Copenhagen: WHO, 1986.

95 Bateman DN. The selected list: diversion rather than threat. *British Medical Journal* 1993;306:1141-2.

96 Reilly A, Brown D, Taylor D *et al.* Effect of the limited list on drugs use. *Pharmaceutical Journal* 1986;19 April:480-82.

97 Ryan M, Birch S. Charging for health care: evidence on the utilisation of the NHS prescribed drugs. *Social Science and Medicine* 1991:33(6):681-87.

98 O'Brien B. The effect of patient charges on the utlization of prescription medicines. *Journal of Health Economics* 1989;8:109-39.

99 Garcia-Alonso G. 'Farmacia': el gasto farmacéutico y su control. In: Navarro C, Cabases JM, Tormo MJ (eds). *La Salud y el Sistema Sanitario en Espana: Informe Sespas 1995.* Barcelona: SG Editores, 1995.

100 Feely J. The influence of pharmacoeconomic factors on prescribing patterns in Ireland. *Pharmacoeconomics* 1992;2(2):99-106.

101 Ferrado C, Henman MC, Corrigan OI. Impact of a nationwide limited prescribing list: preliminary findings. *Drug Intelligence and Clinical Pharmacy* 1987;21:653-58.

102 Freddi G. *The New Pharmaceutical Pricing System in Italy.* Paper presented at a seminar organised by LSE Health, London, February 1995.

103 Gozlan M. French patients will get protease inhibitors. *The Lancet* 1996;347:821.

104 Ministero Della Sanita. Autorizzazione all'immissione in commersio, con procedura centralizzata Europea, della specialita medicinale Betaferon – Interferone beta-1b,

The European Union: References   149

Decreto Ministeriale 5 Febbraio 1996. *Gazzetta Ufficiale Della Repubblica Italiana*. Roma, 19 Febbraio 1996.

105 Sundhedsstyrelsen. *B-interferon Behandling af Patienter med Dissemineret Sklerose: Medicinsk Tecknologivurdering*. København, Januar 1996.

106 NHS Executive. *New Drugs for Multiple Sclerosis*. Leeds: NHS Executive, circular EL(95)97, 1995.

107 NHS Executive. *Clinical Advice from Standing Medical Advisory Committee on the Use of Interferon-Beta-1b in Relapsing–Remitting Multiple Sclerosis in Adults*. Leeds: NHS Executive, 1995.

108 Fink M. The concrete applicability of models for priority-setting (in Danish). Proceedings of a debate on priority-setting in health services, Thursday 22 February 1996. The Danish Council on Ethics and the Association of County Councils in Denmark. Quoted in The Danish Council on Ethics. *Priority Setting in the Health Service. A Report*. Copenhagen: The Danish Council on Ethics, 1996.

109 The Danish Council on Ethics. *Priority Setting in the Health Service. A Report*. Copenhagen: The Danish Council on Ethics, 1996.

110 Obero Hansen P. Experiences from priority-setting at county level (in Danish). Proceedings of a debate on priority-setting in health services, Thursday 22 February 1996. The Danish Council on Ethics and the Association of County Councils in Denmark. Quoted in The Danish Council on Ethics. *Priority Setting in the Health Service. A Report*. Copenhagen: The Danish Council on Ethics, 1996.

111 Advisory Council for Concerted Action in Health Care, Health Care and Health Insurance 2000. *Individual Responsibility, Subsidiarity and Solidarity in a Changing Environment*. (expert opinion report). Bonn, 1994.

112 Advisory Council for Concerted Action in Health Care, Health Care and Health Insurance 2000. *A Closer Orientation towards Results, Higher Quality Services and Greater Economic Efficiency*. (Summary and recommendations of the special expert report). Bonn, 1995.

113 Cabasés JM. The guaranteed health care entitlement in Spain. In: Meneu R, Ortún V (eds). *Política Gestión Sanitaria: La Agenda Explícita*. Barcelona: SG Editores, 1996, pp. 277–94.

114 Direction Générale de la Santé. *Les Priorités Nationales en Santé Publiques: Etûde Delphi*. Paris: Dossier Documentaire, 1995.

115 Have ten AMJH. Choosing core health services in the Netherlands. *Health Care Analysis* 1993;1:43–7.

116 Government Committee on Choices in Health Care. *Choices in Health Care*. Zoetermeer, 1992.

117 Zwart H. Rationing in the Netherlands: the liberal and the communitarian perspective. *Health Care Analysis* 1993;1:53–6.

118 National Research and Development Centre for Welfare and Health (STAKES). *From Values to Choices: Report of the Working Group on Health Care Prioritisation*. Helsinki: STAKES, 1995.

119 Swedish Parliamentary Priorities Commission. *Priorities in Health Care: Ethics, Economy, Implementation*. Stockholm: Swedish Government Official Reports, 1995.

150 *Health Care and Cost Containment in the European Union*

120 Rumeau-Rouquette C, Breat G. Decision-making in health policy in France. In: Holland W, Mossialos E with Belcher P and Merkel B (eds). *Priority Setting in Public Health in the EU Member States*. Aldershot: Ashgate, in press.

121 Schwartz FW, Haase I, Busse R. Erfolgsorientierung – eine neue Dimension in der Vergütungsdiskussion. *Arbeit & Sozialpolitik* 1995;49(5/6):29–34

122 Gunning-Schepers L. Public health and health policy in the Netherlands. In: Holland W, Mossialos E with Belcher P and Merkel B (eds). *Priority Setting in Public Health in the EU Member States*. Aldershot: Ashgate, in press.

123 Hermerén, G. After the priority-setting statement. The Swedish experience (in Swedish). Proceedings of a debate on priority-setting in health services, Thursday 22 February 1996. The Danish Council on Ethics and the Association of County Councils in Denmark. Quoted in The Danish Council on Ethics. *Priority Setting in the Health Service A Report.* Copenhagen: The Danish Council on Ethics, 1996.

124 Essinger K. Hospitals in Sweden. In: Standing Committee of the Hospitals of the European Union. *European Citizens' Rights and Health*. Brussels: BelgoHope, 1996.

125 Calltorp J. Public Health and Priority Setting in Sweden. In: Holland W, Mossialos E, with Belcher P and Merkel B (eds). *Priority Setting in Public Health in the EU Member States*. Aldershot: Ashgate, in press.

126 OECD. *OECD Economic Surveys: Austria 1997*. Paris: OECD, 1997.

127 Olivarius NF, Jensen FI, Pedersen PA. Epidemiological study of persons having Group 2 insurance in Denmark. *Ugeskr Laeger* 1990;142(20):143–6.

128 Laing W. *Private Health Care in the UK*. London: Laing and Buisson, 1994.

129 Buck G, Jenkins P, Leonard A. *Strategic Analysis of UK Non-life Insurance*. London: FT Financial Publishing, 1997.

130 Fenn P. Sickness and disability insurance in the public and private sectors. In: Association of British Insurers (ABI). *Risk, Insurance and Welfare*. London: ABI, 1995.

131 92/49/EEC Third Council Directive on the coordination of laws, regulations and administrative provisions relating to direct insurance other than life insurance and amending Directives 73/239/EEC and 88/357/EEC.

132 Freeman S. Health Care Provision in the EC. *AIDA Information Bulletin* 1994;47:120–22.

133 Mossialos E, McKee M. The European Union and health: past, present and future. In: Harrison A. *Health Care UK 1997/98*. London: King's Fund, 1997.

134 Comité Européen Des Assurances. *Indirect Taxation on Insurance Contracts in Europe in 1996*. Paris: Comité Européen Des Assurances, 1996.

135 Sixma JJ. Chairman, Health Council, The Netherlands, *personal communication*.

136 Abel-Smith B, Calltorp J, Dixon M, Dunning A, Evans R, Jarman B, Holland W, Mossialos E. *Report on the Greek Health Services*. Athens: Ministry of Health, 1994.

137 Cordts B. The containment of cost of health care. *Acta Chirurgica Belgica et Acta Orthopaedica Belgica* 1996;96(2):56–8.

138 Albert S. Le service public hospitalier. In: La Documentation Française. *La Protection Sociale en France*. Paris: La Documentation Française, 1995.

The European Union: References 151

139 Redmon P, Yakoboski P. The nominal and real effects of hospital budgets in France. *Inquiry - The Journal of Health Care Organization Provision and Financing* 1995;32: 174–83.

140 Nolan B. *Charging for Public Health Services in Ireland: Why and How?* Dublin: The Economic and Social Research Institute, Policy Research Series, Paper No. 19, 1993.

141 Yakoboski PJ, Ratner J, Gross DJ. The effectiveness of budget targets and caps in the German ambulatory sector. *Benefits Quarterly* 1994;10:31–7.

142 Busse R, Schwartz FW. Financing reforms in the German hospital sector: from full cost cover principle to prospective case fees. *Medical Care* 1997;35(10 suppl):OS40–9.

143 Busse R, Wismar M. Health care reform in Germany: the end of cost containment? *Eurohealth* 1997;3(2):32–4.

144 O'Donoghue N. Pricing and reimbursement of medicines: the Irish experience. In: Mossialos E, Ranos C, Abel-Smith B (eds). *Cost Containment, Pricing and Financing of Pharmaceuticals in the European Community: The Policy-makers' View.* Athens: LSE Health and Pharmetrica SA, 1994.

145 Goodwin N. General practitioner fundholding. In: Le Grand J, Mays N, Mulligan J (eds). *Learning from the NHS Internal Market.* London: King's Fund, 1998.

146 Harris CM, Scrivener G. Fundholders' prescribing costs: the first five years. *British Medical Journal* 1996;313:1531–4.

147 Schulenburg VD, Graf J-M, Schoffski O. *Implications of the Structural Reform of Healthcare Act on the Referral and Hospital Admission Practice of Primary Health Care Physicians.* Hanover: University of Hanover, 1993.

148 Audit Commission. *A Prescription for Improvement: Towards More Rational Prescribing in General Practice.* London: HMSO, 1994.

149 Le Grand J, Bartlett W. *Quasi-Markets and Social Policy.* Basingstoke: Macmillan Press, 1993.

150 Glennerster H, Matsaganis M. The English and the Swedish health care reforms. *International Journal of Health Services* 1994;24(3)231–51.

151 Saltman R, Figueras J. *European Health Care Reform: Analysis of Current Strategies.* Copenhagen: WHO, 1997.

152 Kröger T. Policy-makers in social services in Finland: the municipality and the state. *Scandinavian Journal of Social Welfare* 1996;5:62–8.

153 Maisonneuve H, Cordier H, Durocher A, Matillon Y. The French clinical guidelines and medical references programme: development of 48 guidelines for private practice over a period of 18 months. *Journal of Evaluation in Clinical Practice* 1997;3(1):3–13.

154 Sloan FA, Grabowski HG. Introduction and overview. *Social Science and Medicine* 1997;45(4):507–12.

155 Froehlich P, Morgon A. Impact of clinical guidelines. *The Lancet* 1996;346:1039–40.

156 Le Fur P, Sermet C. *Medical References: The Impact on Pharmaceutical Prescriptions.* Paris: CREDES-CES, 1996,

157 De Vos C. Financing of medicines in the Netherlands. In: Mossialos E., Ranos C, Abel-Smith B. (eds). *Cost Containment, Pricing and Financing of Pharmaceuticals in the European Community: The Policy-makers' View.* Athens: LSE Health and

152 Health Care and Cost Containment in the European Union

Pharmetrica SA, 1994.

158 Pugner K. *Cost Containment in the German Health Care System: The Pharmaceutical Sector*. London: University of London (MSc dissertation), 1995.

159 Klauber J. Entwicklung des Fertigarzneimittelmarktes 1983 bis 1993. In: Schwabe U, Paffrath D (eds). *Arzneiverordnungs-Report 1994*. Stuttgart: Gustav Fischer Verlag, 1994.

160 Zammit-Lucia J. Dasgupta R. Reference pricing: the European experience. *Health Policy Review* No 10. Imperial College, University of London, 1995.

161 Pineal R *et al*. Randomized clinical trial of one-day surgery. *Medical Care* 1985;23(2): 171–82.

162 Burn JM. Responsible use of resources: day surgery. *British Medical Journal* 1983;286: 492–3.

163 Beech R, Larkinson J. *Estimating the Financial Savings from Maintaining the Level of Acute Services with Fewer Hospital Beds*. London: Department of Community Medicine, St Thomas' Campus, 1989.

164 Audit Commission. *A Short Cut to Better Services. Day surgery in England and Wales*. London: HMSO, 1990.

165 Morgan M. Variations in length of stay at district level. In: Ham C (ed.). *Health Care Variations: Assessing the Evidence*. London: King's Fund, 1988.

166 Morgan M, Beech R. Variations in lengths of stay and rates of day case surgery: implications for the efficiency of surgical management. *Journal of Epidemiology and Community Health* 1990;44(2):90–105.

167 Cleary PD, Greenfield S, Mulley AG *et al*. Variations in length of stay and outcomes for six medical and surgical conditions in Massachusetts and California. *Journal of the American Medical Association* 1991;266(1):73–9.

168 Barrow S, Fisher AD, Seex DM *et al*. General practitioner attitudes to day surgery. *Journal of Public Health Medicine* 1994;16(3):318–20.

169 Fagnani F, Moatti JP, Weill C. The diffusion and use of diagnostic imaging equipment in France. *International Journal of Technology Assessment in Health Care* 1987;3: 531–43.

170 Banta D. Coordination of health technology assessment in Europe. *Eurohealth* 1996; 2(4):11–13

171 Cranovsky R, Matillon Y, Banta D. EUR-ASSESS project subgroup report on coverage. *International Journal of Technology Assessment in Health Care* 1997;13(2)287–332.

172 Le Pen C. Pharmaceutical economy and the economic assessment of drugs in France. *Social Science and Medicine* 1997:45(4):637–46.

173 Schulenburg VD, Graf JM. Economic evaluation of medical technologies: from theory to practice – the German perspective. *Social Science and Medicine* 1997:45(4):623–6.

174 Elsinga E, Rutten FFM. Economic evaluation in support of national health policy: the case of the Netherlands. *Social Science and Medicine* 1997:45(4):607–22.

175 Drummond M, Cooke J, Walley T. Economic evaluation under managed competition: evidence from the UK. *Social Science and Medicine* 1997:45(4):585–98.

176 Wennberg JE, Freeman JL, Culp WJ. Are hospital services rationed in New Haven or over-utilised in Boston? *The Lancet* 1987;1:1185–9.

177 Grol R. Development of guidelines for general practice care. *British Journal of General Practice* 1993;43:146–51.

178 Sackett DL. Evaluation of clinical method. In: Weatherall DJ, Ledingham JGG, Warrell DA (eds). *Oxford Textbook of Medicine*. Oxford: Oxford University Press, 1996 (third edition).

179 Frostick SP, Radford PJ, Wallace WA (eds). *Medical Audit; Rationale and Practicalities*. Cambridge: Cambridge University Press, 1993.

180 Honigsbaum F, Ham C. *Improving Clinical Effectiveness: The Development of Clinical Guidelines in the West Midlands* (report commissioned by the West Midlands Health Authority). University of Birmingham, 1996.

181 Hopkins A, Solomon JK. Can contracts drive clinical care? *British Medical Journal* 1996;313:477–8.

182 British Medical Association. *Managed Care and Disease Management Packages*. London: BMA, 1995 (Briefing Note No.4).

183 Anon. UK DoH issues new DM circular. *Scrip Magazine* 5 November 1996;2178.

184 Deutsche Gesellschaft für Innere Medizin. *Rationelle Diagnostik und Therapie in der Inneren Medizin*. Munich: Urban and Schwarzenberg, 1996.

185 Vogel H. Managed care: (k)eine Lösung für das Deutsche Gesundheitswesen? *Deutsche Apotheken Zeitung* 1996;27:2523–4.

186 Thomas S. Standard setting in the Netherlands: impact of the human factor on guideline development. *British Journal of General Practice* 1994;44(383):242–3.

187 Grol R. National standard setting for quality of care in general practice: attitudes of general practitioners and response to a set of standards. *British Journal of General Practice* 1990;40:361–4.

188 Proper C. Agency and incentives in the NHS internal market. *Social Science and Medicine* 1995;40(12):1683–90.

189 Maynard A. Can competition enhance efficiency in health care? Lessons from the reform of the UK National Health Service. *Social Science and Medicine* 1994;39(10):1433–45.

190 Goodman KW. Outcomes, futility and health policy research. In: Goodman KW (ed.). *Ethics, Computing and Medicine*. Cambridge: Cambridge University Press, 1998.

191 Lomas J, Haynes RB. A taxonomy and critical review of tested strategies for the application of clinical practice recommendations: from official to individual clinical policy. *American Journal of Preventive Medicine* 1988;4(supplement):77–94.

192 Grimshaw J, Eccles M, Russell I. Developing clinically valid practice guidelines. *Journal of Evaluation in Clinical Practice* 1995;1(1):37–48.

193 Avgerou C, Cornford T, Mossialos E. Information systems for the management of medical drug use: a European perspective. *Information Infrastructure and Policy* 1996;5(3):169–234.

194 Holland WW. Achieving an ethical health service: the need for information. *Journal of the Royal College of Physicians of London* 1995;29(4):325–33.

154 *Health Care and Cost Containment in the European Union*

195 Venot A, Kostrewski B, Harding N *et al. OPADE: Optimization of drug prescription using advanced informatics.* AIM project A2027, 1992.

196 Pernice A. *International Harmonisation of Health Cards: EU and G-7 Initiatives.* Brussels: European Commission – DG XIII, September 1996.

197 Schwartz FW, Glennerster H, Saltman R. *Fixing Health Budgets.* Chichester: Wiley, 1996.

198 Mossialos E. Citizens' views on health care systems in the 15 Member States of the European Union. *Health Economics* 1997;6(2):109–16.

199 Pelzman S. Towards a more general theory of regulation. *Journal of Law and Economics* 1976;19:211–40.

200 Evans RG. Illusions of necessity: evading responsibility for choice in health care. *Journal of Health Politics, Policy and Law* 1985;10(3):439–67.

201 Lohr KN, Yordy KD, Thier SO. Current issues in quality of care. *Health Affairs* 1998; 7(1):5–18.

202 Övretveit J. Developing public health service management in Europe. *European Journal of Public Health* 1998;8:87–8.

203 Centro Studi Investimenti Sociali/CENSIS. *Italy Today: Social Picture and Trends, 1996.* Milan: Franco Agneli, 1997.

2 Cost containment and health expenditure in the EU: a macroeconomic perspective

PANOS KANAVOS AND JOHN YFANTOPOULOS

2.1 Introduction

Following the rapid escalation of health care costs throughout the EU cost containment and the search for macroefficiency have been two of the cornerstones of health care reform in Member States, perhaps with the exception of the UK.[1,2] Many hypotheses have been put forward in an attempt to explain the reasons for the escalation of health care costs, including the ageing of the population,[3] the impact of new technology,[4] the intensity of the services provided,[5] and also the relationship between income and the demand for health.[6,7]

This chapter analyses a number of underlying factors that contribute to the objective of cost containment within EU Member States from a macroeconomic perspective. In doing so, it investigates the extent to which economic, organizational, technological, demographic and lifestyle factors play a role in explaining levels of spending on health in individual Member States. By examining the relationship between these variables and health spending over a period of time, it also aims to unveil the dynamics of factors influencing health spending. Furthermore, it aims to identify whether the same factors have similar effects across the EU, thus seeking to measure the impact of national cost-containment policies.

In the following sections, a macroeconomic model of the demand for health is proposed and tested econometrically. The investigation departs from other empirical analyses of this kind in several ways. First, it looks at potential determinants of health care expenditures on a country-by-country, time series basis, thereby avoiding the methodological caveats of cross-section and pooled cross-section analysis, particularly in what concerns the

156 *Health Care and Cost Containment in the European Union*

treatment of income, macroeconomic foundations and health system structure;[*] secondly, by examining countries separately, it avoids the debate over what is a correct conversion factor – a rather contentious issue in the literature;[**] and thirdly, it brings into the debate the short-term dynamics affecting variations in health spending, by looking at the impact of income growth rates, technology intensity and demographic structure on health spending.

Section 2.2 looks into the pressures on health spending in EU Member States and identifies macroeconomic factors, changes in the delivery of health care and health challenges, as the most important pressures. Section 2.3 analyses the theoretical framework in which the treatment of health care spending in individual EU Member States takes place. Section 2.4 presents the model and identifies the variables to be used in econometric analysis, and section 2.5 presents the results of the empirical analysis. Finally, section 2.6 draws the main conclusions.

2.2 Pressures on health spending

Within the EU, pressures on health spending come largely from three different sources. The first is the general macroeconomic constraint, its relation to individual aspects of health systems and the provision of health services. The second is the pressures on publicly funded welfare systems (particularly social security) that most EU countries face; and the third is the incidence of health challenges. Therefore, the improvement in health status of European populations resembles a constrained maximization problem as shown in Box 2.1, where the maximization of health status is subject to three constraints: first, a resource constraint, stemming from macroeconomic budgetary limitations; secondly, a welfare system constraint, arising from difficult choices in allocating scarce resources between critical components of welfare systems which present equally pressing needs (e.g. pensions and education); and thirdly a health challenges constraint, originating from evolving patterns in lifestyles and the incidence of disease.

Health systems in the EU are facing considerable macroeconomic con-

---

[*] For a methodological exposition, see Kanavos P, Mossialos E, 1997.[8]

[**] See for instance, the debate regarding the choice between exchange rates and purchasing power parities in section 2.3.2.

Box 2.1 The problem of further improving the health status of EU populations

MAXIMIZING HEALTH STATUS

subject to:

(a) macroeconomic constraint

(b) welfare system constraint, excluding health

(c) health challenges constraint

straints that may restrict the ability of publicly funded health systems to keep pace with rising health care costs in the near future. Over the past 30 years, demand for health services has been increasing consistently more than national income in real terms, while real GDP growth rates have fallen considerably in the 1980s and 1990s compared with the 1960s and 1970s (Table 2.1 overleaf). The differences in the expansionary process of health care expenditures in conjunction with GDP growth, are reflected in income elasticities of demand for health care. In Europe during the period from 1960 to 1970 this elasticity was 1.37, implying faster expansion of the health sector in comparison with the average economic growth. This was also combined with strong economic growth in all European countries. In the 1970s the two oil shocks and the ensuing recession contributed to the average income elasticity of demand for health care in Europe falling to 1.25. Finally, the 1980s brought a new era in the international health systems by imposing cost control and cost-containment policies. The expansionary process of health expenditures was further curtailed in Europe where the corresponding income elasticity of demand averaged 1.08.[9] Meeting, therefore, an ever-increasing demand for health services from a total pool of resources which does not grow as fast, contributes to the national economies' budget deficits and overall indebtedness.

The macroeconomic constraint is directly linked with the limitations of health systems in providing care for ever-increasing need. For many health systems, the 1960s and 1970s were the decades of expansion with universal coverage introduced in several Member States while extending coverage and introducing further choice in others.[2] Alongside such issues as increasing coverage and attempts to increase responsiveness of health systems to population needs, there also came the need to contain costs since the demand for health kept rising faster than the rate of increase in total income

158 *Health Care and Cost Containment in the European Union*

Table 2.1 Average annual growth rates (AAGR) in GDP, health spending and pharmaceutical spending in EU Member States, 1980–94

Country	1980–84			1985–89			1990–94		
	AAGR in GDP	AAGR in health expend.	AAGR in pharma expend.	AAGR in GDP	AAGR in health expend.	AAGR in pharma expend.	AAGR in GDP	AAGR in health expend.[1]	AAGR in pharma expend.[1]
Austria	1.03	0.40	2.70	2.67	2.27	3.22	2.07	2.80	4.81
Belgium	0.80	2.52	-0.64	2.89	3.78	4.31	1.15	2.20	6.53
Denmark	2.24	0.19	0.55	1.41	1.95	1.23	2.01	2.23	14.14[2]
Finland	2.71	2.76	1.11	4.25	4.10	3.3	-2.02	-3.25	0.29
France	1.44	5.66	7.96	3.14	4.74	7.78	0.83	4.20	5.99
Germany	1.23	0.23	-1.63	3.03	2.24	0.93	5.14	9.25	5.14
Greece	0.90	4.54	2.43	2.39	4.83	-2.26	1.10	0.56	5.37[2]
Ireland	2.42	-1.79	-5.36	3.62	-2.07	8.27	3.98	2.87	4.04
Italy	1.10	1.88	10.82	3.27	4.12	11.27	0.72	1.70	3.55
Luxembourg	2.41	2.82	-2.38	5.01	3.56	8.03	2.05	3.79	n/a
Netherlands	0.82	1.33	3.12	2.86	3.27	5.10	1.80	2.92	8.81
Portugal	0.42	-1.28	n/a	5.30	8.69	n/a	0.70	6.46	n/a
Spain	1.27	1.45	n/a	4.68	10.05	n/a	0.96	3.84	8.9[2]
Sweden	1.69	2.36	0.68	2.52	2.05	9.13	-0.62	-5.48	7.76
UK	1.56	2.02	6.12	4.07	1.78	5.06	0.86	1.87	10.00

Notes: 1. 1990–93. 2. 1990–92.
Source: OECD Health Data, 1996.[10]

in most EU Member States. Consequently, cost containment has been one of the most important thrusts in health policy-making over the last 15 years and, as a result, health care in most EU Member States has become more 'managed'.[11] Reform measures have included the introduction of budgets both for the whole of the health service and parts of it (for instance hospitals), the monitoring of the authorizing behaviour of doctors (who are increasingly being remunerated on a capitation basis), the introduction of priority-setting methodologies, and a growing debate on what is appropriate care through guidelines, economic evaluation of new technologies and evidence-based medicine.

A further source of macroeconomic pressure stems from the determination by most Member States to participate in Economic and Monetary Union (EMU). Admission into EMU presupposes the fulfilment of a number of macroeconomic performance criteria, set out in the Maastricht Treaty: first, inflation convergence, namely that inflation rates must not exceed the three best performing Member States by more than 1.5 per cent; secondly, budgetary convergence, which requires that the current government deficit should not exceed 3 per cent of GDP and the overall debt should not exceed 60 per cent of GDP; and thirdly, interest rate convergence, which requires that long-term interest rates in a Member State must not exceed the three best performing Member States by more than 1.5 per cent.

It is generally accepted that most Member States are still far from meeting the above criteria (Table 2.2 overleaf). As a result, all are currently implementing tight fiscal policies in order to reduce their general government deficits, or overall debt levels, or both; whilst, at the same time trying to achieve and maintain price stability. As health systems in the EU are publicly financed, rising health costs impose additional pressures on national budgets, the deficits of which need to be curbed and kept consistently low. Additionally, low growth rates will limit national governments' flexibility to tackle such problems because of the existing constraints, whereas the onset of a recession in key European economies may limit policy choices even further.

There are lateral pressures on publicly funded health systems, particularly those arising from the funding of other welfare services which are part of the national budget and have seen their share of GDP increase over time. Public pensions are an interesting case in this respect because they will almost certainly exert considerable pressure on national resources in the

160 *Health Care and Cost Containment in the European Union*

Table 2.2 Maastricht Convergence Criteria, 1994 and 1996

	Budget deficit as % of GDP		Debt as % of GDP		Annual inflation rate	
	1994	*1996*	*1994*	*1996*	*1994*	*1996*
Austria	-4.4	-5.0	65.2	71.3	3.0	1.7
Belgium	-5.3	-3.1	136.0	130.0	3.0	1.8
Denmark	-3.8	-2.2	75.6	72.0	1.0	2.2
Finland	-6.3	-3.6	59.8	62.0	1.3	1.2
France	-6.0	-4.5	48.4	54.0	1.8	2.2
Germany	-2.6	-4.0	50.2	61.5	2.7	1.8
Greece	-11.4	-8.0	113.0	117.0	10.8	8.3
Ireland	-2.1	-1.8	91.1	84.0	2.7	3.0
Italy	-9.0	-6.7	125.4	123.0	4.8	4.0
Luxembourg	+2.2	+1.1	5.9	6.8	2.4	2.1
Netherlands	-3.2	-2.8	78.0	72.0	2.4	2.1
Portugal	-5.7	-4.6	69.4	71.0	5.5	3.3
Spain	-6.6	-5.2	63.0	65.5	4.9	4.0
Sweden	-10.8	-4.2	79.3	82	3.1	1.2
UK	-6.8	-3.5	50.3	53.0	2.5	2.4

Source: International Financial Statistics, IMF.[12]

near future for two reasons: firstly, because the ratio of contributors to beneficiaries in public pension schemes is changing as populations age in the EU, and this questions the sustainability of current schemes and their modes of funding; secondly, the generosity of public pension systems, which varies hugely among Member States, will imply that for similar benefits to accrue to future pensioners, contribution rates will have to rise considerably (see Figure 2.1), with severe implications for wage bills, employment rates and national competitiveness. It has been estimated that most industrialized nations will be in need of considerably higher contribution rates to sustain current patterns of benefits.[13]

Health challenges are less compelling, but nevertheless quite important. The EU, in line with other developed countries, faces a number of evolving patterns in the causes of disease and death, which could impact on the ability of health services to deliver care in the near future. There are three such challenges. First, infectious diseases such as HIV pose a considerable threat to the extent that there are no effective treatments that cure the disease. In addition, there are many other known conditions/infections that are resistant

Figure 2.1 The burden of public pensions as a percentage of GDP, selected countries

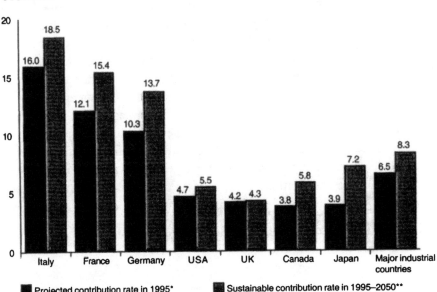

■ Projected contribution rate in 1995*   ■ Sustainable contribution rate in 1995–2050**

Notes:
* Including net budget transfers
** Defined as the constant contribution rate over 1995–2050 that equalises the net asset position in 1995.
Source: IMF staff estimates.

to many (or most) of the known antibiotics, for instance: methicillin resistant staphyllococus aureous (MRSA), strains of tuberculosis resistant to many antibiotics (MDR-TB), the case of Group A Beta-haemolytic streptococcus, and trimethoprim-resistant salmonella. Antibiotic resistance is not new, but what is new is that many more bacteria have developed resistance, and to a larger number of antibiotics.[14] The cost implications of these developments lie in the administration of more costly antibiotics, the need for additional drug testing, and for more prolonged hospital stays, as well as the use of non-antibiotic management, such as isolation techniques. Secondly, conditions such as diabetes and conditions of the central nervous system are gaining in importance. These conditions are to a certain extent associated with age (Alzheimer's), or psycho-social factors (depression, schizophrenia), and contribute considerably to the cost of treating patients[15–21] as

162 *Health Care and Cost Containment in the European Union*

European populations age gradually and available treatments are more palliative than curative. Thirdly, diseases related to diet, habits and lifestyle, impose a further economic burden which is not strictly related to the health sector *per se*, but bring further spillover effects to the family and the social system. Cardiovascular deaths are epidemiologically more apparent in the wealthier EU countries and are closely related to economic development and prosperity, arising partly from diet patterns rich in animal fat. Various types of cancers which are evidently associated with smoking are higher in the less developed EU countries where smoking among young and female populations is increasing and public health measures such as anti-smoking campaigns seem to have little or no effect. Traffic accidents present a major cause of death in the age groups of 25–44 years.[22] Among the European countries, Greece and Portugal present death rates which are three to four times higher than the rest of the Northern European countries. A considerable proportion of these deaths could be prevented if the ambulatory system could function more effectively.

2.3 Theoretical and empirical remarks on the health economics literature

The empirical evidence on the determinants of health spending so far relies exclusively on measurements that are of questionable theoretical foundations. This empirical work, based on cross-section and, more recently, on panel data analysis, puts together data from a number of OECD countries and implicitly makes a number of theoretical assumptions about health systems and the allocation of resources, which are not necessarily compatible with economic theory.

2.3.1. Theoretical remarks

There has been a confusion between macroeconomic and microeconomic approaches without defining whether the so-called demand for health refers to an aggregate approach based on macroeconomic thinking, or is simply derived from utility maximization based on the Grossman hypothesis, subsequently aggregating individual preferences and demands.

The macro-economic foundation The early studies by Abel Smith[6,7] Kleiman[23] and Newhouse[24] adopted an aggregate macro-economic approach based on public finance and international economics. The law of increasing expansion of the public sector and particularly state activities was defined by Wagner in 1883, and was subsequently known as 'Wagner's Law'. He estimated a statistical model based on a time series sample from a number of western industrializing countries:

$$G/Y = a + b \{ Y/N \}$$

where
G/Y = Government share
G = Government spending
Y = Income
N = Population
a and b are parametres to be tested

Musgrave[25,26] further elaborated Wagner's law by suggesting a number of hypotheses, in particular, changes in the share of government during different phases of socio-economic development. He attempted several empirical tests in order to explain the evolution of government expenditures.[26] Similar analyses have been carried out by several other authors.[27-30]

Although Abel Smith[6,7] Kleiman[23] and Newhouse[24] and others do not explicitly refer to Wagner's Law and Musgrave's work, the basic research question remains the same, namely to identify the causes and factors that contribute to the expansion of the health sector. Abel Smith, Kleiman and Newhouse highlighted the relationship between per capita health expenditure and per capita GDP, by the use of a limited number of statistical observations based on a sample selection of around 15 countries.

Abel Smith[7] illustrates this relationship in scatter diagrams for a sample of 15 countries, including developed (USA, Canada, Sweden), less developed (Tanganyka, Ceylon) and Eastern European countries (Yugoslavia, Czechoslovakia). He approximates the Engel Curve by estimating various forms of the following model:

Total health expenditure/national income = F (per capita income in US $)

The analysis is restricted to a fitted regression line and a scatter diagram without making reference to the estimated parametres.

164   *Health Care and Cost Containment in the European Union*

Kleiman[23] followed Abel Smith and used a sample of 16 developed and less developed countries for a single year (1969). The relationship between per capita health expenditures on per capita income was estimated, and a high coefficient of determination was found (R-square = 0.96), revealing that 96 per cent of the per capita variation of health expenditures across the Kleiman's sample could be explained just by the use of per capita income. Similarly, Newhouse[24] made use of a sample of 13 countries and also found a significant relationship. The estimated income elasticity is 1.31 showing that health is a luxury good.

The literature on the determinants of health care expenditures developed further during the 1970s and 1980s, revealing that after adjustment for inflation, exchange rates and population, GDP per capita remained the main determinant of health expenditure.

The micro-economic foundation In the micro-economic framework the evolution of health expenditures is explained by making reference to the theory of consumer utility maximization and demand analysis. Grossman[31] provided a theoretical framework to explain that the demand for health care is derived from the demand for health, which is the outcome of a health production process influenced by education, habits, diet and other lifestyle variables. Thus the consumer of health services is also a producer of a certain level of health status. The estimation and interpretation of income elasticities and other parameters related to the determinants of health expenditure become a difficult task because although it is feasible to derive micro-economic implications from aggregate analysis, the relevant assumptions are extremely restrictive.

In the subsequent analysis some critical remarks are presented on the basic micro-economic hypotheses which are frequently ignored or even violated in a large number of empirical studies. The first economic assumption made by applied researchers is that utility functions are homothetic. Homotheticity of utility functions implies that there are identical individual preferences across countries; it also implies that the marginal rate of substitution between two different bundles of commodities ($x1$ and $x2$) is identical across countries with different initial conditions, hence for instance $(dx1/dx2)_{greece} = (dx1/dx2)_{france}$. Assuming that $x1$ is ambulatory care and $x2$ is hospital care, homotheticity implies that the rate of sacrifice of hospital care in order to get an extra unit of primary care – while keeping utility constant – is the same across all countries. In practice, however, the devel-

Health Expenditure in the EU: A Macroeconomic Perspective 165

opment of ambulatory and hospital care across countries is not the same and the spectrum of services within both primary and secondary care varies significantly. Hence, goods x1 and x2 are not homogeneous across countries, and the rate of substitution is not really comparable.

Secondly, it is implicitly assumed that the proportions of various types of services (for instance hospital care and primary care) are fixed, namely the ratio of Q_{hi}/Q_{pi} is fixed in all countries involved in statistical analysis (where Q_{hi} is the amount of hospital care in country i and Q_{pi} is the amount of primary care in country i). However, allocation of resources is far from being the same in different countries. This implies different utilization of services and, furthermore, different operation of the health system in different countries. Thus, the relative development of primary and secondary care varies across countries and within the European Union, emphasis has been given to secondary care in the Southern Member States, and primary care in the Northern Member States. Epidemiological evidence also reveals that certain cases of morbidity in some countries are treated at primary level and in others at secondary level. Hence the rate of substitution between the two cannot remain identical between all countries. In addition, there are different levels of institutional versus household care in different EU countries, which in a cross-section or pooled data analysis remain unaccounted for. Again, the North–South divide within the EU highlights the differences, with the Northern Member States having more developed institutional care, while the Southern Member States rely more on household care.

A corollary of homothetic utility functions is that technology is given, hence decisions are taken in a (health) technology neutral environment where technological advances remain unaccounted for. The intensity in the use of technology as well as technological advances vary significantly among the Member States. Furthermore, the technology of producing different types of inputs such as doctors and nurses varies, and this can be attributed to different educational standards across countries. Thus, for instance, the augmented human capital in nursing personnel is very different among Member States. In northern Member States nurses there are highly qualified whereas in the southern Member States this may not be the case. This is also depicted in the differences of the educational curricula both at the preclinical and clinical levels. In addition, the rate of substitution among professionals varies due to differences in the production processes of health services. In certain countries the nursing profession substitutes for some areas of the medical profession's functions, while in others it has a purely

166 *Health Care and Cost Containment in the European Union*

auxiliary function.

Fourthly, it is assumed that relative prices are fixed (for instance *hospital care prices* and *primary care prices* are fixed) and price ratios are the same in different countries. Thus, the relative shares of expenditure are assumed to be fixed, so that, for instance, the ratio of $\mathbf{P_{hi}Q_{hi}/P_{pi}Q_{pi}}$ (where $\mathbf{P_{hi}Q_{hi}}$ is hospital expenditure in country i, and $\mathbf{P_{pi}Q_{pi}}$ is primary care expenditure in country i) is the same in all countries. Fixed relative prices imply that the ratio of prices remains the same across countries; this is based on the assumption that the markets of all health goods and services are identical, which means that there is the same degree of competitiveness as well as the same degree of unionization among professions; however, there are considerable differences among countries based on: first, the monopsonistic power of the state which purchases goods and services offered by the health sector; secondly, the monopolistic power of the medical profession, which varies across countries; and thirdly, in the southern European countries there is a significant underground health economy, where a considerable amount of health transactions especially in surgery are taking the form of underground payment.* This influences not only the absolute level of fees given to specialists, but also the price ratio of different inputs since there are no such noticeable payments to other health professionals, e.g. nurses. Thus, health care is not a homogeneous good but a largely heterogeneous one and this is something the empirical literature has largely ignored.

Fifthly, the distribution of income is assumed to be the same within and among all countries. However, income distribution varies within each country. Consequently, the spread of social need can be accordingly higher in countries where income distribution is better. Countries with larger poverty rates have higher needs for medical services and larger unfulfilled needs due to structural problems in the health service. Informational asymmetries also feature very strongly in this debate. Those in poverty are the less educated and the elderly who are potentially the largest users of health care. Equally, they do not consume the 'expected' amount either because there are problems of accessibility in the system or lack of information, or the system itself is not well established so as to diffuse information adequately.

There are a number of problems associated with the non-inclusion of

---

* This is the case in Greece and Spain. For Greece, see Abel-Smith B *et al.*, 1994;[32] for Spain, see De Miguel J M, Guillen M F, 1989.[33]

income distribution. Thus, the existence of different income groups within a country implies that for some income groups certain aspects of health care provision are luxuries, whereas for other income groups the same aspects are necessities. This relates to Newhouse's observation that in countries with higher health expenditure, each marginal unit of health services is more likely to improve subjective health status rather than decrease mortality or morbidity, and that lower social groups (also having lower incomes) have been found to have higher mortality rates and worse disease patterns in comparison with higher social/income groups.[34-37]

Methodologically, the issue of income inequality requires single country analysis. As Atkinson points out,[38] figures on the degree of income inequality are not comparable across countries. One can draw no conclusions from the relative degree of inequality in different countries. Usually, and for each individual country, figures are drawn from national studies of income inequality which are not designed for the purposes of international comparison, and they are not necessarily based on the same concepts of income or method of calculation. If cross-country comparisons are to make sense issues such as type of income (gross versus disposable), or household size, should be standardized across countries.

Finally, there is little or no reference to stock variables, diet, habits, nor the maturity of the health system, in the countries of reference. The incidence of diet and habits is quite important and may affect the level of health spending. However, the way this relationship works is not a straightforward one. There is a considerable lag between the current level of health spending and the impact of diet or smoking and alcohol, in that habits and poor diet may affect someone's health at some point in the future. Yet, the exact incidence is unknown, therefore the literature which has examined the relationship in levels between health spending and diet or habits is severely flawed.[39]

2.3.2 Empirical remarks

The literature on the determinants of health care expenditures has focused a great deal of attention on the aggregate relationship between gross domestic product (GDP) and the level of health spending. The early literature in the area[6,7] showed that, after adjustment for inflation, exchange rates and population, GDP per capita is a determinant of health expenditure and that

168 *Health Care and Cost Containment in the European Union*

most of the variation in health spending was attributable to variations in real per capita income. The above proposition was tested econometrically by many authors and it was confirmed that, in aggregate terms, spending on health rises faster than national income.[24,40,41] Thus the income elasticity of demand for health care is greater than unity, thereby implying that health care is a luxury good. The empirical literature has hovered around this relationship and examined a number of variations based on different methodological perceptions. There are three main stylized facts which summarize the research effort so far, relating to the analytical methodology, the attempts to standardize data from different countries, and the type of model used to analyse the variation in health care expenditures.

A large number of studies have examined the relationship between health spending and income, occasionally adding other variables on a cross-sectional basis, namely for a number of countries at a specific point in time.[24,39,41-44] Other studies followed the route of pooled cross-section analysis, namely by looking at the above relationship for a number of countries and for a number of years.[39,45-47] Finally, very few studies exist to date that look at the determinants of health expenditures on a time-series basis for individual countries.* The main result so far is, on aggregate, a confirmation of the earlier empirical finding that health care is a luxury good across countries (see Table 2.3) – both in the developed and the developing world[50-54] – and that health spending is largely determined by national income. However, the result does not appear to be robust and, at times the choice of year has shown that health care may not be a luxury good.[43] In addition, all empirical research to date has ignored the high correlation between health spending and GDP, particularly since the former is a component of the latter and in this respect health spending may Granger-cause GDP. The high correlation between these two macroeconomic indicators poses questions about the credibility of the existing empirical results.

The type of empirical analysis conducted (cross-section and pooled cross-section) has implied that all economic variables in the different countries have had to be translated into a common denominator. Two approaches have been adopted, namely the use of exchange rates to translate all types of expenditures into a common currency, and US$ Purchasing Power

---

* The only notable exceptions to date are Murillo C, Piatecki C, Saez M, 1993 [48] and Saez M, Murillo C, 1994.[49]

Table 2.3 Estimates of income elasticities of health care expenditures

Benchmark year	Author	Source	No. of observations	Form	Income Elasticity
A. Cross Section Analysis					
1960	Abel-Smith	WHO	15	Linear	Luxury
mid-1960s	Massell and Heyer	Household survey data (Kenya)	n.a.	Linear	Luxury
1968	Musgrove	Latin America	10	n.a.	Luxury
1974	Musgrove	Brazil	n.a.	n.a.	Luxury
1968/9	Kleiman	UN	16	Linear, Logarithmic	Luxury
1972	Newhouse	UN	13	Linear, Logarithmic	Luxury
1974	Leu	OECD	19	Logarithmic	Luxury
1975	Summers	OECD	34	Linear, Logarithmic	Luxury
1980	Parkin et al	OECD	18	Linear	L*
			18	Semi-log	N**
			18	Exponential	L
				Double-log	L
1982	Culyer	OECD	20	Linear, Logarithmic	Luxury
1985	Gerdtham and Joensson	OECD	22	Logarithmic	Luxury
1985	Gerdtham et al	OECD	19	Linear, Logarithmic	Luxury
1985	Murthy	OECD	22	Linear, Logarithmic	Luxury

Table 2.3 (continued) Estimates of income elasticities of health care expenditures

Benchmark year	Author	Source	No. of observations	Form	Income Elasticity
1985	Milne et al	EC	20	Logarithmic	Luxury
1987	Gerdtham	OECD	19	Logarithmic	Luxury
1990	Murray et al	Various	138	Logarithmic	Luxury
B. Pooled Data					
1960–87	Hitiris et al	OECD	560	Loglinear	Luxury
1974, 1980, 1987	Gerdtham et al	OECD and World Bank	57	Logarithmic	Luxury
1972–87	Gerdtham et al	OECD	396	Logarithmic	Luxury
1995	Gerdtham et al	OECD	484	Logarithmic	Normal
C. Time Series					
1960-90	Murillo et al	OECD	11 countries 30 years each	OLS, ML, Co-integration	Luxury

Notes: • This column shows elasticities with exchange rate conversions;
•• This column shows elasticities with PPP conversions.
L implies Luxury good; N implies Normal good.

Source: Kanavos P, Mossialos E, 1997.[8]

Parities. The debate around the appropriateness of either measure has been quite intense,[43,47–49,55–61] and it seems that on methodological grounds the use of PPPs has prevailed due to their ability to better evaluate the true volume of health care expenditure and income.[59] Consequently, it is considered to be the most appropriate method to measure variations in income and expenditure across countries. However, the choice of denominator has been found to alter the extent to which health care is a luxury good or a necessity.[29,43,45,46] For instance it has been shown that the use of PPPs as deflators causes the income elasticity to drop below unity, compared with the case when exchange rates are used.[43] In all the cases, the use of the PPPs weakens the intercountry variations. Other results contradict the above and assert that the use of exchange rates to convert health care expenditure in various countries into a common currency exaggerates the discrepancies between real health care expenditure in those countries.[58]

The empirical research has added other variables in an attempt to explain more fully the variation in health care expenditures across countries. Thus, the relationship between health care expenditure and those variables which represent the characteristics of the various national health care systems has been found to be statistically significant.[41,47] Nevertheless, the impact of those other non-income variables is of minor quantitative importance with respect to GNP. These results are consistent with the assertion that the differences in health care expenditures between countries cannot be entirely attributed to differences in financing the national health system. The same result persists when other potential determinants such as variables representing socio-demographic conditions (for instance, age structure of the population), supplier-induced demand, institutional factors, and habits are added.[39,45]

In the majority of the empirical exercises there has been statistical trial without theoretical foundation. Yet, economic theory may help explain more clearly the factors affecting both demand for health, and hence health spending, as well as whether health spending can abide by a certain theoretical framework. Identifying the theoretical foundations would help recognize the right model and, in turn, test it accordingly. The literature on the variations of health care expenditures, with the exception of a very small number of studies, has made a number of strong economic assumptions regarding the operation of health services across countries. The fact that these assumptions have been made may help partly explain why the results of the empirical analysis may be subject to review. Furthermore, the empir-

172   *Health Care and Cost Containment in the European Union*

ical literature does not provide an adequate explanation about why health expenditures are rising in most tax-, social insurance-, and voluntary insurance-financed systems. Whether the share of national income devoted to health care will continue to rise without limit is an issue left unaddressed.

2.4 The demand for health expenditures

2.4.1 The model

The pressures that health systems face in the European Union are related to the financing of the health sector in the light of technological innovation, change in the structure of the population, increasing demand following higher incomes, and indeed, a number of health challenges that populations face. These for instance were the effects of tobacco consumption, the incidence of infectious diseases such as tuberculosis and HIV and the effects of traffic accidents and the pressures they impose on health care costs, particularly in the southern Member States.[62] In addition, European health systems face the constraint of slow growth and efforts to reduce budget deficits by most European governments in order to qualify for membership in EMU. It is hypothesized that all the above factors have a role to play in determining the level of health spending.

A model was therefore built and subsequently tested in order to establish the exact relationship between health spending and factors hitherto mentioned. The model stipulates that at time t and for country i, the demand for health, proxied by total health spending (HEX), must be determined by a set of variables including demographic patterns (DEM) in country i, health status (HS), the advances in technology (TEC), the organization of the health care system (OR), the impact of the macroeconomy (MACRO), the dietary patterns and habits of the population (DIET), and prices of various inputs (PRICE). Thus, the intertemporal model of the demand for health care is as follows:

$$\text{HEX}_{it} = f(\text{DEM}_{it}, \text{HS}_{it}, \text{TEC}_{it}, \text{OR}_{it}, \text{MACRO}_{it}, \text{DIET}_{it}, \text{PRICE}_{it}), \quad t \leq 1 \quad (1)$$

The analysis presented below deviates from the existing literature of the determinants of health care expenditures in a number of ways. First, the

Health Expenditure in the EU: A Macroeconomic Perspective 173

time series approach has been adopted to analyse the determinants of health expenditures on a country-by-country basis. This follows a limited number of similar previous attempts in the literature.[48] A time-series approach would enable the examination of dynamic patterns arising in the relationship between the dependent and independent variables, particularly the impact that change (in population structure, technology, GDP growth) has on health spending. It will identify such patterns over a long period of time that would hold for a specific country, rather than patterns that hold for a specific year across a number of countries, which may be subject to change because of a different reference year or a monetary denominator.

Secondly, the methodology suggested looks at the health production function within each individual country over a predetermined period without converting economic variables into a common currency. It therefore avoids the methodological problems for both macroeconomic and health indicators that both the use of exchange rates and Purchasing Power Parities (PPPs) present in similar analyses,[8] without sacrificing the possibility of comparing results across countries for similar variables. It also avoids the methodological problems arising from the same variables being collected and/or reported under different guidelines in different countries.*

Thirdly, the proposed analysis analyses the impact of the macroeconomy on health spending by investigating whether the *rate of growth* of national income (proxied by year-on-year change in GDP) has any influence on the demand for health.

Finally, it recognizes that the lag structure of the model is not sufficient to test for the impact of diet (fat or vegetable consumption) or habits such as tobacco and alcohol consumption on health spending. In addition, there are no adequate variables to test this relationship. The analysis is conducted at the macroeconomic level and recognizes that omitted variables such as the distribution of income in each country and the level of the parallel economy may determine some of the variation in health expenditures. Due to difficulties in accounting for these variables, their impact is deduced from the error term structure of each model.

---

*See for instance, the differences in the collection of GDP in EU Member States in Commission of the European Communities, 1996[63] and for differences in collecting health indicators, see OECD, 1993.[64]

174 *Health Care and Cost Containment in the European Union*

2.4.2 The variables

A number of variables have been identified and used in statistical analysis. All variables are expressed in natural logarithms and for those involving monetary values, logarithms of values in constant national currencies (at constant 1990 prices) are used. In this way, the estimated coefficients represent elasticities. The variables are as follows.

Health Spending Total spending on health (LHEX) and the rate of growth in health spending (D(LHEX)) are the dependent variables. Health spending in each country is expressed in national currency units at constant 1990 prices. Although differences exist among Member States regarding the measurement of total health spending,[8] these differences do not affect single-country analysis.

Independent variables that have been included in the analysis are as follows:

Technology A common feature throughout the health sectors of the industrialized world is the increased use of new medical technology and its rising cost. New and expensive devices, drugs and surgical procedures, in addition to their already costly acquisition and implementation by health authorities, seem to need more skilled manpower to operate them.[65] Although health care technology has received a lot of attention in the literature, most attempts to actually measure its impact have failed to do so. This is partly because of the non-availability of credible data and, as a result, technology is one of the non-estimated factors that appear in the residual of econometric investigation; or at the micro level, for instance, looking at the growth in hospital costs.[66–71] This chapter does not attempt to evaluate technology, but in acknowledging its contribution to health care costs, it incorporates it as a flow variable in the model. Given the lack of an adequate global variable, a proxy of technological advance is pharmaceutical consumption (LPHARMA). This variable can be used as a proxy for the organization of the health care system in each of the countries analysed. However, because of the high correlation between the level of health pharmaceutical expenditures in each Member State, the growth rate in pharmaceutical spending (D(LPHARMA)) is used in the regression analysis.

Demography Demography enters the model from a macroeconomic per-

Health Expenditure in the EU: A Macroeconomic Perspective 175

spective, that is, through Wagner's Law. In this analysis two alternative aspects of demography which capture the impact of different parts of the population on expenditure are included. Firstly, much has been written about the effects of the ageing population.[72–80] For instance, it has been shown that medical expenses in France and Belgium are over three times greater for men aged 65 to 74 than for men aged 15 to 44. And expenses double for men over age 75 compared with the age group 65 to 74.[81] On the other hand, the average annual effect of demographic change in Britain has been calculated as less than 0.3 per cent per annum for the next 35 years.[82] In the past also, the effect has been far too small to account for more than a small part of the rising costs of health care in the developed world. However, the fact remains that populations in Europe are ageing and, although the relative distribution of population varies from country to country, the median has shifted towards higher ages. The ageing issue deserves further investigation and the share of individuals aged 65 and above (LOAP) has been included in the model. Secondly, male (LLIFEM) and female (LLIFEF) life expectancy are also included in order to investigate whether improvements in life expectancy, attributed to reduction in infant mortality or care of the elderly, have contributed significantly to the escalation of health care costs.

Health status The health-status variable has important theoretical implications for both macro and micro analysis. In a macro-economic thinking it is important to know whether governments in their expansionary process take into account the 'Aggregate or societal level of health status'. There is no detailed information on this issue (i.e. the formation and priority setting of health objectives from a public management point of view). Furthermore, the estimated coefficient presents the relative effectiveness of the health care system, i.e. to what extent health expenditures have influenced the improvements of health and the reduction of avoidable deaths.

Health status in micro-economic thinking is the outcome of the health-production process. The marginal productivity of health services as well as the diet, habits, and lifestyle parameters can be evaluated on the margin. From the point of view of a single individual, positive marginal productivities could be attained in the consumer's health-production process, by improving the lifestyle and living a healthier life. At the aggregate level, resource allocation could be directed more towards prevention and health education than over-supplying more hospital beds with a limited or even negative productivity upon individual health status.

176   *Health Care and Cost Containment in the European Union*

Infant mortality in each country (LMORTAL) is therefore included as the health-status variable with a view to establishing whether improvements explain part of the variation in health expenditures.

Macroeconomic factors   The macroeconomy exerts considerable pressure on the level and the rate of growth of health care expenditures. In recognizing this, two macroeconomic variables are included in the statistical analysis. The first is the (annual) level of GDP in each country (LGDP); all the empirical literature to date has used GDP and has found it to be the most significant variable in explaining the variation in health spending. The paper evaluates its importance from an individual country perspective. Its inclusion, therefore, reflects the need to establish the type of interaction between GDP and other independent variables. The second variable is the year-on-year rate of growth of GDP (D(LGDP)). It is thought that this may be closely related to health spending, since it is really the change in national income that may determine the extent to which the resources devoted to health rise or not.

Hospital variables   Hospitals absorb a considerable part of total health spending in all EU countries ranging from 32 per cent in Luxembourg (1994) to 61 per cent in Denmark (1994). Dramatic changes have taken place over the past 30 years in the delivery of in-patient care in most European countries, and as a result a reduction not only in the length of stay but also in the number of beds has taken place, both in the total number and those in acute care. It is important to determine whether these changes have impacted the level of health expenditures and, if so, to what extent and in which countries. The analysis therefore includes two variables that may be of interest, namely the number of in-patient care beds in each country (BEDIN) and the average length of stay in in-patient care (ALOSIN). The hypothesis to be tested here is that average length of stay and number of beds are positively related to health spending.

Prices   Health services are a non-tradable public good and as a result the pricing of health services does not necessarily reflect market conditions. The literature on pricing health services, although extensive, has not come to a conclusion as to an appropriate methodology that would give credible prices over a specific time period. In recognizing the importance of prices and their change over time, we have taken as a proxy, the level of relative

Health Expenditure in the EU: A Macroeconomic Perspective   177

wage (WAGE) in the health sector in each country. It is expected that the change in the relative wage (D(WAGE)), may also embody technological innovation in the health service, as higher real wages reflect productivity rises and higher skills due to technical progress. This variable is expected to have a significant positive impact on health spending.

Population Instead of using per capita figures in the regression analysis that follows in the next section, population has been used as an explanatory variable (POP). The rationale behind using aggregate macroeconomic data, and not per capita figures, lies in the fact that population in EU Member States has been stationary over the last 35 years (perhaps with the exception of Ireland) and if it has a significant impact that will probably be shown from its treatment as an independent variable. Generally, a positive relationship would be expected between population and health spending.

Medical profession The literature has suggested that the number of medical doctors per capita may be an important determinant of health care costs. By contrast, its predictive power has not proved to be significant. The total number of practising doctors in each country (DOCS) is included as an explanatory variable on the understanding that it is not able to reveal anything about the authorizing behaviour of doctors in different countries. However, in countries where the number of doctors per capita is high, there may be a positive strong association with health spending, as doctors compete for custom and are prepared to authorize more.

2.4.3 The data

The data used in the empirical analysis are those of the OECD Health Database, which provide a 35 year period for each of the European Union countries.[10] Use is made of both macro and micro elements of the theoretical analysis and variables are included which represent both micro and macro parts of the analysis. Problems of measurement, aggregation and representativeness of individual preferences remain, and this can be attributed to the nature of the available aggregate data. Results are reported for each of the EU Member States with the exception of Luxembourg, for which a comparable dataset could not be obtained. The analysis uses aggregate data for all the above variables, rather than per capita figures.

178   *Health Care and Cost Containment in the European Union*

2.5 Empirical results

The results of the regression analysis are presented in Tables 2.4 and 2.5 overleaf, for each EU Member State with the exception of Luxembourg. For each country a set of equations is shown where the dependent variable is the total spending on health. The period covered by the statistical analysis ranges from 1960 to 1994 for each country. The tables show the values of coefficients and the t-statistics in brackets. Linear regression analysis is applied, the method of estimation being a second-order autoregressive process (AR(2)), or a first-order autoregressive moving average process (ARMA(1,1)). All variables are expressed in logarithms, and those variables involving monetary values are expressed in local currencies and are in 1990 constant prices. The logarithms of these values are subsequently taken. Since population in the 14 Member States has been stationary over the past 34 years, the analysis has avoided values of both the dependent and independent variables expressed in per capita terms; this would avoid incidence of multicollinearity in the models. Various specification and diagnostic tests have been applied to all reported equations, including those for higher order (2nd and 4th respectively) autocorrelation, autoregressive conditional heteroskedasticity (ARCH), White heteroskedasticity, and normality.

Relationship between income and health spending For a number of countries the hypothesis that national income, proxied by GDP explains (at least partly), variations in health expenditures is rejected. The evidence for this is presented in Table 2.4, where, in a simple regression over time, and with both aggregate and per capita figures expressed in national currencies and in constant terms, GDP fails to explain any variation in health expenditures in 7 of the 14 EU Member States. Furthermore, as the value of the income elasticity of demand for health care is significantly below unity, it is shown that health is not a luxury good, but a necessity.

The equations presented in Table 2.5 test the extent to which income, expressed in terms of GDP in national currencies in constant 1990 prices, is among other variables, a determinant of health spending in each of the 14 EU Member States. They also attempt to show how income interacts with other potential determinants of health spending. The linear relationship has been tested against the total spending on health. The evidence suggests that the relationship between national income and health spending is far more complicated than it was originally thought to be, and it certainly contrasts

Health Expenditure in the EU: A Macroeconomic Perspective   179

Table 2.4 Regression results of constant per capita health spending on constant GDP per capita with respect to values expressed in exchange rates, PPPs and national currencies, 1960—93 (t-statistics in brackets)

Country (estimation method)[1]	NCUs[2]		GDP per capita in constant 1990 prices ERs (US$)[3]		PPPs (US$)[4]	
Austria (AR(1))	1.02 (10.5)*	R^2=0.98 DW=1.92	1.02 (24.5)*	R^2=0.995 DW=1.92	1.03 (14.05)*	R^2=0.993 DW=1.92
Belgium	-0.64 (1.51) (ARMA(1,1))	R^2=0.994 DW=1.83	0.97 (12.2)* (AR(1))	R^2=0.994 DW=1.8	0.25 (0.89) (AR(2))	R^2=0.994 DW=1.6
Denmark (AR(1))	1.17 (5.74)*	R^2=0.986 DW=2.17	1.02 (13.9)*	R^2=0.988 DW=2.28	1.05 (3.89)*	R^2=0.929 DW=2.25
Finland (ARMA(1,1))	0.31 (1.61)	R^2=0.997 DW=1.73	0.93 (13.4)*	R^2=0.993 DW=2.12	0.58 (3.81)*	R^2=0.986 DW=1.91
France	-0.29 (0.91) (AR(1))	R^2=0.998 DW=2.16	0.99 (20.7)* (AR(1))	R^2=0.997 DW=1.86	0.55 (3.3)* (AR(2))	R^2=0.996 DW=1.99
Germany (AR(2))	0.46 (2.82)*	R^2=0.993 DW=1.94	0.97 (15.6)*	R^2=0.997 DW=1.89	0.63 (4.38)*	R^2=0.996 DW=1.88
Greece (AR(2))	0.32 (0.94)	R^2=0.99 DW=1.94	0.91 (12.46)*	R^2=0.99 DW=2.06	0.86 (9.77)*	R^2=0.985 DW=2.01
Ireland (AR(2))	0.07 (0.14)	R^2=0.987 DW=2.08	1.19 (9.27)*	R^2=0.965 DW=2.03	0.6 (2.38)**	R^2=0.933 DW=2.01
Italy (AR(2))	1.74 (35.4)*	R^2=0.997 DW=2.01	1.03 (25.9)*	R^2=0.993 DW=1.93	1.04 (9.57)*	R^2=0.986 DW=2.07
Netherlands (AR(2))	0.46 (1.79)***	R^2=0.992 DW=2.06	0.96 (19.3)*	R^2=0.997 DW=1.84	0.97 (8.07)*	R^2=0.993 DW=1.86
Portugal	1.84 (12.3)* (AR(2))	R^2=0.94 DW=2.18	1.2 (8.6)* (AR(1))	R^2=0.968 DW=2.01	0.72 (8.4)* (AR(1))	R^2=0.96 DW=1.98
Spain	1.94 (24.9)* (AR(1))	R^2=0.994 DW=1.92	0.93 (12.9)* (AR(2))	R^2=0.99 DW=1.91	1.07 (5.32)* (AR(2))	R^2=0.96 DW=1.88
Sweden (AR(1))	0.64 (1.46)	R^2=0.989 DW=1.74	0.94 (13.4)*	R^2=0.988 DW=1.67	0.94 (4.38)*	R^2=0.97 DW=1.76
UK (ARMA(1,1))	1.83 (7.73)*	R^2=0.94 DW=2.02	0.73 (2.9)*	R^2=0.796 DW=2.27	0.33 (0.85)	R^2=0.62 DW=2.16

Notes: 1. Estimation method in brackets; estimation method may vary; if uniform, reported under country name; if not uniform, reported under each equation.

2. NCUs: national currency units.

3. ERs: exchange rates (US $).

4. PPPs: purchasing power parities (in US $).

*Significant at 1% level   **Significant at 5% level   ***Significant at 10% level

with the results of the empirical literature to date.

The results concerning the performance of national income, expressed in GDP at 1990 constant prices, can be summarized as follows. First, in seven countries, income was shown to be not at all significant in explaining any of the variation in health spending (Austria, Belgium, Denmark, France, Ireland, Sweden, UK). This result was robust and suggests that other variables play an important role in determining health spending. In all other cases, GDP was found to be statistically significant, but the value of the coefficient varied considerably between countries, from significantly lower than unity (Finland, Germany), to approximately equal to unity (Spain, Greece), to higher than unity (Italy, Netherlands). In those country-cases where GDP was found to be statistically significant, its inclusion in the econometric analysis had no impact on the performance of other variables. This contradicts most of the empirical literature to date, which has concluded that the income elasticity of spending for health care exceeds unity or is near unity.

Second, following the weak performance of income in current levels, the relationship between current levels of health spending with previous levels of income (LGDP(-1)) was tested, based on the hypothesis that current income could determine future expenditure on health. The analysis rejected the above hypothesis and the results (coefficient values and significance) that were obtained for lagged values of GDP were similar to those for current values.

Third, in order to test the hypothesis that income growth rates determine the extent of spending on health rather than levels of income the rate of growth of income was also included in the empirical analysis. It emerged that income growth is a significant variable in 6 of the 14 EU countries, although its association with health spending is negative in four cases (Germany, Greece, Netherlands, and Sweden), contrary to what was expected, and positive in two (Denmark, Portugal). The negative relationship was found to be robust and can be interpreted to imply countercyclical effects in the financing of health services related to the nature of the macroeconomic (business) cycle. The income growth rate was significant particularly when it was included in the analysis together with the income variable in level terms, although its negative sign takes away some of the importance of income and indicates that in some countries health financing follows the macroeconomic cycle with an annual lag.

Finally, income proved to be more closely associated with total health

Health Expenditure in the EU: A Macroeconomic Perspective   181

Table 2.5 Determinants of health expenditure in EU Member States

Variable	Austria Total Spending			Belgium Total Spending			Denmark Total Spending		
	Eq. 1	Eq. 2	Eq. 3	Eq. 1	Eq. 2	Eq. 3	Eq. 1	Eq. 2	Eq. 3
GDP	0.22 (0.47)			0.7 (1.13)			-0.62 (2.98)*		
D(GDP)	-0.65 (1.5)			-0.35 (0.62)			0.72 (2.42)**		
GDP(-1)									
D(GDP(-1))									
DOC	-0.21 (0.75)			-0.08 (0.43)	-0.14 (0.77)		0.04 (0.42)	0.13 (1.12)	
D(DOC)		0.26 (1.16)							
OAP	0.62 (1.12)	0.96 (1.84)***	0.65 (1.06)	-0.85 (1.17)	-0.48 (0.8)		-0.05 (0.1)		
MORTAL	-0.18 (1.1)	-0.11 (1.16)	-0.23 (2.8)*	-0.49 (2.1)**	-0.64 (3.33)*	-0.85 (4.18)*	0.23 (1.7)***	0.1 (1.22)	
PHARMA	0.3 (1.2)	0.39 (3.03)*		0.38 (1.89)***	0.59 (4.69)*	0.37 (2.85)*	0.64 (6.45)*	0.36 (4.57)*	0.48 (7.11)*
LIFEF							13.2 (4.62)*	5.26 (2.55)**	
LIFEM									
ALOSIN						-0.4 (4.5)*		-0.12 (2.01)**	
BEDIN							-0.48 (5.21)*		-0.16 (3.41)*
WAGE		0.79 (3.44)*				0.84 (4.21)*			0.18 (1.05)
D(WAGE)									
POP		-2.83 (2.1)**				-0.84 (2.97)*			
D(POP)									-11.4 (3.02)*
R^2	0.987	0.987	0.989	0.995	0.995	0.997	0.992	0.986	0.98
DW	2.02	1.99	1.93	1.66	1.79	1.74	2.11	2.24	2.1
SSR	0.03	0.04	0.03	0.04	0.04	0.01	0.02	0.03	0.02
F	282	411	508	727	1162	1461	158	249	198

Notes: *Significance at 1% level.   **Significance at 5% level.   ***Significance at 10% level.

182 Health Care and Cost Containment in the European Union

Table 2.5 (continued) Determinants of Health Expenditure in EU Member States

Variable	Finland Total Spending			France Total Spending			Germany Total Spending		
	Eq. 1	Eq. 2	Eq. 3	Eq. 1	Eq. 2	Eq. 3	Eq. 1	Eq. 2	Eq. 3
GDP	0.62		0.61	-0.12			0.41	0.59	
	(4.32)*		(5.01)*	(0.75)			(3.47)*	(3.44)*	
D(GDP)							-0.41	-0.59	-0.42
							(4.37)*	(4.41)*	(3.61)*
GDP(-1)									
D(GDP(-1))					-0.08				
					(0.39)				
DOC	-0.25		-0.043	0.39			0.17	0.23	
	(1.89)***		(0.29)	(3.9)*			(2.19)**	(2.5)**	
OAP	0.22		0.07				0.08	0.055	
	(0.44)		(0.12				(3.7)*	(2.12)**	
MORTAL	0.0002		-0.084		-0.4	-0.5		0.04	-0.09
	(0.002)		(0.87)		(5.00)*	(6.29)*		(0.82)	(2.87)*
PHARMA	0.93	0.67	0.8	0.51	0.56	0.31	0.4	0.4	0.4
	(9.46)*	(5.27)*	(6.77)*	(6.72)*	(11.2)*	(2.27)**	(9.36)*	(8.92)*	(7.15)*
LIFEF			3.97	12.5					
			(2.04)**	(4.97)*					
LIFEM			-5.5	-10.2					
			(3.37)*	(4.43)*					
ALOSIN					0.11	0.27			
					(1.71)***	(3.56)*			
BEDIN	0.15	0.38		0.27	0.33			0.45	
	(1.94)***	(2.41)**		(2.24)**	(2.43)*			(1.3)	
WAGE		0.65				-0.17			0.59
		(3.55)*				(1.1)			(3.1)*
D(WAGE)									
POP		0.78				3.9			0.56
		(0.51)				(1.53)			(9.89)*
D(POP)									
R^2	0.998	0.997	0.998	0.999	0.999	0.999	0.998	0.998	0.997
DW	2.06	1.72	2.13	2.1	1.87	1.78	1.87	2.00	1.91
SSR	0.02	0.02	0.02	0.01	0.02	0.006	0.01	0.01	0.002
F	2164	2324	1856	5651	4665	7241	1597	1186	1128

Notes: *Significance at 1% level. **Significance at 5% level. ***Significance at 10% level.

Table 2.5 (continued) Determinants of Health Expenditure in EU Member States

Variable	Greece Total Spending			Ireland Total Spending			Italy Total Spending		
	Eq. 1	Eq. 2	Eq. 3	Eq. 1	Eq. 2	Eq. 3	Eq. 1	Eq. 2	Eq. 3
GDP	0.91 (2.42)**				0.8 (1.36)		1.45 (6.1)*	1.04 (5.05)*	1.13 (4.61)*
D(GDP)	-0.86 (2.48)**	-0.69 (2.33)**			-0.17 (0.45)		-0.35 (1.43)		
GDP(-1)									
D(GDP(-1))									
DOC		-0.67 (4.01)*		0.78 (2.11)**	0.42 (1.22)		0.08 (0.9)		0.083 (0.93)
OAP	-0.43 (0.8)			-2.49 (1.2)			0.41 (1.33)		0.72 (2.1)**
MORTAL	-0.25 (2.00)**		-0.34 (8.59)*	-0.21 (1.55)	-0.16 (1.24)				-0.11 (0.68)
PHARMA	0.28 (2.23)**	0.5 (23.7)*	0.54 (12.6)*	0.15 (2.59)**	0.42 (3.17)*	0.05 (0.45)	-0.03 (0.63)		-0.04 (0.51)
LIFEF					-12.3 (2.29)**				
LIFEM		16.8 (6.38)*			6.11 (2.41)**				
ALOSIN		-0.08 (0.65)							
BEDIN				0.54 (2.01)**	0.85 (2.84)**	1.13 (4.2)*		-0.09 (0.75)	
WAGE			0.15 (1.72)***			2.17 (3.68)*		0.39 (1.74)***	
D(WAGE)									
POP						1.88 (1.76)***		2.46 (1.55)	
D(POP)			-8.7 (3.77)*						
R^2	0.994	0.996	0.995	0.971	0.984	0.975	0.998	0.998	0.998
DW	2.01	2.08	1.99	2.15	2.3	1.76	1.79	2.12	2.12
SSR	0.05	0.04	0.05	0.03	0.01	0.02	0.03	0.01	0.03
F	696	994	949	68	69	93	2066	3781	1707

Notes: *Significance at 1% level.   **Significance at 5% level.   ***Significance at 10% level.

184 *Health Care and Cost Containment in the European Union*

Table 2.5 (continued) Determinants of Health Expenditure in EU Member States

Variable	Netherlands Total Spending			Sweden Total Spending			UK Total Spending		
	Eq. 1	Eq. 2	Eq. 3	Eq. 1	Eq. 2	Eq. 3	Eq. 1	Eq. 2	Eq. 3
GDP	1.28 (6.9)*	0.92 (5.22)*		-0.14 (0.55)			0.34 (1.52)		
D(GDP)	-0.43 (2.1)**			-0.52 (1.75)***		-0.6 (1.95)***	-0.21 (1.02)		
GDP(-1)									
D(GDP(-1))									
DOC			-0.28 (1.59)***	0.21 (1.56)		0.33 (2.2)**	-0.085 (0.31)		0.3 (3.1)*
OAP		-2.49 (3.87)*	1.45 (2.5)**	1.62 (3.34)*		1.5 (3.06)*	0.16 (0.25)	0.65 (3.61)*	1.12 (6.54)*
MORTAL	0.098 (1.02)		-0.03 (0.21)	0.16 (1.89)***	-0.45 (12.5)*	0.24 (3.2)*	-0.37 (2.74)*	-0.36 (4.7)*	-0.21 (2.75)*
PHARMA		-0.11 (1.96)***	0.11 (3.44)*	0.07 (2.44)**	-0.01 (0.29)	0.06 (1.92)***	-0.08 (1.2)	-0.16 (2.13)**	-0.03 (0.56)
LIFEF	-1.8 (0.81)								
LIFEM	0.72 (0.4)								
ALOSIN						0.31 (8.25)*			
BEDIN			-0.62 (2.31)**	0.36 (9.3)*	0.7 (29.5)*				
WAGE		-0.55 (7.25)*			-0.27 (5.48)*			0.27 (2.49)**	
D(WAGE)									
POP		8.45 (4.65)*			7.98 (9.32)*				
D(POP)								6.32 (2.47)**	
R^2	0.995	0.992	0.988	0.993	0.991	0.991	0.995	0.995	0.994
DW	2.27	1.74	1.75	1.94	2.14	2.28	2.18	2.35	2.25
SSR	0.023	0.003	0.008	0.002	0.002	0.015	0.01	0.001	0.01
F	764	310	310	231	230	205	340	421	451

Notes: *Significance at 1% level.   **Significance at 5% level.   ***Significance at 10% level.

Table 2.5 (continued) Determinants of Health Expenditure in EU Member States

Variable	Portugal Total Spending			Spain Total Spending		
	Eq. 1	Eq. 2	Eq. 3	Eq. 1	Eq. 2	Eq. 3
GDP				1.03 (4.26)*	0.98 (3.83)*	1.02 (3.83)*
D(GDP)	2.5 (2.94)*	1.96 (3.24)*		-0.37 (0.85)		
GDP(-1)						
D(GDP(-1))						
DOC	-0.82 (1.88)***	-0.41 (1.22)		-0.31 (1.87)***	-0.26 (1.83)***	
OAP	0.49 (1.02)	0.84 (2.05)**		1.24 (1.96)***	1.75 (3.09)*	1.64 (3.41)*
MORTAL	-0.91 (5.33)*	-0.93 (3.74)*		-0.21 (1.36)		
PHARMA						
LIFEF		10.9 (2.56)**				
LIFEM		-11.3 (2.85)*				
ALOSIN		0.52 (1.34)				
BEDIN			-1.47 (5.43)*		0.11 (0.52)	
WAGE			1.66 (8.24)*			0.62 (2.09)**
D(WAGE)						
POP			0.42 (0.73)			-4.28 (2.73)*
D(POP)						
R^2	0.948	0.98	0.96	0.997	0.996	0.997
DW	2.00	2.08	1.85	2.07	1.83	1.71
SSR	0.07	0.05	0.02	0.03	0.03	0.04
F	37	45	50	1138	1077	1919

Notes: *Significance at 1% level. **Significance at 5% level. ***Significance at 10% level.

186 Health Care and Cost Containment in the European Union

spending than public spending on health. When the relationship between income and public spending on health was tested it was found to be very weak and statistically non-significant in all cases; as a result it is not reported in Table 2.5. This indicates that GDP is associated with the level of total health spending only.

In conclusion, the individual country analysis has shown that the aggregate relationship between income and health spending has been exaggerated in the literature and that other variables are responsible for the continuous escalation of health spending. The rate of growth of income is an important variable but its relationship with health spending was found to be negative in many cases.

Impact of demography and health status variables Over the past 35 years all EU Member States have experienced considerable improvements in health status, as expressed by both life expectancy and infant mortality. Based on the OECD's Health Data statistics, infant mortality has decreased by an average of 78 per cent in all EU countries between 1960 and 1994.[10] Some Member States experienced great improvements (Portugal, 89 per cent; Austria, Spain, Italy, Germany, 83 per cent; Ireland, Greece, 80 per cent) while others showed smaller improvements (Netherlands, 66 per cent; Sweden, UK, 71 per cent). At the same time, infant mortality rates varied considerably among countries, and fell from high values (Portugal 7.75 per 1000 live lifes; Italy, 4.39; Spain, 4.37; Greece, 4.01) or were already low (Sweden, 1.66; Netherlands, 1.79). The importance of public health systems in reducing infant mortality is well documented as the u-shaped age-expenditure curve demonstrated. The hypothesis, therefore was that reductions in infant mortality would contribute to rising health care costs, hence a negative relationship between the two was anticipated.

The increases in life expectancy (varying in different Member States) can also be associated, among others, with the provision of better care; hence the hypothesis is that increased life expectancy may contribute to high health care costs.

However, as life expectancy has increased, infant mortality decreased, and fertility rates fell. The share of elderly (aged 65 and above) has increased sharply in all EU countries between 1960 and 1994, particularly in Germany (rise by 50 per cent between 1960 and 1994), Italy (57 per cent), Spain (65 per cent), Portugal (74 per cent), Greece (80 per cent) and Finland (84 per cent). All other Member States have experienced increases in the

Health Expenditure in the EU: A Macroeconomic Perspective   187

share of elderly in the population by less than 50 per cent. It is therefore expected that if a relationship exists between ageing and health spending, this should be positive. Furthermore, this relationship is expected to be stronger in countries that have experienced rapid ageing over the past 30 years. The statistical analysis cannot take into account the considerable differences that exist in care for the elderly patterns across the EU, with institutional care more predominant in the north of Europe and family care in the south; neither can it account for differences in budgeting for health services for the elderly. In Sweden for instance, long-term care, having long being a vital part of the health budget, was recently shifted to the social security budget. On a time-series basis, however, this is not expected to show up.*

As all the above demographic variables may have high correlation rates, mortality and age are included together in the analysis without life expectancy, in order to capture the possible effect of the two extremes in the age–expenditure curve. The impact of life expectancy was tested separately.

With these remarks in mind, the statistical analysis has shown that age is an important push factor of health care costs and is positively and significantly associated with total costs in Austria, Portugal, Germany, Spain, Italy, Netherlands, Sweden and the UK. In all other countries the relationship was rather weak and not statistically significant. This included countries such as Finland and Greece where the share of aged population has increased quite considerably over the last 35 years. The only explanation for ageing not showing a significant association with health costs in these countries is that other factors are important, or indeed family care substitutes for institutional care.

Improvements in the mortality rates of individual countries clearly show a negative statistically significant association with the levels of total health spending in seven EU Member States (Austria, France, UK, Belgium, Germany, Greece and Portugal), implying that reductions in infant mortality contribute to health care cost increases over time. The negative relationship was robust in all seven cases, also indicated by the size of the coefficient. By contrast, the relationship between mortality and health expenditures is positive and significant in Sweden and Denmark, two countries that

---

* This does not affect the analysis for Sweden, since the change in budgeting took place after the endpoint of the current dataset.

188 *Health Care and Cost Containment in the European Union*

experienced decreases in mortality rates over the 1960–95 period. Nevertheless, their mortality rates in the early 1960s were considerably lower than any other EU Member State. In all other EU countries improvements in mortality over time do not appear to have been a determinant of health care costs.

Life expectancy is in several cases related with health spending, although the results are very often confusing; when male (or female) life expectancy is included on its own in statistical analysis, its association with health spending is not significant in most cases. When both female and male life expectancy are included in the analysis, many of the results are statistically significant, for instance in Denmark, Finland, Portugal, France, Greece and Ireland. In most cases, however, the sign of coefficients is opposite to what is expected. Thus, there is a tendency for male life expectancy to be negatively associated and for female life expectancy to be positively associated with health care costs.

Impact of medical profession Doctors as gatekeepers and prescribers are key in the determination of health care costs. In addition, the method of paying doctors may lead to escalation of health care costs.

As expected, the sign is positive and the coefficient significant for the cases of Germany, France, Ireland, UK, and Sweden. However, in Finland, Portugal, Greece, and Spain the association between doctors and health spending is negative. In all other countries (Austria, Belgium, Denmark, Italy, the Netherlands), the number of doctors has no impact on health care costs.

In all cases the statistical relationship found was not very robust. In addition, countries with the highest number of doctors per capita, which at the same time have experienced large increases in medical personnel (Spain, Portugal, Greece, Finland), showed a negative association with health care costs, implying that the more doctors there are, the cheaper the system. This further implies an underutilization of medical staff, at least in the formal sector. Furthermore, the weak statistical performance can be explained by the fact that the current variable picks the effect of the total number of doctors within a country, rather than what or how much they authorize.

In Austria the relationship between doctors and health spending proved to be non-significant, whereas in the cases of Belgium and Spain, there is a mixture of results that vary from a positive sign and significant t-ratio, to a negative sign and non-significance.

Health Expenditure in the EU: A Macroeconomic Perspective 189

These results contrast with some of the results in the existing literature, such as Gerdtham *et al*[42] and Saez *et al*,[49] which appear to be conclusive on the positive impact of the medical profession.

Impact of technology Technology has been proxied by pharmaceutical expenditure and the rate of growth in spending for medicines.

Pharmaceutical expenditure has produced robust positive results in all countries except in Italy and the UK where it was found to be non-significant. Due to lack of availability of data, no results have been obtained for Spain and Portugal. The value of the coefficients was in most cases quite high, at times approaching unity. Thus, the rate of growth of pharmaceutical expenditure is a significant determinant of health care expenditures in most Member States.

Hospital variables The rate of utilization of hospital services has been incorporated through the average length of stay in in-patient care and the number of beds in in-patient care. The objective was to determine whether the reduction in the average length of stay in in-patient care observed in most EU Member States (with the exception of the Netherlands and Germany) and the reduction in the total number of beds in in-patient care has had any impact on total health care costs over time. Although a reduction in the length of stay could contribute to the reduction of total costs of using the health service, this is by no means a necessary and sufficient condition. This would depend on the nature of the technology used, the intensity of bed utilization and the method of paying hospital services.

There is no clear trend emerging from the inclusion of the above hospital variables in the statistical analysis. In several cases, their impact is non-significant, implying that average length of stay and beds in in-patient care cannot explain any of the variation in health expenditures (Austria, Germany, Greece, Italy, Portugal, Spain). In four cases the relationship between the above variables and health spending was found to be positive (Finland, France, Ireland, Sweden) and one could infer from this that the net effect of reducing the length of stay or the total number of beds in in-patient care produces savings to the aggregate health budget, which may be due to a number of reasons (e.g. more efficient utilization) not captured by the model. Finally, in the cases of Belgium, Denmark, and the UK, reducing the length of stay or the total number of beds in in-patient care has contributed to the escalation in health care costs (for instance due to more intensive uti-

190 *Health Care and Cost Containment in the European Union*

lization, or more technology-intensive care over time).

Prices The pricing of health services was proxied by the relative average wage of health employees in the health sector (measured in constant 1990 prices) and by the change in the above relative average wage. The growth in average wages to the extent that it is higher than the rate of growth of health spending would contribute significantly to the rise in health care costs, hence a positive relationship was expected. This hypothesis was confirmed in Austria, Belgium, Finland, Portugal, Germany, Greece, Ireland, Italy, the UK and Spain. In most cases it was the lagged value of the price variable that was significant, confirming that price changes take at least a year to feed through the system.

Population Most econometric studies have investigated potential determinants of health spending by denominating all variables in per capita terms. In this study we seek to determine the impact of total population as well as its growth rate over time as a potential determinant of health care costs. The analysis has shown that population and its growth rate do not explain any of the variation in health care spending in four cases (Finland, France, Italy, Portugal). However, population is positively related with health spending and in fact contribute to its rising trend in five cases (Germany, Ireland, Netherlands, Sweden, UK), and is negatively related in Austria, Belgium, Denmark, Greece and Spain.

2.6 Conclusions

This chapter provided the theoretical arguments for the treatment of health care systems and the determinants of health care expenditures on an individual and intertemporal basis. It also highlighted the limitations of the empirical literature in explaining the intertemporal variation in health care expenditures and suggested a number of alternatives which were subsequently tested in each of the 14 EU Member States for a 35-year period. The analytical methodology therefore pursued a country-by-country investigation on a time-series basis.

Conclusive evidence is provided on the limited importance of GDP in explaining part of the variation in health care spending over time. While the

Health Expenditure in the EU: A Macroeconomic Perspective 191

available empirical evidence suggests that GDP is an important determinant of health spending, the present investigation concluded that its significance has been at best overrated, and in many countries fails to explain any of the variation in health spending over time. A similar result is drawn for the rate of growth of GDP. Both results question the appropriateness of GDP in (partly) explaining health spending and stress the need for an alternative macroeconomic variable, theoretically more relevant to the health care sector.

The study confirms a number of observations and arrives at a number of conclusions in relation to policy-making for cost containment in European health systems. As expected, the results vary by country, which is an effect of different organization and delivery mechanisms as well as different needs across the EU. However, some major trends have been identified.

First, technology and, in particular, pharmaceuticals, is an important cost-push factor across the EU; the consumption of medicines does not appear to have a significant impact on hospital costs across the board, although the results obtained were rather mixed.

Secondly, the reduction in the length of stay and the total number of beds in in-patient care would lead to lower total health costs *ceteris paribus* in some Member States, whereas in others the opposite result was found. The latter may be due to more intensive use of resources or more high-technology care provision.

Thirdly, with respect to the demographic structure of the EU populations, it appears that improvements in mortality rates over time have contributed significantly to health care costs in all EU Member States. On the other hand, ageing has produced mixed results which, *ceteris paribus*, point at an exaggeration of its importance over time. The impact of ageing is, however, difficult to isolate, partly because it is related to specific parts of the health budget. For instance, when combined with pharmaceutical spending, it is clearly shown that the elderly consume a high proportion of medicines. Moreover, care for the elderly may be provided by social services budgets, in which case the overall impact is unknown.

Fourthly, the cost of human resources versus the cost of technology has been evaluated with the use of average wages in the health sector. *Ceteris paribus,* average wages have exerted a significant upward pressure on health care costs in most countries, with the exception of a few. In the former, the positive contribution of wages to health care costs is associated with a rela-

Health Care and Cost Containment in the European Union

tive reduction in hospital costs, possibly indicating a cost-saving technology; in the latter, the static downward pressure of wages on health care costs is associated with a relative increase in hospital costs, indicating cost-increasing technology and the preponderance of technology over human resources.

Despite the results obtained from the above analysis, the chapter also highlighted the limits of the available data sources, particularly the OECD databank in actually conducting comparative research for a number of reasons. First, because the methodologies applied in the collection of data vary by country. Second, it is impossible to assess the impact of lifestyles (diet and habits such as alcohol consumption) due to the limitations in the lag structure of the data. Third, it appears that health care has lateral budget relationships with other parts of (public) expenditure which need to be taken into consideration. Finally, further research (both theoretical and empirical) is needed into which aspects of the macroeconomy are most suitable to explain the variations in health care spending.

References

1   OECD. *The Reform of Health Care: A Comparative Analysis of Seven OECD Countries* (OECD Health Policy Studies No. 2). Paris: OECD, 1992.

2   OECD. *The Reform of Health Care: A Review of Seventeen OECD Countries* (OECD Health Policy Studies No. 5). Paris: OECD, 1994.

3   Abel-Smith B. The escalation of health care costs: how did we get there? In: *OECD. Health Care Reform: The Will to Change*. Paris, 1996.

4   Evans RW. Health care technology and the inevitability of resource allocation and rationing decisions – part II. *Journal of the American Medical Association* 1983;249 (16).

5   Congress of the United States. *Long-Term Budgetary Pressures and Policy Options* (report to the Senate and House Committees on the Budget). Washington DC: Congressional Budget Office, March 1997.

6   Abel-Smith B. *Paying for Health Services: A Study of the Costs and Sources of Finance in Six Countries* (Public Health Paper No. 17). Geneva: World Health Organisation, 1963.

7   Abel-Smith B. *An International Study of Health Expenditure and its Relevance for Health Planning* (Public Health Paper No. 32). Geneva: World Health Organisation, 1967.

Health Expenditure in the EU: A Macroeconomic Perspective   193

8   Kanavos P, Mossialos E. *The Methodology of International Comparisons of Health Care Expenditures: Any Lessons for Health Policy?* (LSE Health Discussion Paper No. 3). London: London School of Economics and Political Science, February 1997.

9   OECD. *New Directions in Health Care Policy* (OECD Health Policy Studies No. 6). Paris: OECD, 1995.

10 OECD. *OECD Health Data.* Paris: OECD, 1996.

11 Mossialos E, Kanavos P, Abel-Smith B. Will managed care work in Europe? *PharmacoEconomics* 1997;11(4).

12 International Monetary Fund (IMF). *International Financial Statistics, 1997 Yearbook.* Washington DC: International Monetary Fund, 1997.

13 Chand SK, Jaeger A. *Ageing Populations and Public Pension Schemes* (Occasional Paper 147). Washington DC: International Monetary Fund, December 1996.

14 Orton P. Resistant organisms: a dilemma for primary care? (Editorial). *British Journal of General Practice* July 1997, pp. 415–16.

15 Gray A, Fenn P. Alzheimer's disease: the burden of the illness in England. *Health Trends* 1993;25(1):31–37.

16 Gray AM. The economic impact of Alzheimer's disease. *Review of Contemporary Pharmacotherapy* 1995;6:327–34.

17 Chisholm D, Knapp M *et al.* The mental health residential care study: predicting costs from resident characteristics. *British Journal of Psychiatry* 1997;170:37–42.

18 Freer C. Care of the elderly: old myths, *The Lancet* 1985;1(8423):268–69.

19 Kind P, Sorensen J. The costs of depression. *International Clinical Psychopharmacology* 1993;7:191–95.

20 McCrone P, Weich S. Mental health care costs: paucity of measurement. *Social Psychiatry & Epidemiology* 1993;31:70–7.

21 Torgerson D, Donaldson C et al. Private versus social opportunity cost of time: valuing time in the demand for health care. *Health Economics* 1994;3:149–55.

22 Holland WW. *European Community Atlas of Avoidable Deaths 1997.* Commission of the European Communities, Oxford University Press, 1997.

23 Kleiman E. The determinants of national outlay on health. In: Perlman M (ed). *The Economics of Health and Medical Care.* London: Macmillan, 1974.

24 Newhouse JP. Medical care expenditure: a cross-national survey. *Journal of Human Resources* 1977;12:115–25.

25 Musgrave RA. *Fiscal Systems.* New Haven: Yale University Press, 1969.

26 Musgrave RA. Excess buys and the nature of budget growth. *Journal of Public Economics* 1985;28(3).

27 Rao R. Causality between income and government expenditure: a broad international perspective. *Public Finance* 1986;41.

28 Rao R. Wagner's hypothesis in time series and cross section perspectives: evidence from real data from 115 countries. *Review of Economics and Statistics* 1987;LXIX:194–204.

29 Wagner R. Revenue structure, fiscal illusion and budgetary choice. *Public Choice* 1976:45–61.

194 *Health Care and Cost Containment in the European Union*

30 Peacock A, Wiseman G. *The Growth of Public Expenditure in the UK*. Princeton, New Jersey: Princeton University Press, 1961.

31 Grossman M. *The Demand for Health: A Theoretical and Empirical Investigation*. New York: National Bureau of Economic Research, 1972.

32 Abel-Smith B *et al. Report on the Greek Health Services*. Athens: Pharmetrica, June 1994.

33 De Miguel JM, Guillen MF. The health system in Spain. In: Field MG (ed.). *Success and Crisis in National Health Systems: A Comparative Approach*. London: Routledge, 1989.

34 Le Grand J. Inequalities in health: some international comparisons. *European Economic Review* 1987;31:182–91.

35 Le Grand J, Illsey R. The measurement of inequalities in health. In: Williams A (ed). *Economics and Health*. London: Macmillan, 1987.

36 Benzeval M, Judge K, Whitehead M. *Tackling Inequalities in Health: An Agenda for Action*. London: Kings Fund, 1995.

37 Feinstein J. The relationship between socio-economic status and health: a review of the literature. *Milbank Quarterly* 1993;71:279–321.

38 Atkinson AB. Seeking to explain the distribution of income. In: Hills J. (ed). *New Inequalities: The Changing Distribution of Income and Wealth in the United Kingdom*. Cambridge: Cambridge University Press, 1996.

39 Gerdtham U-G, Joensson B. Factors affecting health spending: a cross-country econometric analyses. In: *New Directions in Health Policy* (OECD Health Policy Studies No. 7). Paris: OECD, 1995.

40 Maxwell RJ. *Health and Wealth: An International Study of Health Spending*. Lexington: Lexington Books, 1981.

41 Leu R. The public–private mix and international health care costs. In: Culyer A, Joensson B (eds). *The Public–Private Mix of Health Services*. Oxford: Blackwell, 1986.

42 Gerdtham U-G, et al. *Econometric Analysis of Health Care Expenditures: A Cross-section Study of the OECD Countries*. Linkoping: Center for Medical Technology, University of Linkoping, 1988.

43 Parkin D, McGuire A, Yul B. Aggregate health care expenditures and national income: is health care a luxury good? *Journal of Health Economics* 1987;6:109–7.

44 Newhouse JP. Cross national differences in health spending: what do they mean? *Journal of Health Economics* (editorial) 1987;6:159–62.

45 Gerdtham U-G. *Essays on International Comparisons of Health Care Expenditure, Linkoeping Studies in Arts & Science No. 66*. Linkoeping: TEMA, 1991, ch. 2,3 and 4.

46 McGuire A, Parkin D, Hughes D, Gerard K. Econometric analyses of national health expenditures: can positive economics help to answer normative questions? *Health Economics* 1993;2:113–16.

47 Hitiris T, Posnett J. The determinants and effects of health expenditure in developed countries. *Journal of Health Economics* 1992;11:173–81.

48 Murillo C, Piatecki C, Saez M. Health care expenditure and income in Europe. *Health Economics* 1993;2:127–38.

49 Saez M, Murillo C. Shared 'features' in prices: income and price elasticities for health

Health Expenditure in the EU: A Macroeconomic Perspective   195

care expenditures *Health Economics* 1994;3;267–79.

50 Dunlop DW, Martins JM (eds). *An International Assessment of Health Care Financing: Lessons for Developing Countries* (EDI Seminar Series). Washington DC: The World Bank, 1995.

51 Massell B, Heyer J. Household expenditure in Nairobi: a statistical analysis of consumer behaviour. *Economic Development and Cultural Change* 1969;12(1).

52 Griffin C. *Health Sector Financing in Asia: Comparative Study of Cost and Financing.* Washington DC: World Bank, 1992.

53 Musgrove P. Family health spending in Latin America. *Journal of Health Economics* 1983;2:245–57.

54 Musgrove P. The economic crisis and its impact on health and health care in Latin America and the Caribbean. *International Journal of Health Services* 1987;17(3):411–41.

55 Gerdtham U-G, Joensson B. Conversion factor instability in international comparisons of health care expenditure. *Journal of Health Economics* 1991;10:227–34.

56 Gerdtham U-G, Joensson B. Price and quantity in international comparisons of health care expenditure. *Applied Economics* 1991;23:1519–28.

57 Murthy VNR. Conversion factor instability in international comparisons of health care expenditure: some econometric comments. *Journal of Health Economics* 1992;11:183–87.

58 Gerdtham U-G, Joensson B. International comparisons of health care expenditure – conversion factor instability, heteroscedasticity, outliers and robust estimators. *Journal of Health Economics* 1992;11:189–97.

59 Kravis I, Heston A, Summers R. Real GDP per capita for more than 100 countries. *Economic Journal* 1978;88:215–42.

60 Milne R, Molana H. On the effect of relative price on demand for health care: EC evidence. *Applied Economics* 1991;23:1221–26.

61 Karatzas G. On the effect of relative price on demand for health care – the EEC evidence: a comment. *Applied Economics* 1992;24:1251–53.

62 Kanavos P, McKee M. Macroeconomic and health challenges in European health systems. In: Saltman R, Figueras J (eds). *Critical Challenges for European Health Systems.* Buckingham: Open University Press, forthcoming.

63 Commission of the European Communities. *The Application of the Council Directive on the Compilation of Gross National Product at Market Prices* (report from the Commission to the Council and the European Parliament, COM(96) 124 final). Brussels, 27 March 1996.

64 OECD. *OECD Health Systems: The Socio-Economic Environment – Statistical References: Volume II* (Health Policy Studies No. 3). Paris: OECD, 1993.

65 Abel-Smith B. *How to Contain Health Care Costs: An International Dilemma.* 1994 Stamp Memorial Lecture, University of London, 1994.

66 Altman SH, Blendon RJ (eds). *Medical Technology: The Culprit behind Health Care Costs?* Washington DC: Government Printing Office, 1979.

67 Moloney TW, Rogers DE. Medical technology: a different view of the contentious

196 *Health Care and Cost Containment in the European Union*

debate over costs. *The New England Journal of Medicine* 1979;301:1413–19.

68 Klarman HE, Rice DP, Cooper BS. Accounting for the rise in selected medical care expenditures: 1929–1969. *American Journal of Public Health* 1970;60:1023–39.

69 Freeland M, Schendler C. National health expenditure growth in the 1980s: an ageing population, new technologies and increasing competition. *Health Care Financing Review* 1983;3:1–58.

70 Scitovsky A. Changes in the cost of treatment of selected illnesses, 1971–1981. *Medical Care* 1985;23:1345–57.

71 Showstack JA, Schroeder SA. Use of medical technologies 1972–77: a study of 10 inpatient diagnoses. *The New England Journal of Medicine* 1982;306:706–12.

72 Busse R, Schwartz FW. Hospital utilisation per year of life is not increasing with higher life expectancy – results from a 7 year cohort study in Germany (submitted to the *British Medical Journal*, July 1997).

73 Fuchs V. Though much is taken. *The Milbank Quarterly* 1984;62.

74 Scitovsky AA. Medical care in the last twelve months of life. *The Milbank Quarterly* 1988;66.

75 Harrison A, Dixon J, New B, Judge K. Funding the NHS: can the NHS cope in future? *British Medical Journal* 1997;314:139–42.

76 Friers J. Aging, natural death, and the compression of morbidity. *New England Journal of Medicine* 1980;303:130–36.

77 Oslansky SJ, Carnes BA, Cassell C. In search of Methusselah; estimating the upper limits of human longevity. *Science* 1990;250:634–40.

78 Manton KG, Tolley DH. Rectangularisation of the survival curve: implications of an ill-posed question. *Journal of Ageing and Health* 1991;3:172–93.

79 Himes C, Preston S, Conrad G. A relational model of mortality at older ages in low mortality countries. *Population Studies* 1994;48:269–91.

80 Preston SH. *Older Male Mortality and Cigarette Smoking.* Berkeley Institute of International Studies, 1970.

81 Sandier S. *Le vieillissement de la population en Europe et le cout des soins medicaux.* Paris: CREDES, 1987.

82 Costain D, Wolfson G. Don't blame the elderly. *Times Health Summary* October 1994, p. 4, quoted by Abel-Smith, Stamp Memorial Lecture, 1994.

3 Is there convergence in the health expenditures of the EU Member States?

ADELINA COMAS-HERRERA*

3.1 Introduction

Since the end of the 1970s most European countries have implemented important health care reforms, mainly aimed at containing their public health expenditure. As pointed out by Abel-Smith *et al.*,[1] there has been considerable convergence in the policies adopted.

This chapter examines whether the fact that European countries are tending to make their health systems more similar, and that they have all faced a similar economic reality (especially the oil crisis, the crisis at the beginning of the 1990s, and now the requirements of the Maastricht treaty and rising unemployment), is having an effect on the proportion of income that each country devotes to public health expenditures. In particular, it raises the question as to whether these factors bring about convergence in this respect, towards a similar proportion of GDP spent on health. Or whether the same type of reforms and circumstances are having different effects on expenditure, perhaps as a consequence of the different characteristics of the original health systems.

The chapter concentrates on public health expenditures as this is where most cost containment measures have been targeted. It begins by examining the arguments for convergence in section 3.2, (internal and external factors)

---

* I would like to thank Julian Le Grand and Siem J Koopman for guidance and supervision, Begoña Alvarez and Geoff Shuetrim for their help with computer programming and Elias Mossialos, Jeremy Kendall, Irini Moustaki, Giovanni Fattore and Howard Glennerster for their comments on various stages of this chapter. Any errors remain the responsibility of the author alone.

198   *Health Care and Cost Containment in the European Union*

and continues with the arguments against in section 3.3. In section 3.4 there is an explanation of the methodological approach taken; in section 3.5 information about the data utilized, in section 3.6 the results are presented and discussed; in section 3.7 the conclusions are presented, and finally there is a technical appendix.

3.2 Arguments in favour of convergence

Several authors have argued that there is convergence in health expenditures[2,3] in European health systems[4] and in welfare systems,[5] in a context of European integration and more general economic convergence. In discussing these arguments, it is useful to distinguish between the internal factors that might bring countries to similar levels of public health expenditure through their own policies; and the external factors (those driven by factors that are not controllable by the governments of each individual country) such as the international situation, the interaction between countries, technology and demographic trends.

3.2.1 Internal factors leading to convergence

3.2.1.1 Similar objectives The first argument for convergence would be that EU countries broadly share similar objectives for their health systems:[6,7] adequacy and equity in access to some minimum of health care for all citizens; macro-economic efficiency (the costs of health care should not exceed an acceptable share of national resources); and micro-economic efficiency (the mix of services chosen should secure maximum health gains and consumer satisfaction at minimum cost). At present we observe both that countries with higher levels of expenditures are trying to contain their costs, and that the Southern countries with traditionally lower levels of expenditures are approaching the general level of expenditures.[8] We could expect these two opposite trends to tend towards some convergence.

In fact, the OECD review of 17 countries[7] claims that since most countries have achieved nearly universal health coverage, their central concern is now macro-economic efficiency, or more specifically, the containment of costs.

Is there Convergence in the Health Expenditures of the EU Member States? 199

3.2.1.2 *Reforms tending to make health systems less diverse* When describing the reforms taking place recently in Europe, most authors emphasize the current trend of convergence in terms of the way that countries are reforming their public health systems. There seems to be a tendency to move towards a public contract model[1] – also called planned markets[9] or quasi-markets[10] – with fixed budgets for all expenditure, or for large parts of it. This convergence in the organization of public health systems could be pictured as a process in which countries with more 'market-like' systems have been introducing budgets, while countries with an NHS type of system have been moving to a quasi-markets approach.

It is still too early to tell whether the trend towards similar forms of organization also leads to similar levels of expenditures, because the effect of the reforms in each country is not yet clear (and some countries have not yet completed the implementation of approved reforms). However, as discussed below, we certainly observe a considerable consensus among countries in many aspects of the organization of a health system.

As pointed out by Abel-Smith *et al.*,[1] the establishment of budgets for health care has been shown to be the most effective means of containing costs. Budgets also seem to be the most extended cost-containment device: they are inherent to integrated and tax-based systems (and maintained when market-oriented reforms are introduced), and are increasingly adopted by insurance-based countries. We might expect their proliferation to add momentum towards convergence.

There are other cost-containment measures that have also been undertaken in most European countries. These include the development of alternatives to hospital care; cost-sharing in order to try to reduce demand; attempts to influence the authorizing behaviour of doctors (in referring and prescribing) and dentists by changing the method of payment; attempts to control expensive medical equipment; and controls on the prices or profits of the pharmaceutical industry.[4] Again, it might be expected that these similar measures should lead to some convergence in expenditures.

3.2.1.3 *Welfare convergence* Some of the generic literature on welfare has also pointed to a process of convergence in welfare systems. For example, Taylor-Gooby[5] argues that we can observe some convergence in both the forms of organization and financing, and in the expenditures level, although substantial differences still remain because of adaptation difficulties. He argues that the main converging forces would reflect the lowest funded sys-

200 Health Care and Cost Containment in the European Union

tems' continued development. In the financing level, he points out how social insurance based systems are now also being funded by taxation, along with a tendency towards decentralization.

3.2.2 External pressures

3.2.2.1 Similar economic benchmark and pressures (Maastricht Treaty)
The actual economic benchmark is very similar for most European countries: recent economic recessions have affected almost all to a greater or lesser extent; Europe as a whole is seeing its competitiveness threatened by the lower costs of production in many non-European countries; and, of course, progress in the process of European integration – especially the requirements in order to enter EMU – have introduced pressure towards similar economic policies.

The generosity (and expensiveness) of the European welfare states is seen as a threat to employment, particularly to unskilled workers. This is because, in a context of ever more globalized economies, employers have started looking elsewhere for cheaper labour. As Esping-Andersen points out,[11] we may be facing a difficult trade-off between unemployment and welfare provision.

Furthermore, the Maastricht Treaty requirements, designed to ensure budgetary discipline (deficits smaller than 3 per cent of GDP, and the goal of having government debt no greater than 60 per cent of GDP) are of obvious relevance for public expenditures. As governments start facing restrictions in their ability to stretch expenditure further than income, they may be forced to take unpopular decisions that they would otherwise try to postpone repeatedly for electoral reasons. This may not be entirely involuntary as far as those governments are concerned. They may feel that they can 'pass the buck' for the difficult decisions by putting blame on Europe. In some countries, the ability to join the EMU may even be presented as a matter of national pride.

There is also a theoretical argument (probably behind the selection of the Maastricht criteria) to explain why efforts to balance the budget are becoming so important. As many authors have pointed out, the tolerance of budget deficits observed since the postwar period was very much influenced by the predominance of Keynesian macroeconomic models, which have now been discredited (see for example, Tyrie).[12]

This change of attitude towards debt and economic policy, together

Is there Convergence in the Health Expenditures of the EU Member States? 201

with the high levels of unemployment and ageing (and aggravated by difficulties in adapting the welfare state to a more gloomy economic environment from the one in which it was created) have introduced great pressure towards control public expenditure, making the actual growth rates of health care expenditures (at a higher rate than GDP) unlikely to be sustainable in many countries. This pressure is very likely to result in changes in the institutions to make them more controllable. And the fact that this is happening all over Europe gives yet another argument in favour of convergence.

3.2.2.2 Migration of policies Another factor that should not be underestimated is the fact that countries seem to be observing the reforms undertaken by others very carefully, as well as investigating the huge amounts of literature on different health care reforms and their consequences. Some countries seem to try to learn from the experience of others. For example, the 1991 reforms of the British NHS have been followed closely by health policy experts from many countries. As Fattore points out in Chapter 18, those reforms are considered as large social experiments that have an enormous influence on many other European countries whose reforms are still under political discussion or have not yet been implemented.

We should also take into account, as Defever highlights,[13] the influence of international agencies such as the World Bank, the WHO, the OECD, and the European Commission, by actively promoting 'health-policy exportation' and acting as a discussion forum.

This is an especially important factor for the 'latecomers' (the countries that started developing their health systems later), which are using the experiences of other countries as reference for their own reforms.

3.2.2.3 Technology Schwartz[14] argued that health care expenditures are mainly driven by population growth, rising real input prices, and increased intensity of services (caused mainly by technological innovation and its diffusion); and that most cost-containment strategies are likely to have only a short-term impact on expenditures. As population growth and input prices are not controllable, Schwartz claims that the essence of cost containment is based on the limitation of the introduction and diffusion of beneficial technology.

Technology is becoming more and more international and its diffusion has become extremely fast. Doctors are rapidly becoming aware of the innovations produced in other countries and naturally want to introduce them in

202　*Health Care and Cost Containment in the European Union*

their own practices. Also, the health technology assessment initiatives at a European level are very likely to make an important contribution to a standardization of health technology. Since technology is such an important determinant of the level of expenditures, we would expect its speed of diffusion and the cooperation in assessment to be a converging drive.

3.3 Arguments against convergence

3.3.1 Differences in the financing and organization of health systems

The main argument against convergence would be the extent to which the original health systems differed in all aspects of their organization (from financing to delivery) before the reforms started, and how these differences profoundly affect the possibility of changes or, for example, can make the same type of reform have different effects in different countries. This means that, despite all the similar developments mentioned above, we may find that expenditures continue to be divergent. This perspective is expressed most clearly by Esping-Andersen.[11] He argues that institutional legacies, inherited system characteristics, and the interests that these cultivate strongly influence the adaptability of welfare states.

In an analysis of the relationship between health expenditures and the main macroeconomic indicators in the United States, Getzen[2] finds that there is an important lag in the adaptation of health expenditures to the macroeconomic environment. He argues that this lag would be caused by the lack of adaptability of the health system due to its institutional complexity.

There is more evidence of the importance of institutional factors in the health care field. Schwartz *et al.*,[15] in a study of the experience of different countries in fixing health budgets, conclude that insurance-based systems find more difficulties in setting budget limits and actually holding the different agents to them. They also conclude that the costs of the central European health systems have proved to be very difficult to contain, while in countries where services are paid out of taxation, political pressures allow for much bigger spending control, as is discussed below. One of the explanations for the different degrees of success that they point to, is the complexity of Central European health systems, with the great number of social partners involved and the wide dispersion of responsibilities.

A clear example of a particularly difficult-to-reform system because of its institutional legacy is France, where the principle of 'never to revoke a right previously granted'[16] is deeply embedded and 'virtually inviolate'. The attempts of the government to move to a universal health scheme instead of the present system of separated funds have been strongly contested, particularly as trade unions have seen it as an attempt to curtail their power. Germany instead, seems to find change a bit easier using its 'consensual' tradition. The United Kingdom has undergone very radical changes with surprising ease, despite the resistance from the medical profession and from the opposition. Klein[17] has argued that this may ultimately reflect the particular character of the UK constitution, in which an extremely powerful central state can push through reforms if it has the political will to do so.

3.3.2 Different roles of the public sector

Not all European countries are following the same health strategies. One of the fundamental differences is the role of the private and the public sector, and where the boundary is drawn between them. In some countries the private sector plays a basically complementary role, while in other countries its role is more as a substitute. Among the 'latecomers', for example, while some countries are actively following the developments of successful countries in cost containment, other countries are following new and different strategies. Portugal for example, instead of investing in the development of a public NHS system in the way Spain is doing, is actively encouraging the growth of the private sector. The option of opting out of the public health system when covered by private insurance is being considered by Portugal, and has been debated in Italy, although it was not finally implemented.

3.3.3 'Expenditure clubs'

Simple observation of public health expenditures as a percentage of GDP in most EU countries suggests that in 1994 we find two clear levels of expenditures depending on how the health systems are financed. In Figure 3.1 overleaf, we can observe:

- a group with a higher level of expenditures that coincides strongly with

Figure 3.1 Public health expenditure as a percentage of GDP in EU countries, 1994

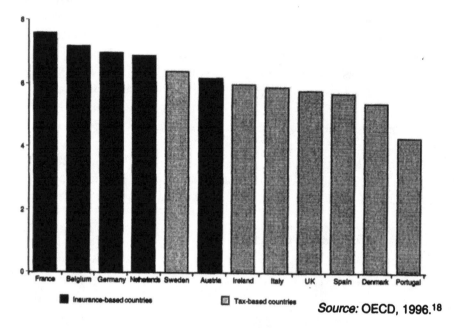

Source: OECD, 1996.[18]

the countries with a predominantly insurance-based system (with the exception of Austria that has relatively low share of public health expenditure); and

- a group with a lower level of expenditures coinciding with the countries with tax-based systems and where health expenditures have to compete with all the other expenditures financed through taxation (Figure 3.1).

The existence of these groupings appears inconsistent with the hypothesis of public health expenditures converging over time to a similar percentage of GDP. But the fact that the countries naturally appear to group on this basis according to a relevant characteristic of health systems, suggests that it may be enlightening to test whether this in fact represents convergence at two different levels as a consequence of the different forms of financing the health systems.

In conclusion, despite the general view of convergence in the various types of reforms, there are substantial aspects of the health systems that remain remarkably different and that are unlikely to change quickly. The

Is there Convergence in the Health Expenditures of the EU Member States?

way in which the level of expenditures is determined is very complex, especially in the less integrated health systems which involve many partners. Also, it seems to be too early to determine whether reforms that are similar in principle and that have common aims will have a similar effect in the levels of expenditures, and, in case they do have an effect, whether it will be stronger in the countries with the highest levels of expenditures so that it produces convergence.

3.4 Methodological approach to testing for convergence

The question therefore arises: has there been convergence over time or not? This is not easy to answer. One approach is simply to observe the percentages of GDP and their changes over time (see Figure 3.2). However, as is apparent from the figure, it is difficult to draw any sensible conclusion from this approach.

Another approach would be to look at the coefficient of variation (or

Figure 3.2 Public health expenditure as a percentage of GDP in EU countries, 1960–92

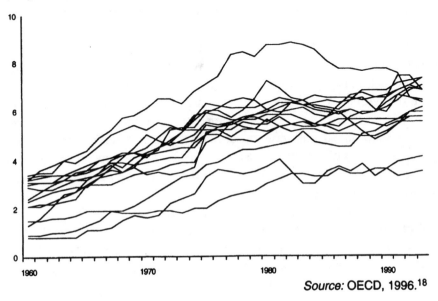

Source: OECD, 1996.[18]

206 *Health Care and Cost Containment in the European Union*

some other measure of dispersion) and see, as in Leidl,[3] if there is a decrease in dispersion. However, there are a number of difficulties with the coefficient of variation approach.

The coefficient of variation can be affected by shocks in particular countries that do not respond to their general trends. If for example, each country had a shock (or an outlier value) in a different year but then returned to the previous trend, a measure of convergence based on the coefficient of variation would be taking into account those shocks as affecting the overall degree of convergence or divergence.

The alternative approach proposed here is to use a convergence test based in structural time series analysis. This type of analysis is very useful to find the 'underlying trend' of the time series data. The trend can be 'smoothed' by separating its 'true' components (the level and the slope) from its irregular component. This provides a much better picture of where the series 'is going' and how it is 'getting there', and makes any test based on the smoothed (or estimated) trends much more robust.

3.4.1 A convergence test

What we want to test in the actual context of reforms is whether, as a consequence of all the factors mentioned above, countries are tending to spend the same or a similar proportion of their GDP in public health expenditures. That is, we test if all the series are tending to meet in one point.

The basic idea of the test we are going to use consists in determining whether the realizations we observe in two different variables (for two different countries) are statistically different or not. (The greater the number of countries with the same level of expenditures, the closer we are to seeing all countries meeting in one point.) In order to test whether the levels of two countries are statistically different or not, we estimate confidence intervals around the trend of the time series. Then, each time two countries intersect in their confidence intervals, we can say that they have a statistically non-different level of expenditure.

We define a *convergence indicator*, C_t (see the appendix for the formal definition). C_t is, for every year, the number of actual intersections, divided by the number of all possible intersections. C_t will therefore have a value of 1 if we find *total convergence* (the situation in which all the series for all the countries will share their confidence intervals) and 0 when we find *total* *divergence. C_t* taking the value 1 would mean that we can say statistically that all countries spend the same proportion of their GDP in health.

We will also define a *converging process* as that in which C_t increases over time (i.e. has a positive slope), and as a *diverging process*, one in which C_t decreases over time (i.e. has a negative slope). Since we are interested in finding whether there has been convergence in recent years, our results will be given as the evolution of C_t over time. We will test whether C_t has a significant slope, and whether it is positive or negative.

3.4.2 Structural time series models

In order to obtain the confidence intervals we have estimated the trend for each series using structural time series models. These consist of regression models in which the explanatory variables are functions of time and the parameters are time-varying. These models, instead of intending to represent the underlying data generation process, aim to present the 'stylized facts' of a series. The basic way the models work is by decomposing the time series into components such as the trend, seasonality, cycles, and an irregular component, and to model them in the way that captures best the evolution of a particular variable. A clear explanation of structural time series models and some of their applications is given in Harvey and Koopman [19] and there is a short summary of the specific models used for this chapter in the appendix.

In the case of health expenditures, the annual data utilized has, as relevant components, only a trend and an irregular component, the seasonality and cyclical components are not significant. This makes the analysis very straightforward.

The estimation of the trend, then, is done by modelling its subcomponents, the level and the slope. We then use the Root Mean Square Errors (RMSE) obtained from this estimation to calculate our confidence intervals. This analysis has been done using the package developed by Koopman *et al.*, STAMP 5.0.,[20] and we have worked with a 0.9986 probability (with this probability, all the values that fall within the same confidence interval are statistically non-different).

Once we have obtained an interval for each country and year, the next step is to check, for every year, how many intersections occur. We have done that with a specially constructed programme. With this programme we

208 *Health Care and Cost Containment in the European Union*

obtain a matrix with a 1 whenever there is an intersection between two countries and 0 otherwise, for every year. Adding up the number of 1s, we obtain the number of intersections for every year; this we normalize to obtain the convergence indicator, C_t. As a result we obtain a time series for C_t that, in the case of having a positive slope would mean that we are looking at a converging process. In case of finding a negative slope, then it would be a diverging process.

The final step, then, is to analyse the time series C_t to determine whether it has a positive or a negative slope. Again, we will estimate a structural time series model for C_t, and this will tell us whether there is a significative slope, and whether it is positive or negative (that is to say, whether we have a *converging* or a *diverging process*).

3.4.3 Propositions tested

First, we test whether there is convergence among all countries, and afterwards whether there is convergence among the insurance-based countries and among the predominantly tax-based countries. The mainly insurance-based group includes Belgium, France, Germany, the Netherlands and Austria. The tax-based group includes Denmark, Ireland, Sweden, the United Kingdom, Italy, Portugal and Spain.

3.5 The data

The data utilized are public health expenditures as a percentage of GDP for 12 European Community countries. They have been obtained from the OECD Health Database 1996,[18] and cover the period from 1960 to 1994.

We have chosen to work with public health expenditures as a percentage of GDP for two reasons: the first is that this avoids all the problems that derive from converting the data to a common unit. As Kanavos and Mossialos explain, the results of most comparative health expenditure studies seem to be strongly influenced by the conversion instruments utilized.[21] The second reason is that this involves an implicit comparison between the level of GDP and the level of public health expenditures which, in the future, may be useful to derive some theoretical conclusions about the demand for health at a macroeconomic level.

Is there Convergence in the Health Expenditures of the EU Member States?

We have not been able to include Finland, Luxembourg or Greece. There are problems with the validity and statistical behaviour of the Greek data that make the estimations unreliable. Luxembourg has not been included because the data was only available from 1975 and this makes the sample too small to be able to make a good estimation of its trend. There have been problems in obtaining a good estimation of the Finnish trend due to the contrast between a very stable trend during most years, and a sharp change at the end of the sample (due to changes in the GDP in these last years).

3.6 Results and discussion

3.6.1 Analysis of the results

3.6.1.1 For all countries The test does not give evidence of convergence among all the countries. C_t has an average value of 0.28, an initial value of 0.36 in 1960, and a final value of 0.36 in 1994 (see Figure 3.3 for a plot of the time series). This seems to suggest that it has a positive slope, but the results of the estimation of the trend show that, although there is a small

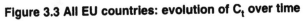

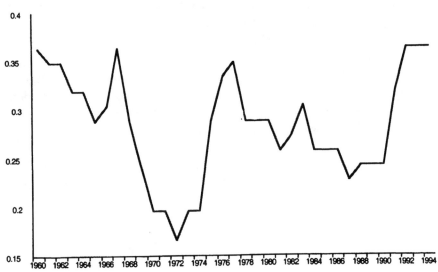

Figure 3.3 All EU countries: evolution of C_t over time

Figure 3.4 Tax-based EU countries: evolution of C_t over time

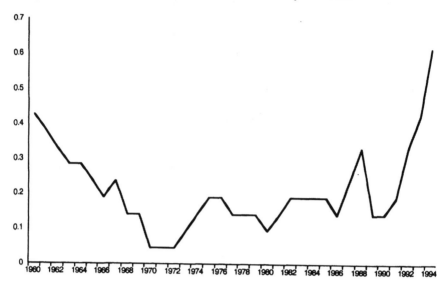

positive slope, it is not significant.

The best estimate of the trend has been obtained by transforming C_t into differences of its logarithm. Since we are estimating the differentiated series, a significant positive level would give evidence of a significant slope in the original series. The results though, give a coefficient for the level of 0.0472 (t-value = 1.0453), and a coefficient for the slope of 0.0029 (t-value = 1.2161). The estimated hyperparameters for the level and the slope are 0, which also means that the level and the slope have no explanatory value (see the appendix).

In conclusion, although C_t has a small positive trend it is not significant. Thus we cannot conclude that there is convergence among all countries. So, despite all the arguments that would suggest general convergence, the test does not show empirical evidence of it.

3.6.1.2 For the tax-based countries There is clear evidence of convergence within this group of countries (see Figure 3.4). C_t has an average value of

---

* This intervention consists of a dummy variable that takes the values 1,2,3,... starting in the period after 1990. It is also called a 'staircase' intervention.[22]

Is there Convergence in the Health Expenditures of the EU Member States? 211

Figure 3.5 Insurance-based EU countries: evolution of C_t over time

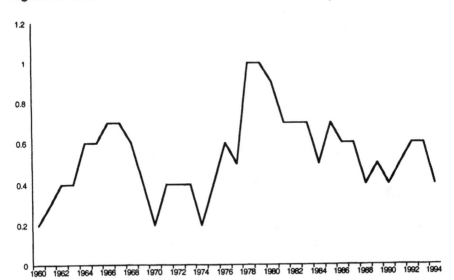

0.21, an initial value of 0.43 in 1960, and a final value of 0.62 in 1994. Also, C_t has a significant positive slope for the overall series, and, furthermore, there is evidence of a structural change from 1990 in the form of an important increase in the slope.

The best estimation of the trend has been obtained estimating the original values with an 'intervention'* in the slope for 1990. The coefficient for the level is 0.5897 (t-value = 19.112), the coefficient for the slope is 0.1342 (t-value = 4.0221), and the coefficient for the intervention variable is 0.1434 (t-value = 3.2713). So both the level and the slope are positive and significant, and there has been a structural break in the evolution of the trend in 1990, in the form of an increase in the slope.

Thus, we can say that there is strong evidence of convergence among the tax-based group of countries, especially from 1990.

3.6.1.3 For the insurance-based countries The results for the insurance-based group (Figure 3.5) are less clear. Because we are dealing with a small group of countries, a change in trend of only one of them produces a huge impact in the level of convergence in the whole group. C_t has an average value of 0.54, an initial value of 0.2 in 1960, and a final value of 0.4 in 1994.

The best estimation of C_t has been obtained by transforming it into dif-

212 *Health Care and Cost Containment in the European Union*

ferences of its logarithm. The estimated level is -0.0799 (t-value = 0.6803), and the estimated slope is -0061 (t-value = -0.9934). So there is a negative slope, but it is not significant, which means that this group of countries is neither converging nor diverging.

3.6.2 Possible explanations It is interesting to speculate as to the possible factors that could help explain the evidence presented. We will structure the possible explanations in two parts. First of all, we will concentrate on why we do not find convergence amongst all countries. Then we will try to find an explanation as to why countries with a tax-based system show a strong converging behaviour while countries with an insurance-based system, if anything, tend to diverge.

3.6.2.1 Non-convergence among all EU countries Here, the arguments of section 3.3 against convergence must be considered. In particular, we could interpret the evidence as consistent with differential impacts of what Esping-Andersen (1996) refers to as 'institutional legacies'. Health systems are very complex, so we would expect that they take long to adapt. Also, the process from approval to complete implementation of a reform is long, and, although some reforms are widely discussed in international fora, they have not yet been implemented.

3.6.2.2 Convergence among tax-based EU countries Tax-based countries have converged very strongly since 1990. They seem to have been able to respond more quickly to the economic environment and to tolerate reforms more easily. One very important cost-containment instrument available to these countries is tax-resistance. Mossialos, in his analysis of the Eurobarometer/LSE health survey[23] remarks that public opinion is divided on whether there should be more public spending on health, but finds that the majority of those favouring more spending are opposed to raising taxes or health insurance contributions and would like governments to spend less in other sectors.

This resistance is likely to be more acute in tax-based systems. Seeing a big chunk of one's income 'disappearing' into the public purse (as in tax-based countries) is more likely to create public hostility than knowing specifically what part of it is going to finance health as in insurance-based countries. The fact that tax-based systems show lower levels of expenditures could be the result of a failure from their governments to reproduce the public preferences in the allocation of resources between different sectors. While in insurance-based systems the preference for higher spending in health would be easier to translate in higher insurance contributions.

In addition, the 'command-and-control' tradition of originally highly integrated systems is playing an important role in the ability to implement and hold budgets, or any other type of reform. It has proved easier to move from a highly centralized and hierarchical system to a new structure giving more autonomy to all the layers than to try to reverse decision rights previously acquired.

3.6.2.3 Non-convergence among insurance-based systems It does appear that similar types of reforms may have different effects in different countries when these countries finance health care through insurance. While some of the five countries seem to accept reforms and change, others appear to find extremely serious difficulties of implementation. As argued above, in insurance-based systems the move towards a more centrally controlled system involves some participants losing rights and discretion previously enjoyed. In Germany, for example, expenditure growth has been comparatively slow in recent years, probably because the reunification effort has helped creating a consensus for the necessity of the application of budgets. In a completely different situation, we find that in France all reforming efforts have been fiercely contested, and public health expenditures have kept growing.

3.7 Conclusion

European public health care expenditures have not converged, neither have they diverged from 1960 to 1994. However, we have found evidence of an important convergence movement since 1990 for countries with a tax-based system, unlike the countries with an insurance-based model.

This can be interpreted as suggesting that, for tax-based countries the same type of reforms have had a similar effect, while in insurance-based countries, the success of cost containment measures has been less uniform; confirming the findings of Schwartz *et al.*[15] The relative success of the former could be at least in part linked to tax resistance effects and the impact of competition for a variety of other demands on total public expenditure. Within insurance-based countries, the disparate outcomes may, we specu-

214   *Health Care and Cost Containment in the European Union*

late, be linked to the fact that institutional legacies have a marked impact on countries' ability to push through reforms in each case. Overall, much of the non-convergence of public health expenditures in the European Union seems to be mostly explained by the fact that more fragmented and 'interests-conflicting' institutions are taking longer to adapt.

Further research could be done in the direction of testing the convergence hypotheses for total expenditures in health as a percentage of GDP because – especially in insurance-based systems – the classification of private/public may not be that clear (and the complementarity or substitution relationship between the two types of expenditures seems to change from country to country). It will be very interesting to test for convergence again in some years, when the reforms will be further on the road of completion, and to try further possibilities of the methodology used here.

References

1   Abel-Smith B, Figueras J, Holland W, McKee M, Mossialos E. *Choices in Health Policy: An Agenda for the European Union.* Dartmouth, 1995.

2   Getzen T. *Health Economics: Fundamentals and Flows of Funds.* Wiley, 1997.

3   Leidl R. European integration, economic growth and health care expenditure. In: Leidl R (ed). *Health Care and its Financing in the Single European Market.* Amsterdam: IOS Press, 1997.

4   Abel-Smith B, Mossialos E. Cost containment and health care reform. A study of the European Union. *Health Policy* 1994;28(2):89–134.

5   Taylor-Gooby P. The response of government: fragile convergence? In: George V, Taylor-Gooby P. *Squaring the Welfare Circle, European Welfare Policy.* Macmillan, 1996.

6   OECD. The reform of health care: a comparative analysis of seven OECD countries, *Health Policy Studies No.2.* Paris: OECD, 1992.

7   OECD. The reform of health care: a comparative analysis of seventeen OECD countries, *Health Policy Studies No.5.* Paris: OECD, 1994.

8   WHO. *European Health Care Reforms. Analysis of Current Strategies.* Copenhagen: WHO, Regional Office for Europe, 1996.

9   Saltman RB. Thinking about planned markets and fixed budgets. In: Schwartz FW, Glennerster H, Saltman RB, Busse R (eds.) *Fixing Health Budgets, Experience from Europe and North America.* Wiley, 1996.

10   Le Grand J and Bartlett. *Quasi-Markets and Social Policy.* London: Macmillan, 1993.

11   Esping-Andersen G. *Welfare State in Transition: National Adaptations in Global Economies.* SAGE, 1996.

Is there Convergence in the Health Expenditures of the EU Member States? 215

12 Tyrie A. *The Prospects for Public Spending.* London: Social Market Foundation, 1996.

13 Defever M. Health care reforms: the unfinished agenda. *Health Policy* 1995;34:1–7.

14 Schwartz WB. The inevitable failure of current cost-containment strategies. Why they can provide only temporary relief. *The Journal of the American Medical Association* 1987;257(2):220–24.

15 Schwartz FW, Glennerster H, Saltman RB, Busse R (eds.) *Fixing Health Budgets, Experience from Europe and North America.* Wiley, 1996.

16 Fielding JE, Lancry PJ. Lessons from France – 'vive la différence'. *The Journal of the American Medical Association* 11 August 1993;270(6):748–56.

17 Klein R. Big bang health care reform – does it work? The case of Britain's 1991 National Health Service reforms. *The Milbank Quarterly* 1995;73:(3):299–337.

18 OECD. *Health Data Base.* Paris: OECD, 1996.

19 Harvey AC, Koopman SJ. Structural time series models in medicine. *Statistical Methods in Medical Research* 1996;5:23–49.

20 Koopman SJ, Harvey AC, Doornik JA, Shephard N. *STAMP 5.0 Structural Time Series Analyser, Modeller and Predictor.* London: Chapman and Hall, 1995.

21 Kanavos P, Mossialos E. *The Methodology of International Comparisons of Health Care Expenditures: Any Lessons for Health Policy?* Discussion Paper No.3, LSE Health, 1996.

22 Koopman SJ, Harvey AC, Doornik JA, Shephard N. *STAMP 5.0 Structural Time Series Analyser, Modeller and Predictor, Tutorial Guide.* London: Chapman and Hall, 1995.

23 Mossialos E. Citizens' views on health care systems in the 15 Member States of the European Union. *Health Economics* 1997;6(1):109–16.

216 *Health Care and Cost Containment in the European Union*

Appendix

Structural time series models

Structural time series models have been used for a variety of problems in economics and other areas. This class of models consists of regression models in which the explanatory variables are functions of time and the parameters are time-varying.

The general model is

$$y_t = \mu_t + \epsilon_t \quad (1)$$

where y_t is the variable of interest (in this case, public health care expenditures), μ_t is the underlying trend, and ϵ_t is the disturbance term which is normal independent distributed, with zero mean and variance σ_ϵ^2.

Determination of the trend:

The special case of a deterministic trend is given by

$$\mu_t = \alpha + \beta t \quad (2)$$

where we define α as the constant (or level), β as the slope of the trend and t is time.

We can allow the trend to be stochastic by writing (2) as

$$\mu_t = \mu_{t-1} + \beta_t + \eta_t \quad (3)$$

with $\mu_0 = \alpha$, and where η_t allows the level to change over time. The disturbance η_t is normal independent distributed with mean 0 and variance σ_η^2.

Furthermore, the slope, β_t can also be allowed to vary over time:

$$\beta_t = \beta_{t-1} + \xi_t \quad (4)$$

Is there Convergence in the Health Expenditures of the EU Member States? 217

where ξ_t is normal independent distributed with mean 0 and variance σ_ξ^2.

The extent to which the level, μ_t, and the slope, β_t , change over time is governed by the relative hyperparameters,

$$q_\eta = \frac{\sigma_\eta^2}{\sigma_\epsilon^2} \text{ and } \frac{\sigma_\xi^2}{\sigma_\epsilon^2} .$$

In the limiting case when both relative hyperparameters are zero, the deterministic trend model is obtained with $\alpha = \mu_0$, as in (2).

The computer package STAMP 5.0 of Koopman *et al.*[20] enables the estimation of the hyperparameters by putting the model in state space form and applying the Kalman Filter to calculate the exact likelihood function. STAMP estimates the hyperparameters by maximum likelihood, which basically entails minimizing the sum of squares of the one-step ahead prediction errors throughout the sample.

The minimum mean square estimates of the trend μ_t (that we will call $\hat{\mu}_t$), together with the root mean square error (*RMSE*) are then obtained from specific smoothing algorithms implemented in the STAMP package.

Convergence test:

Once $\hat{\mu}_t$ and the *RMSE* have been obtained, we can proceed to calculate the upper and lower bounds of the confidence intervals for the trend. (We have worked with 0.9986 probability.)

For every year ($t = 1,...,T$), and for all countries ($i = 1,...,n$), we define:

$$\hat{\mu}_t + 3 \times RMSE = u_t$$

which is the upper bound of the confidence interval, and

$$\hat{\mu}_t - 3 \times RMSE = l_t$$

the lower bound of the confidence interval.

218   *Health Care and Cost Containment in the European Union*

Then we proceed to check whether the confidence intervals intersect, and to count how many intersections have there been per year. This has been done by writing a program on GAUSS. The procedure is as follows:

First we define the index function $I_{ij,t}$ for every country and year, where

$$I_{ij,t} = \begin{cases} 1 \text{ if } [l_{i,t}, u_{i,t}] \cap [l_{j,t}, u_{j,t}] \neq \emptyset, \text{ for } i \neq j \\ 0 \text{ otherwise} \end{cases}$$

We then calculate B_t (the observed number of intersections) as:

$$\forall_t, B_t = \sum_{i=1}^{n} \sum_{j=1}^{n} I_{ij,t}$$

And, finally, we define the *convergence indicator*, C_t as the ratio of B_t and the total number of possible intersections $\left(\dfrac{n^2 - n}{2} \right)$:

$$C_t = \frac{B_t}{\frac{n^2 - n}{2}}$$

C_t takes values between 1 and 0, being 1 in case of total convergence, and 0 in case of total divergence. If C_t increases over time, then we have a *converging process*. If it decreases over time, a *diverging process*.

4 Cost containment and health care reform in Belgium

DAVID CRAINICH AND MARIE-CHRISTINE CLOSON*

4.1 Introduction

In 1945, Belgium established a compulsory health insurance system. This covers employees and their dependents (85 per cent of the population) for major and minor risks, and the self-employed and their dependents (15 per cent of the population) for major risks.** Health insurance is managed and administered by the following: INAMI (Institut National d'Assurance Maladie Invalidité); the '*Mutualités*' (insurance funds which act as representatives for patients); and the providers' representatives. The latter negotiate the main features of compulsory health insurance within INAMI, including coverage and doctors' fees. The function of central government in health care is limited to the regulation and part financing of the system. The Belgian health care system has wide public support, mainly because the social contributions raised to finance it relate to individuals' income rather than health status. The system is also considered equitable in terms of access to care, with 99.9 per cent of the Belgian population insured against health care expenses. However, there has been a large increase in direct (out-of-pocket) payments over the last few years, which has made health care increasingly unaffordable for low income groups.

Delivery of health care in Belgium is mainly private and based on the principle of 'liberal medicine' (*médecine libérale*). This includes an independent medical practice, free choice of doctor and fee-for-service payments. Access to any level of care is direct.

---

* The authors would like to thank Elias Mossialos for his helpful comments and reviews of earlier drafts of this chapter.

** Major risks include in-patient care and special technical services (diagnostics and therapeutics) while out-patient care, medicines, dental care etc. are considered minor risks.

220 *Health Care and Cost Containment in the European Union*

While Belgian health care expenditure is relatively low when compared with neighbouring countries, representing around 8 per cent of Gross Domestic Product (GDP) in 1994, the system seems nevertheless to be responsive to the needs of patients. However, since the mid-1980s successive Belgian governments have felt the need for various reforms designed to increase the efficiency of the system, which hitherto lacked any mechanisms for checking quality and standards of care and monitoring the behaviour of care providers. It may also be the case that the particular structure of the Belgian system, characterized by the marriage of extended insurance cover

Table 4.1 Evolution of per capita total expenditure on health at current prices and annual expenditure growth rate, 1984–94

| Year | Total expenditure on health per capita – current prices $ PPPs | | | | | | |
	Belgium	France	UK	Germany	Netherlands	Italy	Ireland
1984	849	1,045	633	1,097	893	758	554
1985	887	1,091	670	1,164	932	827	586
	4.4	4.4	5.8	6.1	4.3	9.1	5.7
1986	938	1,140	720	1,210	990	862	590
	5.7	4.4	7.4	3.9	6.2	4.2	0.6
1987	998	1,198	775	1,282	1,046	971	611
	6.3	5.0	7.6	5.9	5.6	12.6	3.5
1988	1,086	1,301	840	1,402	1,101	1,080	632
	8.8	8.5	8.3	9.3	5.2	11.2	3.4
1989	1,159	1,422	887	1,419	1,226	1,170	664
	6.7	9.3	5.5	1.2	11.3	8.3	5.0
1990	1,247	1,539	957	1,519	1,331	1,318	748
	7.5	8.2	7.8	7.0	8.5	12.6	12.6
1991	1,375	1,649	1,006	1,534	1,416	1,439	832
	10.2	7.1	5.1	0.9	6.3	9.1	11.2
1992	1,537	1,808	1,170	1,750	1,559	1,564	975
	11.7	9.6	16	1.0	10	8.6	17.1
1993	1,600	1,838	1,165	1,726	1,601	1,522	1,025
	4 .0	1.6	-0.4	-1.3	2.6	-2.6	5.1
1994	1,653	1,866	1,211	1,869	1,641	1,561	1,201
	3.3	1.5	3.9	8.2	2.4	2.5	17.1

Source: OECD Health Data, 1996.[1]

on the demand-side with a private system of delivery of care on the supply-side, leads inexorably to high health care costs. Whatever the earlier reasons for reform, by the early 1990s this was deemed more necessary than ever, as the growth of Belgian health care expenditure rose to become one of the highest in the EU (see Table 4.1).

The structure of this chapter is as follows: section 4.2 summarizes the historical background of the Belgian health care system while section 4.3 explains how the system works in terms of the decision-making process, statutory insurance and the supply and financing of medical care. Section 4.4 deals with the various reforms of the system, focusing initially on those aimed at increasing the financial responsibility of its various stakeholders. Among these are the reform of hospital financing, linking a hospital's funding with its activities and performance, and the reform of statutory health insurance, signified by the adoption of a fixed budget system for each sub-sector covered by insurance and for the total revenue allocated to health insurance. Decreases in the coverage and reimbursement of health care services in 1993 and 1994 are also discussed. This section also outlines how the government has attempted to make sickness funds financially accountable through the progressive introduction of a risk-adjustment formula, which the sickness funds are required to incorporate into their revenue structure. The chapter then provides an overview of the Belgian government's cost-containment measures. These have been aimed primarily at altering the structure of supply, and include the recent decisions to reduce the number of doctors by limiting access to medical schools (the 'numerous clausus'), and modifying the hospital structure through the closure, concentration and conversion of acute hospital beds. Finally, section 4.5 discusses the impact of these reforms and looks at the issues likely to face Belgian health care in the near future.

4.2 Historical background

The foundations of the Belgian health care system were laid at the end of the last century. Industrialization brought with it new forms of poverty which gave birth to health insurance associations (*Mutualités*), trade unions and (more recently) political organizations drawn from the labour movement. The *Mutualités* were established as simple funds of mutual assistance,

222 *Health Care and Cost Containment in the European Union*

with the objective of offering temporary financial help in case of illness, injury or physical disability. The financial viability of these organizations was, however, weak.

Significant improvements in health care provision have been made throughout this century, including an increase in the number of beneficiaries of health insurance and a general extension of the benefits covered. The first major turning point in the social security system occurred during the Second World War, when secret meetings of representatives of employers and trade unions led to the agreement of a project of social solidarity (*Projet d'accord de solidarité sociale*). This agreement advocated equal representation in negotiations between employers and trade unions, universalized access to social insurance, created a centralized structure for raising contributions (the National Organization of Social Security, ONSS, *Office National de Sécurité Sociale*) and made health and unemployment insurance compulsory (the three latter principles applying only to salaried workers). The government enacted these proposals through an '*Arrêté loi de pouvoirs spéciaux*' on 28 December 1944.

The main features of the current Belgian health care system were settled in 1963 through the '*Leburton Law*', which led to the creation of INAMI, responsible for administering the system of compulsory health insurance, the introduction of fee-for-service payment to providers, and the definition of a new category of beneficiaries – VIPOs (widows, the disabled, pensioners and orphans) – no longer charged for care services.*

The social security and health care system developed during a period of economic growth which saw not only the expansion of health care coverage to new social categories (by 1969 health insurance covered the entire population) but also continual improvements to this coverage. Health insurance was only extended to the self-employed in 1964. According to Reman[2] one of the reasons for this late development was a decision taken by representatives of the self-employed to develop a system based on subsidized rather than compulsory insurance. This also explains why the care coverage of this group is less extensive than that of salaried workers.

However, the advances in health care coverage, made possible by surg-

---

* This category currently pays only small co-payments, for example, 7.6 per cent of the cost (30 per cent for all other beneficiaries) for a general practitioner consultation, 7.9 per cent of the cost (35 per cent for all other beneficiaries) for a home visit by a doctor and 8.5 per cent of the cost (40 per cent for all other beneficiaries) of a specialist consultation.

Cost Containment and Health Care Reform in Belgium 223

ing economic expansion, could not last forever. The economic crisis of the 1970s highlighted the need for Belgian health care reforms and led to the initiation of research aimed at developing a more efficient resource allocation within the system. This was reinforced by successive governments who sought to reduce the large public deficit during the 1980s. It was in this climate that strategies designed to make the health care system less expensive, while keeping it accessible, were developed, and led to the series of health care reforms outlined in this chapter.

4.3 Organisation of the system

4.3.1 The decision-making process

Decision-making in Belgian health care is decentralized and based on consultation between all groups involved in health-related policy development. The main bodies responsible for health policy formation are the Ministry for Social Affairs, Public Health and the Environment, regional governments, INAMI, the '*Mutualités*', medical doctors organizations and the National Board of Hospital Establishments.

4.3.1.1. The Ministry for Social Affairs* The Ministry for Social Affairs supervises ONSS, which is the public body responsible for raising social security contributions. The level of contributions to the social security system – negotiated between representatives of employers and trade unions – is subject to the approval of the Minister for Social Affairs.

The Minister for Social Affairs also supervises the functioning of INAMI, the public body responsible for health insurance policy. The 1993 INAMI reform increased the Minister's powers by granting him/her the right to take unilateral action when fixed budgets are exceeded.

---

* The Ministry for Social Affairs and the Ministry for Public Health merged on 1 October 1995, to constitute the Ministry for Social Affairs, Public Health and Environment. However, the merger is currently only administrative. As their main functions and areas of responsibility remain separate, the functions of the two former ministries will be discussed separately in this chapter.

224　*Health Care and Cost Containment in the European Union*

4.3.1.2 The Ministry for Public Health　The former Ministry for Public Health established the protection of patients as its primary health policy. To this end, the Ministry issues edicts for health providers regarding such issues as hospital planning, control over training posts for hospital specialists and the accreditation of medical personnel.*

The Ministry also defines and partly finances the daily running costs of hospitals. These include accommodation and nursing costs, as well as part of the cost of hospital capital investment.

4.3.1.3 Regional governments　In 1991 the Belgian political structure was decentralized. Important functions were shifted from the national level to either the three regions (Flanders, Brussels and Wallonia) or the three Communities (Flemish, French and German). Three functions, directly affecting the health care system, were devolved to the Communities:

(a) the application of standard norms (decided at the federal level) relating to the planning of high technology facilities and the accreditation of services. The Communities must also partly finance investment in these processes;

(b) public health services; and

(c) education programmes.

To finance their activities, Communities and Regions receive subsidies from the federal government, which constitute their main source of income as their ability to raise local taxes is very limited. The Communities receive a lump sum and can allocate resources to different programmes according to their own criteria.

4.3.1.4 INAMI　The management and regulation of financing health insurance is the responsibility of INAMI. It finances medical services through the *Mutualités* and guarantees a unified system through the pooling of surpluses and deficits. The administrative structure of health insurance reflects the

---

* Medical undergraduate education is not within the competence of the Ministry for Public Health, but is the responsibility of the Ministries of Education of the Communities. However, the Ministry for Public Health has the right to intervene and to regulate the market of practising doctors. When the Ministry for Public Health plans to introduce reforms to regulate the health care supply through medical education (as was the case for the *numerus clausus* reform), an agreement with the Ministries of Education of the Communities must be reached.

political will to reconcile cost containment policies with independent medical practices. Fundamentally, INAMI is a place of negotiation between all the stakeholders in the health care system.

4.3.1.5 Health insurance funds (Mutualités) An important feature of the Belgian health care system is the management power of the not-for-profit private insurance organizations, the *Mutualités*. The pivotal role of these *Mutualités* can be explained by their ideological affiliation to political parties. This is certainly the case with the Christian and Socialist *Mutualités*. These two types of association dominate the market of statutory health insurance, covering about 45 per cent and 29 per cent of the population respectively. The *Mutualités* act as the defenders of patients' rights within INAMI.

4.3.1.6 Doctors' organizations Doctors are represented by the Medical Council which deals with ethical issues relating to the medical profession. With statutory powers, it investigates malpractice or over-prescribing on the part of doctors, and imposes penalties in cases of 'unethical' behaviour, including the advertising or offering of services at prices below the agreed level. The negotiation of agreements and contracts between doctors and the *Mutualités* is, however, the responsibility of the profession's trade unions.

4.3.1.7 The National Board of Hospital Establishments (NBHE) Despite having only an advisory role, the NBHE plays an important part in the formation of Belgian health care policy. The board advises the Minister for Public Health on issues related to hospital planning, standards and financing.

4.3.2 The organization and financing of statutory health insurance

Figure 4.1 overleaf shows the organization and financing of primary health care in Belgium.

According to Hurst[3] the financing of primary health care in Belgium can be classified as a public reimbursement model. Patients pay providers on a fee-for-service basis. Social-security contributions are compulsory and income-related, with no upper or lower limits except in the case of the self-employed, where the latter applies. Non-price competition exists between

Figure 4.1 Primary health care: financing and delivery

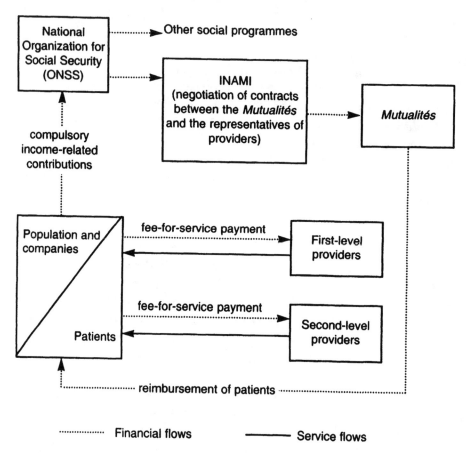

the *Mutualités*. Patients are not reimbursed fully for services since they have to make co-payments, however, they retain the right to choose both their insurance fund and medical provider. Within INAMI, representatives of *Mutualités* and doctors' trade unions negotiate annual contracts which define doctors' fees for each service provided.

Figure 4.2 illustrates the organization and financing of statutory health insurance at the level of in-patient care:

Again, according to Hurst's[3] classification, the financing of hospital in-patient care in Belgium can be characterized as a public contract model. This differs primarily from the public reimbursement model in that

Figure 4.2 Hospital care: financing and delivery

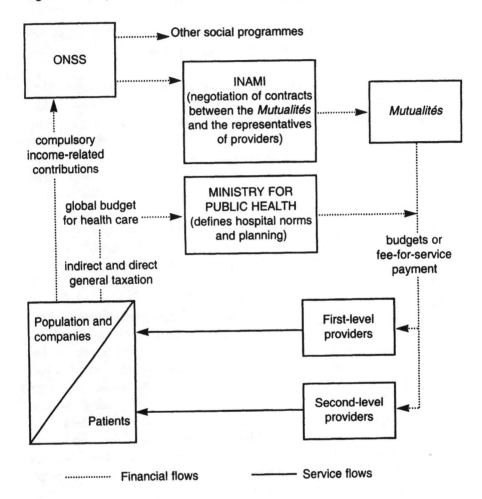

providers are paid directly; both by the *Mutualités* and in the form of co-payments from patients. Patients can make their own choice of hospital. The public contract model is applicable to the arrangements for in-patient care because the fee-for-service revenue that hospitals receive is determined following negotiations between representatives of providers *and* of *Mutualités*. Furthermore, hospitals must meet certain standards (defined by the Ministry for Public Health) in order to be reimbursed for their services.

228   *Health Care and Cost Containment in the European Union*

4.3.3 The health care delivery system

Since there is no referral system in Belgium, specialists and hospitals often form the first point of contact between patients and the health service.

4.3.3.1 Primary health care In Belgium there are few salaried doctors (less than 1 per cent of the total),* and primary health care is mainly provided by self-employed doctors. The market for general practitioners is highly competitive. Entry to medical schools has, so far, not been restricted. The application of a *numerus clausus* in medical schools applied from the academic year 1996–97. However, access to the profession for specialists is more restricted. According to Nonneman and Van Doorslaer,[4] specialist trainees work under the supervision of a specialist practitioner who pays his trainees out of fees from services delivered to patients. Consequently, new entries depend upon the number of clinical training posts in teaching hospitals, the volume of which is largely controlled by established specialists.

Specialized primary medical care is either supplied at the specialist's practice or at a hospital out-patient department. Specialist doctors working in hospital out-patient departments have contractual agreements with the hospital, and are paid on a fee-for-service basis. The hospital retains part of the specialist's fees in return for providing access to its facilities. Similar agreements apply to private hospitals. The extent of fee-sharing is variable and depends on several elements, foremost of which are the balance of power between hospital managers and the number of specialists. In addition to their basic salary, specialists receive a pre-negotiated share of 'pooled' fees.

The functions and roles of health care personnel have not been clearly defined. A prime example of this is the lack of distinction between the roles of GPs and specialists.** Patients have free choice of first contact doctor, and can change their doctor at any time.

The average number of patients per general practitioner and specialist

---

* These salaried doctors mainly work in medical practices which are owned and managed by themselves. Salaried doctors are paid according to a capitation payment for each patient they treat. They also provide other medical and social services such as preventive care, and may work in hospitals (teaching hospitals or public hospitals).

** For instance, there is no difference in the fee for a general practitioner consultation and a specialist consultation (for the same service provided). The reimbursement rate for the patient is, however, slightly higher for a general practitioner consultation.

Cost Containment and Health Care Reform in Belgium   229

Table 4.2 Population per practising doctor, 1977–95

Year	Population per active general practitioner	Population per practising specialist
1977	1,015	1,172
1980	899	1,026
1981	893	980
1982	857	937
1983	799	910
1984	759	893
1985	707	888
1986	706	828
1987	699	797
1988	691	765
1989	685	743
1990	685	722
1991	679	704
1992	675	685
1993	672	674
1994	662	643
1995	660	630

Source: IBES, 1996.[5]

has been declining over the last ten years, as shown by Table 4.2. This trend can be explained by the increasing number of medical students exploiting the policy of free access to medical school (this applied until 1997), and also by the relatively low cost of studying. These two factors have led to the current plethora of both general practitioners and specialists, which recently forced the government to restrict access to medical schools.

4.3.3.2 Secondary care In Belgium, 63 per cent of hospital beds belong to private, not-for-profit hospitals (there are only two for-profit hospitals). The remaining 37 per cent belong to public hospitals managed by cities (municipalities), towns or district authorities (*intercommunales*).*

---

* In 1995 there were 47,550 beds in private not-for-profit hospitals and 27,810 beds in public hospitals. Public hospitals are administered (including hospital planning and appointment of personnel) by the municipalities, which also cover all financial deficits.

230 *Health Care and Cost Containment in the European Union*

The method of financing the two types of hospitals is the same,* the only difference being that as public hospitals are usually required to admit all patients, their administrative rules tend to be more restrictive. Patients who depend on the Public Centres for Social Assistance (CPAS)** use public hospitals to receive health care. As a result these hospitals often have a higher proportion of low-income patients than private ones.

In terms of treatment, there are only two categories of hospitals – general and psychiatric. However, care is also provided in rest homes, combined rest and nursing homes and psychiatric care houses. User-charges in these institutions are much higher than in hospitals, since patients must bear the total cost of board and lodging themselves.***

Rest and combined rest and nursing homes differ in that nursing-intensive cases are only treated within the latter, which fall between rest homes and hospitals. Psychiatric cases can be treated in psychiatric departments within general hospitals (short stays only), in psychiatric hospitals (long stays) or in psychiatric care homes (where less serious cases are treated).

4.3.3.3 Community care Elderly people over 60 may be cared for in either rest homes or in combined rest and nursing homes, with the less severe cases being treated in the former. A daily lump sum payment, calculated according to the patient's degree of dependence, is allocated to rest homes and rest and nursing homes by INAMI for each patient residing within these institutions.

Children suffering from mental disorders are treated in special medical and social institutions. The care they receive is paid by health insurance, while accommodation costs are financed by regional governments. However, care for such children ceases to be financed once a hospital stay has exceeded 90 days. After this time, user charges for hospital treatment are significant and the only solution is to (continuously) change hospital. Due to a lack of sufficient funding, there is a shortage of rehabilitation centres for such cases, and the effectiveness of those which do exist is variable.

---

* The way of financing capital investment is the only exception. See section 4.3.4.3.

** CPAS: Public Centres for Social Assistance (*Centre Public d'Aide Sociale*). Each Belgian town has a CPAS. These institutions provide social, medical, psychological and income support.

*** See Table 4.10 for the difference between what patients are charged in general hospitals, psychiatric hospitals, rest and nursing homes, rest homes and psychiatric care homes.

Cost Containment and Health Care Reform in Belgium 231

4.3.3.4 Dental care The provision of dental services is private. Dentists are paid on a fee-for-service tariff which is negotiated annually within INAMI between the *Mutualités* and representatives of the profession. Dental care reimbursement rates are also defined by INAMI. Currently, reimbursement is available for preventive care (only one consultation a year for those under 18), surgical extractions and orthodontic treatments.

Table 4.3 shows the evolution of dental care expenditure (at current prices) reimbursed by health insurance between 1983 and 1996. The public cost of dental care did not increase significantly between 1991 and 1996. The budgetary targets for dental care were met in 1994, 1995 and 1996. However, during this period co-payments for dental care increased significantly, and some dental treatments and interventions lost health insurance coverage.

Table 4.3 Total public dental care expenditure care at current prices, 1983–96

Year	Dental care expenditure at current prices in both primary and secondary care settings (BEF million)
1983	4,560
1984	4,878
1985	5,265
1986	6,613
1987	7,188
1988	7,474
1989	8,480
1990	9,278
1991	10,275
1992	12,438
1993	11,766
1994	11,801
1995	13,164
1996	13,026

Source: Alliance Nationale des Mutualités Chrétiennes (personal communication).

232   *Health Care and Cost Containment in the European Union*

4.3.4 Financing of the system

4.3.4.1. Sources of financing   Table 4.4 gives a breakdown of total health care revenue by source of funding in 1987 and 1994.

Total health care expenditure in 1994 amounted to BEF 624.6 billion. This has been financed by:[5]

Social security (38 per cent).

General taxation (38 per cent): since the 1981 'Dhoore Law', the Belgian government allocates part of general taxation to health insurance to subsidize the contributions of the unemployed and low income groups. It also partly finances public health services, CPAS and hospital capital investment.

Out-of-pocket payments (17 per cent): Patients pay a fixed proportion of the cost of health care. The co-payment rate depends on the type of service provided.

Other resources (9 per cent): These include voluntary health insurance (VHI) premiums, a levy on car insurance premiums, hypothecated taxes and a tax on the sales of pharmaceutical companies.

Voluntary health insurance covers minor risks (out-patient care, medicines, dental care) for the self-employed (about 70 per cent of them take out VHI insurance), co-payments and some additional services (private rooms in hospitals, and extra billing by doctors). Voluntary health insurance is provided by the *Mutualités* (only for their affiliated members) and by private profit-making insurance companies which each offer different services at different rates. In 1994 Voluntary Health Insurance paid BEF 125 billion for health services. This amount covered co-payments (about BEF 56 billion), non-reimbursed medicines (about BEF 42 billion), additional services

Table 4.4 Sources of funding of health services in 1987 and 1994

Year	Social security	General taxation	Out-of-pocket payments	Other
1987	36%	39%	12%	13%
1994	36%	38%	17%	9%

Sources: Hurst, 1992;[3] Kesenne, 1995.[6]

Table 4.5 Health care expenditure (at current prices) between 1980 and 1995

| Year | Total expenditure (BEF billion) | | | Per capita expenditure (BEF) | | | Percentage of GDP | | |
	Total	Public	Private	Total	Public	Private	Total	Public	Private
1980	229.3	191.1	38.2	23,278	19,405	4233	6.6	5.5	1.1
1981	256.5	209.1	47.4	26,025	21,218	4807	7.2	5.8	1.4
1982	287.2	246.8	40.4	29,129	25,035	4094	7.4	6.3	1.1
1983	311.7	256.5	55.2	31,631	26,033	5598	7.6	6.2	1.4
1984	329.1	273.1	56.0	33,383	27,698	5685	7.4	6.2	1.2
1985	352.6	288.3	64.3	35,760	29,247	6513	7.4	6.1	1.3
1986	378.2	300.2	78.0	38,339	30,432	7907	7.6	6.0	1.6
1987	399.4	322.0	77.4	40,446	33,617	6829	7.7	6.4	1.3
1988	427.3	380.8	46.5	43,042	38,360	4682	7.7	6.8	0.9
1989	459.7	408.7	51.0	46,208	41,086	5122	7.6	6.8	0.8
1990	490.3	436.9	53.4	49,091	43,649	6042	7.6	6.8	0.8
1991	541.1	476.5	64.6	53,991	47,545	6446	8.0	7.1	0.9
1992	575.9	512.0	63.9	57,201	50,854	6347	8.1	7.2	0.9
1993	602.0	535.2	66.8	59,598	52,985	6613	8.3	7.4	0.9
1994	624.6	549.1	75.5	61,655	54,202	7453	8.2	7.2	1.0
1995	635.0	557.4	77.6	62,604	54,954	7650	8.0	7.0	1.0

Source: IBES, 1996.[5]

234 *Health Care and Cost Containment in the European Union*

Table 4.6 Total health care expenditure (at constant 1985 prices) between 1985 and 1995

Year	Health care expenditure (BEF billion)			Per capita expenditure (BEF)		
	Total	Public	Private	Total	Public	Private
1985	352.6	288.3	64.3	35,760	29,247	6513
1986	364.3	289.2	75.1	36,932	29,315	7617
1987	376.0	312.5	63.5	38,075	31,647	6428
1988	394.1	351.2	42.9	39,692	35,375	4317
1989	405.8	360.8	45.0	40,790	36,268	4522
1990	420.1	373.6	46.5	42,068	37,405	4663
1991	451.6	397.7	53.9	45,066	39,685	5381
1992	464.3	412.8	51.5	46,119	41,002	5117
1993	474.5	421.9	52.6	46,980	41,767	5213
1994	472.2	415.1	57.1	46,609	40,609	6000
1995	470.2	412.7	57.5	46,353	40,688	5665

Source: IBES, 1996.[5]

(about BEF 17.7 billion) and self-employed minor risks (BEF 10 billion).* There are no tax incentives to join a private insurance scheme.

Tables 4.5 (previous page) and 4.6 show the evolution of total health care expenditure over the last 15 years (at current prices and constant 1985 prices), and illustrate public and private health expenditure trends. Table 4.5 shows that since 1993 the rising cost of health care has been restrained, following the introduction of several cost-containment measures. Health expenditure reached 8.3 per cent of Gross Domestic Product (GDP) in 1993, but declined to 8 per cent in 1995. Table 4.6 shows that real total expenditure on health even decreased at constant 1985 prices since 1993. Private health expenditure rose due to increases in co-payments and the exclusion of certain services from insurance coverage.

The data presented in Tables 4.5 and 4.6 were collected by the private health economics research centre IBES. There are no comprehensive offi-

---

* Estimates: *Alliance Nationale des Mutualités Chrétiennes* (personal communication).

Cost Containment and Health Care Reform in Belgium 235

cial statistics on health expenditure trends in Belgium. It is highly probable that private expenditure on health (including out-of-pocket payments and voluntary health insurance premiums) is much higher than reported. As Table 4.4 indicates, these two taken together amounted to more than 20 per cent of total health care expenditure in 1994.

4.3.4.2 Budget allocation There is no fixed overall budget for health care in Belgium, but there are both sectoral target budgets and a fixed budget for health insurance expenditure. Figure 4.3 overleaf shows which parts of public health expenditure are limited and which are not. The budget allocation takes place at different levels. Local governments have responsibility for some health matters (applications for and financing of capital investment, medical and paramedical education, health protection and promotion) and therefore allocate resources according to their own policy objectives.

The part of the health care budget allocated by the federal government is cash-limited, and includes the financing of both capital investment and health insurance. For example, in 1997 the Ministry for Public Health allocated BEF 103 million for the financing of capital investment. These resources are allocated to different regions following a distribution formula established in 1988, which takes into account the needs of each Community. The amount allocated to health insurance for 1997 was BEF 428.3 billion. This budget is not allocated on a regional basis, but rather to different sectors within INAMI according to the following procedure.[7]

- Separate sectoral budgets for pharmaceuticals, dental care, hospitals, and primary care are established, based on the recommendations of the Contracts and Agreements Commissions, which negotiate the allocation of funding for each sector.*

- Partial annual budgetary targets** and a global budget for health insurance*** are proposed by the Insurance Committee for Health Care and

---

* It has to be noted that not all these funds are determined within INAMI. For example, the Ministry for Public Health fixes the budget allocated to clinical biology.

** Budgets are intended to cover the expenses of each health care sub-sector and are discussed and proposed by the Contracts and Agreements Commissions.

*** This must include 75 per cent of hospitals' per diem rates financed by the health insurance and defined by the Ministry for Public Health.

Figure 4.3 Health care budgets in 1997

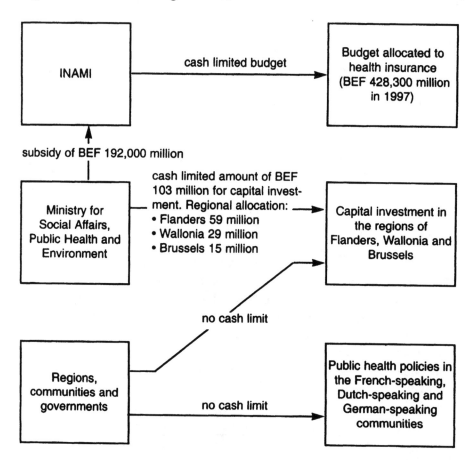

are forwarded to the General Board for Health Care Insurance. Since 1994, the Belgian government has fixed the maximum annual growth rate of the global budget for health at 1.5 per cent, excluding inflation.*

- The General Board for Health Insurance approves the annual budgetary objectives (taking into consideration the advice of the

---

* This limit of 1.5 per cent has been assessed by the Planning Office ("Plan Bureau') and corresponds to an assessment of the likely evolution of the population's health care needs in the near future. It can be broken down into two factors: medical technology evolution (1 per cent) and the ageing population (0.5 per cent).

Commission of Budgetary Control) and forwards its suggestions on to the government. If the General Board for Health Insurance does not agree with the proposals made by the Insurance Committee for Health Care, it notifies the Ministry for Social Affairs. The Council of Ministers may then fix the global budget for health insurance as well as the sectoral budgets. The Minister for Social Affairs communicates the government's decision to the Insurance Committee for Health Care which then fixes annual sectoral budgetary objectives.

- Depending on the availability of funds, Contracts and Agreements Commissions finalise the fees-for-services. The final agreement must include fiscal mechanisms to prevent over-expenditure.

- If expenditure looks likely to exceed the fixed budgets, these mechanisms will be implemented. Thereafter, if expenditure continues to rise, the Minister for Social Affairs, as final decision-maker, may impose more stringent mechanisms to ensure that the fixed budgets are adhered to.

In 1994 and 1995 expenditure on health insurance was contained within the targeted budget. However, limits were exceeded in 1996, resulting in central government intervention. The government terminated the agreement reached by the *Mutualités* and the representatives of providers in December 1995, when it unilaterally reduced the negotiated fees by 3 per cent. These new fees applied in 1996 and 1997.

4.3.4.3 The financing of capital investment Capital investment is financed by the Regions and the Communities* (through the subsidies they receive from the federal government) at 60 per cent for private hospitals and 70 per cent for public hospitals. The remainder is financed directly from the federal government up to a certain limit depending on the project. Capital investments in buildings, operating theatres, and heavy medical equipment are covered by hospitals via part of their per diem charge over a 33-year period for buildings, a 10-year period for other non-medical material, and

---

* The Communities are responsible for the financing of investment and the application of planning norms for university hospitals (as the latter are linked to education, which is a responsibility of the Communities) while the Regions are responsible for these matters in other hospitals.

238   *Health Care and Cost Containment in the European Union*

a 5-year period for heavy medical equipment. Other medical equipment is financed from fees for medical services.

However, this system has led to the duplication of medical treatments – whether justified or not – by hospitals attempting to benefit from economies of scale vis-à-vis costly equipment. In an attempt to curb this practice, there is currently a trend towards the disassociation of fixed costs (which are financed through the per diem charges) from variable costs (which are financed through fees for medical services for capital-intensive equipment). Evidence of this pattern has been witnessed in the case of radiotherapy and nuclear magnetic resonance equipment, which were originally fully financed from medical fees.

In order to control capital expenditure, a national limit to the amount paid off through the per diem charge is fixed. The Ministry for Public Health, which only finances 25 per cent of the per diem charge dedicates an annual average of approximately BEF 103 million to capital investment funding.* Capital investment projects cannot, however, be undertaken by regional governments whenever they choose. In 1989, a construction schedule covering a seven-year period was drawn up to prevent projects being started at the same time. This schedule has also served as a political tool. By fixing the amount of funds available for each type of hospital, the schedule directs funds according to federal government priorities. For example, the 1989 building schedule promoted investments in psychiatric hospitals. This has proved an effective method of control on the part of central government, since only those investments included in the building schedule may be paid off out of daily charge revenue.

Moreover, not all investment projects proposed by hospitals are accepted for public subsidy. Programming and approval rules for capital investment projects have been established by the Ministry for Public Health, based on advice given by the 'National Board of Hospital Establishments'. The Communities are, however, responsible for the application of these rules, since it is they who determine which investment projects meet the criteria. These programming and approval standards are designed to meet the needs of the population through improved efficiency and quality. Factors that are considered include: the type of specialization within a hospital; a

---

* This figure only represents 30 per cent (or 40 per cent for public hospitals) of the total amount dedicated to capital investment, including buildings and heavy equipment.

department's capacity; equipment; geographical distribution; co-ordination in the use of equipment and so on.

Traditionally, two sets of factors have been considered in applications for capital investment funding: the number of beds (number of beds in total and number of beds in each department) and the planning of the capital-intensive equipment (either because of their high prices or because they require highly qualified staff). These either affect the general organization of the institutions (such as total capacity, infrastructure, and number and type of hospitals' department) or the organization and the workings of each department (such as minimal capacity, minimal equipment, function and qualification of the staff).[8]

However, the philosophy behind funding approval has recently changed, and no longer relates solely to hospital infrastructure (i.e. number of beds). Now, more emphasis is placed on the nature of a hospital's medical and nursing activities. There has been a move away from considering the planning of costly equipment towards the recognition of services provided. While it was previously sufficient for a hospital to meet some *quantitative* structural norms (i.e. number of beds, size of the hospital) approval now concerns the department where the equipment is to be installed, which now must meet some *qualitative* criteria (nursing activity, presence of specialists within the department, and case-mix).

These changes are in accordance with the second article of the '*Law of hospitals*' which is formulated in terms of mission (to be worked out by the hospital) rather than in terms of infrastructure. According to this philosophy, approval of investment funding must increasingly be based on hospital activity, expressed in the form of a programme focusing on well-defined patient groups, rather than on static data based on hospital technology. Assessment is conducted through the mechanism of peer reviews that attempt to establish in detail, each department's activities. Peer reviews are considered to facilitate a more concrete evaluation, even if they are based on subjective judgements. However, implementation of this mechanism has been both progressive and cautious.

4.3.4.4 Payment of hospitals The running costs of both public and private hospitals are financed through a mixed formula of fee-for-service and *per diem* fees. Hospitals receive two kinds of revenue.

240 *Health Care and Cost Containment in the European Union*

(1) The revenue from per diem charges

The funding of the daily cost of all hospitals is included within a prospective global budget fixed annually. The standard cost per day is appraised by the Ministry for Public Health which takes on 25 per cent of these expenses, while the remaining 75 per cent is financed by health insurance.

(a) The budgets for hospital 'hotel' and clinical services represent 90 per cent of the revenue from daily hospital charges.

   A cost comparison method has recently been established to reduce the amount spent on hotel costs. Under this system, hospitals are grouped according to size and revenue is progressively adjusted according to the average hotel costs of the group. This system allows efficient hospitals to benefit most and inefficient ones least.

(b) The clinical service budget.

   This budget pays for such clinical services as nursing staff, medical supplies and medicines. The budget for each hospital is fixed according to its structure (i.e. the number of beds and specialization), its nursing requirements and medical activities. This is made possible through a system that clusters nursing activities into 'care units' based on different types of activity. Points are then allocated to activity-related staff costs.

Medical activities are easily recorded because the fee-for-service method of payment contributes to the accurate recording of data. The observed value of medical activities for equivalent services in the whole country is estimated, and additional points are allocated to hospitals according to their position within the distribution. The adaptation of this theoretical budget to the real budget is progressive. In the past, the Ministry for Public Health established quotas of in-patient days by setting a target occupancy rate for each hospital department (for example, 80 per cent in surgery, 70 per cent in paediatrics and 70 per cent in gynaecology). The revenue cost per day was then identified by dividing a hospital's prospective annual budget by the quota. A hospital that went beyond its quota received 30 per cent of the daily charge for each additional day, while one that failed to reach its quota did not receive any compensation. However, this method of setting in-patient day quotas failed to take into account efficiency gains, and effectively penalized hospitals which reduced average length of stay and rewarded hospitals that had more in-patient days.

New measures have now been introduced to promote efficiency and redistribute resources from poorly performing hospitals to more efficient ones. Performance is now measured by analysing the difference between the number of in-patient days recorded by the hospital and the average in-patient days by diagnosis-related group (All Patients Diagnosis Related Groups, APDRGs), sub-divided according to the patient age (under or over 75 years). Since 1996, a specific diagnosis-related group has existed for patients over 75 years with co-morbidities, who have spent at least ten days in a geriatric unit.

An assessment of the extent to which each hospital uses day-care services (as a substitute to in-patient care) is made for each diagnosis-related group. The number of in-patient days saved (or wasted) by each hospital and for each diagnosis-related group can then be evaluated and an estimate made of the respective financial awards or penalties to different hospitals.

Thus, according to this, criteria are based on comparisons between hospitals:

- there are neither penalties nor rewards for differences ranging from between -2 and +2 per cent of the average in-patient day performance;

- for differences ranging between +2 and +10 per cent of the average performance, hospitals lose 50 per cent of the budget allocated to the additional days; and

- if differences are greater than 10 per cent, hospitals lose 25 per cent of the budget allocated to the additional days.

The savings are then redistributed to hospitals whose differences are less than -2 per cent of the average.

The fact that the penalty decreases as the deviation from the average increases (below and above 10 per cent), may appear strange. This is explained by the fact that the government wanted to avoid the closure of some hospitals before an evaluation establishing the causes of their poor performance had been carried out. Since 1996, maximum losses or gains cannot exceed 3 per cent of hospitals' global budgets. This means that in practice differences of above 8 per cent will never be paid back, as the loss of the budget related to these days always leads to a loss exceeding 3 per cent of the budget.

The financial penalties are expected to become stricter in the future. From 1999 changes in implementation of the rules will mean that:

242   *Health Care and Cost Containment in the European Union*

- penalties and awards will be implemented if there is a difference between the number of in-patient days at the hospital and the average in-patient days performance, even if this difference lies within the range of -2 and +2 per cent;

- the hospitals will lose an increasing percentage (over time) of their budget allocated to the additional days (compared to average performance);

- the savings will then be redistributed to better performing hospitals; and

- a limit for the penalties will be fixed at 2.5 per cent of the hospital budget for a hospital with a difference over 5 per cent from the average.

(2) Fee-for-service revenue
In-patient medical services (including surgical operations) are paid on a fee-for-service basis, the level of fees having been set by INAMI. Unfortunately, this system acts as an incentive to over-supply medical services, and expenditure on laboratory testing and radiology has thus increased significantly. In response, a different financing system, based partly (82 per cent) on lump sum payments calculated according to the case-mix of the hospital, and partly (18 per cent) on payment by act (fee-for-service), has been used in clinical biology since 1988 (see section 4.4.1.2).

4.3.4.5 Medical technology   A technical board composed of the representatives of providers, *Mutualités* and university experts, evaluate the efficacy and effectiveness of new medical technologies, taking into account both therapeutic and social criteria. This board also advises on whether old technologies should be replaced by more modern ones. A Commission (including representatives of providers and *Mutualités*), then determines reimbursement levels, taking into account the advice of the technical board, the cost of the technology and the prices set in other countries. The National Board of Hospital Establishments must give an opinion about the planning and the financing of major equipment (i.e. radiotherapy, dialysis). Thus both the assessment and financing of new technologies is made on the basis of negotiation, taking account of the fixed budget. In Belgium the impact of new technologies on the cost of health care has not yet been estimated.

The diffusion of new technology is controlled through installation regulations, enacted by the planning department of the Ministry for Public Health, which must be adhered to by hospitals if they want their investment

Cost Containment and Health Care Reform in Belgium   243

reimbursed. The key role in planning the investment in new technologies is played by central government, thereby avoiding any unnecessary and costly duplication of functions. Nevertheless, continual demands from pressure groups and political parties, which tend to favour investment in hospitals with which they are linked, makes the task of controlling investments in new technologies difficult.

4.3.4.6 Payment of doctors   All Belgian doctors, including both general practitioners and specialists, are paid on a fee-for-service basis. Taking account of budget limitations, a fee schedule is established annually, following negotiations between the *Mutualités* and representatives of health care providers. However, this schedule can only be enforced once it has received the approval of central government. Moreover, an agreement is not implemented if it is rejected by more than 40 per cent of practitioners.* In this situation, the government has three options: to submit an alternative draft agreement to practitioners; to unilaterally impose fees for some or all of the services; or to fix only the reimbursement levels, leaving practitioners free to set their own fees.[3]

If the second option is chosen, doctors have 30 days after the publication of the Royal Decree (reducing the level of fees) to decide whether or not to accept the government's decision. There is a strong incentive for doctors to agree to the fee schedule, even if it has been imposed by the government, since failure to do so may weaken their social and political position and jeopardize certain employment advantages – notably the state contributions to their pensions. This said, competition between doctors is so stiff in Belgium that they usually adhere willingly to the schedule agreements. If the government opts to fix reimbursement levels, it may be the case that those doctors who disagree with the negotiated fee schedule will try to rally public support by claiming that standards of care will suffer.

Thus it can be seen that government involvement in the process of establishing the fee schedule has grown since 1993. If the in-built mechanisms designed to limit the growth of health insurance expenditure fail to produce adequate results, the Ministry for Social Affairs is allowed to reduce unilaterally doctor's fees and patient's reimbursement rates, as occurred in December 1996.

---

* The agreement is not implemented if it is rejected by more than 50 per cent of practitioners in any one of the two sub-groups (general practitioners and specialists).

244 *Health Care and Cost Containment in the European Union*

4.3.4.7 Pharmaceuticals In 1994, about 16 per cent, or BEF 62.1 billion, of the health insurance budget was spent on pharmaceuticals. According to Annemans *et al.*[9] the total market value for pharmaceuticals reached BEF 117 billion for the same year (calculated at retail price level). Retail pharmacies have a monopoly on dispensing medicines and account for approximately 85 per cent of total pharmaceutical sales. If one compares total pharmaceutical sales (BEF 117 billion) with the government's pharmaceutical bill (BEF 62.1 billion), it becomes evident that patients contribute 46.3 per cent to the cost of drugs in Belgium.

Pharmaceutical prices are fixed by the Ministry for Economic Affairs. The Ministry's Pricing Commission for Pharmaceutical Specialities seeks advice from the Transparency Commission of the Ministry for Public Health regarding a drug's therapeutic importance, package size in relation to dose, and the package with regard to health care cost.[9] On the basis of this technical advice, the Pricing Commission sets a *maximum* price at which pharmaceutical firms are allowed to sell medicines in Belgium. However, the final retail prices of medicines are negotiated between INAMI and the various pharmaceutical companies. Acting on the advice of its Technical Council for Pharmaceutical Specialities, which considers the prices of different products, INAMI sets pharmaceutical reimbursement levels. Once these levels are decided, INAMI then sits down to the negotiating table.

Belgian doctors, including both GPs and specialists, are able to prescribe most drugs, except in the case of extremely expensive medicines, when the consent of the medical adviser of the *Mutualités* is first required. Out of a total of 6,000 drugs available in Belgium, currently around 2,500 drugs are reimbursed by INAMI. The extent of reimbursement, and thus of patient co-payment, depends upon the therapeutic value of a given drug. Accordingly, each drug is classified into one of five reimbursement categories:

(a) Drugs used for the treatment or care of serious diseases such as epilepsy or diabetes, are classified into category A. These drugs are fully reimbursed.

(b) Category B includes effective but high-cost drugs. They are reimbursed at a rate of 75 per cent (85 per cent for VIPOs) with a co-payment ceiling of BEF 345 (BEF 230 for VIPOs) per prescription.

(c) Category C drugs are reimbursed at a rate of 50 per cent. There is a co-payment ceiling of BEF 575 (BEF 345 for VIPOs) per prescription.

Table 4.7 Trends in pharmaceutical expenditure in primary care at current prices, 1985–95

Year	Expenditure		Reimbursed pharmaceutical consumption Packs of drugs (million)	Average expenditure per drug		Average patient contribution per drug	
	Total (BEF million)	Reimbursed (BEF million)		Total (BEF)	Reimbursed (BEF)	Amount (BEF)	% of total expenditure
1985	28,541	20,986	84.9	336	247	89	26.5
1986	31,396	23,311	88.5	355	263	92	25.9
1987	33,945	25,402	90.7	374	280	94	25.1
1988	37,357	28,254	96.0	389	294	95	24.4
1989	41,745	31,112	98.7	423	315	108	25.5
1990	47,122	34,727	103.9	454	334	120	26.4
1991	52,660	39,078	108.5	485	360	125	25.8
1992	56,333	41,904	99.2	568	422	146	25.7
1993	57,571	42,454	94.1	612	451	161	26.3
1994	60,671	45,004	94.3	644	477	166	25.8
1995	65,679	48,981	97.7	672	501	171	25.4

Sources: IBES, 1996.[5]

246 *Health Care and Cost Containment in the European Union*

(d) Category Cs includes drugs of limited effectiveness or ones that are not used on a regular basis. They are reimbursed at a rate of 40 per cent. There is no co-payment ceiling.

(e) Category Cx is a transition category. New drugs are initially included in this category, pending their evaluation and a final decision on reimbursement.

Generic drugs are subject to a lump-sum payment. If the original version is not reimbursed, then the generic is also excluded from reimbursement. Partly because it is perceived that the price of brand-name drugs is low, pharmaceutical policy towards generics has not been developed in Belgium.

Overspending by the drug sub-sector in 1994 led to the implementation of corrective fiscal measures. These included the introduction of budgets in hospitals for the use of antibiotics before surgical operations. This budget is now allocated depending on the number of surgical operations in each hospital. The government intends to extend the principle of in-hospital budget controls to other categories of medicines. The co-payment for in-patient pharmaceutical care is BEF 25 per day.

Table 4.7 on the previous page shows the trends in pharmaceutical expenditure in primary care at current prices between 1985 and 1995. The table also presents trends in reimbursed pharmaceutical expenditure, the number of drug packs reimbursed by INAMI, the cost per drug, and the co-payment per drug.

Similarly, Table 4.8 shows the trends in reimbursed pharmaceutical expenditure in hospitals and the amounts reimbursed at current prices.

4.4 Health care reforms in Belgium

The central rationale behind the introduction of health care reforms in Belgium in the 1980s was the rise in health care costs, combined with a reduction in revenue (caused by increasing unemployment) and a growing public deficit. Although compared to other European countries, Belgian health care expenditure comprises a relatively low share of GDP, its growth rose quite rapidly at the end of the 1980s and particularly in the early 1990s. Few incentives exist for consumers to reduce their demand and providers, paid on a fee-for-service basis, are largely motivated to *increase* it.*

Cost Containment and Health Care Reform in Belgium 247

Table 4.8 Trends in pharmaceutical expenditure in hospitals at current prices, 1985–95

Year	In-patient care*		Out-patient hospital departments	
	Reimbursed amounts (BEF million)	Annual growth rate (%)	Reimbursed amounts (BEF million)	Annual growth rate (%)
1985	4,880	-2.0	294	27.3
1986	6,331	29.7	573	94.9
1987	7,564	19.5	1,202	109.8
1988	7,868	4.0	1,401	16.6
1989	8,103	3.0	1,004	-28.3
1990	9,156	13.0	1,356	35.1
1991	10,346	13.0	1,842	35.8
1992	11,316	9.4	2,345	27.3
1993	12,320	8.9	2,720	16.0
1994	13,132	6.6	3,080	13.2
1995	13,592	3.5	3,262	5.9

* Amounts exclude the in-patient co-payment of BEF 25 per day.

Sources: IBES, 1996.[5]

Health care reforms implemented during the last 15 years have been aimed at containing the system's costs without forsaking its more positive characteristics. The Belgian public debt, growing social-security expenditure, problems associated with increasing social contributions and patient co-payments, all contributed to the need for significant cost-containment measures.

The reforms of the Belgian health care system, which arise from the need to contain spiralling costs, have been twofold. Firstly, by adapting the financial mechanisms of the system, the reforms have been aimed at devolv-

---

* There are no Belgian studies providing evidence of induced demand. In 1993 the General Board of Management of INAMI was charged with the responsibility of publishing a report on the uniform application of statutory health insurance in the whole country, including an assessment of non-justified practice variations and proposals of measures to tackle these. The first report was published in 1996 (which includes 1994 data) and pointed out that per capita medical consumption was highest in the Region of Brussels, where the medical supply is also the highest in the country.

248 *Health Care and Cost Containment in the European Union*

ing responsibility for Belgian health care to the system's various stakeholders. This has been done by progressively moving away from a *retrospective* financial system (based on the payment of costs, and treatments undertaken) to a *prospective* system, focused on needs, risks and performance indicators. Secondly, the Belgian government has implemented reforms which focus on the supply-side of the system.

4.4.1 Financial accountability transferred to different sectors

4.4.1.1 Reforms in hospital financing The central thrust of the reforms in hospital financing has been to build a new financial structure based on a hospital's function, needs and performance, rather than one base solely on medical treatments provided and costs incurred. The adjustment of hospital financing to such a case-mix system has made it necessary to collect clinical information concerning patients. Since 1990, the systematic collection of a 'minimal clinical summary' (*Résumé clinique minimum*) – describing the patient's clinical situation – and a selective collection of a 'minimal nursing summary'(*Résumé infirmier minimum*) – outlining nursing activity by unit of service – have been introduced to enable better identification of effective and ineffective hospitals (in terms of length of stay) by the Ministry for Public Health.

However such an ambitious programme of changing the method by which hospitals are financed also implies adapting the structure of those institutions responsible for financing hospitals. The objective of building a financial system based on needs and risks is difficult to realise when the information required to do so is widely dispersed among various financial players (see Figure 4.4).

Under the current system, case-mix-related data are submitted to the Ministry for Public Health, while data relating to the consumption of medical services and products are submitted to INAMI through the *Mutualités*. To resolve the problems inherent in such a decentralized decision structure, the Ministry for Public Health has proposed the following measures to encourage better integration of the financing system with assessment of medical activity.

(a) Creation of a consultation structure
This consultation structure gathers together all parties involved in the health

Figure 4.4 Distribution of information related to hospitals

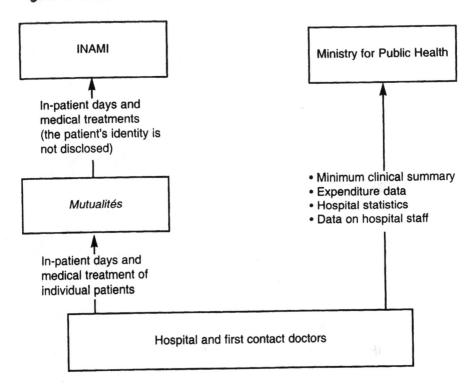

care system (the Ministry for Public Health, Evaluation Commissions (see below), INAMI, hospitals, *Mutualités*, medical organizations etc.) under the aegis of the Ministry for Public Health. The aim of the consultation structure is to establish a financing system that focuses on the patient.

(b) Creation of a central data bank
The creation of a central databank for medical information is currently underway. Within this structure, data will be collected from the Ministry for Public Health (i.e. minimal clinical summaries, accounting data) and from INAMI (invoicing data). The bank will then facilitate the flow of useful information between the system's various players.

In addition to assisting in the adaptation of the system's financial structure, the central databank will also allow hospitals to compare their performance with other hospitals classified in the same category.

250 *Health Care and Cost Containment in the European Union*

(c) Creation of Evaluation Commissions

The difficulties inherent in evaluating both the quantity *and quality* of medical care provided by each hospital have necessitated the creation of Evaluation Commissions. The Commissions are responsible for evaluating both the quality and efficiency of new technologies and the provision of care.

4.4.1.2 Financing the reforms in clinical biology Clinical biology used to be financed on a fee-for-service basis. However, this led to the considerable over-production of laboratory testing. In 1985, the Minister for Public Health (within the framework of the agreement concluded between doctors and *Mutualités*) introduced a single national budget devoted to clinical biology in both primary care and hospitals. The Minister retained the right to unilaterally cut fees should this budget be exceeded. However, far from curtailing the widespread practice of over-prescribing, these reforms encouraged many doctors to act as 'free-riders' and the number of prescriptions rocketed. This led the Minister for Public Health to reduce prices of laboratory tests by 30 per cent in 1988.

Following the failure of the 1985 reforms, the government employed a new strategy in 1988. The new strategy combined a fixed national budget for clinical biology with a new financing mechanism based partly on patient co-payments and partly on the increased accountability of laboratories.[10] In the case of primary care services, each laboratory is now required to repay a certain percentage of funds if the national budget is exceeded. The amount repayable is calculated (according to laboratory size) and collected by INAMI, which holds information on the clinical biology expenses of all laboratories. INAMI then passes these recovered funds back to the government, whereupon they are used to decrease the budget deficit.

In the case of hospital in-patient care, the 1988 reforms replaced the method of payment per test with a daily rate which is added to the admission fee. These daily rates are partly calculated on the basis of historical expenses (from 1987) and partly on an evaluation of a hospital's case-mix structure (assessed on the basis of invoicing data); thus they vary greatly from one hospital to another. The compulsory collection of minimal clinical summaries since 1990 should paint a more precise picture of the case-mix structure within each hospital. The payment by act for clinical biology services have been maintained at the rate of 18 per cent of their value since 1988.

Table 4.9 Expenditure on clinical biology at current prices, 1983–96

Year	Expenditure on clinical biology at current prices for primary and in-patient care (BEF million)
1983	21,810
1984	25,191
1985	25,686
1986	28,881
1987	30,784
1988	28,587
1989	26,955
1990	27,499
1991	29,513
1992	30,138
1993	25,127
1994	24,157
1995	24,004
1996	25,860

Source: Alliance Nationale des Mutualités Chrétiennes (personal communication).

To strengthen the strategy of devolving financial responsibility an agreement was reached in 1992 between the *Mutualités* and doctors which introduced an element of financial accountability into the prescription of laboratory tests. As a result, doctors' prescribing practices are now closely monitored; those who may be over-prescribing are investigated and, after one warning, their reimbursement is decreased. This cost-containment measure has proved particularly effective and expenditure on primary care clinical biology fell by 25–30 per cent between 1992 and 1993.[10] Table 4.9 shows this trend in expenditure in clinical biology over the last three years.

4.4.1.3 The control of drug expenditure The Belgian government has initiated several measures aimed at controlling drug expenditure. According to Annemans *et al.*,[9] these cost containment strategies were as follows:

- The downgrading of some drugs from a higher to a lower category of reimbursement in 1992.

252 *Health Care and Cost Containment in the European Union*

- Increasing co-payments for category B medicines from BEF 300 to BEF 345 per prescription (from BEF 200 to BEF 230 for VIPOs) and for category C medicines, from BEF 500 to BEF 575 per prescription (from BEF 300 to BEF 345 for VIPOs).

- Increasing co-payments from 75 per cent to 80 per cent for category Cx medicines.

- Freezing at 1996 levels the prices of all reimbursable medicines;

- Decreasing the price of branded generics in order to promote their use (by 20 per cent since 1996).

- Levying a 2 per cent tax on the sales of reimbursed pharmaceutical products.

The government has also achieved some volume controls by restricting reimbursement of some drugs to specific diagnoses and groups. Moreover, reimbursement of certain drugs is now subject to a limited period and granted only after the agreement of the medical advisor of the respective *Mutualité*.

More efficient mechanisms for financing pharmaceuticals are in the process of being developed under several projects. Among these are: the development of prescription profiles by doctor within INAMI, both for primary and in-patient care; the creation of a prescription practice evaluation committee to analyse the data and convene peer review committees on prescription practices; and the development of price-volume contracts for new drugs.

4.4.1.4 INAMI reforms The INAMI reforms created fixed budgets for each sub-sector of health care, as well as establishing a global budget. They also set in place mechanisms for issuing penalties when expenditure exceeds fixed limits. The reforms give the system a legal framework and extend the control of central government. Since 1994, the government has capped the growth of expenditure devoted to health insurance at 1.5 per cent above general inflation.

These reforms represent a fundamental change in government policy towards health care. The previous funding strategy was demand-led and based on the *ex-post* recording of health care expenses determined by the workload of providers. This has been replaced by an *ex-ante* system that

Cost Containment and Health Care Reform in Belgium   253

assesses the available public resources and determines how much is necessary to meet the health needs of the population. In 1994 the target budget for health insurance was BEF 387 billion; in fact only BEF 380 billion was spent. However, as noted by Robert[11] these savings were achieved largely through a substantial increase in patient co-payments which totalled around BEF 8.5 billion in that year.

Again, in 1995 the budget target of BEF 407 billion* was achieved, with actual expenditure totalling BEF 400 billion. A breakdown of expenditure for that year reveals that most sub-sectors stayed within their budgets. This was the case for psychiatric institutions (-21.3 per cent), clinical biology (-7.7 per cent), doctors (-4.5 per cent) and dentists (-6.6 per cent). However, certain sub-sectors went into the red, most notably; implants (+9.7 per cent), rest and nursing homes (+3.6 per cent), dialysis (+17.1 per cent) and medicines (+3.5 per cent).[11]

However, as the 1996 budget was exceeded these budgetary successes were relatively short-lived. In 1996 the budget was set at BEF 418 billion but in fact reached BEF 442 billion. Although a fee-for service increase of 1.3 per cent had been negotiated in an attempt to counter the predicted over-expenditure, the Belgian government instead chose to reduce fees by 3 per cent in December 1996. This unilateral action prompted a backlash from medical providers in January 1997, who responded by *putting up* fees by 2 per cent for consultations, and maintained fees at the 1996 level for technical acts. This fee increase was expected to be at the expense of patients who were then to pay the difference, as the amounts reimbursed by the *Mutualités* would not increase. However, this was not the case. Doctors did not in fact set excessive fees, and the government made significant efforts to ensure that a new agreement between the *Mutualités* and the representatives of the providers was reached, such that an additional amount of money was allocated to cover for increases in doctors' fees. The fee schedule was fixed for 1998 with a proportional increase of both doctors' fees and reimbursement levels.

4.4.1.5 Patient cost-sharing As mentioned in the previous section, the effort to control health care expenditure has led to a dramatic increase in patient

---

* It has to be noted that in fact the annual budgetary target for the health insurance exceeds the 1.5 per cent increase over the previous year as this norm does not take into account the inflation rate.

254 *Health Care and Cost Containment in the European Union*

cost-sharing. This is one of the most commonly deployed cost-containment measures and is expected to reduce the demand for health care, as well as achieving direct savings by cutting the government's share of the cost.

Three changes in patient cost-sharing were introduced in the 1990s:

(a) The conversion of acute and chronic hospital beds into beds for rest and nursing homes and into beds for psychiatric care homes. This produces savings for health insurance as the share of the cost borne by patients in these institutions is much higher.

Table 4.10 gives the different user charges in general hospitals, psychiatric hospitals and psychiatric care homes. Patients pay a lump-sum payment which, in the case of psychiatric care houses, includes all services (medical services, board and lodging etc.) but which excludes medical fees in both general and psychiatric hospitals. User charges in rest and nursing homes are fixed by each institution according to the facilities provided. These charges have, however, to be approved by the Minister for Economic Affairs. Patients have to pay for medical services according to the fee-schedule in general hospitals, psychiatric hospitals, rest homes and in rest and nursing homes. Patients in private beds may be charged extra in hospitals, where they are also liable for a daily lump sum payment of BEF 25 for pharmaceuticals.

(b) The downgrading of some medicines in 1992 from a higher to a lower category of reimbursement. (see section 4.4.1.3).

(c) Increasing co-payments. These measures were implemented in two stages. In October 1993, co-insurance rates and lump sum payments for in-patient care were increased. These included co-payment for the first in-patient day, lump sum payment for clinical biology and co-payment for some special medico-technical treatments in the case of out-patient care. Then in January 1994, co-payments for home visits and consultations were increased (except for VIPOs). Table 4.11 overleaf, illustrates the differences in prices paid by patients for three standard medical services between October 1993 and January 1995.

These co-payment increases were followed by the introduction of a social and fiscal exemption mechanism in 1994, designed to protect the patient from excessive charges. These exemptions establish a certain cut-off point above which health care services are fully reimbursed. Social exemption applies to the long-term unemployed (who are head of a household), the disabled, those on very low incomes and VIPOs. In the case of patients whose total annual health care bill exceeds BEF 15,000, co-payments are fully reimbursed under this mechanism. Under the fiscal exemption mechanism, households are able to deduct co-payments from their annual income tax bill, up to a certain limit dictated by their income bracket. Table 4.12 shows these limits and the related revenues.

Table 4.10 User charges per in-patient day paid by patients in various medical institutions in 1997

	VIPOs (BEF)	Other categories (BEF)
General hospital		
1st in-patient day	156	1366
2nd to 8th in-patient day	156	366
after the 9th in-patient day	103	259
after the 90th in-patient day	226	490
Psychiatric hospital		
1st in-patient day	156	1366
2nd to 8th in-patient day	156	366
9th to 365th in-patient day	103	259
1st to 5th year	193	456
Psychiatric care homes		
Daily lump-sum payment	672	872
(including care and accommodation costs)		
Rest and nursing homes	Prices are fixed by each home and approved by the Ministry for Economic Affairs	
Rest homes		

Source: Fédération des Institutions Hospitalières de Wallonie; Union Nationale des Mutualités Libres (personal communication).

256 *Health Care and Cost Containment in the European Union*

Table 4.11 Fee-for-service, reimbursement and co-payments for selected medical services

	Fee-for-service	VIPOs		Other categories	
		Reimbursement	Co-payment	Reimbursement	Co-payment
GP consultation					
before October 1993	504	465	39	401	103
after October 1993	520	480	40	364	156
after January 1995	550	508	42	385	165
% change 1993–95	+9.1%	+9.2%	+7.7%	- 4.0%	+60.2%
GP visit					
before October 1993	648	597	51	482	166
after October 1993	656	604	52	427	229
after January 1995	671	618	53	437	234
% change 1993–95	+3.5%	+3.5%	+3.5%	-9.3%	+41.0%
Specialist consultation					
before October 1993	810	741	69	608	202
after October 1993	827	757	70	497	330
after January 1995	840	769	71	504	336
% change 1993–95	+3.7%	+3.8%	+2.9%	-17.1%	+66.3%

Source: Alliance Nationale des Mutualités Chrétiennes, 1995.[12]

Table 4.12 Income brackets and co-payment ceilings as at January 1994

Taxable annual income bracket	Ceiling to the amount of co-payment by income bracket
BEF 0 – 537,999	BEF 15,000
BEF 538,000 – 828,999	BEF 20,000
BEF 829,000 – 1,119,999	BEF 30,000
BEF 1,120,000 – 1,410,999	BEF 40,000

Source: Alliance Nationale des Mutualités Chrétiennes, 1994.[13]

Cost Containment and Health Care Reform in Belgium   257

Neither co-payments for supplementary expenses in the case of hospital care nor drugs, are taken into account in the calculations of social and fiscal exemption limits.

4.4.1.6 Reform of the Mutualités   Although in theory the *Mutualités* enjoy financial autonomy enshrined under Belgian law since 1963, in practice their funds have always been underwritten by the state. The way the system worked was that the surpluses and deficits of all the individual *Mutualités* were pooled and then redistributed between the funds according to need; thus the surpluses and deficits of any one *Mutualité* (i.e. the difference between subscribers' contributions and their health care consumption) were largely theoretical. As pointed out by Kesenne,[5] this system of pooling meant that Socialist *Mutualités* consistently received more than their statutory share (BEF 54.2 billion between 1963 and 1991) and the Christian *Mutualités* received less (BEF 31.5 billion over the same period). This distribution can be explained by the social make-up of the two types of *Mutualités*. The former traditionally include more workers, with lower average earnings and (frequently) poorer health status than members of the higher social classes, who tend towards membership of other funds, particularly the Christian *Mutualités*. However, while this system was redistributive it failed to promote an efficient allocation of resources. For this reason, the Christian *Mutualités* proposed to reform the way in which *Mutualités* were financed.

The legislation enacting these reforms is dealt with in the first article of the Royal Decree of 12 August 1994, which covers the distribution of resources between the *Mutualités*. Under these reforms, the principle of redistribution based on the social contributions paid by members of each *Mutualité* is replaced by a double distribution key taking account of real expenses (historical key) on the one hand, and the risks borne by each *Mutualité* (normative key) on the other.* It is intended that this system will be implemented progressively, with funding being allocated less on an his-

---

* This allocation formula, resulting from research carried out by economists and statisticians of the Dutch-speaking university, Katholieke Universiteit van Leuven and the French-speaking Université Libre de Bruxelles, takes into account: age, sex, mortality rates, unemployment rate, income, family composition and rate of urbanization. It is crucial that the influence of these factors is assessed as accurately as possible, otherwise the system could cause adverse selection.

258 *Health Care and Cost Containment in the European Union*

torical basis and more on a normative basis *over time*. In 1995 and 1996 the allocation was 90 per cent historical and 10 per cent normative. In 1997 and 1998 this shifted to 80 per cent and 20 per cent respectively, and is expected to move still further to 70 per cent and 30 per cent by 1999. The maximum amount of funds allowed to be allocated according to the risks will be 40 per cent.

Once the *Mutualités* revenues are determined, each is individually accountable for a certain proportion of the resources allocated to them under the normative allocation (15 per cent in 1996). The remainder is subject to collective accountability. If the whole system exceeds the fixed budget, the *Mutualités* (individually or collectively) will only be liable for the first 2 per cent of the budget deficit. It will then be up to the Board of Directors of INAMI to decide how to finance the remaining deficit.

The central weakness of the Royal Decree is that it does not consider the most efficient way of implementing these expenditure controls. Indeed, as pointed out by Poucet,[14] it even failed to improve upon the currently inadequate mechanisms for negotiations between the insurance funds and central government.

One further method of cost containment that has been suggested is to abandon the principle of free choice of doctor for patients, and free choice of treatment for doctors.

4.4.1.7 The funding of capital investment As discussed earlier in this chapter, the system is progressively switching away from a mechanism of investment programming to accrediting individual departments. While the former (based on structural criteria such as size and number of beds) is rather static, the latter is more dynamic and patient-centred, taking account of, among other factors, the presence of medical and paramedical staff within the department and patient case-mix. It is envisaged that the expansion of this scheme could facilitate a closer relationship between the supply of services and the population's medical needs.

4.4.1.8 The accreditation formula The basic idea behind the accreditation system (proposed in 1994 and applied from 1 July 1995) is the improvement of health care standards by increasing the quality, efficiency and effectiveness of doctors. Accreditation is granted to those doctors who satisfy certain quality requirements. These include: communicating well with other health care providers; producing a medical brief for each patient treated, continu-

Cost Containment and Health Care Reform in Belgium   259

ing to attend education courses (20 hours a year including health economics and ethics courses); maintaining effective and efficient prescriptive and therapeutic practices; and finally, consulting a high number of patients. Since fees-for-services and patient reimbursement rates are higher for a consultation with an accredited doctor, the system offers both financial incentives for doctors and quality incentives for patients.

4.4.1.9 The introduction of bar code prescriptions Introduced in July 1994, bar code prescriptions are designed to generate a greater supply of information concerning the prescriptive behaviour of doctors. Until 1994, health insurance reimbursed pharmacists – through the *Mutualités* – for their total expenditure. Although all prescriptions carried the prescribing doctor's name, doctors were not identified under this procedure. Bar code prescriptions now enable prescribers to be identified systematically. The objective of this reform, however, was not to penalize heavy prescribers, but to increase data on prescribing practices.

4.4.2 Restructuring supply

The second set of health care reforms instituted by the Belgian government aims to limit the supply of medical services. The reforms offer incentives to health care providers to reduce unnecessary in-patient days, consultations, and prescriptions.

4.4.2.1 The numerus clausus To tackle the problem related to the plethora of medical students, the *numerus clausus* reform was enacted in June 1995, with the effect of limiting entry to medical schools (this commenced in the academic year 1996–97). Since Communities are responsible for educational programmes, they have implemented this reform. Therefore each Community had already been assigned a fixed number of students.

A Royal Decree has fixed the authorized number of candidates at 700 in 2004,* 650 in 2005 and 600 in 2006. These figures are shared between the French-speaking Community (280 in 2004, 260 in 2005 and 240 in 2006) and the Dutch-speaking Community (420 in 2004, 390 in 2005 and

---

* This restriction was implemented at the beginning of the academic year 1997/1998 as (at least) seven years are usually required to study medicine in Belgium.

260　*Health Care and Cost Containment in the European Union*

360 in 2006).

4.4.2.2 Hospitals A policy of bed reduction has applied since the introduction of a moratorium stating that the number of beds counted on 1 July 1982 could not be exceeded from that date. The government intended to reduce the number of in-patient days through these cuts. Financial incentives have also been introduced to promote the policy of bed-reduction, in the form of compensation being granted for the non-execution of building projects already authorized, and the closure or failure to open hospitals and geriatric departments. In this way the government expects to reduce the number of beds by 5000.

Moreover, incentives to reduce investments have also been introduced. Communities now have the option of reducing their contributions from 60 per cent to 30 per cent for investments that cut the number of beds in a hospital by at least 25 per cent (the remaining 30 per cent being paid by health insurance). Taken together, these reforms have substantially reduced the number of hospital beds over the past two decades (Table 4.13).

Table 4.14 shows that policies aimed at reducing the total number of hospital beds have (*inter alia*) led to a reduction in the average length of hospital

Table 4.13 Number of hospital beds, 1979–94

	General hospitals	Psychiatric hospitals	Total
1979	65,654	24,637	90,291
1984	69,418	22,220	91,638
1987	67,341	21,213	88,554
1990	61,178	19,371	80,549
1994	58,283	17,077	75,360

Source: Ministry for Social Affairs, Public Health and Environment, 1995.[15]

stay, and have cut the total number of in-patient days. These factors also influence hospital financing, since, as discussed above, hospitals are now either rewarded or penalized for their level of efficiency in terms of in-patient stays.

The Belgian government has also implemented a policy of bed concen-

Cost Containment and Health Care Reform in Belgium   261

Table 4.14 Indicators of in-patient stays, 1990–94

	Average length of stay	Total number of in-patient days
1990	13.74	25,417,607
1991	12.99	24,917,496
1992	12.27	24,048,711
1993	11.96	23,681,507
1994	11.65	23,072,313
Change 1990–94 (%)	-15.2	-9.2

Source: Ministry for Social Affairs, Public Health and Environment, 1995.[16]

tration. Under this policy, a hospital must contain a minimum number of 150 beds, spread across at least three departments. The Ministry for Public Health has forced hospitals that do not contain the requisite number of beds to either merge with other hospitals or to close altogether. Until the 1980s, the Belgian hospital structure was characterized by the existence of a considerable number of small hospitals. However, these measures have led to an increase in the average size of hospitals and a concomitant reduction in the number of small institutions (see Table 4.15 overleaf).*

At the same time, specialised geriatric departments (G services) have been established in some hospitals and financial incentives granted to convert acute beds into geriatric beds, beds for rest and nursing homes and beds for rest homes. These tactics are designed not only to produce savings – because all accommodation costs in the latter institutions are covered by patients (as discussed earlier) – but also because in these institutions staff pay agreements are more flexible, and therefore pay levels are likely to be lower. Hurst [3] has calculated that by the end of 1989 nearly 18000 places had been created in rest and nursing homes as a result of the closure of

---

* The sudden and temporary increase in the number of small hospitals in 1985 is explained by the fact that V services (which includes care of long-term patients) have been accounted separately since that year. Most of these beds were thereafter transformed into beds for rest homes and beds for rest and nursing homes. This explains the increase of this category of beds after 1985.

262 *Health Care and Cost Containment in the European Union*

Table 4.15 Number and size of hospitals, 1980–93

Year	Number of hospitals					Average size (beds)
	Total	<150 beds	150–299 beds	300–499 beds	>500 beds	
1980	521	317	127	41	36	177
1981	531	319	133	42	37	175
1982	432	204	142	47	39	213
1983	425	195	140	50	40	216
1984	414	190	135	48	41	219
1985	449	231	137	43	37	200
1986	440	222	137	45	36	201
1987	385	165	143	41	36	216
1988	378	156	144	44	34	217
1989	379	158	149	40	32	213
1990	374	156	145	43	30	212
1991	368	151	147	43	27	211
1992	366	149	147	42	28	212
1993	363	129	147	56	31	213

Source: IBES, 1996.[5]

wards in acute hospitals. Table 4.16 shows the number of beds in rest homes and rest and nursing homes.

Since 1990, measures intended to convert acute hospital beds into beds in psychiatric care homes have also been implemented by the government. Belgian law stipulated that 6,000 acute hospital beds were to be replaced by less expensive beds over a five-year period. Thus, the number of beds for long-term hospital care has been reduced, psychiatric hospital beds have been converted to psychiatric nursing home beds (where patients pay for accommodation costs) and the financial contribution of patients residing for longer than five years in psychiatric hospitals has been increased.

Cost Containment and Health Care Reform in Belgium   263

Table 4.16 Number of beds in rest homes and rest and nursing homes, 1970–95

Year	Beds in rest homes	Beds in rest and nursing homes*
1970	55,087	n.a.
1975	63,980	n.a.
1980	69,368	n.a.
1984	n.a.	2,304
1985	85,708	3,837
1986	88,321	4,779
1987	91,170	12,874
1988	93,906	13,789
1989	96,693	15,305
1990	93,377	17,264
1991	94,700	17,877
1992	98,593	18,593
1993	91,182	18,753
1994	n.a.	19,240
1995	96,465	19, 475

* higher level of patient dependency.

Note: n.a. = not available.

Source: IBES, 1996.[5]

4.5 Conclusion

The central components of the recent cost-containment reforms in Belgium are twofold: first, financial responsibility for health care has been devolved to the system's stakeholders who are made accountable for their budgets, while the fixing of both global and sectoral budgets by central government has increased. The spirit of these reforms has been captured by Hurst[3] who describes the result as follows:

> The government may assume full responsibility for macro-economic efficiency – or the overall control of health expenditure –

264   *Health Care and Cost Containment in the European Union*

and leave the patients, insurers and providers to pursue micro-economic efficiency within a firm framework of solidarity and global budgets.

Secondly, in its efforts to curb health care expenditure, the Belgian government has aimed to control the supply of medical services. In addition to introducing the '*numerus clausus*', the government has restructured the supply of hospital care, and provided incentives to limit unnecessary treatment and in-patient stays.

More generally, the Belgian health care system is switching away from a system of finance based simply on the reimbursement of costs – whether justified or not – to a financing mechanism based on the needs, risks and performance criteria of each actor/sector. Nevertheless, since the assessment of these factors is far from straightforward, both the implementation of the reforms and the changes they are designed to produce are relatively slow.

Further cost-containment measures are under discussion but are encountering resistance from some health sector groups. However, the increasing pressure of a financial deficit will no doubt add impetus to the cost-containment process. Indeed, the current competitive environment makes the reduction of public expenditure a necessity.

It seems that the containment of expenditure through fixed budgets will not be an easy process. The 1.5 per cent maximum growth rate of expenditure devoted to health insurance is considered by patients' groups and representatives of the *Mutualités* to be inadequate. This assessment may be correct if the efficiency savings gained through the new reforms are not taken into account. However, if these savings are included, the current growth allowance appears more substantial. Unfortunately, with the likelihood of increased demands being made on the system – through technological advancement and a growing elderly population – further increases in co-payments are nevertheless likely in the future.

The probability of increasing health care expenditure has led to further suggestions as to methods of cost containment. Two ideas currently being discussed are worth noting here: the first explores the possibility of complete devolution of all health matters from the federal level to Regional and Community control. Political pressure for this option comes from the Flemish region, and arises partly from a desire for greater autonomy and partly from a refusal to be associated too closely with the South (Walloon Community). This is because the redistribution element is regarded as too costly. Such a change would require a modification of the Constitution so that this issue could be on the agenda after the 1999 general election, provided that a Constitutional reform is introduced. The second set of proposed reforms involves a reassessment of the current system of managed care and the role of the State and of the 'Mutualités' within the health care system. Such a reform would involve detailed negotiations between numerous interest groups and is unlikely, therefore, to be implemented in the near future.

References

1   OECD. *OECD Health Data.* Paris: OECD, 1996.

2   Reman P. *Politiques Sociales: Théories, Acteurs et Régulation.* Faculté Ouverte de Politique Economique et Sociale, Université Catholique de Louvain, Louvain-la-Neuve, 1994.

3   Hurst J. The reform of health care. A comparative analysis of seven OECD countries. *Health Policy Studies No.2* Paris: OECD, 1992.

4   Nonneman W, Van Doorslaer E. The role of the sickness funds in the Belgian health care market. *Social Science and Medicine* 1994;39(10)1483–95.

5   IBES Institut Belge d'Économique de la Santé. *Compendium des Statistiques de Santé.* Brussels, 1996.

6   Kesenne J. Health care reform and risk structure compensation: the case of Belgium. In: *Risk Structure Compensation – Financing Health Care: Sharing Risks, Preserving Solidarity* (proceedings of an AIM workshop, Maastricht, 11 October 1995). Brussels, Alliance Nationale des Mutualités Chrétiennes, 1996.

7   Moorthamer L, Hermesse J. Reforme de l'AMI. Loi instituant et organisant un régime d'assurance obligatoire soins de santé et indemnités. Brussels: Alliance Nationale des Mutualités Chrétiennes. *M-informations* February 1993;156:2–10.

8   Closon M.-C. The Health Care system in Belgium. Université Catholique de Louvrain, unpublished paper, 1995.

9   Annemans L, Crott R, De Clercq H, Huybrechts M, Peys F, Robays H, Steen I, Vanschoubroek K, Winderickx P. Pricing and reimbursement of Pharmaceuticals in Belgium. *Pharmacoeconomics* 1997;11(3):203–9.

10 Hermesse J. Les réformes de financement et d'organisation des soins de santé en Belgique. *Solidarité Santé – Etudes économiques* 1993;2.

11 Robert B. L'évolution des dépenses soins de santé en 1994. Un bilan contrasté. Brussels: Alliance Nationale des Mutualités Chrétiennes. *M-informations* June 1995;166:2–3.

12 Alliance Nationale des Mutualités Chrétiennes. Effet des mesures récentes sur les tarifs. *M-informations* June 1995;166:13

13 Alliance Nationale des Mutualités Chrétiennes. Remboursement des soins de santé et franchise. *En Marche* March 1994;1074:2.

266 Health Care and Cost Containment in the European Union

14 Poucet T. L'assurance Maladie-Invalidité en 1994: le train-train des tensions en gare de triage? *L'Année Sociale 1994*. Brussels: Université Libre de Bruxelles, Institute of Sociology, 1995, pp 214–25.

15 Ministère des Affaires Sociales, Santé Publique et de l'Environment. *Annuaire Statistique des Hôpitaux – Partie 2: Rapport Annuel 1995*. Brussels, 1995.

16 Ministère des Affaires Sociales, Santé Publique et de l'Environment. *Annuaire Statistique des Hôpitaux – Partie 3: Activités dans les Hôpitaux*. Brussels, 1995.

5 Health care and cost containment in Denmark

TERKEL CHRISTIANSEN, ULRIKA ENEMARK,
JØRGEN CLAUSEN AND PETER BO POULSEN

5.1 Introduction

The Danish health care system is characterized by the absence of major reforms over the last 25 years. Minor adjustments are, however, made continuously. The Danish health care sector is mainly public, and its organization is decentralized within 15 administrative units (14 counties and 1 hospital authority: the latter was established in 1995 and is based on a system of cooperation between municipalities in the metropolitan areas).[1] The counties are responsible for the delivery of health care. Hospitals are generally owned by the counties, while general practitioners and practising specialists are privately organized. The services of the latter two groups are financed through the Public Health Insurance, managed by the counties.

The most important cost-containment measures – some of which were introduced several decades ago, while others were introduced recently – can be summarized as follows.

- GPs act as gate-keepers to hospitals and to specialist treatment (with some exceptions). Patients should be treated at the lowest level of care (cost-wise) at which effective treatment is possible.

- GPs have a limited economic incentive to treat, as only part of their income comes from fee-for-service payments, and the rest from capitation fees.

- A limit has been put on the number of GPs per 1000 population and on the number of specialists who are allowed to practice and bill the Public Health Insurance.

- Total expenditure on GP services, as well as the growth rate of this expenditure, is decided in a collective agreement between the Association of GPs and the Public Health Insurance. Expenditures and activities of GPs are monitored locally.

268 *Health Care and Cost Containment in the European Union*

- A cooperative initiative between the state government and the local authorities has produced annual budgets that ensure an overall ceiling on expenditures of the municipalities and counties. Health care expenditure amounts to 60 per cent of the total expenditure of the counties, so there has not been much room for re-allocating budgets to health care from other tasks.

- Use of global budgets for hospitals has kept the cost of running the hospitals within agreed limits.

- The cost of using pharmaceutical products has been limited by various measures over the last decade, namely: limits on the number of drugs eligible for public reimbursement (by either 50 per cent, 75 per cent or 100 per cent), or removal of drugs to a lower reimbursement level; use of a deductible (introduced, and abolished again); use of generic prescription; use of reference prices; tolerance of parallel imports ; and price agreements used as a cost controlling measure.

5.2 Financing of health care

The main sources for the financing of the Danish health care sector are shown in Table 5.1. Taxation includes all kinds of local and state government taxes. No earmarked taxes are used.

Table 5.1 Main sources of financing in the Danish health care sector, 1985, 1990 and 1995 (%)

	1985	1990	1995
General taxation	85.0	82.2	82.8
Private insurance	1.0	1.6	1.7
Out-of-pocket payment	14.0	16.2	15.5
Total (%)	100.0	100.0	100.0
Total, billion DKK	40.3	51.7	61.6

Sources: Danmarks Statistik: Statistisk Årbog (Statistical Yearbook), various years.[2] Facts. MEFA, various years.[3]

Health Care and Cost Containment in Denmark 269

More than 80 per cent of the total expenditure is financed through general taxation while a minor share is financed through user charges and insurance premiums. As seen in Figure 5.1 overleaf, the counties are responsible for about three-quarters of the total expenditure.

State taxes were used to finance both the highly specialized National Hospital (except in 1995 when it was transferred to the regional level) and the state block grants to counties and municipalities to supplement their general budgets. Figure 5.1 illustrates the flows of payments for one year (1994). For each kind of payment, the share of total health care expenditure has been estimated.[2,3]

A minor share of county expenditure on health care is financed from state block grants, while the rest is financed through county taxation. On the assumption of a pro rata distribution of general grants to health care and other county activities, the general grants accounted for about 19 per cent of the total health care expenditure in 1994. Using the same assumption, general state grants to municipalities amounted to about 1 per cent of the total health care expenditure.

County and municipality taxes consist of taxes on income, levied proportionately, and taxes on real estate. The average county income tax rate * in 1994 was 9.7 per cent, and the average municipal tax rate was 19.7 per cent. County income tax rates in 1994 varied between 8.9 and 10.4 per cent, while municipality income tax rates varied between 13.5 and 22.3 per cent. County real estate tax is 10 per thousand, while it varied between municipalities with an average of 13.6 per thousand.

General state grants are financed through government taxes which include both a personal, progressive tax on income and property and numerous indirect taxes.

User charges finance about 17 per cent of total health care expenditure. Insurance plays a minor role and serves mainly to cover user charges.

Expenditure on health care is shown in Table 5.2 overleaf. Private expenditure consists mainly of payment of user charges. The total amount of user charges is based on estimates.

Due to cooperation on setting budgets between the government and local authorities, combined with global budgeting for hospitals, health care expenditure has been kept almost stable for a decade, and the percentage of GDP used for health care purposes is below the OECD average.

---

* Exclusive of the municipalities of Copenhagen and Frederiksberg

Figure 5.1 Financing health care in Denmark, 1994

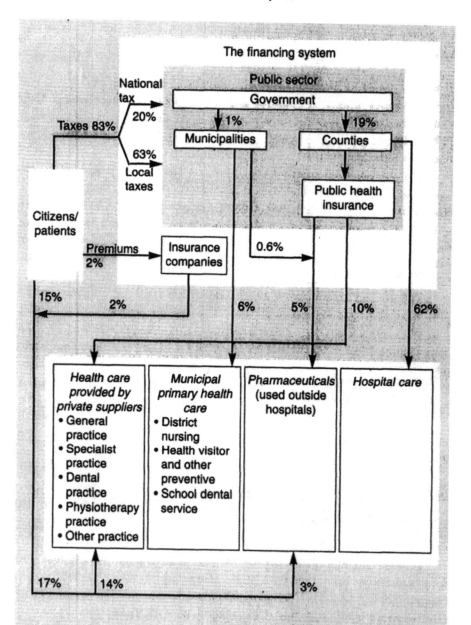

Percentages refer to the share of total health care expenditure in 1994 (DKK 61.3 billion)

Table 5.2 Public and private expenditure on health care (construction costs excluded), 1985 and 1994 (%)

Year	Public %	Private %	Total %	Billion DKK	Percentage of GDP
1985	84.5	15.5	100.0	40.288	6.6
1994	82.6	17.4	100.0	59.631	6.4

Note: With construction costs included the total expenditure as a percentage of GDP increases to 6.8 (1985) and 6.5 (1994).

Sources: Danmarks Statistik: Statistisk Årbog (Statistical Yearbook), various years.[2]
Facts. MEFA, various years.[3]

5.3 Overall budgets for the health sector

As illustrated in Figure 5.1, counties are responsible for the financing of hospitals. Providers who practise privately outside the hospitals (general practitioners, specialists, dentists, physiotherapists), may get a billing number from the Public Health Insurance in the local county, which allows them to bill the Public Health Insurance. Billing numbers are limited by reference to an agreed number of suppliers per capita. Municipalities are responsible for district nursing, health visitors and other preventive services, such as the school dental service. These activities are financed from municipal budgets.

The administrative structure is illustrated in Figure 5.2, overleaf. Each county and municipality has a council consisting of elected politicians. The councils establish a number of committees for various tasks. Most counties have a committee on health and social affairs which is responsible for these tasks under the Public Health Insurance Act, and a hospital committee responsible for running the hospitals. The committees are supported by an administration. Some counties have merged the two committees into one, called a health committee. Municipalities have a similar administrative structure; among the municipal sub-committees is a committee on social and health affairs.

The budgets and hence the activities in the health care sector, are decentralized. Each year, a total budget (and hence the taxation rate) is decided upon by each local government (municipality or county).

Figure 5.2 Budgets and the political–administrative system in the health care sector in Denmark

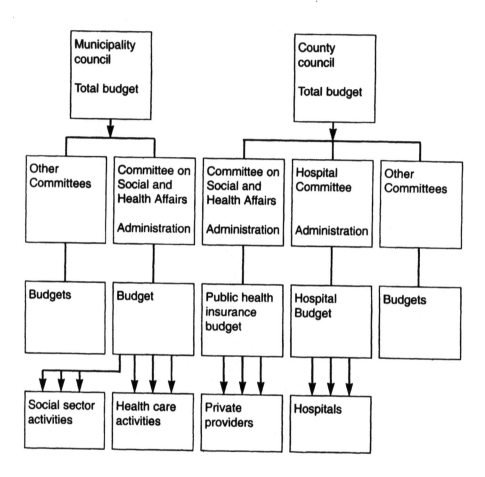

The total budget of a local government is divided into budgets for separate committees, each of which is then responsible for its own budget. In principle, the budgets should be adhered to. If the budget is exceeded, the local council may grant an additional amount during the year (if reserves are available) or activities may be slowed down (e.g. a hospital department may stop intake from a waiting list during the last month(s) of a fiscal year).

Each county has a budget for the operation costs of hospitals and a budget for Public Health Insurance services. Investments over a certain amount are granted separately. The extent of decentralization varies among the counties; several counties allocate a budget to each separate hospital which is then responsible for its own budget. A hospital may in turn allocate individual budgets to separate departments, which are then responsible for their budget *vis-à-vis* the hospital management. In principle, the hospital budget is a fixed budget as the size of the budget is determined by the beginning of the year, and changed activity does not automatically change the budget. In contrast, the budget under the Public Health Insurance is in principle an open-ended budget, as the total expenditure depends on the activity in the practice sector (consultations, prescriptions, etc.) There is, however, a ceiling on the total expenditure on fees due to collective agreements and the continous monitoring of activities in the sector by the Public Health Insurance administration. The total budget for Public Health Insurance covers both primary health care and pharmaceuticals.

The budgeting principle is typical marginal budgeting; each budget is based on previous years and modified on the margin to account for new activities, changes in tasks, and areas of specific need.

In spite of the decentralization of the health sector, the state government has some power to control the overall budget and growth rate. To ensure an overall policy on public expenditure, the overall budget is negotiated each year in a Budget Cooperation between the state government and the local governments, represented by the County Council Association and the Association of Municipalities.[1] In this cooperation, an overall ceiling of growth in the local tax rate is agreed upon and the level of state block grants is negotiated. Special areas needing additional resources are highlighted and extraordinary state grants may be given (e.g. to reduce waiting time for operations and to expand psychiatric care), although there has been a clear policy to reduce the block grant from the state over time. Between 1990 and 1994, an unchanged overall tax level was agreed upon in relation to a tightened fiscal policy. Generally, the growth rate has been limited. During the period 1980–95, hospital expenditure has only increased by 10 per cent in fixed prices. In Denmark, the budget mechanism based on negotiation functions well from a cost-containment point of view.

In 1994, an agreement was made between the government and the association of counties with respect to the development of hospital services for the following four years. According to this agreement, the hospital sector is to be gradually allocated increased budgets. The government guaranteed that the counties will have the necessary economic means to

274 *Health Care and Cost Containment in the European Union*

carry through an expansion of hospital capacity and an improvement of their services, no matter how the economies of the counties might develop. General state grants were significantly increased in 1994. In return, the expanded capacity must be negotiated each year in connection with the economic negotiations.

The expanded capacity and improved services include *inter alia* (1) increased operation capacity, especially increased capacity to perform heart operations, (2) increased efforts to care for mental patients, (3) improved patient information. According to the last point, counties were obliged to set goals for each hospital concerning information to patients as to when examination and treatment of a referred patient can take place, the expected waiting time from referral to examination, and from examination to treatment.[4]

Before the 1995 budget year it was agreed that tax rates should be kept stable from 1994 to 1995. The rates were, however, increased slightly on average. Before 1996, an average tax rate increase of 0.5 per cent was negotiated. Besides the change in tax rates, the increased economic activity in society was assumed to increase the tax revenue each year and thereby the economic means of running the health care sector.

During recent years, there has been consistent overspending – or underbudgeting, depending on the point of view – in the counties, due mainly to higher health care spending. As a consequence, the liquidity of the counties has decreased in recent years. For the three years 1993–95, the average deviation between hospital budgets and actual expenditure was 2.5 per cent. For the Public Health Insurance, the average deviation was about 2 per cent.[5]

It is the responsibility of hospital managements to ensure that budget ceilings are respected. Hospital budgets are normally not allowed to exceed the appropriated sum. If the activity has been above average during the beginning of a budget year, a reduction in the activity is usually required during the remaining period. Typically, the intake from a waiting list has been reduced.

In order to solve some of the specific problems causing the high running costs of hospitals in the Copenhagen area, a new hospital authority, the Copenhagen Hospital Cooperation, was created in 1995. The Cooperation has its own board and directors. It owns the hospitals in its area (The National Hospital – which was formerly owned by the state – plus six hospitals in the municipalities of Copenhagen and Frederiksberg). Hospitals on the outskirts of the capital were not included, however, and they are still run by Copenhagen County. The Cooperation is financed from the two municipalities in its area, the state, and from user charges paid by the home county of guest patients who use the hospitals of the Cooperation. The Cooperation has greater freedom of running the hospitals as compared to the political committees in the counties. One of the tasks of the Cooperation has been to reorganize the supply of hospital care, e.g. through amalgamation of identical specialties. As a consequence, the closure of one of the larger hospitals has been decided.

Although the Cooperation has secured a better coordination of supply through reorganization, there still remains some coordination problems between the hospitals belonging to the Cooperation and the nearby hospitals belonging to Copenhagen County.

Non-hospital services are financed through the Public Health Insurance. Providers are paid on a fee-for-service basis (GPs only partly, however) and expenditure depends on the number of services provided. Similarly, drug costs depend on the level of consumption. Hence, the budget is by nature open-ended. For the cost-containment measures, the reader is referred to the sections below on primary health care and drugs.

5.4 Administrative costs

Administrative costs amounted to DKK 600 million in 1994, constituting about 1 per cent of total health care expenditure.[6,7] It is, however, important to note that this figure is an underestimate, because it only includes expenditure with respect to budgeting, financing and planning tasks in the Ministry of Health, the National Board of Health and the health divisions in the counties and municipalities. Administrative costs at the level of provision are not included.

5.5 Hospitals

5.5.1 Public hospital budgets

Since the early 1980s, hospital budgets are determined by each hospital authority (county) as global budgets. Until 1993, the total hospital budget within a county was fixed from the beginning of a budget year. Counties which do not own a highly specialized, regional hospital pay for treatment of their patients at these hospitals when referred. With the introduction of free choice of hospital for patients, an uncontrollable element has been introduced into the counties' budgets, as the home county of a patient must pay for treatment when the patient has chosen a hospital outside his or her home county. Each patient is paid for by the home county at a rate of DKK 2200 per day (1996). An additional amount is paid in cases where the patient receives a very expensive treatment. The payment is received by the county in which the patient is treated, and the treating hospitals do not necessarily receive any reimbursement for the cost of treatment of these guest patients. In practice, most of the patients are acute, and among the non-acute patients it seems that most choose their local hospital (see section 5.9 on Patients' choices).

The size of the county global budgets is heavily influenced by the limits on the total expenditure in each county due to the budget coordination between the state and the local governments. The budgets for the hospital sector and, within this, individual hospitals, are determined through a political negotiation process. Global budgets replaced the former highly specified budget for each hospital. This change took place along with an increased decentralization of economic responsibility. The hospital sector's share of the total health care budget has declined from about 66 to 61 per cent over the period 1985 to 1995.[2]

Capital investments are controlled by various means. Greater investments are made on the basis of a specific appropriation by the county. Smaller investments are made out of the current budget.

Since 1993, the counties have gradually introduced contracts between the county and individual hospitals.[8] The contracts supplement the global budgets and involve management by objectives, but they do not imply any competition among hospitals. The agreed contract includes a specification of objectives, global budget and underlying conditions. The individual hospital may in turn make contracts with each of its departments.

Contracts vary between the counties where they have been introduced. A contract may include the following main elements:[8]

- general objectives of the county and additional general objectives of the individual hospital;

- specific objectives with respect to quantity and quality of production, size of the global budget, and underlying conditions;

- general and specific conditions;

- an appendix specifying departmental activity and set priorities if the number of acute cases changes during the budget year.

The stated quality objectives are related to the production process rather than the outcome of treatment, e.g. statements about maximum waiting times.

The introduction of departmental budgeting was recommended by some public reports in the 1980s. The aim was to increase the association between professional and economic responsibility at the departmental level. However, the introduction of departmental budgets has been relatively slow.

Global budgets do not provide an incentive to increase productivity as such. Due to changes in both input and output, it is uncertain whether productivity has increased during recent years. An agreement in 1993 between the employers and the various unions of professionals resulted in greater flexibility with respect to the planning of the daily running of the hospitals, compared to the former agreement which – with modifications – dated back to 1981. The increased flexibility results from the agreement on the composition of the working hours (normal working hours and duty on call). The agreement implied that more time would be spent during normal working hours and less on duty on call by the young doctors. This is considered to be an improvement for doctors under education as well as for the patients.

The DRG system has not been used in Denmark. A report from the first experiment using DRG for comparing hospital productivity was published in 1996,[9] and a final report in 1996.[10] Whether a case-mix system (like the DRG system) will be introduced to measure and compare hospital productivity will be decided upon by the Ministry of Health.

5.5.2 Public hospitals

In 1994 Denmark had 96 hospitals, including 13 psychiatric hospitals. Among the Danish hospitals 24 are classified as highly specialized hospitals – some with a national or regional coverage of specialties. The rest are 59 local hospitals providing only basic services. Each county has at least one central hospital plus a number of minor hospitals.

Admission to a hospital requires – apart from emergency cases – that the patient is referred from a practising doctor (general practitioner or specialist). When referred, patients have a free choice of hospital within the same level of specialization in the whole country.

During the period 1974–94 there was a steady decrease in bed-days at

278   *Health Care and Cost Containment in the European Union*

Table 5.3 Hospital activity statistics, somatic hospitals, 1974–94

	Bed-days per 1,000 population	Discharges per 1,000 population	Ambulatory visits per 1,000 population	Average length of stay days
1974/75	1,835	166	533 *	11.0 **
1984	1,647	191	675	8.3
1994	1,420	214	871	6.6
Change (%)	-22.6	28.9	63.4	-40.0

* Data from 1975/76. ** Estimated.

Source: Sundhedsstyrelsen: Virksomheden ved sygehusene.[11]

Table 5.4 Hospital activity statistics, psychiatric hospitals, 1974–94

	Bed-days per 1,000 population	Discharges per 1,000 population	Ambulatory visits per 1,000 population
1974/75	703	4.8	15.6 *
1984	485	4.5	16.4
1994	143	2.5	25.7
Change (%)	-79.7	-47.9	60.7

* Data for 1977.

Source: Sundhedsstyrelsen: Virksomheden ved sygehusene.[11]

Table 5.5 Hospitals and hospital beds, 1975–94

	Somatic Hospitals	Beds 1,000 population	Psychiatric Hospitals	Beds 1,000 population
1975	119	6.500	17	1.473
1984	104	5.813	16	0.945
1994	83	4.593	13	0.435
Change (%)	-30.5	-29.9	-23.5	-70.5

Note: Includes private hospitals.

Source: Sundhedsstyrelsen: Virksomheden ved sygehusene.[11]

somatic hospitals, while the number of discharges and ambulatory visits has increased (Table 5.3). A similar, but even more pronounced pattern can be observed in case of psychiatric hospitals (Table 5.4).

The decrease in bed-days follows a decrease in the number of hospitals and hospital beds (Table 5.5). The reduction has taken place primarily in the case of small hospitals with less than three clinical departments, often in the form of hospital mergers with other hospitals in the region, resulting in reduced or changed activities. As a principle, the hospital service in each county should be viewed as a unity, with the possibility of dividing tasks between the hospitals. The period 1974–94 has seen an increased specialization among hospitals. Some local hospitals have specialized in rehabilitation or surgery. The trend is expected to continue.

Decreased length of stay has made room for new patients. Since the lost days are typically less resource-intensive, hospital activities have become more intensive.

Hospital admissions have to a certain extent been substituted by day care or ambulatory care in hospitals, or by private practising specialists. Day care is defined as admissions where monitoring is necessary and available for up to 12 hours. Due to long waiting times for some categories of elective surgery, the focus for development of day care has mainly been within surgery. Of all surgical patients, 82 per cent were admitted to hospitals as in-patients, 6 per cent were admitted as day-care patients, and 12 per cent received ambulatory care in the hospital (1995).[12] The increase in day care admissions and ambulatory care has been especially pronounced for patients within the specialties of ear-nose-throat surgery, orthopaedic surgery and gynaecology.

Registrations of ambulatory and day care activity have frequently been incomplete and the two labels often used for the same activities. As of 1995, the counties have had to report on ambulatory activities. Two-thirds of these concern surgical patients.[12] Among almost 500,000 ambulatory cases in the first half of 1995, 10 per cent required surgery. Ambulatory surgery is used for smaller ex-post treatment and for some acute care. However, operations like eye cataract surgery, knee surgery, sterilization and hernia operations are also undertaken in ambulatory or day care.[12]

The decrease in hospital bed-days has also been accompanied by an increased effort to supply care for discharged patients in the community, in order to allow the earlier discharge of patients to nursing homes or to their own homes, with assistance from visiting nurses. A shortage of community

280 *Health Care and Cost Containment in the European Union*

care remains, however, and there is still need for improvement.

5.5.3 Manpower control

As it is the responsibility of the counties to run the hospitals, and they are given global budgets, there is no explicit manpower control. The supply of manpower is influenced by the limited number of training places for specific professions (doctors, dentists, nurses). Temporary shortages of nurses and some specialists occur.

5.5.4 Waiting lists

Official waiting lists were not established until 1995. Consequently, it is impossible to know whether overall waiting lists have changed over the last few years.

Waiting lists for a number of surgical procedures have been in focus for a number of years. Some extra block grants from the government to the counties have been given with the aim of reducing waiting lists. However, this does not appear to have happened, possibly due to a change in the criteria for being eligible for treatment.

A waiting time guarantee was introduced in 1995 for two types of surgery: knee operations and operations for a slipped disc. If not treated within the time limit, the patient had a right to be treated at another hospital. As a consequence, the rebound effect meant that the waiting time for hip operations increased. The guarantee was abandoned by the end of 1996, as it did not function as expected.

It was expected that a patient's free choice of hospital, introduced in 1995 (see below), would cause a certain levelling out of the lengths of waiting lists across hospitals. Relatively few patients have used this option, however. Various ways of improving the information have been tried. For example in the county of Funen, waiting time for surgical procedures, along with other information on the addresses and opening hours of various services, is available to the GP in an electronic database which is supplied on a computer diskette and regularly updated.

5.5.5 Planning of specialties

The National Board of Health issues guidelines for the planning of specialties.[13] It defines which specialties have the character of national or

Health Care and Cost Containment in Denmark 281

regional specialties, and it determines their location. It is the responsibility of each county to plan hospital services, including the mix of specialties, and to take care of the daily running of hospitals.

The tight economic frames have given the counties an incentive to treat patients in the home county, instead of paying for highly specialized treatment outside the county, and this has led to some duplication of expertise. Thus it has been claimed that at the national level there is some unnecessary duplication of specialties as a consequence of a decentralized system. For example, Denmark has two heart and four kidney transplantation centres. The number of centres could possibly be reduced.[14]

In 1996, an initiative was taken to merge overlapping specialties in the Copenhagen area through an organizational reform made by the Copenhagen Hospital Cooperation. In other counties, some local hospitals have reduced acute medical services outside normal working hours. Currently, some rationalizations are made in the counties to avoid duplication, for example through cooperation between local hospitals. With the aim of coordinating the planning of specialties, such cooperation has been established between counties in three greater areas in Denmark.

5.5.6 Investments in public hospitals

Private investments are not made in the public hospital sector, although some equipment has been donated privately. A report[15] has shown that a substantial part of the medico-technical equipment of hospitals is old, due to low investment in the past (the gap is estimated to DKK 1.8 billion). For the period 1996–2001, the report estimates that the need for investment in medico-technical equipment will be, on average, around DKK 505 million a year, or 1.7 per cent of the total running costs of the hospitals.

But what are the reasons for the past under-investment in new technologies at the hospital level, and an apparently slower rate of adoption of such technologies in Denmark compared to other countries in Europe and the USA? In one governmental report, experts claim that the Danish health care system is conservative in the adoption of new technologies and treatments.[16] The use of global budgeting at the departmental level might be one reason for this conservatism. Studies comparing the diffusion of CT and MRI scanners in the Nordic countries showed this tendency in Denmark and put it down to conservatism among physicians.[15] Furthermore, it could be argued that factors such as the centralization of treatments and technologies, the trend towards fewer and larger hospitals, and the lack of technology as

282   *Health Care and Cost Containment in the European Union*

a parameter of competition in the sector, could explain this apparent lack of innovation.

5.5.7 Private hospitals

There are currently six private hospitals and an additional 16, in which only cosmetic surgery is performed. In total, the private hospitals have 130 beds corresponding to 0.5 per cent of the total number of beds in Danish hospitals. In addition, patient organizations run seven non-profit specialized hospitals with approximately 400 beds.[17] Whereas the counties appear to be somewhat reluctant to collaborate closely with the private hospitals, the non-profit hospitals are well integrated in the public system.

Like the public hospitals, private hospitals are subject to a quality control by the National Board of Health. There is no specific regulation of the private hospital sector.

5.6 Alternatives to hospital care

5.6.1 Private practising specialists

Services provided by the private practising specialists are, as previously mentioned, financed by Public Health Insurance. In 1994, expenditure on these services amounted to 13 per cent of the total Public Health Insurance expenditure.[18] Through the early 1990s, the real growth in expenditure for private practising specialists was greater than that for general practitioners. Over the period 1989–93 the real growth rate for specialist care was 15.5 per cent whereas it was only 7.5 per cent for general practice care.[19]

The county has the responsibility for developing a coordinated plan of all ambulatory specialist services in the county, i.e. provided in hospitals as well as in private practices. For private practising specialists, full remuneration of services is paid up to a certain level of turnover. Beyond this level additional remuneration is reduced by a percentage. The percentage reduction increases with increasing turnover. A maximum ceiling is set, for which no additional payment will be given from the Public Health Insurance, but the ceiling is seldom reached. Further significant deviations from the county or national average in the number of services per patient attending the practice, will lead to an investigation and may result in more specific ceilings being imposed on the number of services or on the

Health Care and Cost Containment in Denmark   283

repayment of fees. In practice, this is very rare.

The number of full-time surgeons in private practice has increased, whereas the number of full-time psychiatrists has decreased.[19] The number of part-time practices has also decreased. These practices are primarily run by physicians who work mainly in hospitals and are often open only a few hours a week. This development is in line with stated policy objectives.

Private practising specialists are increasingly undertaking ambulatory surgery. The number of operations performed by private practising specialists has increased by 24 per cent over the period 1990 to 1995.[18,19] While the increase in the 1980s was primarily in eye surgery, the largest increase in the 1990s has been in orthopaedic surgery and ear, nose and throat surgery.

5.6.2 Community mental health services

For psychiatric patients, community mental health services were established as a complement to, and substitute for, hospital treatment and care in the early 1990s. The services are decentralized and managed by a multi-disciplinary team of professionals whose scope of work is treatment and social work. The reform of the supply of psychiatric treatment and care has been criticized. It is claimed that the capacity of community psychiatric health care is too small to make up for the decrease in psychiatric hospital beds. As the decrease in beds began before the establishment of the community mental health services, there has not really been time to properly develop these services.

5.6.3 Visiting nurses and nursing homes

A well-established visiting nurse organization in the municipalities makes early discharge from hospital possible and may prevent the hospitalization or institutionalization of frailer patients such as the elderly. The municipalities have the responsibility for the provision of care by visiting nurses, nursing homes and other facilities for the elderly. As of 1992, the municipality may choose to delegate the operation of existing facilities to others, who are then accountable to the municipality. The municipality is responsible for the provision of services and for supervising the service provided.

The division of responsibilities between the municipalities which mainly run the social services system, and the counties which run the health care

284 *Health Care and Cost Containment in the European Union*

system, has created some adverse incentives. Some estimated 600–800 patients in hospitals cannot be discharged due to a shortage of nursing homes and other facilities financed by the municipalities.[20] On the other hand, municipalities pay sickness benefits for some patients waiting for hospital treatment. In 1992, the counties were allowed to demand payment from municipalities for somatic patients who could not be discharged due to a shortage of suitable municipal services. From 1992 to 1994 a reduction in the number of non-dischargable somatic patients occurred.[20] The maximum payment allowed was increased in 1995, and at the same time the right to demand payment was expanded to psychiatric patients.

Since 1994 each county and its municipalities are required to develop a health plan every fourth year. The objective is to have common rules concerning cooperation and planning for all parts of the municipal and county health care service, preventive as well as curative.

5.7 Primary health care sector

General practitioners are the gatekeepers to the health care system and, in principle, the coordinators of patient care. Information on treatment and discharge from higher levels of care should therefore be sent to and kept by the GP. Patients cannot in general choose the level of care at which they receive treatment, although there are some possibilities for opting out (see section below on Patients' choices). GPs can refer patients to hospital or to a private practising specialist.

The GPs work in private practices, on their own or in small group practices. The capacity of the primary care system is regulated through practice planning. The number of practices allowed to bill the Public Health Insurance is tightly controlled and is regulated by the population per GP within fairly small geographical areas.[21] The average population per GP has been fairly stable, around 1600 during the early 1990s.[19]

While hospital physicians are paid a salary and private practising specialists are paid a fee-for-service, general practitioners are paid partly by capitation and partly through fees-for-service. Capitation fees are paid for all patients listed with the GP. Until 1996 children were listed together with one of their parents with no additional capitation fee. Since 1996 children have been listed separately and capitation fees gradually adjusted so that the total capitation payment per capita remains unchanged. The income from capitation fees amounts to approximately one-third of a GP's total income.[19] Every contact between patient and GP results in a fee-for-service payment. Basic fees are paid according to the type of contact (consultation, telephone, home visit) and supplementary fees are paid for additional services depending on the nature of the visit.

Collective agreements, including payment for non-hospital care, are negotiated between the Public Health Insurance and the provider organizations regularly. Expenditures and activities of GPs are monitored by a committee which represents the county and the GPs.[21] Deviations from the county average, in terms of expenditure per patient, by 25 per cent, or in terms of services per patient, by 40 per cent, lead to an investigation which may result in a ceiling for the Public Health Insurance payment to the practice. Less than 1 per cent of practices are subject to these sanctions.[22]

5.8 Changes in the GP agreements

Until 1987, the GPs in the city of Copenhagen were paid purely on a capitation basis, whereas GPs in the rest of the country were paid according to the combined capitation and fee-for-service system described above. Since 1987 the latter remuneration method has been used in the whole country. The effects have been described elsewhere.[22,23] The changes in services provided by GPs in the city of Copenhagen were measured and compared to the changes in the surrounding county of Copenhagen (which was not affected by the payment system change). The number of prescription renewals and referrals to secondary care decreased significantly more in the city than in the county. The number of diagnostic services provided increased significantly more in the city, as did the number of curative services. The latter, however, stabilized after a year.[22,23]

In 1991, the agreement between the Public Health Insurance and the Organisation of General Practitioners in Denmark (PLO) included some major changes in the relative price structure, in the limitations of expenditure, and in out-of-hours services.[24]

In the agreement, priority was given to face-to-face rather than telephone contact, and remuneration for renewals of prescriptions was discarded. The price structure for basic services was changed as presented in Table 5.6, overleaf.

In light of the changes in the fee structure, the parties agreed on a 4 per cent limit to the growth in consultation expenditure at county level. Also, the total expenditure for the years 1991–93 was frozen at the 1990-level

286 *Health Care and Cost Containment in the European Union*

Table 5.6 Strucure of basic fees for GPs, 1988 and 1991

	Fee in DKK		Fee relative to consultation fee	
	1988	*1991*	*1988*	*1991*
Consultations	33	80	1.0	1.0
Telephone consultations	19	20	0.6	0.25
Renewal of prescriptions	15	0	0.45	0.0
Home visits (within 4 km)*	59	114	1.79	1.42

* The fee increases with increasing distance.

Sources: Praktiserende Lægers Organisation. *Landsoverenskomsten,* 1991 and 1988.[24,25]

Table 5.7 Distribution of services in terms of type of contact, 1989 and 1993

	Million Services	
	1989	*1993*
Consultations	13.4	15.2
Telephone consultations	9.7	10.9
Renewal of prescriptions	3.1	—
Home visits (within 4 km)*	1.9	2.6
Total	28.1	28.7

Sources: Sygesikringens Forhandlingsudvalg. Personal communication.[18]
Sygesikringsstatistik 1991. Sygesikringens Forhandlingsudvalg.[26]

with adjustment for demographical changes, price index regulation of fees and transfer of services to general practice due to activity changes in municipalities and counties. If these limits were exceeded without justification, negotiations for repayment were to be undertaken at county level.

Despite the removal of the fee-for-prescription renewals – and hence the registration of the activity as a service – the total number of services registered did not change except for a slight increase from 28.2 million to 28.7 million (1989–93) as presented in Table 5.7.[18,19] The removal of this fee was intended to create a disincentive to needless renewals in favour of a more thorough review.

Due to the change in fees, a shift in the distribution of services in terms of the nature of visits, towards relatively more consultations is likely. In 1989 consultations amounted to 48 per cent of all services, whereas that share had increased to 53 per cent by 1993. Renewals in 1989 may be categorized with telephone consultations, in which case the structure is seen to have changed as expected towards relatively more consultations, slightly more home visits and fewer telephone consultations. Home visits changed from being almost only home visits to being half that and half telephone consultations followed by home visits. The shift away from the cheaper telephone consultations and prescription renewals tended to increase the cost of the system.

The maximum yearly growth rate of 4 per cent in consultations was exceeded in 1992 and 1993 by a total of about DKK 70 million.[21] The renegotiations resulted in the partial repayment of 50 per cent of this amount, as the GPs were able to give several justifying reasons for the excessive increase: increases in tasks transferred from the hospitals to general practices in terms of pre-admission tests and follow-up controls, increases in early discharges from hospitals and ambulatory care, and unusually severe epidemics during the winter of 1992/93. The validity of these arguments is difficult to determine.

Finally, the out-of-hours services were also changed dramatically from 1992. Before that, the out-of-hours services were usually organized within smaller areas of up to 10,000 patients. In addition to service fees there was an hourly payment dependent on population size. In some cities, larger areas of up to 48,000 patients were covered in an organization which included a visitation system with an hourly payment for the visiting doctor.[25]

In the 1991 agreement between the Public Health Insurance and the Organization of General Practioners in Denmark, the system of larger organizations for out-of-hours services with visitation was generally expanded to the whole country. The place of service was centralized and was often placed at a hospital. The number of GPs on duty outside normal hours was dramatically reduced. The hourly payment was removed. The fees-for-services provided out-of-hours were largely unchanged, except for home visits for which the fee was increased by 50 per cent (due to greater distances).

However, the objective of shifting contacts towards the daytime does

288 *Health Care and Cost Containment in the European Union*

not appear to have been successful. The number of basic services provided outside of normal hours was 9 per cent of total basic services in 1989.[19] This percentage had increased to 12 per cent by 1994.[18] Relatively, home visits have been reduced and telephone consultations increased.

There are several explanations for the increase in out-of-hours services. There is some evidence that the distribution of work between emergency units and general practices has shifted towards more treatments in general practices outside normal opening hours.[27,28] The marginal cost of treating the patient immediately, rather than referring him of her for treatment by a personal GP the next day, has decreased for GPs on duty (the GP is placed in a central unit when on call rather than at home) and the marginal benefit of doing so has increased. The fee contributes relatively more to income, since the hourly payment is discarded, and the likelihood that the patient can be referred to his or her own practice for treatment the following day has decreased.

5.9 Patients' choices

Patients are free to choose between two types of public health plans. The Group 1 health plan allows treatment in general practice at no charge. The choice of general practitioner is limited to a restricted, geographically-determined set of providers. After a minimum enlistment of six months, patients can change their GP. Not many patients do, however. The loyalty towards the family doctor appears to be considerable. Free treatment at a private practising specialist requires referral from a GP. When referred, the patient can choose any specialist who has an agreement with the Public Health Insurance. Services by a physician who does not have an agreement with the Public Health Insurance is paid solely by the patient. The Group 2 health plan allows free choice of both GP and private practising specialist. Payment for services is only partly reimbursed by the Public Health Insurance and physicians are allowed to extra-bill. Less than 3 per cent of the population has chosen the latter health plan.[19]

Until 1992 the hospital referral system was characterized by very strict referral rules, depending on geographical location and treatment needs. From 1993, the dependency on geographical location was removed. Except for some highly specialized hospital services, patients may now choose their hospital regardless of catchment area. In practice, consumer choice is, however, only relevant for non-acute referrals by GPs or private practising

Health Care and Cost Containment in Denmark 289

specialists to non-specialized hospitals. Any change due to consumer choice within the county is not registered. In 1994, the non-acute admissions to non-specialized hospitals by GPs and private practising specialists outside home counties amounted to about 1 per cent of all hospital admissions.[29] It may be the case, therefore, that patients are very loyal to their local hospital and that distance to the hospital seems to be a more important determinant of hospital choice than short waiting time.

5.10 Cost sharing in the Danish health care sector

In 1995 Danish patients paid about DKK 10.6 billion in different cost-sharing arrangements, corresponding to 18.4 per cent of total health care expenditure (Table 5.8).

Table 5.8 Estimated cost sharing in Denmark as a percentage of total health care expenditures, 1986–95

	1986	1987	1988	1989	1990	1991	1992	1993	1994	1995
%	14.6	15.9	16.6	17.1	18.0	17.6	18.0	17.3	17.4	18.4

Source: MEFA, various years.[3]

Cost-sharing applies to services that traditionally contain some out-of-pocket payments: pharmaceutical consumption in the primary health care sector, dental care, eye-glasses, auxiliary services and treatments by physiotherapists and chiropractors. No major changes have been made since 1990.

Pensioners, low-income families and disabled persons are, to some degree, exempt from co-payments, particularly with regard to the consumption of pharmaceuticals or dental care. The criteria for exemption or reduced co-payments are income, wealth or illness.

Decisions on who should be exempted from what, are taken by the municipalities according to the social legislation, and are often based on individual criteria. Therefore, variations exist between the municipalities. It is also possible to have individual reimbursement for drugs, after application to the National Board of Health. The common feature for

290   *Health Care and Cost Containment in the European Union*

exemption or reduced co-payments is that there should be a recommendation from either a GP or a dentist.

5.11 Dental care

In Denmark dental care is provided by dentists in private practice. For people below 18 years all dental care is free. These services are financed by the municipalities. For people older than 18 years cost sharing applies in the area of 35 per cent to 100 per cent dependent on the service supplied, Table 5.9.

Table 5.9 Cost-sharing arrangements for dental services

Cost-sharing	Services	Price-setting
100%	X-rays, dentures	Negotiated
35% (18–25 years)	Clinical and some extended diagnostic examinations, some preventive services	
55% (25 years +)	Examinations and scaling	
60%	Other services	
Various according to flat rate reimbursement	Operations, some fillings, surgical periodontal treatments	Free

Source: Rudbeck B *et al.*, 1995.[30]

It follows that cost sharing for dental services depends on the service supplied and the age of the patient. The dentist has the possibility for a free price setting for some services. Prices for other services are negotiated between the Public Health Insurance and the dentists.

Overall, patients financed about 75 per cent of dentist incomes in 1994 while the Public Health Insurance financed about 23 per cent (Table 5.10). Two per cent were financed through other means, e.g. services normally supplied by school dental services covered by the municipalities. The cost sharing has increased gradually since 1978 when patients' co-insurance rate was about 53 per cent.

Health Care and Cost Containment in Denmark 291

Table 5.10 Patients' cost-sharing as a percentage of total turnover by dentists, 1986–94

	1986	1988	1990	1992	1994
Patients' cost-sharing (%)	65.4	66.7	69.6	72.0	74.9
Public Health Insurance (%)	33.3	30.2	26.7	25.0	22.6
Other (%)	1.3	3.1	3.7	3.0	2.5
Total turnover (DKK billion)	–	3.0	–	3.8	4.1

Source: Holt, 1997 [31]

5.12 Drugs

5.12.1 The reimbursement scheme for prescription drugs

As seen from Table 5.11, the total consumption of prescription drugs in primary health care was about DKK 5,000 million in 1995 (including VAT and excluding prescription charges), or about 9 per cent of total health care expenditure. Consumption of pharmaceuticals placed on the reimbursement list receives a proportional public reimbursement rate (co-insurance) of 100,

Table 5.11 Consumption of prescription drugs in primary health care, 1987–95

Reimbursement group	Consumer prices DKK million, including VAT, excluding prescription charges			
	1987	1990	1992	1995
100%*	-	138	144	155
75%	1,993	2,365	2,956	3,003
50%	719	601	849	867
0%	734	964	1,065	979
Total	3,446	4,068	5,014	5,004
Share of total health care expenditure (%)	7.8	7.9	8.8	8.6

* Total public financing of some insulin-products was introduced in 1990.

Source: MEFA, various years.[3]

292 Health Care and Cost Containment in the European Union

75, 50 or 0 per cent. The reimbursement rate breakdown is as follows: 100 per cent for insulin and related products; 75 per cent for products towards the treatment of life-threatening diseases; and 50 per cent for products with a valuable and well-defined therapeutic effect

The general reimbursement scheme administered by the counties finances approximately 72.5 per cent of total consumption of prescription drugs in Denmark. Municipalities finance about 7.7 per cent, as they partly cover the consumption of drugs by pensioners, low-income families and disabled persons according to social legislation. Disregarding reimbursement from private insurance, patients' cost-sharing is about 19.8 per cent for prescription drugs. There is no direct price control of pharmaceuticals in Denmark.

5.12.2 Initiatives regarding the pharmaceutical market

Consumers pay the full price for over-the-counter drugs (about DKK 1,300 million in 1995). This has been in effect since 1984, until when some OTC drugs still received general public reimbursement. During the last decades, efforts have been made to lower the growth in public expenditure on pharmaceuticals by: reducing the number of products allowed for public reimbursement, removing drugs to a lower reimbursement level, and stimulating price competition in the market by introducing reference prices, generic prescription and the parallel importation of drugs.

A *deductible* was introduced in July 1989. Consumption of prescription drugs below a yearly payment of DKK 800 was no longer reimbursed. The effect was public savings of approximately DKK 800 million per year. The deductible was abolished in January 1991 due to public resistance.

Generic prescription as another measure to control public expenditures on pharmaceuticals was introduced in 1991. Generic prescription in Denmark means that GPs add the letter G to the prescription, and the pharmacy is then responsible for finding the cheapest product within a certain price range. The GPs are consequently more aware of drug prices, but very often already prescribe the cheapest products.[32,33]

Reference prices were introduced into the Danish reimbursement scheme in 1993. The reference price in Denmark is the average of the two cheapest drugs in a group of synonymous products, defined according to ATC-level

Health Care and Cost Containment in Denmark   293

five (Anatomical Therapeutic Chemical Classification System). This means that if consumers want more expensive drugs they have to pay a relatively larger out-of-pocket amount. In 1993 about 389 of 2256 registered drugs were influenced by reference prices (31 per cent of total turnover). The effect is reflected by the price changes in 1993: prices for 48 per cent of all packets decreased, 40 per cent were unchanged and only 12 per cent showed increased prices.[34]

The parallel importation of drugs has been allowed in Denmark since 1990. The parallel import of drugs is affected by several factors. First, drug prices in Denmark are relatively high compared with other European countries with direct public price controls. Secondly, initiatives like generic prescribing and reference prices give incentives to import drugs from low price countries. Thirdly, general cost containment strategies influence the demand towards the cheapest (synonymous) drugs.

Price agreements are also used as a cost-controlling measure. A voluntary agreement was established between the Danish Ministry of Health and the pharmaceutical organizations not to raise prices over a period of 15 months (between January 1994 and April 1995). Another agreement of general reductions in prices of 5 per cent for pharmaceuticals with public reimbursement and 2 per cent for all other drugs followed (May 1995 to April 1997). One reason for these agreements was that following the introduction of the reference price system in 1993, prices increased for drugs not regulated by the reference prices, e.g. OTC drugs and products with no direct generic substitutes.

Overall, there is no doubt about the price reducing mechanism in the reference price system. Since 1990, consumer prices have fallen by 15 per cent. Generic prescriptions and parallel imported drugs may also have contributed to the same pattern. As different mechanisms are working at the same time, it is difficult to separate the individual effects.

5.13 Private health insurance

Private health insurance plays a minor role in Denmark. Only one private health insurance organization exists – Sygeforsikringen 'Danmark' – which, as a non-actuarial and non-profit-making organization, provides supplemen-

294 *Health Care and Cost Containment in the European Union*

tary insurance to a varying degree, for most patient co-payments. In 1995 'Danmark' had 1.4 million members [35] – 27 per cent of the total population. A study of the members of 'Danmark' has clearly shown a positive correlation between income and membership.[36] The funds come from fixed individual contributions without the possibility of tax allowance. Due to the large amount of patient co-payment in Denmark there are obvious insurance incentives to join 'Danmark'. However 'Danmark's' share of the total population's co-payment was only 12 per cent on average in 1993.[37] One reason for this minor share of co-payment is that 'Danmark' has many healthy members (patients with chronic disease cannot become members unless they were enrolled before the onset of their disease). Another explanation is that the coverage varies depending on which of the insurance groups the member belongs to. More than two-thirds are members of insurance group five, which only secures a coverage rate of half the co-payment on prescription drugs. By not interfering in the negotiation between the Public Health Insurance and the suppliers, 'danmark' has not had any direct impact on cost-containment initiatives.

5.14 New technology

Evaluation of technologies already in use in Denmark is not required. With respect to new technologies, a systematic (clinical) evaluation of the technology (efficacy and safety) is only required in the approval for the market of new pharmaceuticals. Medical devices are only regulated by the gradual implementation of a European Commission Directive focusing on safety.[38] An indirect control of hospital equipment occurs through the national guidelines for specialty planning.

Economic evaluations are not yet a part of the systematic assessment policy regarding medical technologies. However, some sparse and uncoordinated economic evaluations are performed. In 1995, an expert group [39] recommended that, if a cost-effectiveness criterion should be part of the future reimbursement decisions of new drugs, then a set of evaluation guidelines is needed. Economic evaluations, however, were not recommended for use in the public regulation of drug prices.

Health technology assessment (HTA) in Denmark was first discussed in 1980,[40] and several HTA-committees have been established since then. A breakthrough, however, did not occur until 1994 when the Health Technology Assessment Committee of the Danish Board of Health was

Health Care and Cost Containment in Denmark   295

established. In 1996 the committee launched a national strategy for HTA.[41] As a result, a national HTA institute under the National Board of Health – the Danish Institute for Health Technology Assessment (DIHTA) – was created in 1997 with an annual budget of DKK 25 million.[42] The aim of DIHTA is to initiate and support HTAs as well as to create an early warning system for emerging health technologies.

It is important to emphasize that HTA in Denmark does not solely focus upon cost issues. The definition of HTA is broader than this single economic issue, as it is considered to be a comprehensive and systematic assessment that includes clinical issues as well as organizational and patient-related questions. This is consistent with the purpose of HTA in Denmark as a planning and priority-setting tool aiming to secure the use of technologies that are evidence-based and accepted by the health professionals as well as by the public.

In the future it is likely that a wider dissemination of economic evaluation and HTA in decision-making will be seen.

5.15 Quality assurance – practice guidelines

A national Strategy for Continuous Quality Development was formulated in 1993. According to the recommendations, the counties and municipalities must include quality measures in their goals for their health plans. Moreover, the plans must include guidelines for the fulfilment of the goals.[43]

The National Board of Health has developed prototypes of practice guidelines (Reference Programmes) with the purpose of achieving decentralized implementation and use of these guidelines.[44] Furthermore, the medical societies have promoted and developed practice guidelines.

5.16 Equity issues

The emphasis on free and equal access to health care is a fundamental value in Danish health policy. Thus, there is global health insurance for all permanent residents of the country. No fee is paid for visiting a GP or – when referred – for treatment by a practising specialist or hospital treatment. There are, however, substantial user-charges for prescribed medicine, dental care and physiotherapy. In general, user-charges weigh relatively heavily on lower income groups. The overall financing in

296 *Health Care and Cost Containment in the European Union*

Denmark is, however, almost neutral as total payment to health care is about proportional to income.[45] Equal geographical access to basic as well as specialist treatment have also been targeted.

5.17 Recent proposals

Hospital service and efficiency has been publicly debated for a long time in Denmark. In late 1995 the government appointed a Hospital Commission with the task of evaluating the present system and recommending changes that would improve the quality and efficiency of services. A report was published in January 1997.[46] Among the problems and challenges found in the hospital sector were management and control, organization of the daily work and borderlines between professions, problems related to the clinical education of doctors, long waiting times and unsatisfactory coherence in the treatment of patients, and need for an increase in the number of hospital services in the future. Some of the major recommendations of the Commission will briefly be presented in following.

Global budgeting should remain but be supplemented with both financial and non-financial incentives for clinical departments and/or individuals to improve activity. Free choice of hospital, as an incentive to improve services, should be expanded to the highly specialized hospitals. The capacity of these hospitals should, however, not be expanded on this account. Contracts as a supplement to global budgets should be further developed and should, for example, specify punishments for breaking the contract. More experiences should also be sought with a supplier-provider split which gives hospitals more freedom in daily planning and operation.

Fees for patients who are receiving treatment outside their home county should be based on treatment episodes rather than per diem, and they should be differentiated according to diagnosis. Basic treatment fees should correspond to average variable costs, while fees for treatment at a highly specialized level should also include fixed costs, because hospital capacity is planned to allow treatment of patients from other counties. Current work on the development of a Danish case-mix system (a DRG system) should be continued with the purpose of obtaining differentiated fees for episodes of treatment.

The required number of beds is expected to decrease in the future due to increased use of ambulatory services. Some of the highly specialized functions should be combined to ensure high quality service, and quality considerations should be emphasized when it comes to choosing between centralizing or decentralizing highly specialized treatments.

A better division of work and better coordination between counties may also improve the system. Whether or not to maintain the relatively high number of departments in some of the larger hospitals must be reconsidered. The number of smaller hospitals cannot be maintained in their present form. Surgical functions at minor hospitals may be changed to elective surgery only, or such hospitals may be transformed to centres for rehabilitation or local health centres. Acute duty for the general population is currently taken care of by GPs on call and hospital emergency departments; these two functions should be merged.

Some decentralization of management to the departmental level has taken place, but effective information systems to support this decentralization have not yet been developed to a satisfactory extent and require further development.

Municipalities should increase their capacity to care for patients, e.g. through acute beds in nursing homes. This may reduce the number of hospitalizations and also speed up hospital discharges. Counties should be able to take part in the financing of such activities.

To avoid unacceptable waiting times, differentiation with respect to maximum waiting times for different types of patients is recommended. Generally, the gravity of a patient's condition, possibly together with capacity considerations, should be reflected. Use of a booking system is also recommended. Coherence of treatment episodes between all levels of care, i.e. within a hospital as well as between different providers, is emphasized. The task force refers to 'the patient focused hospital' where each patient is allocated a personal doctor and nurse. For professionals involved with surgical departments, working hours should, within certain limits, be variable without prior warning, so that planned operations are not cancelled.

During the 1980s, investment in health care was low, and should now be increased, particularly as much of the equipment is worn out and in need of renewal. Health technology assessment should be used to a greater extent.

Various counties have already tried a number of these suggestions on an experimental basis. The Commission recommends that such experiments are further expanded. The general conclusion is that by employing a broad range of initiatives, there is a good chance of improving the level of quality and service, while at the same time increasing efficiency. Although there are certain areas where problems can be identified, Danish hospitals currently

298 *Health Care and Cost Containment in the European Union*

function in a manner similar to hospitals in most Western European countries.

5.18 Concluding remarks

As it is predominantly tax-financed, the Danish health care system has its merits in terms of equity and access. From a cost-containment point of view the budget cooperation has been a success in spite of a system which is decentralized.

A 1994 public report [47] concluded that although there may be problems of delimitation of the health care sector in international comparisons, Denmark is among the OECD countries who use the smallest share of GNP on this sector. Moreover, in contrast to most other OECD countries, the share in Denmark has been decreasing since the middle of the 1970s. Despite this, when capacity and activity are compared internationally, Denmark does not rank especially low. The reason for this is because of the Danish system of controlling the health care sector: the counties and communities have almost sole responsibility for financing health care. This has made expenditure control through global budgeting possible, in contrast to a system based on the reimbursement of costs.

The government is in the unique position of being able to control costs without being held directly responsible. Priority-setting between the supply of health services and other locally administered services is the responsibility of the local governments. The political cost to the government of constraining the local budgets is relatively low and may have resulted in a relatively higher priority being placed on services for which the government is directly responsible.

In the 1980s, yearly increases in (especially) hospital budgets were replaced by almost constant budgets in fixed prices, with an average increase of about 0.5 per cent per annum. This occurred at a point in time where treatment possibilities increased – some at increasing costs. The stabilization has been perceived by much of the health care personnel and the population as a direct reduction of budgets, and it is fair to say that it has resulted in dissatisfaction, especially among hospital personnel. This dissatisfaction has not, however, been reflected in surveys of patient satisfaction. Nonetheless, despite this long period of almost constant budgets, there is without doubt still room for productivity improvements.

From the patient's point of view, the public hospitals are almost in a

Health Care and Cost Containment in Denmark 299

monopoly situation. Patients on waiting lists for surgery may in principle choose a private hospital. They must, however, pay the total price for treatment (in addition to their tax payment for health care purposes), so this option is only used by a very small percentage of patients. Patients can, however, choose between public hospitals, when referred. The choice is limited to hospitals at the same level of specialization as the one he or she was originally referred to. Within primary health care, patients may choose between doctors within a restricted geographical area. Generally, patients have a fairly free choice within a given level of care, but not between levels of care.

Whether the Danes are spending too little on health care is difficult to determine. The increase in life expectancy has been the lowest among OECD countries in the period 1980–90.[48] A task force concluded that this could be attributed to life style rather than lack of health care.[49] The conclusion has, however, been challenged as it has been shown that health care expenditures have an effect on the mortality rate and hence on the expected length of life.[50]

A recent report by a group of experts[51] was critical of the consequences of the current tight control over expenditure on health care in Denmark. It was pointed out that professional development has been neglected to a certain extent, and it has not been possible to meet demand, as witnessed by the existing length of waiting lists.

References

1 Alban A, Grønvald LF. Health care in Denmark. In: Alban A, Christiansen T (eds). *The Nordic Lights. New Initiatives in Health Care Systems.* Odense University Press, 1995.

2 *Danmarks Statistik: Statistisk Årbog* (Statistical Yearbook). København, various years.

3 MEFA. *Facts.* København: MEFA, various years.

4 Indenrigsministeriet. *Den Kommunale Økonomi 1993–1994–1995.* Skøn. København, 1994.

5 Finansministeriet. *Kommunal Budgetoversigt.* København, 1994 and 1995.

6 Amtsrådsforeningen. *Amternes Økonomi.* Budget '96. København, 1996.

7 Finansministeriet, Budgetdepartementet. *Finansstatistikken 1992.* København, 1992.

8 Alban A, Jeppesen JOS. From global budgets to contracts. In: Alban A, Christiansen T (eds.). *The Nordic Lights. New Initiatives in Health Care Systems.* Odense University Press, 1995.

9 Sundhedsministeriet. *Måling af Produktivitet på Sygehusene.* København, 1996.

300   *Health Care and Cost Containment in the European Union*

10   Sundhedsministeriet. *Måling af Danske Sygehuses Produktivitet.* København, 1996.

11   Sundhedsstyrelsen. *Virksomheden ved Sygehusene.* København, various volumes and years.

12   Sundhedsministeriet. *Månedstal for Sundhedsvæsen.* København, February 1995.

13   Sundhedsstyrelsen. *Specialeplanlægning og Lands- og Landsdelsfunktioner i Sygehus-væsenet.* Vejledning, 1996.

14   Varder J. Interview in *Det Fri Aktuelt* 29.4.1996.

15   Jørgensen T, Danneskiold-Samsøe B. *Investeringer i Sygehusenes Medicinske Udstyr.* Dansk Sygehus Institut. Institut for Sundhedsvæsen. DSI Rapport 95.05. København, 1995.

16   Erhvervsfremmestyrelsen. *Medico/Sundhed – en Erhvervsøkonomisk Analyse.* København, 1993.

17   Lægeforeningens vejviser 1996. *Lægeforeningens Forlag.* København, 1996.

18   Sygesikringens Forhandlingsudvalg. *Personal communication,* 1997.

19   Sygesikringens Forhandlingsudvalg. *Sygesikringsstatistik.* Various volumes.

20   Amtsrådsforeningen. *Personal communication,* 1997.

21   Praktiserende Lægers Organisation. *Landsoverenskomsten.* København, 1995.

22   Johansen AS. Primary Care in Denmark. In: Alban A, Christiansen T (eds). *The Nordic Lights. New Initiatives in Health Care Systems.* Odense University Press, 1995.

23   Krasnik A, Groenewegen PP, Pedersen PA, Scholten Pv, Mooney G, Gottschau A, Flierman HA, Damsgaard MT. Practice observed. Changing remuneration systems: effects on activity in general practice. *British Medical Journal* 1990;300:1698–701.

24   Praktiserende Lægers Organisation. *Landsoverenskomsten.* København, 1991.

25   Praktiserende Lægers Organisation. *Landsoverenskomsten.* København, 1988.

26   *Sygesikringsstatistik 1991.* Sygesikringens Forhandlingsudvalg, København.

27   Hansen TB, Kristensen KA, Breddam Poulsen M, Gravers M, Laursen CN, Ross-Hansen KM. Ændres fordelingen af skadebehandlingen i Ringkøbing Amt mellem almen praksis og skadestue ved etablering af storvagtkredse for alment praktiserende læger? *Ugeskrift for Læger* 156(27);1994:4032–35.

28   Rasmussen SW, Thomsen H, Jensen P, Angermann PP, Appelquist E. Skadestuehenvendelser for og efter ændring af vagtlægeordningen. *Ugeskrift for Læger* 156(35);1994:4968–71.

29   Sundhedsministeriet. *Månedstal for Sundhedsvæsen,* No. 2, 1995.

30   Rudbeck B, Knudsen MS, Gyldmark M, Alban A. *Brugerbetaling i Sundhedsvæsenet - Kortlægning og Analyse.* Dansk Sygehus Institut. København, 1995.

31   Holt C. *Danish Dental Association.* Personal communication, 1997.

32   Nielsen HB. Generisk substitution er en succes. *Ugeskrift for Læger.* 1993;155:134.

33   Neymark N, Jessen HC. *Generisk Substitution – en Spørgeskemaundersøgelse af Praktiserende Lægers og Apotekers Holdninger til og Erfaringer med det nye Ordinationsprincip.* AKF Forlaget. København, 1992.

Health Care and Cost Containment in Denmark 301

34 Finansministeriet. *Udviklingen i Medicinudgifterne.* Finansministeriet, Sundhedsministeriet o.a. København, 1994.

35 Sygeforsikringen 'danmark'. *Årsberetning 1995.* København, 1996.

36 Pedersen KM. Sundhedsøkonomiske grundproblemstillinger; forbindelse med
brugerbetaling. In: Andersen P, Christiansen T (eds). *Brugerbetaling i
Sundhedssektoren. Teori, Viden, Holdninger.* Odense Unversitetsforlag, 1990.

37 Sygeforsikringen 'danmark'. *Kort fortalt.* København, 1995.

38 European Commission Directive (93/42/EEC). 1993.

39 Sundhedsstyrelsen. *Sundhedsøkonomiske Analyser af Lægemidler. - en Gennemgang af
Metoder og Problemstillinger ved Implementering i Beslutningsprocesser.* København,
1995.

40 Buch Andreasen P. *Medicinsk Teknologivurdering. Nyttiggørelse af lægevidenskabelige
forskningsresultater i sundhedsvæsenet. Rapport til Folketingets udvalg angående
videnskabelig forskning.* København, 1980.

41 Sundhedsstyrelsen. *National Strategi for Medicinsk Teknologivurdering.* København,
1996.

42 *Sundhedsministeriets Afsluttende Ændringsforslag til Finanslovforslaget for 1997.*

43 Sundhedsstyrelsen. *National Strategi for Kvalitetsudvikling i Sundhedsvæsenet.* København, 1993.

44 Sundhedsstyrelsen. *Referenceprogrammer - En vej til Kvalitet.* København, 1992.

45 Christiansen T. Denmark. In: van Doorslaer E, Wagstaff A, Rutten F. (eds). *Equity in the
Finance and Delivery of Health Care. An International Perspective.* Oxford Medical
Publications, 1993.

46 Sundhedsministeriet. *Sygehuskommissionens Betænkning.* København, 1997.

47 Sundhedsministeriet. *Rapport fra Udvalget Vedrørende Sygehusenes Økonomi.*
København, 1994.

48 OECD. *OECD Health Data.* Paris: OECD, 1997.

49 Sundhedsministeriet. *Sundhedsministeries Middellevetidsudvalg: Middellevetid og Dø-
delighed.* København, 1994.

50 Søgaard J. *Analyse af Middel- og Restlevetider i OECD Landene 1970 til 1989.* CHS
Arbejdsnotat 1996:8. Odense Universitet.

51 Perdersen KM el al. *Et Bedre Sundhedavæsen – Men Hvordan?* København, 1995.

6 Cost containment in Germany: twenty years experience

REINHARD BUSSE AND CHRIS HOWORTH

6.1 The German system

The German health care system is organized around a tri-partite system of a statutory and social insurance (the so called 'Bismarck system') which covers nearly 90 per cent of the population. The three main groups involved are: the federal government which sets the framework within which the other parties operate and which has recently tried to set overall financial constraints, the state governments which have the decision-making control over investment in the hospital sector, and the corporate bodies representing the sickness funds, the physicians and dentists all of which are constituted under regulations covering public ('corporate') bodies. Additional to this group are the hospitals associations which, although they perform similar representative functions as the other representative bodies, do not enjoy the public incorporation and have limited rights concerning negotiations within the frame of the statutory health insurance (*Gesetzliche Kranken-Versicherung*, GKV). Operational control is exercised through a process of negotiations between the sickness funds and service providers.[1] The structural framework set out by the federal government is mainly contained in the Imperial Insurance Regulation (*Reichs-Versicherungs-Ordnung*, RVO) and later in the Social Code Book V (*Sozial-Gesetz-Buch*, SGB V) which has largely replaced the RVO parts dealing with health insurance since 1989.[2]

The three main actors with which the patient has direct contact (sickness fund, office-based physician and hospital) are sharply separated in contrast to a 'National Health Service' (or Beveridge) model. Office-based specialists provide many of the services which in the NHS system are provided by hospital out-patient departments. Sickness funds as bodies separate from the service providers (only the miners' fund has the right to operate its own health care institutions) result in an automatic purchaser–provider split within the system. These features have impacts both on the methods of cost containment and the areas of expenditure strain. For example, the division between providers and sickness funds has established the principle of negotiation between purchaser and provider, enabling these discussions (although not without some pain) to encompass decisions concerning the benefits' catalogue and pricing of items contained in it more easily than may be the case in a unitary system. At the same time, the split between stationary care and specialist ambulatory care has resulted in a requirement for greater levels of investment in medical technology and a subsequent higher level of diagnostic procedures. A good proportion of diagnostic procedures carried out in the ambulatory sector are also repeated after the patients have become in-patients.

In the late 1960s and early 1970s, a public and political debate came to the conclusion that Germany needed more physicians and a better equipped health system. The foundation of new medical schools and the Hospital Financing Act of 1972 were results of that debate; with the latter regulating hospital investments and remuneration. These measures were successful: Germany had more doctors and more modern hospitals. Of course, health care expenditure increased rapidly as well – from less than 6 per cent of GDP to over 8 per cent, which was largely due to increased expenditure for hospital treatment. The term 'cost explosion' was born, entered into the political vocabulary and led to a series of laws intended to contain sickness fund expenditure since 1977 (see below).

The German health care system has been largely free of any explicit rationing measures, and even now explicit rationing is restricted to the pharmaceutical market (negative list – SGB V §34), and dentistry (cosmetic orthodontics, 'major dental work' and crowns and dentures in the future for the over 18s – SGB V §29 and 30). There are few sections of the population excluded from the health provision package (and these are usually privately insured) and decisions on the benefits package at a central level are inclusive rather than exclusive. At the regional (ambulatory and dental care) or local (hospital) negotiating level, decisions over the services are made between sickness funds and providers on the basis of available skills and equipment rather than rationing criteria. This is evidenced in the fact that waiting lists in Germany are largely confined to transplant surgery where the scarcity of organs for transplant rather than the scarcity of financial resource is the limiting factor. The cost-containment measures in Germany have, then, consisted of organizational reforms designed to rationalize the delivery of services rather than ration them.[2]

6.2 The era of cost containment, 1977-97

The era of cost containment in the German health care system began in 1977 with the Health Insurance Cost Containment Act which was followed by a series of other acts:

Acts affecting all areas of health care	Year
Krankenversicherungs-Kostendämpfungs-Gesetz (KVKG) Health Insurance Cost Containment Act	1977
Kostendämpfungs-Ergänzungs-Gesetz (KVEG) Cost Containment Amendment Act	1981
Haushalts-Begleit-Gesetz 1983 (HBG83) Budget Support Act 1983	1982
Gesundheits-Reform-Gesetz (GRG) Health Care Reform Act	1988
Gesundheits-Struktur-Gesetz (GSG) Health Care Structure Act	1992
Krankenversicherungs-Beitrags-Entlastungs-Gesetz (KVBEG) Health Insurance Contributions Reduction Act	1996

Since 1977, the purchasers and providers of health care have been required to pursue a goal of contribution stability (SGB V §71 section 1 and §141 section 2) which has remained the main goal of cost containment in health care ever since. This requirement is defined as holding increases in contributions level with the rate of rise in contributory income,* and ensuring compliance with the intentions of this legislation is one of the main tasks of the 'Concerted Action in Health Care' (*Konzertierte Aktion im Gesundheitswesen* – RVO §405a, later SGB V §141). Although this constraint is set out in the legal framework for the health system, its efficacy has

---

* Contributory income is that part of an employee's income which is assessed for the purposes of calculating his or her contribution liability into the social insurance funds. There are upper limits, income above which is not liable (for sickness funds in 1997: DEM 6,150/month). If income is below a lower limit, it is not liable for contributions (in 1997: DEM 610/month).

306 *Health Care and Cost Containment in the European Union*

been restricted by the absence of sanctions in the case of failure to adhere to the constraint.

Cost containment in Germany has largely been achieved – or attempted – by the following measures:

- budgets for sectors or individual providers (but not for the whole system, cf. Table 6.1);
- restricting the number of high-cost technology equipment;
- restricting the number of office-based physicians;
- co-payments for an increasing number of services; and
- since 1997, the exclusion of benefits in the dental sector.

The budgets have been of varying forms and efficacy but have been generally more successful in containing costs (details in the relevant sections of this chapter) than any of the other supply or demand-side measures which largely failed.

Table 6.1 Budgets in the German statutory health insurance system, 1990s

Part of system	Type of budget
Overall system	No budget
Ambulatory care	Fixed budget on regional level (negotiated until 1992 and in 1996/97; growth rate set by law 1993–95)
Dental care	Fixed budget on regional level (negotiated until 1992 and in 1996/97; growth rate set by law 1993–95)
Hospitals	Target budgets for individual hospitals until 1992 and from 1997, fixed budgets 1992–96 (growth rate set by law)
Pharmaceuticals	Spending caps 1993–97: in 1993 set by law for West Germany, 1994–97 regional negotiable caps for all 23 physicians' associations
Non-physician care (physiotherapy etc.)	Included in pharmaceutical spending caps
Other (rehabilitation, transport, home nursing etc.)	No budgets

Overall, GKV health expenditure in Germany remained remarkably stable between 1975 and 1995 at between 6 and 7 per cent of GDP when calculated as a percentage of GDP per capita – taking inflation, number of insured persons and GDP growth into account (Figures 6.1 and 6.7).* Due to reasons outside the health care system, however, cost containment was not as successful when comparing it to its primary objective of a stable contribu-

Figure 6.1 Sickness funds' expenditure 1975–95 in current prices, in 1991 constant prices, in constant prices per insured person and as proportion of GDP per capita

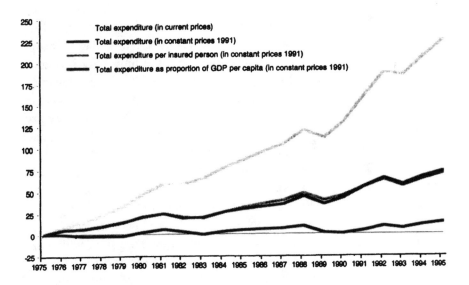

---

* Data in this paper are sourced from official German government statistics [3,4] unless otherwise stated. GDP figures are adjusted to 1991 values and GDP has been calculated on a per capita basis to avoid distortions caused by changes in the percentage of population covered under the GKV over the period discussed. The deflator used to convert into 1991 prices is the standard deflator for national inflation found in the German official statistics. The data cover the western part of Germany (or Old Bundesländer) only, unless otherwise stated.

308 *Health Care and Cost Containment in the European Union*

tion rate.

The following sections examine the most important health care sectors within the statutory health insurance system (ambulatory care, dental care, hospitals, and pharmaceuticals, respectively). Separate sections deal with co-payments within this system and the private health insurance sector. The final section comments on the relationship between health care costs as a proportion of GDP, sickness fund contribution rates, and the proportion of wages compared to GDP.

6.3 Ambulatory physicians

German ambulatory medicine is almost exclusively carried out in private offices of physicians working on their own premises, rather than by hospital out-patient clinics (the only exception being the university hospitals' policlinics). In accounting for one-fifth of total health care spending the ambulatory sector has, therefore, been an important area for cost containment. Between 1975 and 1977 budgetary constraint in the ambulatory sector was achieved through voluntary negotiations between the sickness funds and the physicians' associations. The 1977 KVKG introduced a Uniform Value Scale (*Einheitlicher Bewertungs-Maßstab*, EBM) giving a 'point value' to be used by all sickness funds for calculating reimbursement of fees-for-service (RVO §368g4;[5]). This EBM can be (and is) used in fee-for-service reimbursement in two ways: either with fixed budgets as a relative value for allocating proportional payments out of the budget, or with a pre-determined monetary conversion factor as the basis for direct fee for payment without fixed budget ceilings. In addition, the EBM permits the relative value of one procedure to be changed in relation to others. This enables incentives to change in light of over- or under-use of particular procedures or the introduction of new techniques, without the need to inflate the over-all price of health delivery.

The ability to vary the relative point values was used when a first major revision of the EBM was carried out in 1987. Points for laboratory and radiology services were lowered to provide fewer incentives for these services. While this led to a negligible increase of 7 per cent between 1988 and 1992 in reimbursement for the so-called basic laboratory services (i.e. the ones which do not necessarily have to be referred to a laboratory medicine specialist), expenditure for the special laboratory services was up by 66 per cent in the same period. The same happened in radiography: expenditure for conventional radiography was up by 11 per cent between 1988 and 1992, while NMR experienced an increase of 434 per cent and CT scanning of 66 per cent. In both areas, the respective specialists were the real winners: total remuneration for laboratory specialists and radiologists was 54 per cent and 32 per cent higher in 1992 than in 1988, while the average increased by only 21 per cent and remuneration for general practitioners by only 16 per cent.[6] (For further details concerning the various specialties, see Klose, 1993[7]).

Since 1977 therefore, the ambulatory sector has operated under some form of budgetary constraint and the percentage of GDP per sickness fund insured has remained stable throughout this time at just above 1 per cent (see Figure 6.2), and the percentage of sickness fund expenditure accounted for by ambulatory care fell from 19.4 per cent in 1975 to 16.9 per cent in 1988.[8] In 1989 following the enactment of the 1988 GRG, the voluntary fixing of budgets through negotiation which had contained ambulatory expenditure since 1975 became compulsory (SGB V §85). The sickness funds and physicians' associations were being tasked with negotiating a budget which would ensure contribution rate stability (SGB V §86/2).

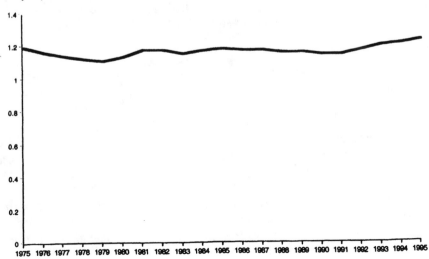

Figure 6.2 Sickness funds' expenditure on ambulatory physicians 1975–95 as a proportion of GDP per capita

310   *Health Care and Cost Containment in the European Union*

The GRG, while setting out the legal requirement of contribution stable budgeting, did not set out rules as to how this was to be done, and some procedures actually remained outside the area of contribution stability in order to promote their use. These included ambulatory surgery and anaesthesia, screening measures against cancer, and the newly introduced preventive 'check-ups'. With the enactment of the GSG all services were included in the calculation of the regional budgets for ambulatory care. The increase in regional budgets was determined by the Federal Minister of Health, using estimates concerning the (expected) increase in contributory incomes as the limit, the only exceptions being ambulatory surgery (including anesthesia) with an additional increase of 10 per cent, and 'check-ups' and screening measures an additional increase of 6 per cent (SGB V §85/3a). These regulations were in force for 1993, 1994 and 1995, after which the 1989 regulations came back into force, i.e. mandatory but negotiated budgets.

Under both negotiated and legally fixed budgets, the number of services rendered increased substantialy, by 32 per cent in the four years between 1988 and 1992 and by 26 per cent in the three years between 1992 and 1995 (Table 6.2). Less than half of this increase was attributable to the rising number of physicians. A good part of the other half may be explained by the 'Prisoner's Dilemma' phenomenon: no matter how the other physicians behave, the individual physician tries to increase his share of the total budget by increasing his or her services. Even though this is a rational behav-

Table 6.2 Changes in the number of physicians, services provided, and remuneration in the German ambulatory care sector (western part)

	1988–92	*1992–95*	*1988–95*
Physicians	+ 12%	+ 15%	+ 29%
Services (incl. new services)	+ 32%	+ 26%	+ 67%
Services (incl. new services)/ physician	+ 18%	+ 10%	+ 30%
Total remuneration (in current prices)	+ 34%	+ 13%	+ 51%
Remuneration/ physician (in current prices)	+ 19%	- 1%	+ 18%
Remuneration/ service (in current prices)	+ 1%	- 10%	- 9%

Own calculations based on Brenner et al, 1994,[6] physician numbers provided by the Federal Chamber of Physicians, and frequency statistics provided by the Federal Association of Physicians (partly estimated due to the inclusion of East-Berlin in official statistics since 1994).

iour for each individual, it contradicts collective rational behaviour which would be to limit the number of services in order to increase the reimbursement per service rendered. Actually, the remuneration per service rendered decreased by 10 per cent (current prices) between 1992 and 1995 where previously it had remained stable. This drop in remuneration per service was even slightly larger than the increase in services per physician, such that total remuneration per physician saw a small drop between 1992 and 1995 (after an increase in the previous four years). This trend led to severe dissatisfaction among office-based physicians. The Federal Association of Physicians tried to counter-act this dissatisfaction by adopting a new Uniform Value Scale.

This revision introduced higher point values for 'pastoral care' and communication with patients (to increase patient satisfaction), and combined frequent single services into single values for a whole range of services. Both measures were intended to increase the remuneration of general practitioners. Additionally, sickness funds and physicians' associations negotiated for 1996 an increase of 1 per cent above the expected rise of contributory incomes to facilitate the changes. (Due to this, ambulatory care expenditure increased by 2.1 per cent per sickness fund member in 1996.)[9] The new EBM was partly successful in this respect, however, the total volume of points rose by nearly 30 per cent in the first quarter of 1996 with a subsequent fall in the value of the points. By mid-1996, both specialists and general practitioners were dissatisfied with the new system (even though neither knew the exact financial effects) and a new system was decided upon, to start in July of 1997. This has created point caps for each practice depending on the number of patients treated in any given quarter. This regulation is intended to hold point values up, though its main foreseeable shortcoming is a lack of any cap for the number of patients. These new regulations may not be confused with capitation, since no minimum or even fixed remuneration is guaranteed. In effect, however, a capitation-like effect may be expected since most physicians will probably reach the point caps.

The RVO gave the physicians' associations and the sickness funds the duty of setting out requirements for ambulatory provision at a state level (RVO §368, later SGB V §99). This duty to develop 'need plans' (*Bedarfspläne*) was not only used to define areas of under provision, but also gave the right to close sub-regions with the aim of encouraging new entrants into areas of under provision (RVO §368r, later SGB V §100). The 1986 Act to Improve Sickness Fund Physician Need Planning (*Gesetz zur*

312 Health Care and Cost Containment in the European Union

Verbesserung der kassenärztlichen Bedarfsplanung) added to these duties and powers the power to declare areas of over provision in which a bar on the entry of new physicians should be made (RVO §368t, later SGB V §101). This regulation concerned the twelve physician specialties with the largest number being ambulatory physicians. The physicians' association, the state sickness fund association, and the state health department were to decide, on the basis of the 1980 federal average for physicians in each speciality, the requirement for physicians in each sub-regional speciality. Should the sub-region reach more than 150 per cent of the 'planned requirement' for physicians of a particular speciality, this region was to be closed to new entrants with this specialization. The GRG legislation ruled that even where a state had reached this situation in all sub-regions, a minimum of 50 per cent of the sub-regions should remain open for each speciality (RVO §368t/4, later SGB V §102) and that closure to new entrants could not be for longer than three years (RVO §368t/8, later SGB V §10/3).

Following the 1992 GSG, the over capacity required before closure of a sub-region was reduced to 110 per cent of the average number of physicians of a specialty in comparable regions (in total, 10 different types from metropolitan areas to rural areas were defined). There is no longer a requirement to keep any region open should this 110 per cent over capacity level be reached in the whole federal republic (SGB V §101). The time limit on closure was removed and replaced with the statement that closures may last only so long as the reasons for this restriction remain (SGB V §103). By the end of 1993, an average of 39 per cent of the regions was still open within the 12 specialities affected by the regulation. By the end of 1994, this number was down to 35 per cent and by the end of 1995 down to 28 per cent; with a range from 36 per cent for orthopaedists to 13 per cent for surgeons. This means that while there was no state in 1995 where all sub-regions were open for all specialities, there were openings for all specialities within the federal republic elsewhere. This is important, as it means that the legality of the SGB V §103 regulation still has to be tested against the German constitution (Article 12/1), which rules that all German citizens have a right to freedom of choice over their profession (the so-called *Berufsfreiheit*). This freedom was confirmed by the ruling of the German constitutional court (*Bundesverfassungsgericht*) on 22 March 1960 which prevented an earlier attempt to restrict new entrants into the ambulatory sector.[10]

The sharp divide in Germany between ambulatory practice and the hospital sector, and the legal priority of the ambulatory sector (SGB V §73/4, which rules that referrals for hospital treatment may only be made if ambulatory treatment will not be effective) has resulted in a high level of 'large (high cost) medical technology' in both the ambulatory and the hospital sectors. The 1981 Hospital Cost Containment Act (*Krankenhaus-Kostendämpfungs-Gesetz*) therefore set out a requirement for the physicians' associations, sickness funds, hospitals and the state health ministries to negotiate a 'need plan' for medical technology (*Gesetz zur wirtschaftlichen Sicherung der Krankenhauspflegesätze* §11a). The GSG (§85 2a) ruled that reimbursement for medical technology could only be provided under the sickness fund reimbursement package when this technology had been included in such a plan. However, the regulation contained an 'amnesty' clause for equipment purchased before the third quarter of 1992 which destroyed almost all of its possible effect.

While the containment of expenditure on ambulatory practice cannot be described as unsuccessful, the graph of GKV expenditure on physicians shows that the most successful periods were the voluntary phase and immediately following the KVKG, while the GRG regulations were less effective.

6.4 Dental care

Although many of the regulations relating to ambulatory physicians (dental EBM, regional fixed budgets) are also relevant to the dental care sector of German health care, there is a major difference. Cost sharing has played a far greater role in the dental sector than the rest of ambulatory practice, with cost shares of up to 50 per cent and exclusion of certain procedures from the service catalogue (see 'Cost-sharing', section 6.7). These more radical policies have resulted in tight control of dental expenditure which has fallen in GDP terms between 1975 and 1990 (Figure 6.3). Since then, it has risen continuously, most pronounced after the expiry of legal budgets in 1996 when expenditure per sickness fund member increased by 7.1 per cent in current prices.[9]

More radical measures (i.e. higher cost sharing and exclusion from benefits for certain persons since 1997; see below) have resulted in GKV expenditure on dental prosthesis falling by 50 per cent in real terms. It has to be taken into account, however, that cost sharing in this area is now approximately 50 per cent, so that real expenditure as a proportion of GDP per capita is ca. 0.5 per cent. These reforms have resulted in the expenditure on dental prosthesis, which in 1975 was equal to that on the rest of dental care, to rise above general dental care in the late 1970s, and thereafter to fall away steadily as an expenditure factor since 1985; except for a pre-GRG 'bounce' as patients and dentists took avoiding action over the forthcoming legislation (Figure 6.3). In 1996, this phenomenon was observed again. Expenditure increased by 10.2 per cent per sickness fund member [9] which was partly caused by the new regulation in effect since 1997.

All legal measures mentioned for ambulatory and dental care are subject to

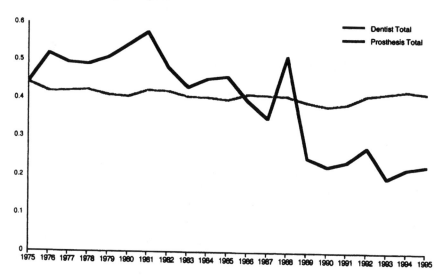

Figure 6.3 Sickness funds' expenditure in the dental sector 1975–95 as a proportion of GDP per capita

the sanction that in the case of the various actors not being able to reach a negotiated agreement within the framework of the regulations, the federal or state health ministry (depending on the level at which the disagreement happens) is empowered to take over the running of the particular organization. Until 1995, this sanction had never been tested, despite lapses in the observance of many of the guidelines. However, in the summer of 1995, following the decision by the dental physicians' association of Lower Saxony not to treat patients in order to increase total reimbursement (and many dentists followed this decision), the state ministry responsible for health exercised its mandate to take control of the dental association for a limited period of time. During this time, a 'state commissioner' signed all necessary contracts with the sickness funds concerning remuneration on behalf of the dental physicians' associations which remained valid after the elected officials returned to their offices.

6.5 Hospitals

In line with most western health systems, the average length of stay in German hospitals has fallen drastically in the last 30 years, while at the same time the number of hospital cases per 1000 population has risen even more markedly (Figure 6.4, overleaf). Both the occupancy rate (83.9 per cent in 1994, 8 per cent less than in 1965) and, possibly more surprisingly, the number of hospital beds have, however, remained relatively stable. In 1965, West Germany had 106.5 hospital beds per 10000 population; in 1975, this number reached its peak at 118.4. In 1980, 1985, 1990 and 1994, the respective figures were 114.8, 110.6, 104.5, and 100.1 (i.e. only 6 per cent fewer than in 1965).* These figures are partly misleading, however, since they include general acute hospitals, specialized hospitals (i.e. psychiatric hospitals) and rehabilitative hospitals.** Especially since 1990, the almost constant number of hospital beds obscures the fact that beds in general and psychiatric hospitals are decreasing and those in preventive and rehabilitative institutions are increasing. In 1990, the composition was 83.6 and 20.8 while in 1994 it had changed to 76.9 (- 8%) and 23.2 (+ 12%). If

---

* In East Germany, in spite of its different health care system, the numbers of hospital beds were very similar even though the peak was earlier (i.e. 1964): 121.0 (1965), 111.3 (1970), 108.3 (1975), 102.7 (1980), 101.5 (1985), and 97.9 (1990). Since re-unification, the eastern part of Germany has experienced a marked decrease to 84.4 in 1994 (about 16 per cent lower than in the West, compared to -6 per cent at unification).[11,12]

** German hospital data over time have to be interpreted carefully since the definition of what constitutes a hospital changed between 1989 and 1990. Formerly, a distinction was made between acute hospitals and special hospitals (including psychiatric and rehabilitative hospitals) while in-patient institutions are now sub-divided into general hospitals, psychiatric hospitals (which are usually combined for statistical purposes) and preventive and rehabilitative institutions.

Figure 6.4 Changes in hospital sector figures 1965–95: beds, cases, average length of stay, and average occupancy rate

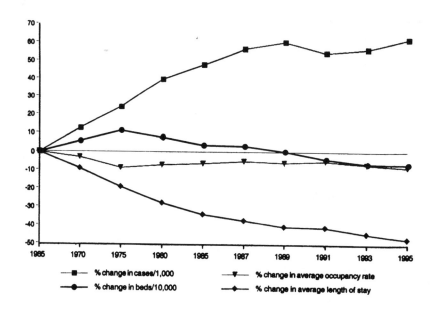

this distinction is made for average length of stay, as well, the fall in the hospitals in the narrow sense becomes steeper as well (from 14.8 in 1990 to 12.7 in 1994) while it has remained virtually constant in preventive and rehabilitative institutions (31.9 in 1990 and 31.3 in 1994).

Expenditure on hospital care in Germany has risen considerably over the last 35 years. The steep rise in hospital expenditure in the early 1970s (data not shown) may be explained by the introduction of hospital planning to address a perceived shortage of hospital beds. However, even when this rise is discounted it may be seen that, since 1975, hospital expenditure is the area of German health care least constrained in its growth with an increase from 1.9 per cent of GDP per capita in 1975 to 2.4 per cent in 1995 (Figure 6.5). This explains almost two-thirds of the increase since 1975 and all of the increase since 1988, i.e. the phase of the two major reform acts GRG and GSG. The responsibility for hospital planning, which is retained by the Länder in Germany, has for a long time resulted in a reluctance to instigate effective cost-containment measures in the hospital sector.

This is the result of the 1972 Hospital Financing Act, which introduced the

Figure 6.5 Sickness funds' expenditure on hospital care 1975-95 as a proportion of GDP per capita

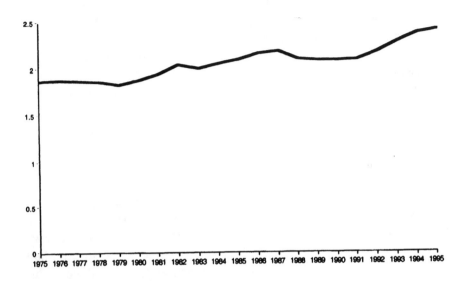

'dual-financing' mechanism, i.e. the coverage of capital costs through the states and the running costs through the sickness funds. Only hospitals enlisted in the hospital plans of the states are eligible for having their investments paid by the states. For the running costs, a full cost cover principle was introduced, with hospital reimbursement through *per-diem* charges which were retrospectively calculated by the states for each hospital. Only minor legislation on hospital services was included in the KVEG, restricting post natal hospital stay to six days, except in the case of medical need for a longer stay, and requiring hospitals to agree purchases of 'large (high cost) medical technology' together with ambulatory physicians. The 1984 Hospital Restructuring Act introduced prospectively negotiated *per-diem* charges which were based upon expected costs. Coverage of excess costs was *de jure* limited, *de-facto*, however, hospitals received a full compensation through adjustments of charges. Additionally, the act opened the possibility of including capital costs in *per-diem* charges if investments would lower running costs in the medium or long term. Since the 1988 GRG, hospital and sickness fund associations are obliged to negotiate contracts concerning quality assurance (which took several years to be put into practice). Additionally, the sickness funds received the right to contract additional

318 *Health Care and Cost Containment in the European Union*

hospitals and, through a complicated mechanism involving the state, to de-contract hospitals.

The 1992 GSG became the first major law in the cost-containment area to affect the hospital sector. This was possible since the Social Democratic Party, being the opposition in the federal parliament but the ruling party in most states, had agreed to this statutory reform. As in the ambulatory care sector, expenditure between 1993 and 1995 was tied to the increase in contributory incomes. Additionally, the full cost-cover principle was abolished, i.e. the hospitals were allowed to make both profits and deficits. The introduction of (prospective) case-fees and procedure-fees for selected treatments from 1996 and the attempt to loosen the strict separation between the ambulatory and hospital sector, i.e. by allowing ambulatory surgery in hospitals, were other measures.

Politically, fixed budgets in the hospital sector were sold as an interim measure until a new prospective payment system would be introduced from 1996. (Hospitals which introduced it on a voluntary basis in 1995 returned to prospective budgets in that year.) Two different kinds of prospective budgets were introduced: case fees which are supposed to cover all costs during a hospital stay, and procedure fees fees which are reimbursed on top of (slightly reduced) *per-diem* charges. Case fees are based on a combination of a certain diagnosis and a specific intervention, procedure fees just on an intervention. The number of points for both the currently more than 70 case fees and the currently almost 150 procedures, are set nationally by the Federal Ministry of Health, while the monetary conversion factor is negotiated at state level. The number of points were calculated by taking real costs of a relatively small sample of patients with these diagnoses/interventions, and assuming a 15 per cent reduction in average length of stay. The percentage of cases paid on a prospective basis is less than a quarter; all other cases are now reimbursed by a two-tier system of *per-diem* charges: a flat hospital wide rate covering non-medical costs and a department-specific charge covering medical costs including nursing, pharmaceuticals, procedures etc.[13]

While hospitals have only been allowed to offer surgery on an ambulatory or day-case basis since 1993, day-case surgery is not new in Germany. Due to the separation of the hospital and the ambulatory care sector, surgeons, ophthalmologists, orthopedic surgeons and other specialists in private practice have performed minor surgery (removal of lumps etc.) for a long time. Since the 1980s, this was supported through the introduction of new items in the Uniform Value Scale, both to cover additional costs of the operating physician (equipment, supporting staff etc.) and to cover necessary anaesthesia. In 1993, additional items for post-operative care were introduced. The frequency of these items may be used to estimate the extent to which ambulatory surgery is taking place in Germany, though they do not allow a distinction between hospital-based and office-based day surgery since remuneration is done under the same norms. By the end of 1994, 28 per cent of all hospitals offered day surgery [14] but this does not allow any conclusions about service frequencies.

According to the frequency statistics of the Federal Association of Physicians (Table 6.3), day surgery increased rapidly in the first half of the 1990s with growth rates higher than anticipated when budgets were fixed. Growth rates are even higher if the volumes of points for the services is taken into account, since procedures with the smallest surcharge increased only by 26.6 per cent while those with the highest surcharges increased by 303.9 per cent between 1990 and 1994. While it is not (yet) possible to calculate whether ambulatory surgery has led to cost containment (and it is doubtful at this time), a recent calculation came to the conclusion that ambu-

Table 6.3 Estimated volume of ambulatory surgery in Germany 1990–94 (western part)

	Surcharge for ambulatory surgery	Ambulatory anesthesia	Post-operative care
1990	DEM 1.56 m	DEM 0.20 m	–
1991	DEM 1.75 m + 12%	DEM 0.28 m + 38%	–
1992	DEM 2.00 m + 14%	DEM 0.38 m + 37%	–
1993	DEM 2.47 m + 24%	DEM 0.57 m + 50%	DEM 0.21 m
1994	DEM 2.54 m + 3%	DEM 0.73 m + 28%	DEM 0.44 m + 109%
1990–94	+ 63%	+ 266%	

Source: Frequency statistics provided by the Federal Association of Physicians, adopted from Busch and Pfaff, 1996.[15]

320 *Health Care and Cost Containment in the European Union*

latory surgery may be expected to save between as little as DEM 7 and as much as DEM 102 per year per sickness fund member, which translates to between 0.02 and 0.25 percentage points of contributions. The most realistic estimation, however, is DEM 20 and 0.05 percentage points.[15]

Altogether, cost containment through fixed budgets in the hospital sector was a failure. Expenditures per sickness fund member increased by 16.5 per cent between 1992 and 1995, while the contributory incomes increased only by 7.4 per cent. Amongst others, two factors led to this failure and the expenditure growth rate, which was even higher than before:

1. the law allowed for several exceptions for extraordinary increases, one of them was even made mandatory through the same law: a new calculation of nursing time per patient;

2. actual negotiations about volume and prices remained at the level of the individual hospital.

In early 1996, a tighter budgeting law – the Hospital Expenditure Stabilizing Act – was passed for the hospital sector only, abolishing most of the exceptions and allowing for an increase only as large as that of the wage increase in the public service (under which conditions almost all hospital employees are paid) and which was less than 0.2 per cent. This law, however, was in force only for 1996 so that the next reform law may be expected sometime in 1997. In 1996, expenditure for hospital treatments actually decreased by 0.7 per cent in current prices.[9] This is, however, not (yet) attributable to prospective payment systems since all hospital budgets are fixed. In the meantime, through the KVBEG, hospital budgets were additionally reduced by 1 per cent each year from 1997 to 1999 to make up for alleged savings through the newly introduced statutory long-term nursing care insurance.

6.6 Pharmaceuticals

Pharmaceutical expenditure is an effectively controlled area of German health care expenditure. GKV expenditure on pharmaceuticals as a proportion of GDP per capita in 1995 was slightly lower than in 1975 (Figure 6.6). The major elements of this ability to control drug expenditure are cost-sharing measures described below. These comprise a short negative list (SGB V §34), reference prices (SGB V §35) introduced in 1989 under the GRG and lastly, and of most impact, the pharmaceutical spending cap (SGB V §84) introduced in 1993.[16]

The idea behind the reference prices was to establish an upper limit for the costs reimbursable through the sickness funds. Reference prices were defined in three phases. First for drugs containing the same substance, then for drugs with similar substances, and finally for drugs with comparable efficacy. Due to reduced prices for drugs previously above the reference price, these regulations led to decreasing prices for reference priced drugs, but the pharmaceutical industry compensated these partly through above average increases for non-reference priced drugs so that the overall effect on costs was very moderate [17] (but still visible in Figure 6.6). For patients, reference prices had two effects. Generally, pharmaceuticals priced at or below the reference price for that substance were co-payment free (until 1992). On the other hand, if a sickness-fund-insured patient wished to use a more expensive alternative, he or she had to pay the difference out of their own pocket. For all prescribed drugs without a reference price, the patient had to pay a co-payment of DEM 3 per package – instead of the previous DEM 2 (SGB V §31). These new regulations led to an increase of co-payments by about one-third, but subsequently – due to the increasing number of refer-

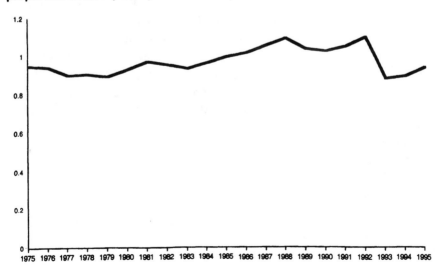

Figure 6.6 Sickness funds' expenditure on pharmaceuticals 1975–95 as a proportion of GDP per capita

322 *Health Care and Cost Containment in the European Union*

ence-priced drugs – it fell to the 1988 level by 1992.[17] While in 1990 refer-ence-priced drugs accounted for only 10 per cent of the drug market, this share increased to about 30 per cent in 1992 and has been calculated to reach more than 60 per cent in 1997.

The spending cap for pharmaceuticals imposed a real reduction of phar-maceutical expenditure which had accounted for DEM 26.7 billion in 1992. Based upon the 1991 expenditure of DEM 24.4 billion, the cap reduced future spending to a maximum of DEM 23.9 billion per year. In the case of overspending in the first year, any excess spending up to DEM 280 million would have been clawed back from the physicians' associations (from physician remuneration) and the pharmaceutical industry. Since 1994, the physicians' associations have been liable for any overspending with no upper limit. This liability is in force for every single association in the case of overspending, even if total pharmaceutical spending remains below the cap. At the same time as introducing the spending cap, the GSG imposed a price cut of 5 per cent for existing drugs not covered by reference pricing and a price freeze for new drugs – both measures applying for 1993 and 1994.

The result of all three cost containment measures in their first year of operation, i.e. price moratorium, new cost-sharing regulations and expendi-ture cap, was a reduction of 18.8 per cent in sickness funds' costs for phar-maceuticals in the ambulatory sector. This represents a reduction for the sickness funds of DEM 5.1 billion from 1992 expenditure, or DEM 2.2 bil-lion more than had been required under the terms of the GSG. Of these sav-ings, around DEM 1 billion was attributable to price reductions, which were 3.9 per cent on average. Another almost DEM 800 million were the result of the new cost-sharing regulations. In spite of the smaller market, this meant a total increase of 66.7 per cent in the patients' direct expenditure. Of expenditure for prescribed pharmaceuticals, cost sharing accounted for 7.8 per cent in 1993, over the 4 per cent in 1992. In other words, only about 60 per cent of the total reduction was attributable to changes in physicians' pre-scribing behaviour.[16]

Physicians reduced the number of prescriptions in western Germany by 10.4 per cent (-13.7 per cent in eastern Germany; average: -11.2 per cent). The average value per prescription in 1993 was 4.6 per cent lower than in 1992 (+30.2 per cent and -0.9 per cent respectively). Most of this decrease was due to the above mentioned 3.9 per cent price reduction (-2.9 per cent and -3.6 per cent respectively). The 'structural composition' of all pharmaceuticals prescribed constituted the remainder. These components include changes between drugs and changes in prescribed strength and package size within one drug. That 'structural components' had a negative effect (-0.8 per cent in western Germany) for the first time was largely due to the increase in the prescribing of generic products. From 1992 to 1993, generic products increased their volume market share from 30.8 per cent to 35.8 per cent, and their value market share from 24.9 per cent to 28.5 per cent.[17] In 1994, pharmaceutical expenditure in the united Germany increased by 4.6 per cent with the number of prescriptions decreasing by 3.1 per cent and the value per prescription increasing by 7.9 per cent. In 1995, expenditure increased by as much as 7.1 per cent with both the number of prescriptions (+ 6.3 per cent) and the value per prescription (+ 0.8 per cent) increasing.[18] In 1996, the increase slowed to 6.4 per cent.[9]

Due to these increases, regional caps were exceeded in some of the 23 regions in 1994; even though national figures remained within the total (hypothetical) spending cap both in 1994 and 1995. The overspending occurred mainly in the eastern states (which were not affected by the 1993 cap) where the increase in pharmaceutical expenditure was so high that per capita expenditure in 1995 was almost 13 per cent higher than in the west. Since the legislation allows overspending in one year to be rectified in the next, no sanctions were imposed in 1995. However, some of the regions also exceeded the 1995 budget and therefore, in September 1996, the sickness funds instigated proceedings to claim back money from nine regions which had overspent their budget by up to 11.3 per cent. The physicians' associations are resisting payment, arguing that they cannot effectively manage overall or physician-specific drug expenditure, due to untimely and unspecified data. Despite these current difficulties with the budget cap and sharper rises in pharmaceutical expenditure in 1996 – when nation-wide spending would have exceeded the cap if there had not been agreements in several states to even things out in coming years - the spending cap has proved to be a very effective method of short-term reduction and a long-term modification of pharmaceutical expenditure. However, it has not altered physicians' prescribing behaviour much in terms of quality.[16]

While there was an initial drop in the prescriptions for disputed or ineffective drugs from DEM 9 billion in 1992 to DEM 7 billion in 1993, this figure has remained at an almost constant percentage since then (in absolute terms it is increasing). Furthermore, the initial reduction was mainly attributable to physicians with an above-average quality of prescribing, while the

324 *Health Care and Cost Containment in the European Union*

others reduced their prescriptions mainly on the basis of price.[16] A recent calculation has shown that more rational prescribing behaviour for 10 drugs alone could save as much as 3 per cent of the total pharmaceutical expenditure (*Arzneimittel-telegramm* 11/96, pp. 110f).

6.7 Cost sharing

Cost-sharing has a long tradition within the German health care system, the most traditional sector being pharmaceuticals. In this area, nominal cost-sharing was increased over the years, but cost-sharing as a percentage of total costs remained stable at less than 5 per cent of pharmaceutical expenditure until 1992 (when it was 3.5 per cent). Through the GSG, cost- sharing was newly regulated in two steps. The first step was new co-payments according to the price of the pack (1993) and the second, new co-payments according to pack size (1994). These measures increased patient cost-sharing to 7.5 per cent in 1993 and to 8.8 per cent in 1994 (in absolute figures from DEM 1.3 billion in 1992 to DEM 2.4 billion in 1993 and DEM 2.9 billion in 1994). The 1996 KVBEG will lead to a further increase to about 12 per cent (DEM 3.6 billion).

In other areas, cost-sharing was reduced in the 1970s by enlarging the benefits catalogue (i.e. denture treatment), but later cost-sharing was increased again. New areas for cost-sharing since the 1980s are charges for in-patient days in hospitals, rehabilitation facilities and ambulance transportation. Most of these were cost containment measures to shift spending from the sickness funds to the patients – they were not intended to reduce overall spending. Patients were told for example that the DEM 5 co-payment in the hospital had to be paid to cover the food.

In the 1988 GRG, cost-sharing was advocated for two purposes: both to raise revenue (to reduce the expenditure for dental care, physiotherapy and transportation and making the patient liable for pharmaceutical costs above the reference prices) and to reward 'responsible behaviour' (again dental treatment) and rewarding good preventive practice with lower co-payments – see Table 6.4). These cost-sharing regulations were part of a complete restructuring of co-payments throughout the GRG, resulting in generally higher cost-sharing than before. While sickness funds' expenditure for dentures fell (see above), the other measures did not alter spending patterns in the respective areas. On the contrary, transportation, stationary preventive spa treatment, and non-physician care have been the areas of the largest increases during the first half of the 1990s: + 42 per cent, + 34 per cent and + 18 per cent between 1992 and 1995 respectively (overall increase: + 10 per cent in current prices).

Except for co-payments for dentures and in-patient treatment, yearly cost-sharing of mandatory sickness funds' members is limited to a maximum of 2 per cent of their gross income for single persons (SGB V §62). For voluntary members with incomes above the upper limit for mandatory membership, the limit is 4 per cent of the gross income for single persons. If two or more persons are dependent on this income the threshold is lower (by 15 per cent per person of the upper limit for mandatory membership for the first and 10 per cent for every subsequent person). In case of very low income, patients are exempted from these co-payments (SGB V §61). For 1997, the limits in the West were DEM 1,708 for one person, DEM 2,348 for two persons, and DEM 427 for every additional person and, in the East, DEM 1,456, DEM 2,002, and DEM 364, respectively. This regulation affects 8 million persons and all 12 million insured children.[19] In effect, these regulations make cost-sharing in Germany for most areas – with dentures being an important exception – both socially tolerable and economically ineffective.

Table 6.4 Cost sharing regulations in Germany (western part) July 1977 – June 1997

Cost sharing for:	Act	Date in force	Level	Reference
Prescription of pharmaceuticals and dressings	KVKG	1.7.77	DEM 1/item	RVO §182a
Prescription of pharmaceuticals and dressings	KVEG	1.1.82	DEM 1.5/item	RVO §182a
Prescription of pharmaceuticals and dressings	HBG83	1.1.83	DEM 2	RVO §182a
Prescription of pharmaceuticals and dressings without reference prices	GRG	1.1.89	DEM 3 or 100% if <DEM 3	SGB V §31/3(1)

326 *Health Care and Cost Containment in the European Union*

Cost sharing for:	Act	Date in force	Level	Reference
Prescription of pharmaceuticals and dressings without reference prices	GRG	1.7.93 (never in force)	15 %/item (min. DEM 1, max. DEM 10)	SGB V §31/3(2)
Pharmaceuticals – up to 30 DEM in price	GSG	1.1.93	DEM 3 or 100% if <DEM 3*	SGB V §31/3
Pharmaceuticals – 30–50 DEM in price	GSG	1.1.93	DEM 5*	SGB V §3/3
Pharmaceuticals – over 50 DEM in price	GSG	1.1.93	DEM 7*	SGB V §31/3
Pharmaceuticals – small pack	GSG	1.1.94	DEM 3 or 100% if <3 DEM*	SGB V §31/4
Pharmaceuticals – medium pack	GSG	1.1.94	DEM 5*	SGB V §31/4
Pharmaceuticals – large pack	GSG	1.1.94	DEM 7*	SGB V §31/4
Pharmaceuticals – small pack	KVBEG	1.1.97	DEM 4 or 100% if <DEM 4*	SGB V §31/3
Pharmaceuticals – medium pack	KVBEG	1.1.97	DEM 6*	SGB V §31/3
Pharmaceuticals – large pack	KVBEG	1.1.97	DEM 8*	SGB V §31/3
Orthodontic, crown and denture treatments (total costs)	KVKG	1.7.77	min. 20%	RVO §182c
Technical portion of crown and denture treatment	KVEG	1.1.82	min. 40%	RVO §182c
Crown and denture treatment (total costs)	GRG	1.1.89	50%	SGB V §30/1
– if insured has had regular yearly check ups for the last 5 years	GRG	1.1.89	40%	SGB V §30/2

* plus 100% of price above reference price.

Cost Containment in Germany: Twenty Years Experience 327

Cost sharing for:	Act	Date in force	Level	Reference
– if insured has had regular yearly check ups for the past 10 years, and has cared for his/her teeth regularly	GRG	1.1.89	35%	SGB V §30/2
Orthodontics (if eating, speaking or breathing is severely limited)	GRG	1.1.89	20%	SGB V §29/1
Major dental work (more than 4 replacement teeth per jaw or more than 3 per side of mouth, excepting multiple single bridges, which may exceed 3)	GSG	1.1.93	100%	SGB V §30/1
Crown and denture treatment (total costs for those born before 1.1.79)	KVBEG	1.1.97	50%/40%/35%	SGB V §30/1
Crown and denture treatment (total costs for those born after 31.12.78)	KVBEG	1.1.97	100 %	SGB V §30/1
Travel costs to and from visit to medical facility	KVKG	1.1.77	DEM 3.5/trip	RVO §194/1
Travel costs to and from visit to medical facility	KVEG	1.1.82	DEM 5/trip	RVO §194/1
Travel costs to hospital for in-patient treatment	GRG	1.1.89	DEM 20/trip	SGB V §60
Travel costs for ambulatory treatment	GRG	1.1.89	100%	SGB V §60
Prescription of 'non-physician care' (physiotherapy etc.)	KVKG	1.7.77	DEM 1	RVO §182a
Prescription of 'non-physician care'	KVEG	1.1.82	DEM 4	RVO §182a
'Non physician care'	GRG	1.1.89	10%	SGB V §32
Spectacles	KVEG	1.1.82	DEM 4	RVO §182a

328 *Health Care and Cost Containment in the European Union*

Cost sharing for:	Act	Date in force	Level	Reference
Spectacles, devices etc.	GRG	1.1.89	100% of costs above reference price	SGB V §33/2
Hospital stay*	HBG83	1.1.83	DEM 5/day	RVO §184/3
Hospital stay*	GRG	1.1.91	DEM 10/day	SGB V §39/4
Hospital stay*	GSG	1.1.93	DEM 11/day	SGB V §39/4
Hospital stay*	GSG	1.1.94	DEM 12/day	SGB V §3/4
Stationary preventive spa treatment	HBG83	1.1.83	DEM 10/day	RVO §187/4
Stationary preventive spa treatment	GSG	1.1.93	DEM 11/day	SGB V §2/6
Stationary preventive spa treatment	GSG	1.1.94	DEM 12/day	SGB V §2/6
Stationary preventive spa treatment	KVBEG	1.1.97	DEM 25/day	SGB V §23/6
Stationary rehabilitative treatment*	GRG	1.1.89	DEM 5/day	SGB V §40/5
Stationary rehabilitative treatment*	GRG	1.1.91	DEM 10/day	SGB V §40/5
Stationary rehabilitative treatment*	GSG	1.1.93	DEM 11/day	SGB V §40/5
Stationary rehabilitative treatment*	GSG	1.1.94	DEM 12/day	SGB V §40/5
Stationary rehabilitative treatment if beginning within 14 days after a hospital stay*	KVBEG	1.1.97	DEM 12/day	SGB V §40/6
Other stationary rehabilitative treatment	KVBEG	1.1.97	DEM 25/day	SGB V §40/5

* charge limited to 14 days per year.

All in all, cost sharing accounted for more than DEM 13 billion in 1995 compared to the total of sickness fund expenditure of DEM 228 billion including monetary benefits such as sick pay. Therefore, cost sharing amounted to 5.5 per cent of total expenditure (or 8.4 per cent if OTC drugs are included in the calculation). Depending on the health care sector, variation in cost-sharing is considerable (Table 6.5).

Cost sharing has increased markedly since the beginning of 1997. Crown and denture treatment has been removed from the benefits catalogue for everyone born after 1978, pharmaceutical co-payments have been increased as well as co-payments for spa treatment and rehabilitation (from DEM 12 to DEM 25/day). Drastic increases will take effect later in 1997 (see below).

Table 6.5 Actual cost sharing for different health care sectors in 1995 (whole Germany)

	DEM billion	As % of total sector expenditure
Ambulatory medical treatment	0	0
Ambulatory dental treatment (excluding crowns and dentures)	0	0
Hospital in-patient treatment	1.4	2
Devices and 'non-physician care'	0.5	3
Preventive spa and rehabilitation	0.4	7
Pharmaceuticals (excl. OTC)	3.1	9
[Pharmaceuticals incl. OTC]	[ca. 10.7]	[ca. 25]
Ambulance transportation	1.1	22
Crown and denture treatment	6.8	48

Source: Authors' reseearch based on data provided by the Federal Ministry of Health.

6.8 Private health insurance

As mentioned before, almost 90 per cent of the population are covered by the statutory health insurance, many of them voluntarily.[2] Part of the reason

330 *Health Care and Cost Containment in the European Union*

why so many persons who have the chance to drop out of the statutory health insurance and become privately insured choose not to do so, are the different growth rates in health care expenditure between the two kinds of health insurance. From the health system analysis point of view, German private health insurance is of special interest, since many regulations affecting the statutory health insurance do not affect private health insurance; so that differences can be related to political cost-containment measures in the former area. Table 6.6 summarizes changes in per capita expenditure for the two areas in four important health care sectors. The greatest differences occur in dental care which is mainly attributable to the cost sharing regulations in the GKV (while private insurances often pay 80 per cent or even 100 per cent). But in ambulatory care, differences are also large since reimbursement for privately insured persons is not budgeted. It may be the case that physicians also increased the number of services for privately insured patients to compensate for smaller increases in the reimbursement for patients with statutory health insurance. For pharmaceuticals, the effects of the expenditure cap which was confined to the GKV is clearly visible (especially in the 1987–93 comparison). The exception in expenditure growth is the hospital sector with roughly even growth rates is *per diem* charges for sickness fund members are valid for privately insured persons as well. The latter are, however, billed for physician services additionally.

Table 6.6 Changes in per capita expenditure (current prices) for statutory health insurance (GKV) and private health insurance (PKV)

Percentage change		1982–88	1982–90	1987–91	1987–93	1987–95
Ambulatory care	GKV	+ 28	+ 44	+ 21	+ 33	+ 41
	PKV	+ 33	+ 72	+ 31	+ 51	+ 71
Dental care	GKV	+ 33	- 1	+ 2	+ 4	+ 15
	PKV	+ 36	+ 92	+ 34	+ 69	+ 78
Pharmaceuticals	GKV	+ 48	+ 58	+ 23	+ 8	+ 21
	PKV	+ 36	+ 62	+ 17	+ 28	+ 35
Hospital care	GKV	+ 35	+ 53	+ 22	+ 39	+ 22
	PKV	+ 39	+ 62	+ 18	+ 31	+ 46

Source: Verband der privaten Krankenversicherung, 1996 and earlier.[20]

Cost Containment in Germany: Twenty Years Experience   331

6.9 Cost containment: successful but politically dead

Germany has achieved remarkable stability in its health care expenditure when compared with GDP, at least pre-unification until 1990.* This stability is attributable to a mixture of negotiation by self-governing 'corporate' bodies and state intervention; the separate effects of which are not always clearly distinguishable. However, all major health care reform acts – which were usually passed when health care expenditure had reached a new peak, i.e. surpassed the level at which the prior law was passed – had a small but noticeable effect on health care expenditure when calculated as a proportion of GDP per capita. The KVKG and the KVEG both lowered that figure by 0.1 per cent, the HBG83 by 0.2 per cent, the GRG by 0.5 per cent and the GSG by 0.1 per cent. Though the effects did not last very long (with the GRG being the most and the GSG the least successful), they ensured a remarkable stability of health care expenditure in the long run which was only weakened in the 1990s due to the additional expenditures needed in the East.

However, since the factor being used by both politicians and employers (and to a much lesser extent, the employees/insured) has been the contribution rate alone, this stability has for a long time not been acknowledged in discussions about health care costs. This rate is increasing slowly but steadily (from 10.4 per cent in 1975 to 13.4 per cent in 1996), with cost-containment measures having only minor and transient effects. Usually overlooked is the fact that rising health care costs (which rise in line with GDP) are not responsible for this. It is primarily the shrinking proportion of GDP used for wages, from which all social insurance contributions are raised (Figure 6.7, overleaf). Thus, larger profits by employers, a higher number of unemployed, and wages increasing less than productivity have led to this situation. The current debate about social costs is dominated by employers and economists who believe that an even smaller percentage of GDP used for wages will be the solution of the current economic crisis with high numbers of unemployed – a questionable belief which is hardly supported by hard

---

* Even though the chapter focuses on the health expenditure by the statutory health insurance, since this is the relevant figure in the German political discussion, the OECD data on total expenditure on health as a percentage of GDP support this conclusion: in 1975, 8.1%; 1980, 8.4%; 1985, 8.7; 1990, 8.3% and 1995, 9.6%. In the pre-unification years until 1990 2% above the sickness funds' expenditure per capita and 2.5% above it since unification.

Figure 6.7 Wages, sickness fund contributions and expenditure in relation to GDP, 1980–95

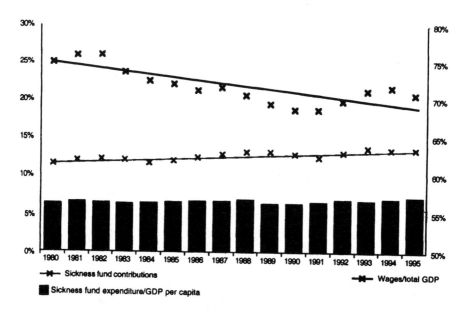

Sources: own calculations based on Kühn, 1995[21]; Statistisches Bundesamt, 1996.[4]

data.

The discussion about health care costs in Germany has changed recently, especially after the Advisory Council published its report on *The Health Care System in Germany: Cost Factor and Branch of the Future* [22] which acknowledged the success of cost containment in the health care sector but also declared the health care sector to be the branch of the future in terms of new jobs. Since then, the Minister of Health, Horst Seehofer, is determined to keep additional costs on labour down for employers, and yet to allow the health care sector to grow. He confirmed this in his speech before the Bundestag on 20 March 1997, when the 2nd Statutory Health Insurance Restructuring Act was passed. He called the German health care system 'one of the best and most social systems in the world' and named three major challenges: (1) international economic competition; (2) rising life expectancy; and (3) the technological advances which should be paid for. In his opinion, budgets would in the end lead to rationing and were not successful, anyway, since providers had developed escape strategies.[19]

The Act abolishes both the budgets for ambulatory care and the spending caps for pharmaceuticals, and replaces them with physician-specific 'targets' which still have to be negotiated between the sickness funds and the physicians' associations. Physicians and dentists will – after 20 years of floating point values – again be guaranteed a certain point value which will only be decreased for services above a pre-determined level. To get more money into health care, all cost-sharing measures (except for preventive spa treatment and rehabilitation) will be raised by DEM 5, i.e. for pharmaceuticals to DEM 9/ 11/ 13 per pack depending on size, for hospital treatments to DEM 17 per day, and for transportation costs to DEM 25 per trip. Cost sharing regulations expressed as a percentage will be raised by 5 per cent except for crowns and dentures. For these, patients will get a flat amount from their sickness fund (if they are not excluded totally under the regulations of the KVBEG) and have to get – and pay for – the treatment as private patients. In his speech, Horst Seehofer announced that the total share of costs borne by patients would increase from 4 per cent to 6 per cent through these measures.[19] If these figures are supposed to include crowns and dentures, they are simply wrong (see above).

In addition to these measures, the 1st Statutory Health Insurance Restructuring Act mandates increases in cost-sharing if sickness funds need to increase their contribution rate. Cost-sharing measures expressed in DEM will increase by DEM 1 for every 0.1 percentage point increase in contribution rates and cost-sharing measures expressed as a percentage will increase by 1 percentage point for every 0.1 percentage point. In effect, a raise by 1 percentage point (not unlikely for several sickness funds) would increase co-payments for pharmaceuticals from DEM 9/ 11/ 13 to 19/ 21/ 23, i.e. to levels where the word 'sharing' loses its meaning since many pharmaceuticals would no longer be covered at all. Compared to the 1996 cost sharing levels, these amounts would be higher by a factor of between 3.3 and 6.3. In the same example, cost-sharing for physiotherapy will increase from 15 to 25 per cent, i.e. by a factor of 2.5 compared to 1996.

The increased cost-sharing mechanisms may not, however, compensate for the effects of the abolition of budgets on health care costs, i.e. sickness funds contributions may have to be raised (leading to even higher cost sharing levels). Health care costs could then again become topical in the 1998 election and cost containment in Germany might experience a renaissance.

The authors would like to thank Sue Holloway for her help on earlier drafts of this chapter.

334 *Health Care and Cost Containment in the European Union*

References

1   Schwartz FW, Busse R. Germany. In: Ham C (ed.) *Health Care Reform – Learning from International Experience*. Buckingham-Philadelphia: Open University Press, 1997. pp. 104–18.

2   Busse R, Howorth C, Schwartz FW. The future development of a rights based approach to health care in Germany: more rights or fewer? In: Lenaghan J (ed.). *Hard Choices in Health Care – Rationing and Rights in Europe*. London: BMJ Publishing Group, 1997, pp. 21–47.

3   BMG (Bundesministerium für Gesundheit) *Daten des Gesundheitswesens – Ausgabe 1995*. Baden-Baden: Nomos, 1995. (published bi-annually).

4   Statistisches Bundesamt *Statistisches Jahrbuch 1996*. Stuttgart: Metzler Poeschel, 1996. (published annually).

5   Henke K-D, Murray MA, Ade C. Global budgeting in Germany: lessons for the United States. *Health Affairs* 1994;13(4):7–21.

6   Brenner G, Heuer J, Pfeiffer A. *Innovation und Strukturwandel in der vertragsärztlichen Versorgung*. Köln: Deutscher Ärzte-Verlag, 1994.

7   Klose J. *Leistungsreport Ärzte*. Stuttgart-Jena: G. Fischer, 1993.

8   Schwartz FW, Busse R. Fixed budgets in the German ambulatory care sector. In: Schwartz FW, Glennerster H, Saltman RB (eds). *Fixing Health Budgets – Experience from Europe and North America*. Chichester: Wiley & Sons, 1996. pp. 93-108.

9   BMG (Bundesministerium für Gesundheit) *96er Finanzergebnisse der GKV besser als erwartet – Zur Entwarnung besteht jedoch kein Anlaß*. Pressemitteilung No. 17:1997. www.bmgesundheit.de/presse/97/17.

10 Hungeling G. Die Jungen sind die Dummen – Neuregelung der Zulassung zur kassenärztlichen Tätigkeit. In: *Jahrbuch für Kritische Medizin* 20. Hamburg: Argument, 1993.

11 Arnold M, Paffrath D. (eds). *Krankenhaus-Report '96*. Stuttgart-Jena: G. Fischer, 1996. (published annually).

12 Statistisches Bundesamt *Gesundheitswesen – Reihe 6.1: Grunddaten der Krankenhäuser und Vorsorge- oder Rehabilitationseinrichtungen 1994*. Stuttgart: Metzler Poeschel, 1996. (published annually).

13 Busse R, Schwartz FW. Financing reforms in the German hospital sector – from full cost cover principle to prospective case fees. *Medical Care* 1997;35(10):OS 40–9.

14 Asmuth M, Müller U. *Entwicklung des ambulanten Operierens im Krankenhaus 1993/94. Ergebnisse einer Repräsentativerhebung das Krankenhaus* 1995;87:377–83.

15 Busch S, Pfaff A. Ambulante Operationen – Eine Möglichkeit zur Kostendämpfung im Gesundheitswesen. In: Düllings J (ed.). *Von der Budgetierung zur Strukturreform im Gesundheitswesen*. Heidelberg: R. v. Decker, 1996. pp. 131–47.

16 Busse R, Howorth C. Fixed budgets in the pharmaceutical sector in Germany: effects on costs and quality. In: Schwartz FW, Glennerster H, Saltman RB (eds). *Fixing Health Budgets – Experience from Europe and North America*. Chichester: Wiley & Sons, 1996. pp. 109–28.

Cost Containment in Germany: Twenty Years Experience 335

17 Klauber J. Entwicklung des Fertigarzneimittelmarktes 1983 bis 1993. In: Schwabe U, Paffrath D (eds). *Arzneiverordnungs-Report '94*. Stuttgart-Jena: G. Fischer, 1994. pp. 465–89.

18 Schwabe U, Paffrath D. (eds). *Arzneiverordnungs-Report '96*. Stuttgart-Jena: G. Fischer, 1996. (published annually).

19 BMG (Bundesministerium für Gesundheit). *Rede von Bundesgesundheitsminister Horst Seehofer anläßlich der 2./3. Lesung des 2. GKV-Neuordnungsgesetzes vor dem Deutschen Bundestag am 20. März 1997*. Pressemitteilung No. 25:1997. www.bmgesundheit.de/presse/97/25.

20 Verband der privaten Krankenversicherung. *Die private Krankenversicherung – Zahlenbericht 1995/96*. Köln, 1996. (published annually).

21 Kühn H. Zwanzig Jahre 'Kostenexplosion' – Anmerkungen zur Makroökonomie einer Gesundheitsreform. In: *Jahrbuch für Kritische Medizin* 24. Hamburg: Argument, 1995.

22 Advisory Council (for the Concerted Action in Health Care). *The Health Care System in Germany: Cost Factor and Branch of the Future. Volume I: Demographics, Morbidity, Efficiency Reserves and Employment*. Special Report 1996 – Summary. Bonn; complete version in German: Sachverständigenrat für die Konzertierte Aktion im Gesundheitswesen, 1996. Gesundheitswesen in Deutschland: Kostenfaktor und Zukunftsbranche. Band 1. Baden-Baden: Nomos, 1996.

N.B.: If references are published regularly, only the latest available edition is mentioned in this section.

Appendix 6.1 Data

Table A6.1 Sickness funds' overall expenditure (in current prices in DEM billion/year), 1975–96

	Ambulatory care	Dental care (excl. dentures)	Dentures	Hospitals/ in-patient care	Pharma-ceuticals	Non-physicians and devices	All other	Total
1975	11.26	4.13	4.18	17.53	8.90	2.58	9.58	58.17
1976	11.92	4.30	5.31	19.26	9.64	3.05	10.10	63.59
1977	12.49	4.61	5.40	20.46	9.85	3.34	10.46	66.61
1978	13.19	4.97	5.76	21.87	10.65	3.84	11.18	71.46
1979	14.12	5.22	6.47	23.25	11.37	4.36	12.64	77.44
1980	15.36	5.52	7.35	25.47	12.57	4.88	14.81	85.96
1981	16.49	5.94	8.11	27.32	13.63	5.27	15.44	92.20
1982	16.92	6.07	6.99	29.57	13.78	5.05	14.31	92.68
1983	17.76	6.28	6.66	30.97	14.45	5.23	14.54	95.90
1984	18.92	6.56	7.34	33.22	15.55	6.06	15.91	103.56
1985	19.66	6.66	7.67	35.05	16.60	6.51	16.56	108.70
1986	20.30	7.17	6.90	37.49	17.63	7.22	17.37	114.06
1987	20.97	7.37	6.28	39.21	18.89	7.85	18.36	118.93
1988	21.65	7.69	9.65	39.49	20.45	8.91	20.22	128.06
1989	22.65	7.69	4.86	40.81	20.22	7.83	19.18	123.24
1990	24.37	8.17	4.84	44.60	21.84	8.43	21.99	134.24
1991	26.74	9.13	5.61	49.12	24.49	9.69	26.86	151.63
1992	28.94	10.16	6.84	53.94	27.08	10.84	30.04	167.85
1993	29.89	10.41	4.91	56.95	21.81	11.32	30.80	166.09
1994	31.07	10.90	5.67	61.36	22.89	12.83	33.71	178.42
1995	32.80	11.19	6.13	64.65	25.06	14.05	35.71	189.59
1996	33.62	12.02	6.78	64.47	26.78	15.36	36.32	195.35

Table A6.2 Sickness funds' overall expenditure (in constant [1991] prices in DEM billion/year), 1975–95

	Ambulatory care	Dental care (excl. dentures)	Dentures	Hospitals/ in-patient care	Pharma-ceuticals	Non-physicians and devices	All other	Total
1975	18.85	6.91	7.00	29.53	14.90	4.32	16.04	97.55
1976	19.26	6.94	8.58	31.11	15.58	4.93	16.32	102.72
1977	19.45	7.18	8.41	31.87	15.34	5.20	16.29	103.75
1978	19.71	7.42	8.60	32.66	15.91	5.74	16.70	106.74
1979	20.33	7.52	9.32	33.47	16.37	6.27	18.19	111.46
1980	21.05	7.56	10.08	34.91	17.24	6.69	20.30	117.84
1981	21.70	7.81	10.67	35.95	17.94	6.94	20.32	121.34
1982	21.32	7.65	8.80	37.26	17.36	6.36	18.03	116.77
1983	21.68	7.67	8.13	37.80	17.63	6.39	17.74	117.03
1984	22.63	7.85	8.77	39.71	18.59	7.25	19.03	123.82
1985	23.03	7.80	8.98	41.06	19.45	7.63	19.40	127.35
1986	23.04	8.14	7.83	42.57	20.01	8.20	19.72	129.51
1987	23.37	8.21	7.00	43.70	21.05	8.75	20.46	132.55
1988	23.77	8.44	10.59	43.35	22.45	9.78	22.20	140.58
1989	24.28	8.25	5.21	43.75	21.67	8.39	20.56	132.11
1990	25.32	8.49	5.03	46.33	22.69	8.75	22.85	139.46
1991	26.74	9.13	5.61	49.12	24.49	9.69	26.86	151.63
1992	27.71	9.73	6.55	51.67	25.94	10.39	28.78	160.77
1993	27.74	9.66	4.56	52.86	20.25	10.50	28.59	154.15
1994	28.27	9.92	5.16	55.83	20.83	11.68	30.68	162.36
1995	29.25	9.98	5.47	57.65	22.35	12.53	31.83	169.05

338 *Health Care and Cost Containment in the European Union*

Table A6.3 Sickness funds' expenditure per insured person (in constant [1991] prices in DEM/year), 1975–95

	Ambulatory care	Dental care (excl. dentures)	Dentures	Hospitals/ in-patient care	Pharma- ceuticals	Non-physicians and devices	All other	Total
1975	333	122	124	518	263	76	283	1719
1976	342	123	152	552	276	87	289	1822
1977	346	128	149	566	273	92	289	1843
1978	351	132	153	581	283	102	297	1898
1979	361	133	165	594	290	111	323	1978
1980	371	133	178	616	304	118	358	2079
1981	384	138	189	635	317	123	359	2144
1982	380	136	157	664	309	113	321	2082
1983	381	135	143	664	310	112	312	2055
1984	400	139	155	701	328	128	336	2186
1985	412	139	161	734	348	136	347	2276
1986	418	148	142	773	363	149	358	2352
1987	424	149	127	793	382	159	371	2406
1988	431	153	192	786	407	177	403	2550
1989	444	151	95	799	396	153	376	2414
1990	454	152	90	830	406	157	409	2498
1991	470	161	99	864	431	170	473	2668
1992	485	170	115	904	454	182	503	2812
1993	483	168	79	920	352	183	497	2682
1994	493	173	90	973	363	204	534	2829
1995	508	173	95	1000	388	217	552	2933

Table A6.4 Sickness funds' expenditure as proportion of GDP per capita (in %), 1975–95

	Ambulatory care	Dental care (excl. dentures)	Dentures	Hospitals/ in-patient care	Pharma- ceuticals	Non-physicians and devices	All other	Total
1975	1.20	0.44	0.45	1.87	0.95	0.27	1.02	6.19
1976	1.16	0.42	0.52	1.88	0.94	0.30	0.99	6.20
1977	1.14	0.42	0.49	1.87	0.90	0.31	0.96	6.08
1978	1.12	0.42	0.49	1.86	0.91	0.33	0.95	6.07
1979	1.11	0.41	0.51	1.82	0.89	0.34	0.99	6.08
1980	1.13	0.41	0.54	1.88	0.93	0.36	1.09	6.34
1981	1.17	0.42	0.58	1.94	0.97	0.37	1.10	6.55
1982	1.17	0.42	0.48	2.05	0.96	0.35	0.99	6.41
1983	1.15	0.41	0.43	2.00	0.93	0.34	0.94	6.20
1984	1.17	0.41	0.45	2.05	0.96	0.37	0.98	6.38
1985	1.18	0.40	0.46	2.10	0.99	0.39	0.99	6.50
1986	1.17	0.41	0.40	2.16	1.01	0.42	1.00	6.56
1987	1.17	0.41	0.35	2.18	1.05	0.44	1.02	6.62
1988	1.15	0.41	0.51	2.10	1.09	0.47	1.08	6.81
1989	1.16	0.39	0.25	2.08	1.03	0.40	0.98	6.28
1990	1.14	0.38	0.23	2.08	1.02	0.39	1.03	6.27
1991	1.14	0.39	0.24	2.09	1.04	0.41	1.14	6.46
1992	1.17	0.41	0.28	2.18	1.09	0.44	1.21	6.77
1993	1.20	0.42	0.20	2.28	0.87	0.45	1.23	6.65
1994	1.20	0.42	0.22	2.38	0.89	0.46	1.31	6.88
1995	1.22	0.42	0.23	2.41	0.93	0.52	1.33	7.06

7 Health care and cost containment in Greece

ARIS SISSOURAS, ANTHONY KAROKIS AND ELIAS MOSSIALOS

7.1 Introduction

It is generally very difficult to discuss cost containment in the Greek health care system, since cost control, as a goal in health policy, was not a major concern in Greece until the early 1990s. On the contrary, health policy during the 1970s and 1980s sought to expand the provision of health services and to increase public health expenditure. Emphasis was more on expansion than on containment.

This chapter will show:

- cost containment has only very recently been discussed in Greek health policy;

- any efforts to implement cost-curtailing measures face problems arising from lack of accurate data, adverse incentives in the operating financing mechanisms, obsolete administrative practices and segmentation of the sources of funding;

- consequently, cost containment measures will not produce any significant results, unless they are taken together with measures for the reorganization of the health care system; and

- the problem is made more difficult by the fact that not only public but private expenditure is growing and, given the current fiscal constraints, it is unlikely that governments will try to curb private spending as long as it acts as a substitute for public financing.

The Greek health care system developed as a system of compulsory social health insurance mainly in the post-war period. After 1974, when the democratic regime in Greece was restored, governments on the whole followed expansionary policies in health care. The main policy objectives in the

342 *Health Care and Cost Containment in the European Union*

1970s and early 1980s were to improve the quality of public hospital services and expand health insurance coverage to segments of the population which until the early 1980s were fully or partially excluded. These goals were adequately justified by the fact that health expenditure in Greece was very low compared with other OECD countries, and had even been reduced significantly during the period of the Colonels' Dictatorship between 1967 and 1974.[1]

Apart from increasing the level of public expenditure on health, an extensive debate was held during the 1970s on whether additional changes in the organization of the health care system were required. The proponents of a more substantial reform of the Greek health insurance system were arguing for the introduction of a national health system based on the British NHS model. This was viewed as a means for combating the existing geographical and income inequalities in health care provision and access, and distinguishing the limits between public and private provision by public doctors.[2, 3]

In the early 1980s the rise of a socialist party in power brought the introduction of a national health system in Greece. This reform gave a further impetus for expansionary expenditure policies. There was a deliberate effort to expand the public health care sector and substitute functions and operations hitherto exercised in the private sector. This trend resulted in an increase in the total amount of health expenditure.[4–6]

This trend has been reversed, albeit slightly, in the 1990s. There have been two main reasons for this. The first is political. The conservative government, which came to power in 1990 deliberately sought to reduce the share of public involvement in the health care field. The second reason is both political and economic. The need to abide by the convergence criteria set for the Maastricht Treaty has created new realities and priorities for government policy. The major targets include the reduction of the inflation rate, the reduction of public deficit as a percentage of GDP, the attainment of stable currency exchange rates and the convergence of long-term interest rates with the EU members. Consequently a convergence programme has been agreed between Greece and the European Commission, covering the period from 1994–99 for the achievement of these targets.

In 1995, the inflation rate fell by 2.7 per cent from the 1994 level to reach 8.1 per cent, and in the spring of 1997 it fell further to around 6 per cent, although this was still high compared to other EU countries. The public sector deficit reached 9.8 per cent of GDP at the end of 1995, while the

Health Care and Cost Containment in Greece   343

public debt reached 117 per cent of GDP at this time.

The fiscal pressures to achieve the convergence targets required for entry into the second round of EMU have forced the government to seek ways to reduce public spending. This is the major driving force in any attempt to contain health expenditure in Greece. Despite these trends for a different approach toward public health financing, no deliberate efforts have been made to control private expenditure on health and to promote a more effective use of health care resources. This is mainly due to the fact that the new cost containment philosophy has not yet acquired a comprehensive view on the problem of health care expenditure.

In the sections that follow, this chapter will outline the following:

- an overview of the cost containment measures planned or implemented in the Greek health care system in the past two decades;
- the policy trends that guided the implementation or absence of cost containment measures;
- an analysis of health care expenditure trends in Greece in various levels of care, in order to assess the efficacy of the cost containment initiatives undertaken;
- the current proposals for health care reform and an assessment of their prospects for implementation, and the future evolution of health expenditure.

The structure of the chapter is as follows. At first the Greek health care system is briefly described. In the following sections the expenditure trends and cost containment measures are discussed, together with an assessment of their effects on the expenditure trends. Finally, the plans for health care reform are presented and the chapter ends with an overall assessment of cost containment measures in Greece.

7.2 The Greek health care system

7.2.1 The Greek health insurance system

The Greek health care system is a system of compulsory public health insurance with strong elements of a national health system and extensive

344   *Health Care and Cost Containment in the European Union*

involvement of the private sector. In terms of the taxonomy proposed by Hurst,[7] it is a mixture of the public contract and public integrated models.[5] Greek citizens are compulsorily insured in one of about 40 social insurance funds that provide coverage against sickness. The choice of fund is based on the occupation of the insured, and it is usual that if a person changes occupation they will also have to change their insurance fund.

The main funds are IKA, which covers salaried workers; OGA, which covers rural workers and TEVE, which covers the self-employed. Together these three funds cover over 80 per cent of the insured population against sickness (Table 7.1). Apart from these funds, a separate scheme operates for public servants, in which about 600,000 people are insured. This is not an autonomous fund but an administrative department in the Ministry of Health and the Ministry of Economy. In reality, accurate figures on the number of people insured under this scheme do not exist. However, the government has recently announced that this department is going to become an autonomous insurance fund, in the hope of achieving stricter administration and better control of resources.

Table 7.1 The major insurance funds in Greece, 1996

Fund	Directly insured	Indirectly insured	Total	% of total insured population
IKA (salaried workers)	2,772,000	2,690,000	5,462,000	50.7
OGA (rural population)	1,894,000	571,000	2,465,000	22.9
TEVE (small businessmen)	506,000	759,000	1,265,000	11.7
TAE (merchants)	181,000	308,000	489,000	4.5
Telecommunications personnel	58,700	91,850	150,550	1.4
Public servants scheme* sioners.	This covers about 600,000 public servants and pen-			

*The scheme for the public servants is not yet an autonomous fund, and is not supervised by the Ministry of Labour and Social Insurance.
Source: Social Budget. Ministry of Labour and Social Security, 1996.[8]

Health Care and Cost Containment in Greece 345

The rest of the funds each cover less than 1 per cent of the insured population. It must be noted that the total number of people insured is larger than the total population of Greece, not withstanding the non-insured population. This is due to the fact that some individuals can be concurrently insured with more than one insurance organization. This may happen if an individual has two occupations covered by different funds or if they are insured directly in one and indirectly (in case of another working member of the family) in another. In such cases an individual is free to choose which insurance organization to use.

According to OECD databases the entire Greek population enjoys some form of insurance coverage against the risk of sickness. In reality, however, a small part of the population still remains uninsured. In a local health inter-

Table 7.2 Health insurance contributions in major insurance funds in Greece, 1997

Fund	Employers' contributions (% of monthly salary)	Employees' contributions (% of monthly salary)	Self-employed contributions	State subsidies	Social contributions
IKA	5.10	2.55	—	Yes	Yes
OGA	—	—	—	Yes, total expenses are financed by the state budget	Yes
TEVE	—	—	14 categories 6,772–27,735 GRD per month*		
TAE	—	—	14 categories 8,900–10,100 GRD per month*		
Telecom. Personnel	13.33	6.67		Yes, 10% of the total fund's revenue	

*The insured chooses the category he or she wishes to be insured under.

Source: Social Budget. Ministry of Labour and Social Security, 1996.[8]

346   *Health Care and Cost Containment in the European Union*

Table 7.3 Services covered by selected insurance funds, 1997

(a) Benefits in kind

	Medical care	Hospital care	Pharmaceutical care	Dental care	Spectacles, laboratory tests etc.	Other benefits
IKA	+	+	+	+	+	+
OGA	+	+	+	-	+	+
TEVE	+	+	+	-	+	+
TAE	+	+	+	-	-	+
Electricity	+	+	+	+	+	+
Banks[a]	+	+	+	+	+	-[a]

(b) Cash benefits

	Income lost due to illness	Accident allowance	Spa treatment	Maternity and birth allowance	Death and funeral expenses
IKA	+	+	+	+	+
OGA	+	+	-	+	+
TEVE	+	-	+	+	+
TAE	-	+	-	+	+
Electricity	-	-	+	-	-
Banks	(-)[b]	-(+)[b]	+	+	+

Notes:
(a) Almost all different funds for banking institutions provide the same range of benefits in kind.
(b) The signs in parentheses mean that the minority of funds in banking institutions provide (+) or do not provide (-) the particular benefit.

Source: Social Budget. Ministry of Labour and Social Security, 1996.[8]

Health Care and Cost Containment in Greece 347

view survey of 2000 households in the district of Achaia, 6 per cent of the respondents stated that they did not enjoy any form of health insurance coverage. A large proportion of those uninsured were young and unemployed individuals.[9] This figure may be slightly exaggerated, since the unemployment rate is higher in that particular district compared to the Greek average. Thus the probable number of uninsured should be less than 5 per cent. To these one should also add the large number of illegal immigrants, most of whom come from the Balkan countries. Their total numbers are unknown, but estimated to be around 400,000.

7.2.2 The level of health insurance contributions The funds are financed mainly by contributions paid by employers and employees, and some of them also receive additional subsidies from the state budget. The level of contributions and the subsidies are determined by the state – as the funds are heavily regulated – and vary widely between the funds (Table 7.2).

7.2.3 Extent of coverage All funds cover hospital care, primary medical care, diagnostic services and pharmaceutical care. There are differences in the coverage for dental care and a number of prosthetic or other services. These differences do not reveal any explicit rationing processes or decisions but are the result of historical developments in health insurance in Greece (Table 7.3).[10]

7.3 Health care provision

7.3.1 Provision of hospital services

As far as hospital care is concerned all funds provide their members with free access to all public hospitals and a large number of private contracted ones. The number of private contracted hospitals differs among the funds depending mainly on the number of insured members and their distribution across the country. Some funds, like IKA, provide some hospital care in their own hospitals, but the majority of the population relies on the services of the public hospital system.

    The uninsured population also has access to public hospitals. Services are provided to local inhabitants free of charge. Otherwise they must pay for

348   *Health Care and Cost Containment in the European Union*

the services provided and are charged with the state-fixed tariffs that social insurance funds are also charged with. Uninsured people also have access to private hospitals and clinics on a willingness and ability to pay basis.

In 1993 there were 384 public hospitals in Greece, accommodating a total of 52,834 beds, of which 10,714 were psychiatric care beds. The number of private hospitals and clinics is 233 (61 per cent of the total) but in terms of the number of beds the public sector prevails with 37,974 beds or 72 per cent of the total.[11] In terms of total number of beds, Greece has a relatively low bed to population ratio among OECD countries.[12] In 1993 there were 5.1 beds per 1,000 inhabitants.

7.3.2 Provision of primary health care services

Primary health care services are provided by rural health centres, doctors contracted by health insurance organizations, health insurance polyclinics and private practice physicians.[13]

There are 196 rural health centres, all in rural and semi-urban areas, which provide free primary medical care to all inhabitants. These centres have been especially beneficial for OGA members (the rural population), since they were primarily targeted for them.

In urban areas, social insurance funds either employ salaried doctors in their own polyclinics (mainly IKA), or contract out private physicians to provide primary health care services to their members (the rest of the funds, except OGA). IKA doctors are paid on a salary basis, whereas contracted physicians are reimbursed by the funds on a fee-for-service basis, alongside state-determined tariffs, which are below market charges.

OGA members have free access to rural health centres and the out-patient departments of public hospitals.

Moreover, primary care physicians (including IKA and contracted doctors) operate their own private practices, where patients have access on an ability-to-pay basis.

Primary health care services are also provided in the out-patient departments of public hospitals on a walk-in or appointment basis. Currently these services are provided only during morning hours, while evenings and nights are reserved for Accident and Emergency services. All Greek inhabitants have access to these services, for which a nominal charge of GRD 1,000 (GBP 2.00) has been set.

Although a multiplicity of primary health care provider services exists, the different organizational arrangements can be a cause for concern for members of the various funds. In general, it is perceived that the funds which offer a wider choice of physicians, and have the largest number of contracted-out doctors, provide better quality coverage than other funds, whose doctors are salaried or are based in polyclinics.[13]

The total number of doctors in Greece in 1992 was 38,738, of which 18,565 were hospital doctors and 20,173 were doctors involved in primary health care provision.[14] Of the latter, less than 1,000 are general practitioners and the rest are specialists. It should be pointed out that Greece has one of the highest doctors to population ratios among the OECD countries. In 1993, there were 3.9 doctors per thousand population, second only to Spain where the rate was 4.1 doctors per thousand inhabitants.[12]

7.3.3 Pharmaceutical care

All insurance funds in Greece cover pharmaceutical care for their members. This was not the case even in the early 1980s, when apart from the medicines provided by sparsely distributed rural doctors, the rural population did not enjoy insurance coverage for pharmaceutical care.[15] With some exceptions, the general co-payment rate for pharmaceuticals in primary health care is 25 per cent of prescription costs. There are no co-payments for pharmaceuticals provided to in-patients, neither is there any formal OTC market for drugs in Greece.

In 1992, there were 7,698 pharmacies in Greece and 130 pharmaceutical wholesalers. For the same year the number of pharmacists stood at 7834, 31 per cent higher than the 1985 figure.[16] Less than 500 pharmacists were employed in the hospital sector. Although the number of pharmacists is high, unemployment in the field is practically non-existent. It is questionable, though, whether so many pharmacies are necessary.[17]

7.3.4 Dental care

Dental care is provided by public hospitals, public rural health centres, doctors employed or contracted by insurance funds and by private dentists. Wide differences exist among insurance funds with regard to coverage for

350 *Health Care and Cost Containment in the European Union*

dental care services. The largest fund, IKA, only covers dental care services provided by doctors employed by the fund. OGA members only have free access to dentists employed in rural health centres, but there are wide gaps in the employment of dentists among health centres.

Some funds, such as the funds for merchants and small businessmen, do not cover dental care at all. Other funds cover care provided by contracted dentists. Most funds cover dental treatment like fillings and extractions. Some funds cover prosthetic services as well, but in the case of the Public Servants Scheme there is a 50 per cent co-payment rate. Preventive dental services are neither covered nor provided, apart from some temporary and uncoordinated initiatives by certain dentists in rural health centres or dentists contracted by the funds for banking personnel.[18]

7.4 Overall health care expenditure and its control

7.4.1 The level of health care expenditure

By international comparison, Greece has always been considered a low spender on health. According to the OECD database, total health expenditure in Greece accounted for 5.9 per cent of GDP in 1996, and per capita health expenditure measured in Purchasing Power Parities was at USD 748, making Greece third from last among OECD countries.[12]

A different picture arises though, if one looks at the figures of the National Accounts of the Greek National Statistical Service. According to these figures, Greece is a moderate to high spender on health, with a significant part of expenditure being private. In Table 7.5 overleaf, the figures from the National Accounts are presented according to the new system of national accounting that was introduced in 1994.

Total health care expenditure in Greece increased significantly during the 1970s; grew steadily but marginally slower during the 1980s; and has been growing at moderate rates during the 1990s. This trend is evident, both in OECD data and the Greek National Accounts data.

The element of expenditure that contributes most to the overall expenditure growth is private expenditure. According to the National Accounts, in 1992 private expenditure on health rose to 42.5 per cent of total expenditure in constant prices, with 57.5 per cent being public expenditure. In 1987 the

Health Care and Cost Containment in Greece 351

Table 7.4 Health expenditure in Greece 1970–96 (according to the OECD database)

Year	PPP (USD)	% GDP	GRD million (current prices)	GRD million (in 1990 prices)*
1970	60	3.4	12,072	218,300
1975	106	3.4	27,382	282,289
1980	191	3.6	74,172	354,043
1981	215	3.7	91,956	370,641
1982	224	3.7	113,756	372,726
1983	243	3.8	142,199	408,853
1984	254	3.8	172,798	422,799
1985	289	4.1	224,526	452,218
1986	330	4.5	295,517	503,093
1987	328	4.3	325,775	502,352
1988	342	4.2	378,619	522,666
1989	370	4.3	451,456	546,094
1990	395	4.3	560,977	560,977
1991	416	4.2	685,262	530,799
1992	480	4.5	836,460	561,533
1993	549	5.0	1,050,000	627,240
1994	634	5.5	1,300,000	—
1995	703	5.8	1,530,000	—
1996	748	5.9	1,750,000	—

Source: OECD Health Data File, 1997.[12]
* Current national total expenditure on health deflated by a weighted health specific deflator.

respective figures were 40 per cent private and 60 per cent public (see Table 7.6 overleaf). However, the estimates of expenditure levels, differ according to the price index employed in the calculation of constant prices (see Tables 7.6, 7.6a, and 7.6b).

In Table 7.6, constant prices were calculated by deflating the figures on public expenditure according to the General Price Index, and the figures on private expenditure according to the Medical Care Price Index (MCPI). This

Table 7.5 Health care expenditure in Greece: current prices, selected years

| | Public expenditure on health | | Private expenditure on health | | Total expenditure on health | Gross Domestic Product | Total expenditure on health |
	GRD million	% of GDP	GRD million	% of GDP	GRD million	GRD million	% of GDP
1970	6,240	2.41%	8,371	3.24%	14,611	258,000	5.66%
1980	58,863	3.86%	42,051	2.75%	100,914	1,523,724	6.62%
1987	244,867	4.46%	163,091	2.97%	407,958	5,478,103	7.44%
1988	298,333	4.50%	183,129	2.76%	481,462	6,619,583	7.27%
1989	371,688	4.74%	213,627	2.72%	585,315	7,838,252	7.46%
1990	442,076	4.79%	263,075	2.85%	705,151	9,218,908	7.64%
1991	531,699	4.80%	338,811	3.06%	870,510	11,071,526	7.86%
1992	610,438	4.87%	429,607	3.42%	1,040,045	12,531,000	8.29%
1993	–	–	529,354	3.68%	–	14,359,000	–
1994	–	–	651,538	4.07%	–	15,979,051	–

Sources: National Statistical Service of Greece, 1992;[19] National Statistical Service of Greece, 1994.[20]

Table 7.6 Health care expenditure in Greece: constant prices (1988 = 100), selected years*

	Public expenditure on health		Private expenditure on health		Total expenditure on health	Gross Domestic Product	Total expenditure on health
	GRD million	% of GDP	GRD million	% of GDP	GRD million	GRD million	% of GDP
1987	277,942	4.46%	192,324	3.09%	470,266	6,218,051	7.56%
1988	298,333	4.50%	183,129	2.76%	481,462	6,619,583	7.27%
1989	326,902	4.74%	188,883	2.73%	515,785	6,893,801	7.48%
1990	322,919	4.79%	197,801	2.93%	520,720	6,734,045	7.73%
1991	324,999	4.80%	214,709	3.17%	539,708	6,767,436	7.97%
1992	322,131	4.87%	238,538	3.60%	560,669	6,612,665	8.47%
1993			244,280	3.68%	—	6,623,155	—
1994			271,927	4.09%	—	6,644,096	—

* Figures on public expenditure have been deflated according to the General Price Index, and figures on private expenditure have been deflated according to the Medical Care Price Index (National Statistical Service of Greece, various years, 1988 = 100).

Sources: National Statistical Service of Greece, 1992;[19] National Statistical Service of Greece, 1994.[20]

Table 7.6a Health care expenditure in Greece: constant prices (1988 = 100), selected years*

	Public expenditure	on health	Private expenditure	on health	Total expenditure on health	Gross Domestic Product	Total expenditure on health
	GRD million	% of GDP	GRD million	% of GDP	GRD million	GRD million	% of GDP
1987	288,758	4.64%	192,324	3.09%	481,082	6,218,051	7.73%
1988	298,333	4.50%	183,129	2.76%	481,462	6,619,583	7.27%
1989	328,637	4.77%	188,883	2.73%	517,520	6,893,801	7.50%
1990	332,387	4.94%	197,801	2.93%	530,188	6,734,045	7.87%
1991	336,944	4.98%	214,709	3.17%	551,693	6,767,436	8.15%
1992	338,944	5.13%	238,538	3.60%	577,482	6,612,665	8.73%
1993	–	–	244,280	3.68%	–	6,623,155	–
1994	–	–	271,927	4.09%	–	6,644,096	–

* Figures on both public and private expenditure have been deflated according to the Medical Care Price Index (National Statistical Service of Greece, various years, 1988 = 100).

Sources: National Statistical Service of Greece, 1992;[19] National Statistical Service of Greece, 1994.[20]

Table 7.6b Health care expenditure in Greece: constant prices (1988 = 100), selected years*

	Public expenditure on health		Private expenditure on health		Total expenditure on health	Gross Domestic Product	Total expenditure on health
	(GRD million	% of GDP	GRD million	% of GDP	GRD million	GRD million	% of GDP
1987	288,758	4.64%	185,210	2.98%	463,062	6,218,051	7.44%
1988	298.333	4.50%	183,129	2.76%	481,462	6,619,583	7.27%
1989	328,637	4.77%	187,886	2.72%	514,788	6,893,801	7.46%
1990	332,387	4.94%	192,166	2.68%	515,085	6,734,045	7.47%
1991	336,944	4.98%	207,097	3.06%	532,096	6,767,436	7.85%
1992	338,944	5.13%	226,705	3.42%	548,836	6,612,665	8.29%
1993	–	–	244,167	3.68%	–	6,623,155	–
1994	–	–	270,910	4.07%	–	6,644,096	–

* Figures on both public and private expenditure have been deflated according to the General Price Index (National Statistical Service of Greece, various years, 1988 = 100).

Sources: National Statistical Service of Greece, 1992;[19] National Statistical Service of Greece, 1994.[20]

356 *Health Care and Cost Containment in the European Union*

approach was assumed to be more appropriate since public expenditure includes payments from the state budget and the social insurance organizations, which follow, in general trends, the priorities of government spending and are thus more sensitive to GDP changes. The MCPI is calculated by estimating private consumption and following the trends presented in the Family Budget Surveys. If the MCPI is employed in calculating constant prices for both public and private expenditure, then overall expenditure seems much higher, since public expenditure overall seems higher than the figures calculated with the general price index (Table 7.6a). If on the other hand, the general price index is used to deflate both public and private expenditures (Table 7.6b), then overall expenditure seems high, but less so than the figures presented in Table 7.6. The reason is that private expenditure is estimated at marginally lower levels. It should be stressed though, that the increase in private expenditure is sharp even with this calculation, and after 1991 private expenditure does seem to increase considerably – at growth rates that exceed those for public expenditure. Another important point to notice in this respect, is that in both Tables 7.6a and 7.6b, public expenditure remains around 58–59 per cent of the total. In general, the facts are that health expenditure in Greece is relatively high and that private expenditure in recent years is growing faster than public expenditure; irrespective of the price index employed.

Another issue is the different expenditure levels between the national accounts and the OECD database. These can be partially attributed to the different calculation methods involved. OECD calculations include private and public consumption on health, as components of health expenditure, excluding the expenditure incurred by the social insurance organizations, which are treated as transfer payments. On the other hand, the Greek National Accounts calculation of public and private consumption underestimates some parts of expenditure, most notably pharmaceutical expenditure. For the latter, public expenditure on pharmaceuticals is not included in the calculations, since it is mainly financed via the expenditure of the social insurance organizations. (A more detailed analysis of the problems and a comparison of the calculation methods of OECD and Greek National Accounts data are provided in Kyriopoulos and Niakas.)[21] In addition, private expenditure is probably underestimated both in OECD data and the National Accounts, as further discussed in section 7.6 below.

Health Care and Cost Containment in Greece   357

Table 7.7 Overall budget ceilings in various levels of health expenditure in Greece, 1997

Level of expenditure	Existence of budget	Enforcement of the budget
Private expenditure	No	
Public expenditure	No overall budget	
State budget expenditure	Yes	No
Public hospital expenditure	Yes	No
Social insurance organization	Yes	No
Pharmaceutical expenditure	Budget for public expenditure, by the social insurance funds	No
Primary health care expenditure	Budgets for expenditure by the rural health centres (via the hospital budgets) and the expenditure of the social insurance organizations	No

7.4.2 Overall health care expenditure controls

It is very difficult to impose a ceiling on overall health expenditure. The first impediment is the large share of private expenditure, which is beyond any control. As far as public health expenditure is concerned, overall ceilings are supposedly agreed at the beginning of each financial year. But the large number of payers, the lack of coordination among them, the absence of adequate financial management and accounting systems and the lack of any monitoring processes allow for the presence of excesses in the budget. As a result, the levels of the annual budgets do not serve as yearly expenditure ceilings and, in most cases, realized expenditure exceeds budget predictions (see Table 7.7). A more detailed discussion on the budgeting processes for state expenditure and the social insurance funds, as well as their effectiveness, will follow in section 7.5 below.

358 *Health Care and Cost Containment in the European Union*

7.4.2.1 Expenditure transferred to public debt requirements Over the next four years about GRD 150 billion of health care expenditure will not be included in the health services budget, but will be added to the general public debt requirements. This will include payments that the government has undertaken as a means to reduce public hospital deficits (see section 7.7.2 below).

7.4.2.2 Expenditure for treatment abroad Another portion of expenditure that is not wholly included in total health expenditure concerns payments for treatment abroad. A large number of Greeks seek treatment abroad, especially for cardiovascular care. The main reason for treatment abroad is heart surgery (49 per cent), and the most commonly visited country is the UK (70.5 per cent of all patients treated abroad).[22] Total expenditure for treatment abroad is presented in Table 7.8.

Table 7.8 Health expenditure for treatment abroad (USD 1,000s),1976–91

Year	Expenditure
1976	5,884
1977	5,735
1978	7,746
1979	11,969
1980	16,231
1981	15,819
1982	22,032
1983	18,195
1984	15,932
1985	18,330
1986	24,787
1987	33,476
1988	51,659
1989	59,322
1990	71,514
1991	76,585

Source: Bessis, 1993.[23]

There are two ways for patients to seek treatment abroad. One is to use the European Union procedures for pre-authorized (form E-112) or emergency treatment (form E-111). The second is to seek treatment via the administrative procedures of the social insurance funds. Kyriopoulos and Geitona[22] have shown that more than 80 per cent of the IKA patients who seek treatment abroad do so using the internal procedures of the fund. These require the certification by at least two doctors that the particular condition cannot be treated in Greece.

Governments in the 1990s have tried to reduce the flow of patients to foreign countries. In 1991, following a Central Council of Health Recommendation, the government decided to allow social insurance funds to contract private hospitals to perform heart surgery for their members. The tariffs were arbitrarily determined at relatively high levels when compared with those for other procedures. However, it seems that this measure has managed to reduce the flow of patients for heart surgery abroad. This is true for IKA and TEVE patients, but less so for the rural population. The adverse effect of this initiative has been that more patients now use private hospitals for heart surgery instead of public ones, thus likely increasing the overall costs.[22]

7.5 Public health expenditure and its controls

7.5.1 Public health expenditure trends

Public health care expenditure in Greece, as a share of GDP, increased considerably during the 1970s and 1980s. In current prices, they rose as a share of GDP from 2.4 per cent in 1970 to 3.8 per cent in 1980, and to 4.79 per cent in 1990 (Table 7.5). Since then they remained stable or were slightly reduced during the 1990s. The trend is similar if one looks at trends of health care expenditure in constant prices as well. As Table 7.6 shows, during the 1990s there has been a growing stabilization of public expenditure in Greece, whereas there has been a marked increase in the share of private expenditure.

The sources of public health funding include income from general direct and indirect taxation, which is distributed via the state budget, and income from social insurance contributions which is then distributed by the

360 *Health Care and Cost Containment in the European Union*

social insurance funds. State budget expenditure includes expenditure for OGA members, subsidies to public hospitals and other health service institutions (i.e. rural health centres), expenditure for health care services provided to the members of the Public Servants Scheme, and expenditure on

Table 7.9 Public health expenditure in Greece, 1987–92

| | State budget expenditure:— | | Social insurance |
	Current prices (GRD million and % of total)	Constant prices (GRD million and % of total)	Current prices (GRD million and % of total)
1987	139,624 57.0	158,483 [1] 57.0	105,243 43.0
	—	164,651 [2] 57.0	—
1988	174,292 58.5	174,292 58.5	124,041 41.5
1989	213,289 57.4	187,589 57.4	158,399 42.6
	—	188,584 57.4	—
1990	259,837 58.8	189,801 58.8	182,239 41.2
	—	195,366 58.8	—
1991	307,343 57.8	187,862 57.8	224,356 42.2
	—	194,767 57.8	—
1992	352,480 58.0	186,005 57.8	257,958 42.0
	—	195,713 57.8	—

(1) The figures in the first row for each respective year have been deflated according to the GDP price index (1988 = 100).
(2) The figures in the second row of each respective year have been deflated according to the Medical Care price index (1988 = 100).

Health Care and Cost Containment in Greece 361

capital investments in public health services. The expenditure on the social insurance funds includes payments for services provided to their members.

As Table 7.9 shows, state budget expenditure consists mainly of public health expenditure, rising to almost 60 per cent of total public expenditure.

funds expenditure Constant prices (GRD million and % of total)	Total public expenditure:	
	Current prices	Constant prices
111,177 [1] 43.0	244,867	277,942 [1]
124,166 [2] 43.0	—	288,758 [2]
124,041 41.5	298,333	298,333
139,313 42.6	371,688	326,902
140,052 42.6	—	328,637
133,118 42.2	442,076	322,919
137,022 42.2	—	332,388
137,137 42.2	531,699	324,999
142,177 42.2	336,945	—
136,126 42.2	610,438	322,131
143,230 42.2	—	338,944

Sources: National Statistical Service of Greece, 1992;[19] National Statistical Service of Greece, 1994.[20]

362 Health Care and Cost Containment in the European Union

7.5.2 Controlling overall public expenditure

7.5.2.1 Trends in public health services policy During the 1980s there was no explicit policy trend or initiative in Greece to control public spending. On the contrary, the introduction of the NHS marked a period where the explicit goal was to increase public sector involvement both in the financing and provision of health care. In 1983 the Socialist government sought to substitute private finance and provision of health care with public services and funding, as a means for improving access to health care for all citizens and reducing the influence of market forces on the financing and provision of health care. Apart from this ideological and political reasoning, two other factors contributed to the increasing emphasis and expansion of the public health sector. The first was the need to modernize the existing public hospitals, and the second was to fill the gaps in the provision of services that existed in the rural areas.[2,5,15]

In ideological and political terms the turning point was 1989. The then-Socialist government lost the election, and after two coalition governments for about a year, the Conservative party came into power in 1990. The Conservatives ended the hostility, at least in policy initiatives, between the public and private sectors and actively sought to encourage the involvement of the latter. In addition, they sought to shift the balance from the state budget to the social insurance funds, albeit with minimum success. The significant characteristic of this period was the demise of the policy trend to expand the public health care sector in order to substitute private health care provision. Nevertheless, even in this period no coherent cost containment initiatives were undertaken.[6,24]

In 1993 the Socialists returned to government. There were two main differences from the 1980s. The first was that the government followed a strict public fiscal policy. The pressures to meet the convergence criteria set by the Maastricht Treaty forced the government to seek ways to reduce overall public spending. The second was that the new Socialist government seemed more receptive to pressures to re-organize the health care system along the lines of the health care reforms that had been introduced in other European health care systems in the late 1980s and early 1990s.

Whether these efforts will succeed is a matter for discussion (see section 7.13 below). In the paragraphs that follow, an assessment of the few cost containment efforts that have been undertaken since the 1980s will be attempted.

Health Care and Cost Containment in Greece 363

7.5.2.2 Imposing an overall budget ceiling Each year an annual budget ceiling is determined with regard to public health expenditure. Ceilings are set both on the expenditure of the state budget and on that of the social insurance organizations. Nevertheless, for a number of reasons these ceilings are not strictly monitored. The main factor is the budgeting process itself.

(a) The budgeting process for government spending The state budget for health care is determined annually each November in the central government expenditure planning process. The components of the state budget include expenditure that is allocated by the budget of the Ministry of Health expenditure allocated via the budgets of the 52 local prefectures. The local prefectures finance subsidies to public hospitals and expenditure for capital developments. They also reimburse providers for services provided to members of the Public Servants Scheme in their prefecture. The total budget supposedly determines the maximum amount of expenditure that should be financed from general taxation revenue.

It can be reasonably argued though, that a better budgeting process would result in a more rational use of resources and evaluation of priorities. Whereas the overall level of the budget is determined according to the government's fiscal priorities, the sub-components of the budget are determined on an historical basis. Under the current public accounting system, the budget is composed of different code numbers, each representing planned expenditure for some purpose. For the state or any other public agent (like the local prefectures, or the public hospitals) to allocate resources to a certain purpose, a code for this purpose should have been included in the budget. In reality, the coding system is based on historic patterns of expenditure and not actual or even ongoing priorities. Thus resources allocated to certain purposes are not spent at all, whereas planned expenditure on other more urgent priorities is often inadequate (see also Kyriopoulos and Niakas).[25]

For example, in the budget of the Ministry of Health there is a code which covers allowances to Hansen disease patients. These resources are never spent during the fiscal year. On the other hand, expenditure on public hospitals is annually determined at a lower level than is needed.

Table 7.10 overleaf shows the actual budget deficits and surpluses that resulted between the years 1992 and 1994. As can be seen, the portion of the budget that is allocated via the Ministry of Health is not totally spent and presents a small surplus at the end of each fiscal year. Meanwhile, the

364 Health Care and Cost Containment in the European Union

Table 7.10 Actual surpluses and deficits in state budget expenditure, 1992–94

Year	Ministry of Health expenditure (GRD)	Local prefecture expenditure (GRD)	Total state budget expenditure (GRD)
1992	+ 45,194,140,043	- 14,631,694,072	+ 30,562,445,971
1993	+ 72,878,517,082	- 64,038,899,605	+ 8,839,617,477
1994	+ 40,671,622,721	- 69,234,721,400	- 28,563,098,679

Note: + = surplus, - = deficit

Source: Ministry of Finance, 1992, 1993, 1994.[26]

expenditure allocated via the local prefectures presents deficits at the end of each year. The deficits are due to real expenditure being higher than planned expenditure in the public sector scheme and to subsidies to public hospitals.

Although the overall picture shows that total expenditure is not completely spent within each fiscal year, it should be emphasized that in practice the funds are not transferred from one budget to the other. Thus whereas some Ministry of Health funds are not totally spent, public hospitals and services in local prefectures are running up budgetary deficits, because there is no transfer between the various budgets. In practice, the expenditure of the local prefectures exceeds their budget, because realized expenditure on hospital subsidies and expenditure for health services to local public servants exceed planned expenditure.

(b) The budgeting process of the social insurance funds The social insurance funds are, in theory, responsible for determining the budgets for primary health care, pharmaceutical care and for the hospital services provided to their members. These budgets are published annually by the Ministry of Labour and Social Security after a consultation process with the insurance funds. The budget for each fund, as well as the subsidies that are given to certain funds, are negotiated on an individual basis between the fund and the Ministry and no coordination between the funds and the providers takes place. Budgets are calculated mainly on an historical basis. In reality, these budgets do not set expenditure limits as the expenditure of the social insurance organizations is demand-led.

Health Care and Cost Containment in Greece 365

Until 1993 most social insurance funds presented overall surpluses in their health insurance accounts, mainly because of the low tariffs with which they reimbursed providers. In 1993, there was a significant increase in the hospital tariffs of the social insurance organizations. As a result the health insurance branches of the social insurance funds presented deficits.[4]

However, it should be realized that the accuracy of the data published in the social budget surveys is limited, and in practice erroneous calculations or imprecise results may be presented. These errors may not change the overall expenditure trends, but show the inadequacy of the planning and evaluation processes used by the social insurance funds. Characteristically, for the same year different figures may be presented in different publications. One example of this was the figure for the expenditure of the biggest insurance fund IKA for 1993. In the 1993 Social Budget, planned expenditure showed an expected deficit of GRD 32,447 million. In the 1995 Social Budget, data on realized expenditure presented a surplus of GRD 27,242 million. For the same year though, the IKA Statistical Booklet shows a deficit of GRD 32,303 million. Thus it is difficult to accurately estimate the expenditure of the social insurance funds by using the data from the social budget surveys. On the other hand, most funds do not publish their own accounts separately. As a result, most figures are estimates.

7.6 Trends in private expenditure

Figures show that health care expenditure in Greece has actually been increasing during the 1990s, mainly due to increases in private consumption. In 1990 it reached 40 per cent of total health expenditure and has shown a constant sharp increase over the decade (Tables 7.5, 7.6, 7.6a and 7.6b).

There are a number of reasons for the increase in private expenditure (see also Bessis):[23]

- The way primary health care provision is structured forces patients to use both public and private services at the same time. In a health interview and utilization survey in the area of Patras, it was shown that 30 per cent of insured patients used both social insurance funds and private doctors' services in the same period.[27] Similar trends were found in surveys of IKA patients.[28]

366 *Health Care and Cost Containment in the European Union*

- Doctors have the ability to transfer patients from social insurance funds to their private practices. Often a patient may visit the private practice of a doctor for a thorough medical examination, and then visit the same doctor in the social insurance clinic for the prescription of medicines.[9]

- Although private practice for public hospital doctors has been forbidden since 1983 (except for university hospital doctors), in practice most doctors in public hospitals also have private practices. It should be emphasized that dual public and private practices of public doctors has been criticized since 1976 as a factor which increases expenditure and causes duplication of services.[3]

- Despite the efforts to diminish the involvement of the private sector in health care provision, the private sector has expanded in the area of diagnostic services (especially in the late 1980s) further contributing to increasing private expenditure.[23,29]

- Dental health care is not adequately covered by most funds and is primarily financed by private expenditure.[18]

- Private health insurance rapidly expanded in the late 1980s and the early 1990s.[30]

A further point is that actual private expenditure may be higher if one considers the extent of the shadow economy in the Greek health care system. The shadow economy stems mainly from the following practices: (a) hidden payments to hospital doctors for in-patient services; (b) hidden payments to hospital doctors for out-patient services; (c) hidden payments to private doctors who overbill patients for primary health care services.

It has been estimated that in 1984 the shadow economy reached about 70 per cent of official health expenditure.[31] Other researchers estimated that in 1988 the shadow economy was either GRD 34 billion[32] or GRD 105 billion.[33]

Whereas it is difficult to precisely estimate the extent of the shadow economy, private expenditure on health from the Family Budget Surveys data show that its extent is significant. These surveys are carried out every four years and calculate the consumption expenditure of Greek households as they are reported by the households themselves. The sample of 6,756 households is representative of the total Greek population. According to the 1992 household budget survey, private expenditure on health reached GRD

Health Care and Cost Containment in Greece   367

Table 7.11 Private expenditure in Greece, 1992

Type of expenditure	% Total private expenditure
Expenditure on pharmaceutical goods	22
Expenditure on primary medical care	28
Expenditure on dental care	34
Expenditure on hospital care	16
Total	100

Source: National Statistical Service of Greece, 1992.[34]

631,783 million in that year. As has been shown in Table 7.5 above, total private expenditure for the same year has been estimated in the National Accounts at the level of GRD 429,607 million. The difference is GRD 202,176 million, which is 47 per cent of the estimated official data. If the picture from the Family Budget Surveys is more accurate, total expenditure is actually much higher in Greece and exceeds 8.5 per cent of GDP. In the same way, private expenditure should be estimated at about 50 per cent of total expenditure.

Table 7.11 presents the percentage distribution of private health expenditure by type of care according to the Family Budget Survey in 1992. As can be seen, private expenditure on health is driven mainly by payments to providers for out-patient and dental care (84 per cent of the total). Dental care expenditure is more than one-third of the total.

7.7 Hospital expenditure and its control

There are two main problems when it comes to assessing cost containment measures in hospital expenditure in Greece. The first is the lack of accurate data. The second is the absence of any real cost containment philosophy in the Greek hospital sector until after 1993.

Data on private hospital expenditure is not published. Accurate data on public hospital expenditure is also difficult to obtain. The main source is the Social Budgets, where the annual public hospital budgets are published.

368 *Health Care and Cost Containment in the European Union*

However, predicted expenditure bears little relationship to actual expenditure. For the latter, accurate data exists only for 1992 and 1993, when the statistical unit of the Central Health Council worked on producing a reliable database on public hospital expenditure. Unfortunately the work of this unit has now ended, since the current administration in the Ministry of Health considered their work unnecessary, and the members of the unit have been transferred to other posts in the Ministry.

7.7.1 Trends in hospital expenditure

Hospital expenditure absorbs the bulk of public health expenditure. In addition, since the expenditure of public rural health centres is channelled via hospital budgets, this part of expenditure is important in shaping nearly all of the publicly-owned or provided health services.

According to the OECD database, hospital expenditure in Greece increased from 44.7 per cent of total health expenditure in 1975 to 59.25 per cent in 1992.[12]

Data from the Central Council of Health[11] on actual public hospital income and expenditure are presented in Table 7.12. Since these also include expenditure for rural health centres, and income from private payments and own properties, actual hospital income reaches about 65–70 per cent of total public expenditure.

State subsidies and social insurance fund reimbursements comprise the majority of hospital income. The rest comes from hospitals' own sources and the fees paid by individuals themselves. The major governmental effort during the 1990s was to alleviate the burden for the state budget and trans-

Table 7.12 Actual public hospital expenditure in Greece, 1992 and 1993 (GRD million, current prices)

Year	Realized income	Realized expenditure	Deficits	Total hospital expenditure
1992	461,668	433,553	50,130	483,683
1993	484,773	483,858	62,627	546,485

Source: Central Council for Health, 1993.[11]

Health Care and Cost Containment in Greece 369

fer it to the social insurance funds. This was done by increasing social insurance tariffs for hospital services by 200 per cent in 1992 and again by 300 per cent in February 1993. As the data show, this effort seems to have produced some effect.

In 1992, state subsidies comprised 86 per cent of actual hospital income. Of this, 95 per cent was allocated to operating expenses and 5 per cent to financing capital expenditure by public hospitals. Social insurance tariffs covered less than 13 per cent of total realized hospital income. In 1993 state subsidies as a percentage of total public hospital income fell to 65 per cent, whereas social insurance contributions rose to 34 per cent of total income.[11] This shift in the burden of financing is the result of the increases in the tariffs paid by the social insurance organizations imposed in 1992.

Whereas this result led to reducing state budget hospital expenditure, it did not have any effect on overall expenditure growth and the absence of any controls on expenditure led to the creation of large deficits in public hospitals. Accumulated hospital deficits rose to GRD 181.5 billion by mid 1996.[35] The estimated hospital expenditure for 1996 was GRD 710 billion, according to the 1996 Social Budget. Thus, the accumulated deficits rose to 26 per cent of estimated hospital expenditure.[35]

7.7.2 Measures to control hospital expenditure

It should be stressed from the outset that no actual measures to reduce overall public expenditure have been coherently initiated by governments during the 1980s and 1990s. Especially after the introduction of the National Health System in 1983, the prevailing philosophy in hospital care was expansion of the public sector in order to substitute or eliminate private provision. At the beginning of the 1990s the approach was to shift the burden of public hospital financing from the state budget to social insurance and to allow for more private involvement in hospital provision. Since 1993, there have been efforts to eliminate the accumulated deficit and to seek ways of rationalizing the hospital financing system in order that cost containment policies become feasible.

7.7.2.1 Imposing an overall budget on hospital expenditure
In theory, expenditure in public hospitals in Greece should be kept within annually

370 *Health Care and Cost Containment in the European Union*

determined budgets, established for each hospital. The budgeting process is a rather complicated one.[4,16,25]

Hospitals determine their annual budgets in January of each year. The budgets are formulated on an historical basis and in most cases take the previous years' figures and adjust them according to estimated inflation rates. They do not take into account the expected use of services or any other priorities. Their budgets must be approved by the Health Directorates of the local prefectures, which also provide hospitals with their major source of income, i.e. state subsidies. The problem is that the budget for hospital subsidies received from the local prefectures is already determined by the Ministry of Health according to the fiscal priorities of the government. Thus, hospitals usually have to readjust their budgets according to the overall state subsidies budget.

As far as social insurance contributions are concerned, Greek hospitals have no communication or negotiation with the social insurance funds, rather they use arbitrary estimates. These are seldom realized for, when in fiscal difficulty, social insurance funds delay payments to hospital providers. The Ministry of Health has estimated that GRD 48 billion (or 27 per cent), of the GRD 181.5 billion total public hospital deficit could be met by the delayed payments of the social insurance funds. Thus the overall budget process with regards to hospital income is based on unrealistic estimates.

Equally unrealistic are the budget forecasts for expenditure. Again these are formulated on an historical basis and without any consideration for expected utilization or any other policy priorities. As a result hospitals often get into financial difficulty because their expenditure is higher and their income lower than planned. In this case they either get more state resources or hospitals themselves delay payments to providers, thus accumulating deficits.

Consequently, although in theory the budget limits should be considered as overall public hospital expenditure ceilings, in practice this is not the case. Their implementation is impossible to follow or monitor by either the Ministry of Health or the social insurance funds, which have no influence on hospital administration.

7.7.2.2 Reducing hospital deficits As mentioned above, total public hospital deficits reached the level of GRD 181.5 billion in June 1996. It should be stressed that the term '*deficit*' refers to delayed payments to hospital suppliers. If the hospitals run out of money, or do not receive enough social

Health Care and Cost Containment in Greece 371

insurance contributions or state subsidies, they delay payments to providers. When resources arrive they are used to pay for the supplies of the previous years. Delays of payments of up to 18 months have been observed.

Almost 80 per cent of total deficit comes from teaching hospitals and the big district hospitals in Athens and Thesaloniki (the two biggest urban centres). As the Committee on Hospital Deficits stressed, 40 per cent of the deficit concerns delayed payments to the pharmaceutical industry for the provision of hospital drugs, and the rest consists mainly of delayed payments for consumable materials and medical technology equipment.[35]

In February 1997, the government passed legislation which provided for the state to undertake payment of hospital debts in the following manner: Suppliers were asked whether they wanted to reduce their claims by up to 20 per cent. Depending on the level of claims reduction by the suppliers, they could receive up to 10 per cent of their claims in cash and the rest of the debt was covered by government bonds of two, three and four years' duration. In the future, hospitals will be obliged to reimburse their suppliers within three months of the purchase of goods, otherwise they will not be allowed to proceed with other supplies.

Whereas this attempt has practically eliminated hospital deficits (by transferring the debt to the general government), nothing has actually been done to improve the management of resources within hospitals. A committee set up by the Ministry of Development in spring 1996 found evidence that large savings could be made in the hospital supplies system if the whole process were rationalized. In the current system, hospitals have no incentives to be economical in their supplies, they lack a basic knowledge of competitive prices of goods in the market and the ability to judge the prices of supplies according to their quality. In addition there is no monitoring of the use of resources once they are purchased.[36]

In response to this committee's findings, the Ministry of Development – which is responsible for monitoring procurement procedures in the public sector – has proposed legislation to create a special private legal entity to carry out the majority of procurements in the public sector, including hospitals. Centralized procurement procedures followed by the Ministry of Development in 1996 showed that large savings could be made in the purchase of consumable goods and medical technology equipment.[36]

Both committees have shown that the major problem is actually the poor efficiency in hospital administration, However, any action on this would require drastic changes to the overall system of hospital management

372 *Health Care and Cost Containment in the European Union*

and financing: such changes are still pending.

7.7.2.3 Improving hospital efficiency Until recently, there has been little or no attempt to improve hospital efficiency. The current system of hospital management is obsolete and provides no incentives to administrators, medical personnel or patients to use resources efficiently and effectively.[4,11,16,25]

Hospitals are run by state appointees with little or no knowledge of hospital management or any experience in administration. There are no specific targets for hospital managers for improving efficiency and there are no controls on provider behaviour. The activities of individual hospitals are not coordinated either at national or local level. No evaluation mechanisms exist on the efficiency, effectiveness or appropriateness of clinical practices. No controls exist from purchasers on hospital outputs and behaviour. There is a complete lack of accountability for all participants in the system. The obsolete current accounting system, the lack of information systems in hospitals and the fact that all hospital employees enjoy permanent tenure as public servants, add difficulties even in the implementation of personal initiatives by some individual hospital administrators.[4,16,37]

In 1993–94 the Ministry of Health planned to introduce a new team of hospital managers with extended responsibilities in order to improve the everyday administration of public hospitals. A number of public servants were given incentives to follow post-graduate studies in hospital management and health economics. Unfortunately the scheme did not succeed as it did not become law, and the current public accounting system does not allow the offering of higher salaries in order to attract competent managers from other sectors of the economy. As a result no actual improvement in the management process has been realized.

In addition, a programme for establishing up-to-date information systems in 68 public hospitals is currently under way but has not produced any results for a number of years. Even if it were successfully completed, its impact would be modest as the information gathered would not influence actors' behaviour, due to the lack of adequate management structures and accountability in the public sector.[16]

In terms of efficiency indicators, average length of stay has been reduced in recent years, but this is mainly due to advances in clinical practice rather than improved operational efficiency. For example, occupancy rates have not improved and have remained at around 70 per cent for public

Health Care and Cost Containment in Greece   373

hospitals during the 1990s (Table 7.13). Moreover no incentives are provided for transferring patients to other 'less expensive' forms of care, such as day surgery, or the provision of services now provided in hospitals by primary care doctors. In 1992, there were only 114 beds available for day surgery, which comprised 0.22 per cent of total hospital beds.

However, data from the Central Council for Health[11] show that mean length of stay in 1992 and 1993 was only 8.4 days (lower than the OECD figure), and that the average occupancy rate for these years was 57.8 per cent and 57 per cent respectively (again lower than those figures given in the OECD data).

Table 7.13 Average length of stay and occupancy rates in Greek hospitals, 1975–96

Year	Average length of stay (days)	Occupancy rate (% of used beds)
1975	14.5	73
1980	13.3	69
1985	11.6	70
1986	12.0	72
1987	11.0	72
1988	11.0	71
1989	9.8	66
1990	9.9	68
1991	9.9	71
1992	9.2	70
1993	7.0	73
1994	6.5	70
1995	6.4	72
1996	6.1	67

Source: OECD Health Data file, 1996[12] and Ministry of health, Greece (unpublished data).

374 *Health Care and Cost Containment in the European Union*

7.7.2.4 Controls on the number of hospital beds During the last two decades the total number of hospital beds in Greece has fallen by almost 15 per cent (Tables 7.14 and 7.15 overleaf). In 1980 there were 60,067 hospital beds whereas by 1992 these had fallen to 51,442. The reduction in the number of beds is due to the large number of hospital closures in the private sector that occurred during the 1990s. About 18,000 beds in private hospitals were closed between 1980 and 1992. In contrast, about 10,000 beds were gained in the public sector (Table 7.15).

This is the result of the policies pursued during the 1990s to substitute private with public hospital provision. After the introduction of the National Health System in 1983, the creation of new private hospital beds was for-

Table 7.14 Evolution of the number of hospital beds and hospital personnel in Greece, 1980–93

	1980	1981	1982	1983	1984	1985	1986
Hospitals							
Public	112	114	116	122	125	127	137
Community health centres	92	92	92	92	92	92	64
Private non-profit	28	27	27	21	22	15	8
Private profit-making	468	455	429	391	356	318	279
Total hospitals	700	688	664	626	595	552	488
Hospital beds							
Public	25905	26733	26853	29705	31838	32646	35448
Community health centres	740	721	731	737	723	725	472
Private non-profit	8347	7881	7996	5428	4860	3300	684
Private profit-making	25075	24579	23358	21626	19660	17767	16260
Total hospital beds	60067	59914	58938	57496	57081	54438	52864
Number of doctors	11871	12350	13040	13617	14134	14256	14067
Number of nurses	18654	1803	21050	21826	21811	24467	26107

Source: National Statistical Service of Greece, various years.[38]

bidden. Large non-profit private hospitals were forced to acquire public hospital status (about 1,000 beds during the 1980s) and three big new regional teaching hospitals were built. In addition to the refurbishment of a large number of existing district hospital beds, new beds were created in some hospitals. Apart from expanding the public hospital sector, the tariff policy followed by the Ministry of Health and the social insurance funds led to the closure of many private clinics, the majority of which had fewer than 40 beds. As the discussion on the trends in hospital expenditure above showed, the reduction in the number of beds did not lead to a reduction in hospital expenditure.

The trend to expand public hospital services has continued during the

1987	1988	1989	1990	1991	1992	1993
136	137	138	140	140	140	140
46	26	9	9	5		
5	5	3	3	3	3	4
267	262	252	244	232	229	224
454	430	402	396	380	372	368
35290	35342	35773	35896	36184	36474	36780
312	183	61	66	34		
243	236	154	153	153	151	270
15900	15826	15460	15214	14926	14797	15094
51745	51587	51448	51329	51297	51422	52144
15205	16769	17335	18787	18390	18565	18492
27454	29850	33071	34582	35715	36505	37211

376 *Health Care and Cost Containment in the European Union*

Table 7.15 Hospital beds in Greece, 1975–93

Year	Total number of beds	Share of public beds (%)	Share of private beds (%)
1975	58,501	46.0	56.0
1980	60,067	44.0	56.0
1981	59,914	45.0	55.0
1982	58,938	46.0	54.0
1983	57,496	52.0	48.0
1984	57,081	56.0	44.0
1985	54,438	61.0	39.0
1986	52,864	68.0	32.0
1987	51,575	68.6	31.4
1988	51,587	68.7	31.3
1989	51,448	68.6	30,4
1990	51,329	70.0	30.0
1991	51,297	70.6	29.6
1992	51,422	70.9	29.1

Source: OECD Health Data File 1996.[12]

1990s. Assisted by resources allocated from the Cohesion Fund of the EU, Greek governments in the 1990s have implemented programmes to refurbish or expand public hospitals. Between 1993 and 1998, the operational plan for the allocation of the 2nd European Union Cohesion Framework (Delors II package), planned the creation or refurbishment of some 5,000 more beds. Apart from expanding provision, this programme is estimated to add about GRD 100 billion in annual operating hospital costs.[39] It is significant that of the GRD 194 billion allocated under the programme for investments in the health sector, 59 per cent will be allocated to the expansion of beds and 15 per cent to the acquisition of medical technology equipment. Only 2 per cent will be allocated to improvements in public health services and 4 per cent to human resource training and education. Most notably,

Health Care and Cost Containment in Greece 377

despite the absence of any form of information systems in public hospitals, no resources are to be allocated for their development which is thus indefinitely postponed.

Moreover, similar trends are found in insurance funds like IKA, TEVE and the funds for banking personnel, which all plan to expand their facilities. IKA and TEVE plan to upgrade their polyclinics while the funds for banking personnel plan to build a new hospital in Athens.

Despite the expansion of hospital facilities, no measures have been taken to coordinate their activities. As a result a large number of patients, mainly those residing in rural areas, bypass their local facilities and seek treatment in the teaching hospitals in Athens, Thesaloniki and certain other major urban centres.[16] Since 1983, successive laws have planned the establishment of regional health authorities to better organize the provision of local services. However, these plans have not been implemented and as a result the system has remained highly centralized with little coordination between the activities of individual hospitals.

7.8 Primary health care expenditure and its control

It is difficult to estimate the level of expenditure for primary health care services in Greece over a number of years. Total expenditure for primary health care includes the expenditure of social insurance funds for services provided to their members, the expenditure of the central government for the finance of primary health care services and individual patients' out-of-pocket payments to private doctors and private diagnostic centres. However, data is available only for the expenditure of the social insurance organizations, although even for these, data on actual expenditure is only available until 1990. Data on the expenditure of health care centres is unavailable because their financing is allocated via hospital budgets and separate figures are not published. Health centres were financed autonomously in 1993 and this is the only year when actual expenditure on health centres is available. Data for private expenditure on ambulatory care is only available if one takes the Family Budget Surveys into account and even then, this data is only included in the 1992 survey.

Karokis and Sissouras[4] have shown that actual expenditure on primary health care by the social insurance organizations reached 17.1 per cent of

378 *Health Care and Cost Containment in the European Union*

the total expenditure on health by insurance funds in 1990. This has generally been the level that primary medical expenditure (including prosthetic services and spa treatment) has operated at in the 1990s, as is shown in the planned expenditure from the Social Budget in 1996.

The evolution of expenditure depends on the various methods of payment to primary care doctors used by each fund. Thus, because the fund employs salaried doctors whose level of remuneration does not depend on the volume of services provided, IKA expenditure on primary medical care has remained relatively stable as a percentage of total health expenditure. As data from the activities of IKA show, the evolution of expenditure on primary medical care is driven more by the use of medical technology than from an increased number of visits. As the *IKA Statistical Bulletin* shows,[40] the average number of visits fell from 6.08 per member in 1970 to 4.39 in 1994. On the other hand the average number of medical technology tests per member rose from 1.03 in 1970 to 1.89 per member in 1994.

The situation varies among the other funds. OGA does not pay for medical care services because its members enjoy free access to primary health care centres and out-patient departments of public hospitals. Members of most of the other funds enjoy free access to contracted primary care doctors who are reimbursed on a fee-for-service basis, fixed at the level of the state. These tariffs are deliberately set much lower than market prices for the same reasons as the tariffs for hospital services, i.e. to keep the social insurance funds within their budgets.

The result of this policy has been that doctors usually overbill patients or transfer them to their private practices, where the patients pay out of their own pockets. The exact level of this private expenditure cannot be accurately calculated. In a local survey in Patras it was, however, shown that about 30 per cent of all insured patients' annual doctor visits are to private physicians, despite the fact that the same patients enjoy full cover for the same services by the social insurance funds. Thus whereas the measures to control expenditure on medical care visits seem to help the budgets of the social insurance funds, they have the effect of transferring the burden of expenditure to the patients themselves.[9] This is why, as shown earlier, private expenditure on health is mainly spent on primary medical care (see section 7.6, Table 7.11).

Apart from controlling reimbursement levels, no other supply-oriented cost containment measures have been effectively taken. There is no control on the prescribing patterns of doctors, on the appropriateness of care provided, and no information systems are fully in operation.

7.9 Cost-sharing

Greek governments have not placed great emphasis on cost-sharing arrangements as a means for controlling health expenditure.

Cost-sharing has mainly been employed in pharmaceutical care. In this sector there are three co-payment levels, which are the same across all funds. The general co-payment rate is 25 per cent, but there are exceptions to this. For example, for pharmaceuticals used in the treatment of certain diseases including Parkinson's Disease, diabetes, heart diseases, rheumatoid arthritis, tuberculosis, Chronic Obstructive Pulmonary Disease, ulcerative colitis and Crohn's disease, liver diseases etc., the co-payment rate is only 10 per cent.

For pharmaceuticals used in the treatment of industrial accidents, obstetric care, cancers and neoplasms, or by chronic patients suffering from diseases such as: insulin-dependent diabetes, thalasaemia, psychiatric disorders, kidney diseases, epilepsy etc., there is no co-payment rate.

The cost containment arrangements have not managed to reduce the overall amount of pharmaceutical expenditure (see section 7.10 below). The pharmaceutical expenditure of patients (from co-payments) reached GRD 103 billion in 1994, or 23 per cent of total pharmaceutical expenditure.

A general 25 per cent co-payment rate exists for the use of diagnostic services and procedures both in the largest social insurance fund IKA, and in most other funds. There are no co-payment rates for visits to medical doctors in ambulatory care.

Since 1992 a flat fee of GRD 1,000 has been charged for visits to the out-patient departments of public hospitals. According to the Central Health Council data, the number of visits to doctors in out-patient departments was 8,660,279 in 1993.[11] If the fee of GRD 1,000 was paid for each visit, the income of public hospitals would be GRD 8.7 billion, still only a minimal part of the GRD 450 billion spent by public hospitals in that year. However, in practice, patients rarely pay this fee because many hospitals do not follow the charging procedures.

380 *Health Care and Cost Containment in the European Union*

Table 7.16 pharmaceutical expenditure in Greece (GRD million, constant prices* 1988 = 100), 1987–95

Year	Hospitals**	Pharmacies	Total
1987	14,058	88,703	102,761
1988	15,545	94,833	110,378
1989	16,569	96,749	113,318
1990	18,822	108,944	127,766
1991	21,097	117,314	138,411
1992	23,957	130,682	154,639
1993	25,044	142,239	167,283
1994	26,781	151,592	178,373
1995	30,078	159,019	189,097

* Prices have been deflated with the Medical Care Price Index.

**Hospital prices are different from retail prices, with which pharmacies sales are calculated.

Source: Pharmetrica, 1997.[41]

Table 7.17 Pharmaceutical expenditure as a percentage of GDP, public and total health care expenditure (current prices), 1991–94

Year	%GDP	% Public health expenditure	% Total health expenditure
1990	1.31	26.15	16.35
1991	1.37	27.25	17.17
1992	1.52	30.89	19.04
1993	1.75	35.15	21.94
1994	1.90	38.96	24.22

Source: Pharmetrica, 1997.[41]

7.10 Controlling pharmaceutical expenditure

Pharmaceutical expenditure in Greece has risen significantly during the 1990s (Table 7.16). Available data shows that expenditure reached 1.90 per cent of GDP in 1994 (at current prices), a figure considered one of the highest in OECD countries (Table 7.17). Expenditure on pharmaceuticals comprises the largest share of the expenditure of the social health insurance funds[42, 43] which are the main sources of funding for pharmaceutical care[42] (Table 7.18). This is due to a lack of effective controls on pharmaceutical prescribing and the fact that other elements of social insurance fund expenditure, i.e. expenditure on medical and hospital care, are heavily subsidized.

Three factors are considered to have caused the rise in pharmaceutical expenditure. These include price increases, increases in the volume of medicines consumed and changes in prescribing patterns. As Table 7.19 overleaf shows, the main cost driver has been changes in prescribing patterns. How exactly prescribing habits have contributed to the increase in expenditure is not known, as no studies on the subject exist. The main reasons given have been the prescribing of new and more expensive products, the introduction

Table 7.18 Evolution of pharmaceutical expenditure by source of funding (GRD million, current prices and percentage of total expenditure), 1990–94

Year	Public Hospitals	Insurance funds	Patients' co-payments	Private expenditure	Total
1990	25 14.7%	92 54.1%	18 10.6%	35 20.6%	170
1991	33 15.1%	112 51.4%	22 10.1%	51 23.4%	218
1992	43 15.5%	148 53.2%	30 10.8%	57 20.5%	278
1993	54 14.9%	187 51.6%	37 10.2%	84 23.2%	362
1994	71 15.9%	228 50.9%	46 10.3%	103 23%	448

Source: Athanasopoulos G, 1995.[44]

382 Health Care and Cost Containment in the European Union

Table 7.19 Factors Influencing the Increase In pharmaceutical expenditure (percentage contribution to total annual expenditure Increase), 1990–94

Year	Increased number of units	Price increases	Changes in prescribing patterns	Total annual expenditure increase
1990	4.7	19.5	8.4	32.6
1991	-0.8	14.5	14.8	28.5
1992	3.3	9.0	15.2	27.5
1993	6.3	2.7	21.2	30.2
1994	0.8	6.5	16.3	23.6

Source: Athanasopoulos G, 1995.[44]

of new treatments with higher costs and the lack of controls on the prescribing behaviour of social insurance contracted doctors.[44] However, in the absence of any relevant documentation or information systems, data from social insurance funds cannot provide an adequate explanation of the factors that contribute to rising pharmaceutical costs.

Apart from cost-sharing, two other measures have been taken to control pharmaceutical expenditure: price controls and the introduction of a positive list of drugs for the major insurance funds.

With regards to pricing controls, a new initiative was adopted by the current government in early 1996 which aimed to reduce overall pharmaceutical expenditure. This initiative was to change the system of pricing pharmaceuticals by determining that the prices of imported drugs, which have acquired a larger market share than locally produced drugs, would be set according to the lower ex-factory price of the same drug in the EU. The government planned to change the prices of all imported drugs according to this method. Prices of locally produced drugs are based mainly on costing estimates by the Ministry of Development.

However, this change in prices was never instituted because the government realized that changing the base price alone would not have a significant effect on the overall level of pharmaceutical expenditure. In June 1997, the government introduced further measures to reduce the prices of the pharmaceutical products as a means of reducing overall spending. According to this new legislation, there are (as before) two pricing schemes, one for imported and one for locally produced drugs.

With regards to imported drugs, prices will be determined according to a formula based on the lowest ex-factory price of the same substance in the EU. Under the previous system, the government subtracted 7 per cent of the ex-factory price, which reflected the charges added to the original ex-factory price and added a 12 per cent profit margin for the importer. Now the whole profit margin is abolished but the government does not subtract the 7 per cent.

Under the previous system a number of charges were added to the lowest ex-factory price, which included wholesaler and pharmacist margins, contributions to social insurance funds and taxes. These charges were calculated in a cumulative way. That is, they were calculated on the sum of the ex-factory price, plus the importers' margin, plus any charges. Thus the retail price was about 100 per cent higher than the original ex-factory price. Under the current system the charges for contributions to social insurance funds and the National Drug Organisation are reduced by almost 40 per cent and are calculated on the ex-factory price alone. In addition the wholesaler and pharmacist margins have not been reduced but whereas, under the previous system, they were calculated on the ex-factory price plus charges for social insurance, they are now calculated on the ex-factory price alone.

The prices of locally produced drugs are determined according to costing data supplied by the industry, although a number of limitations apply. The manufacturer's margin is reduced by 4 per cent. The reductions in surcharge rates outlined above for imported drugs, also apply. Further, the upper limit for the price of any locally produced drug is the lowest price of the same product in the EU. If the price of the drug according to costing estimates is lower than the lowest price for the same drug in the EU, then the lower price of the two will apply. If the costing data leads to a higher price than the lowest price in the EU for the same drug, then the price in the EU will apply.

These prices are considered maximum prices and companies are allowed to sell at lower prices if they so wish. In addition, the government is planning to reduce the level of promotional expenditure that companies can spend annually.

The government estimates that this will lead to an overall reduction in pharmaceutical spending of GRD 100 billion, out of an estimated GRD 600 billion expenditure for 1996. Of this, 40 billion will be income lost for the social insurance funds and the National Drug Organisation. The measures

384 *Health Care and Cost Containment in the European Union*

will also affect the pharmaceutical industry, both because of the abolition or reduction of profit margins and because of the imposition of the rule of the lowest EU price margin. It will also affect the wholesalers and pharmacists since their profit margins will now be calculated on the basis of a lower price.

Despite strong reactions, mainly from the pharmacists' association which immediately went on strike, the government is going ahead with the new measures and published the new price list in autumn 1997. These measures will lead to a short-term reduction in the growth rates of pharmaceutical expenditure but their long-term effect is questionable since they are not followed by prescribing controls.

The only measure in this direction would be to expand the positive list that exists in IKA to all insurance funds, and to introduce a new system for the formulation of a positive list. Under the new system, drugs would be included in the list according to their average daily treatment cost. In July 1997, the government produced a first draft of the new positive list. All major active substances are included in the list. The government has calculated the average daily cost of treatment for each drug according to the defined daily dose scheme produced by the World Health Organization (WHO). Exactly how the list will work, which drugs will be included and what will happen to drugs currently on the list, but which exceed the average daily cost of their class or group, is not yet clear for two reasons. The first is that the list will have to be revised again according to more recent prices. The second is that the criteria for inclusion or exclusion from the list are still not clearly defined.

The practical effect of this new system is difficult to estimate, since the implementation of the list in IKA has not been monitored adequately, nor is there any information system to control providers' behaviour. There is also no guarantee that the prescribing behaviour of doctors will actually be effectively monitored even after the introduction of the positive list.

It is also significant that in the discussion about pharmaceutical expenditure controls, the spectrum of options considered is limited only to pricing regulations, avoiding any consideration of measures to control provider behaviour or the introduction of elements that would take into account the cost-effectiveness of pharmaceutical products. This is a very narrow perspective which cannot adequately be justified in view of the current trends in the EU pharmaceutical market and the limited effectiveness of pricing regulation schemes as a means of controlling pharmaceutical expenditure. [45]

7.11 Controls on capital expenditure and medical technology

7.11.1 Controls on capital expenditure

As has been indicated throughout the chapter, the 1980s were the decade of expansion in the Greek public health care sector. This is reflected in the growth in capital expenditure over the past two decades (Table 7.20).

Table 7.20 Capital expenditure in Greece, 1970–91 (constant prices [1982 = 100] GRD million)

Year	Public expenditure	Private expenditure	Total expenditure	Expenditure on land	Expenditure on medical equipment
1970	203	107	310	175	135
1971	243	112	355	227	128
1972	269	136	405	254	151
1973	404	179	583	371	212
1974	362	252	614	384	230
1975	398	319	717	404	313
1976	367	338	705	303	402
1977	386	339	725	332	393
1978	360	361	721	346	375
1979	476	412	888	378	510
1980	455	385	840	290	550
1981	674	324	996	563	433
1982	411	392	798	352	446
1983	784	301	1085	614	471
1984	980	417	1397	772	625
1985	1466	475	1541	713	828
1986	1222	950	2172	799	1373
1987	965	722	1687	656	1031
1988	933	591	1524	615	909
1989	750	847	1597	499	1098
1990	584	1090	1674	425	1249
1991	623	1227	1850	430	1420

Source: Kyriopoulos, Levet and Niakas, 1994.[29]

386 *Health Care and Cost Containment in the European Union*

Table 7.21 Public capital expenditure in Greece, 1981–89 (GRD million, current prices)

Expenditure	1981	1982	1983	1984
Purchases of land and hospital buildings	250.7	480.2	233.3	131.9
Construction works of hospital buildings	451.8	1,289.0	2,651.1	4,818.6
Studies for the construction of hospital buildings	45.1	55.8	120.5	299.9
Mechanical equipment	421.7	2,65.8	1,074.9	654.9
Supplementary works	72.6	-	50.0	-
Other expenditure	-	-	-	-
Expenditure allocated via the state budget	72.6	2,28.3	210.0	130.0

Source: Government Accounting Office.[46]

As the table shows, public expenditure significantly increased during the 1980s, whereas private expenditure only started to increase after the beginning of the 1990s. In addition, expenditure on medical technology seems to comprise the largest share of capital expenditure at the end of the 1980s and the beginning of the 1990s.

Table 7.21 shows actual capital public expenditure on health from 1981 to 1989. It is evident that expenditure on land, buildings and medical equipment rose sharply during this decade. Indeed, not only were 196 rural health centres built and equipped, but also three new teaching hospitals were built and a number of small district hospitals were refurbished. This data indicates that during the 1980s Greece followed expansionary policies in health.

As has been shown in section 7.7.2.3, expansionary trends in capital expenditure still exist in the 1990s, only now the major source of financing seems to be EU funding via the Cohesion Fund Programmes.[39]

1985	1986	1987	1988	1989
1,092.0	110.5	-	409.9	-
5,527.0	5,214.1	1,206.0	6,015.8	5,671.2
408.2	423.5	367.4	676.0	797.1
1,816.0	1,806.1	1,566.7	3,637.8	3,152.1
-	-	-	-	-
1,250.0	35.0	35.0	133.5	211.7
299.8	2,700.0	2,700.0	2,360.5	-

7.11.2 Controls on medical technology

Although the private sector was restrained during the 1980s it expanded further in the 1990s. Since the mid-1980s, it turned to investment in the provision of diagnostic services as a means to overcome the prohibition for the creation of private clinics. A large number of diagnostic services were created in the late 1980s and early 1990s. Whereas only 21 diagnostic centres were created between 1980 and 1985, 159 were created between 1986 and 1991. The increase has been tremendous and led to an explosion in the provision of expensive diagnostic procedures among the Greek population. In 1991, there were 119 CT-scanners in Greece, of which 97 were in the private sector. Bessis[23] and Kyriopoulos and Niakas,[47] showed that the number of CT-scanners and MRIs in Greece is the highest per thousand of population among OECD countries. In practice this rapid increase in medical

388   *Health Care and Cost Containment in the European Union*

technology has demonstrated the failure of controls on private provision, even during the 1990s. What is more important is that there is still no control on the introduction of new technologies and further expansion is allowed. Many of these private diagnostic centres are contracted by the social insurance funds to provide diagnostic services for their members.

7.12 Private health insurance

Together with the expansion of the private diagnostic sector, private health insurance also expanded in the late 1980s and at the beginning of the 1990s.[48]

Table 7.22 shows the evolution of private health insurance during recent years. The figures represent estimates as it is very difficult to calculate the exact level of private health insurance expenditure. This is because most private insurance companies publish their figures together with life insurance

Table 7.22 Evolution of private health insurance premiums (GRD million, current prices), 1985–94

Year	Health insurance premiums	% Annual change
1985	1,430	
1986	1,879	31.4
1987	2,553	35.9
1988	3,904	53.0
1989	5,829	49.3
1990	8,878	52.3
1991	13,859	56.1
1992	22,295	60.9
1993	33,913	52.1
1994	45,000	32.7

Source: IMOSY, 1996.[49]

Health Care and Cost Containment in Greece 389

expenditure.

Liaropoulos[30,48] argued that dissatisfaction with public health services, the expansion of the private sector in diagnostic services and increases in the charges of private hospitals as a response to the low tariffs paid by social insurance organizations, may account for the rapid growth. It seems that the market has now reached a level of some maturity after a period of rapid expansion, where private insurance companies were competing for custom by offering generous insurance packages without deductibles or co-payment rates. Private health insurance is mainly oriented towards cover for hospital care services. In public hospitals, this covers additional expenses and offers daily allowances to members in excess of social insurance cover. In private hospitals private insurance covers the full cost of treatment. Up to now, apart from isolated initiatives, private health insurance in Greece has not managed to offer a comprehensive package of cover and has focused on the cover of hospital and diagnostic care.[30]

Life and private health insurance premiums and expenditure were exempted from taxation from the late 1980s. Since 1997, however, expenses over GRD 200,000 are taxed.

Private health insurance expenditure is not included in the calculations of private health expenditure for the Family Budget Surveys, because the survey methodology excludes this kind of expenditure from health consumption expenditure.

7.13 Attempts to reform the Greek health care system

Reform of the Greek health care system has been discussed since the introduction of the National Health System in 1983. Until 1989, reform efforts were concentrated on establishing the public character of the National Health System. After the political turmoil in 1989–90 with three general elections taking place within 12 months, the Conservative government which came to power tried to reform the legislation for the National Health System by enacting a new law in 1992. This differed from previous legislation in that it gave more emphasis to the development of the private sector in health care provision and more impetus to the development of health promotion activities and patients' rights. It should be emphasized that this legislation did not pay any particular attention to the introduction of cost

390 *Health Care and Cost Containment in the European Union*

containment measures.

Again, this legislation was only partially implemented and by 1993 the Socialists had returned to power. The new government changed parts of the Conservative legislation and set up a process of consultation, necessary for reform of the National Health System.

This consultation process culminated in the report prepared by a Foreign Experts Committee which was chaired by the late Professor Brian Abel-Smith and included well-known academic and policy consultants in the field of health care reform.[50] The Committee's recommendations were based on a research report prepared by a team of Greek researchers in the Ministry of Health[51] and extensive consultations, interviews, and local visits carried out in Greece.

The Committee's main recommendations included:

1. the necessity for the development of improved public health services, as the existing ones were considered inadequate;

2. the introduction of a general practitioners' scheme, reimbursing GPs on a capitation basis in order to: decrease the differences in ambulatory care provision between social insurance funds, act as gate-keepers to secondary care, limit the movement of patients between public and private doctors and ensure continuity of care;

3. the establishment of a unified insurance fund, which would gather the resources devoted to health care and act as a purchaser of services from public and private services, as this would facilitate the imposition of overall budgets and monitoring systems with regards health expenditure, which the existing fragmented system does not allow;

4. the creation of regional health authorities and the decentralization of the health care system, so as to reduce its bureaucratic character;

5. the development of a health services research strategy in order to acquire adequate and useful information on the system and introduce quality control;

6. the improvement and training of medical personnel; and

7. the improvement of the management of the system, by giving independent status to public hospitals and by abolishing the permanent tenure of hospital personnel.

The Committee's findings were published and discussed. Their assessment of the system and final recommendations were in line with the remarks of many Greek researchers, who had previously advocated the reforms necessary for the health care system.[2,3,5,25,52] They were adopted by a wide range of academics and politicians, across the political spectrum. The Ministry of Health accepted the principles of the report and created three teams of working experts to formulate specific proposals for the implementation of the Report's three major recommendations. These included the creation of the Unified Fund, the improvement of the management of the system and decentralization, and the reform of the primary health care system with the expansion of the general practitioners' scheme.

Unfortunately, the political climate in Greece and the ambivalence of the political authorities allowed neither a thorough discussion of the Committee's recommendations nor, most importantly, the full implementation of its proposals.[53] Reactions came from those who would have been first affected by the recommendations. Hospital doctors' trade unions opposed any reform of the management of the public hospital system because it threatened the permanent tenure status of hospital doctors. Objections also came from those parts of the insurance funds whose bureaucracies were threatened by the new fund and the resulting transfer of power. Both camps employed the argument that the committee's recommendations sought to transfer experience from other countries to the Greek health care system, without taking into account the particularities of the system, and that the reforms would jeopardize the public character of the system. In addition, both the creation of the unified fund and the establishment of some form of management accountability in the system were considered as too radical and thus milder interventions were advocated.[54]

As the more specific recommendations of the Greek experts' Committees that followed the Foreign Experts' report were published,[37,55,56] it became easier to criticize the latter over the former. But the major problem in the implementation of these reports was the political ambivalence which prevailed at the time.

The Minister of Health, who had initially invited the Foreign Experts, prepared draft legislation in 1995 which followed a less radical approach to the reforms. It placed emphasis on improving public health services, introducing hospital managers and the establishment of a coordinating body between the major insurance funds in the place of the unified fund. However, the Prime Minister Andreas Papandreou's death resulted in a new

392 *Health Care and Cost Containment in the European Union*

government in which the Minister of Health was replaced. The new Minister followed the lines of his predecessor and prepared further draft legislation, though on a little more radical basis, which would have abolished permanent tenure and given more impetus to the development of primary health care services. This draft legislation also did not manage to reach Parliament because another general election then took place. Another Minister of Health took over who prepared yet further draft legislation. This draft was debated in Parliament in the summer of 1997, after significant delays.

The main points of this new legislation include the following:

(a) Development of regional health authorities: this is on the agenda once again, despite having been the subject of three successive legislative Acts over the past 15 years.

(b) The improvement of public health services with the development of public health physicians and the creation of regional public health authorities.

(c) The coordination of the social insurance funds in terms of managing health care resources. Instead of creating the Unified Fund, the current government – to counter the reaction of the separate insurance funds, proposes only the creation of a committee composed of the directors of the four major insurance funds.

(d) The law provides for the creation of 'Networks of Primary Health Care' provision and the introduction of a general practitioner's scheme. Instead of concentrating on altering the financing mechanisms of the health care system, the current reform attempts to alter the system of health care provision by unifying the way ambulatory care is provided. Thus, the government is planning to coordinate health care provision among insurance funds so that the same package of services is provided to the members of all funds in a given region, and to ensure access to all types of services for the members of all funds. The networks of care will gradually be staffed by general practitioners. It should be emphasized though, that the status of general practitioner was only introduced in 1987, and currently less than a thousand doctors have this status.

(e) The funds will finance hospitals with a tariff based on the introduction of some form of prospective DRG-like (Diagnosis Related Groups) system of payment, although no mention is given of how this would be developed.

Health Care and Cost Containment in Greece   393

(f) Hospital doctors are to be allowed to work privately within public hospitals, by providing medical care and house visits to patients. This measure contradicts the efforts to develop primary health care networks and gate-keepers to the hospital system.

(g) More emphasis is given to controlling the development of medical technology and a number of agencies are to be created with the purpose of providing health technology assessment.

(h) The possibility of merging public hospitals and wards is mentioned for the first time.

(i) Hospital managers are to be appointed in public hospitals with the aim of providing more effective daily management. Nevertheless, it seems likely that they will lack the real power and accountability necessary to impose their views on the medical and administrative personnel, who still retain their permanent tenure.

7.14 Overall conclusions

A review of the cost containment measures undertaken (or not) in the Greek health care system is presented in Table 7.23 overleaf. As the table shows, health policy in Greece has not tried to employ the large array of cost containment measures which have been used in other countries.[55,57,58] Even those measures that have been initiated have been only partially implemented, and generally with minimal effectiveness.[5,21,50,51]

The reasons for this have been developed throughout the discussion of this chapter. They include policy priorities, lack of continuity in health policy, administrative inefficiencies, prevailing perverse financial incentives, lack of coordination of financing sources and inability to confront vested interests in the Greek health care sector.[21,52]

So is there a future for success in rationalizing the use of health care resources in Greece? This is a difficult question to answer. The current government has shown that it has set as its priority the promotion of efficient mechanisms for the use of public resources. The need to participate in EMU forces the government to seek ways to reduce and rationalize public spending. The Ministry of Health has adopted such principles and is seeking ways to implement them.[37, 55, 56]

394 *Health Care and Cost Containment in the European Union*

Table 7.23 Overview of cost containment measures

Measure	Comments
Overall budget for health expenditure cost-sharing	Mainly for pharmaceuticals, no effect.
Rationing	Some services are covered by certain social insurance funds, no explicit rationing.
Control on capital equipment	No actual controls but expansion. No controls on private expenditure.
Hospital efficiency	No.
Reduction in hospital beds	No, though increases are planned.
Differential pricing	No.
Private beds in public hospitals	No.
Private practice by public hospital doctors	Yes.
Overall hospital budgets	Yes, but not monitored.
Consequences of budgetary excess	None.
Incentives to increase productivity	Currently none. Proposals for management improvement.
DRG payment system	No, a hybrid system is proposed in legislation.
Alternatives to hospital care	No.
Insurers as purchasers	Currently no, proposals for development of contractual agreements with provider.
Manpower control	None for entry into the medical profession. Restrictions on entry to public hospitals, but only because of fiscal problems.
Changes in the ways doctors are paid	No. Fee-for-service dominates. Incentives for additional private payments. Proposals for a general practitioner scheme paid on a capital basis.

Table 7.23 (continued) Overview of cost containment measures

Measure	Comments
Ceiling on incomes of out-of-hospital doctors	No.
Practice guidelines	No.
Medical profiles	No.
Positive list for drugs	Yes.
Reference prices for drugs	Currently none. Planned for the future with regard to the new positive list for drugs.
Patient choice	Yes.
Private health insurance	No cover for co-payments. No taxed premiums.
Quality assurance	No.
Controls on medical technology	No.
Development of information systems	No.

Nevertheless it is doubtful whether these recent initiatives will succeed in transforming the financing mechanisms and incentives prevailing in the Greek health care system. Whereas the general government priority is the reduction of public spending, the trends in health care are to expand public hospital and medical technology facilities, thus creating more demand for increased resources. The attempts to improve the management of hospital facilities have not been successful thus far, and since 1994 the introduction of hospital managers has been discussed but not implemented. Any attempts to change the way hospitals are managed, both organizationally and financially, face negative reactions from the public hospital doctors' trade unions and are considered threats to the public character of the system. The Foreign Experts' Committee report was criticized on these grounds, although it is evident that the Committee's recommendations did not threaten the public character of the system, which in any case does not primarily depend on

396 *Health Care and Cost Containment in the European Union*

whether public hospital doctors enjoy permanent tenure.[59]

As far as primary health care is concerned, the new draft legislation aims to challenge rising costs by changing the structure of health care provision. The 'Networks of Primary Health Care' aim to coordinate the provision of services among insurance funds and health centres. Although this move, if implemented, may equalize the package of services offered to the insured population, it focuses again on provision and not on financing incentives. Given the lack of general practitioners and the difficulties in creating an adequate number of family physicians in the near future, it seems that even this reform will not influence the way resources are managed. Thus it is doubtful whether it will lead to a more efficient use of resources.

Emphasising the reform of health care financing requires, to some degree, the separation of purchasing from provision, the enhancement of the negotiating powers of the insurance funds and the creation of flexible management structures which could combine purchasing decisions with local health needs.[55] The creation of a unified fund is aimed directly at this. But the implementation of this reform seems improbable at the moment, as the current draft legislation provides only for a loose communication structure between the insurance funds. The fragmented approach in health care financing hinders the imposition of budget ceilings and reduces the negotiating power of the social insurance funds.

Even if these proposals become law, it is doubtful whether they will be fully implemented because of the lack of adequate information mechanisms and administrative skills in the Greek health services.[51] Very little attention is being paid to health services research and to human resource training and development. The need to invest in people as well as facilities is imperative.[51]

Thus even if the intentions are good, the prospects are gloomy and much effort is required to establish a culture for the rational use of resources in Greek health care. It seems that the government should take a more decisive approach, in which agreement between all involved parties is necessary.

Until then, public hospital personnel will remain dissatisfied with the current situation in public hospitals, where they have to work under very uncomfortable decisions, and, of all the EU countries, Greek citizens will remain the most dissatisfied with their health care system.[60, 61]

References

1 Ritsatakis A. *Health Planning in Greece* (in Greek). Athens: Center for Planning and Economic Research, 1976.

2 Sissouras A. Backgrounds and development in health care in Greece. In: Casparie AF *et al.* (eds). *Competitive Health Care in Europe: Future Prospects.* Dartmouth, 1990.

3 Center for Planning and Economic Research. *Health: Report of a Special Committee* (in Greek). Athens: Center for Planning and Economic Research, 1976.

4 Karokis A, Sissouras A. Organisational and financial aspects of the Greek health care system (in.Greek). In: *Report on the Planning and Organisation of Health Services.* Athens: Ministry of Health, 1994.

5 Sissouras A, Karokis A, Mossialos E. Greece. In: OECD. *The Reform of Health Care Systems. A Review of Seventeen OECD Countries.* Paris: OECD, 1994.

6 Karokis A, Sissouras A, Mossialos E. Achilles' Heel: Greece's troubled health care system. *Health Service Journal* 1992;102:22–5.

7 Hurst J. *The Reform of Health Care Systems: A Comparative Analysis of Seven OECD Countries.* Paris: OECD, 1992.

8 Ministry of Labour and Social Security. *Social Budget.* Athens: Ministry of Labour and Social Security, 1996.

9 Deligianni Y, Kalomenidis K, Karokis A, Mitropoulos J. *Report on the Health Status of the Population of Patras* (in Greek). Patras: University of Patras, 1995.

10 Matsaganis M. Is health insurance in Greece in need of reform? *Health Policy and Planning* 1991;6(3)271–81

11 Central Council for Health. *Health Statistical Bulletin* (in Greek). Athens: Government Printing Office, 1993.

12 OECD. *OECD Health Data File.* Paris: OECD, 1997.

13 Theodorou M. Primary health care In: Ministry of Health. *Report on the Planning and Organisation of Health Services* (in Greek). Athens, 1994.

14 National Statistical Service of Greece. *Statistics of Social Welfare.* Athens: National Statistical Office, 1994.

15 Yfantopoulos J. *Planning for Health Services in Greece* (in Greek). Athens: National Center for Social Research, 1988.

16 Polyzos N. Secondary-tertiary care. In: Theodorou M, Karokis A, Polyzos N, Roupas T, Sissouras A, Yfantopoulos J (eds). *Report on the Planning and Organisation of Health Services* (in Greek). Athens: Ministry of Health, 1994.

17 Polyzos N. Pharmaceutical care. In: Theodorou M, Karokis A, Polyzos N, Roupas, Sissouras A, Yfantopoulos J (eds). *Report on the Planning and Organisation of Health Services* (in Greek). Athens: Ministry of Health, 1994.

18 Koletsi-Kounari H, Kyriopoulos J. *The Economics of Dental Care in Greece* (in Greek). Athens: Center for Sciences and Health and the Greek Society for Community Dentistry, 1992.

398 *Health Care and Cost Containment in the European Union*

19 National Statistical Service of Greece. *National Accounts.* Athens: National Statistical Service of Greece, 1992.

20 National Statistical Service of Greece. *National Accounts.* Athens: National Statistical Service of Greece, 1994.

21 Kyriopoulos J, Niakas D. *Aspects of Health Economics and Policy* (in Greek). Athens: Center for Social Sciences and Health, 1994.

22 Kyriopoulos J, Geitona M. *Cross-border Flow of Patients in Greece and Europe* (in Greek). Athens: Exantas, 1995.

23 Bessis N. *Private Health Expenditure* (in Greek). Athens: Institute for Economic and Industrial Research, 1993.

24 Mossialos E, Karokis A. Greece: health care reforms. *The Lancet* 1992;340:41–2.

25 Kyriopoulos J, Niakas D. *Financing Health Services in Greece* (in Greek). Athens: Center for Social Sciences and Health, 1991.

26 Ministry of Finance. *National Budget.* Athens: Ministry of Finance, 1992, 1993, 1994.

27 Karokis A. *Demand for Primary Health Care and the Creation of the Unified Fund in Greece* (in Greek). Paper presented at the 5th Hellenic Conference on Health Economics: The Prospects for a Unified Fund in Greece, 1996.

28 Theodorou M. *Primary Health Care in IKA* (in Greek). Athens: IMOSY, 1993.

29 Kyriopoulos J, Levet J, Niakas D (eds). *Management of Biomedical Technology in Greece* (in Greek). Athens: Center for Social Sciences and Health, 1994.

30 Liaropoulos L. Health services financing in Greece: a role for the private health insurance. *Health Policy* 1995;34:53–62

31 Pavlopoulos P. *The Underground Economy in Greece* (in Greek). Athens: Institute for Economic and Industrial Research, 1987.

32 Kanellopoulos G. *The Underground Economy. What the Official Data Show.* Athens: Center for Planning and Economic Research, 1992.

33 Niakas D, Kyriopoulos J, Georgoussi E. Investigation of the hidden economy in the Greek health sector: a first quantitative approximation (in Greek). *Health Review* 1990;6:42–5.

34 National Statistical Service of Greece. *Family Budget Survey 1991–1992.* Athens: National Statistical Service of Greece, 1992.

35 Ministry of Health and Social Welfare. *Report on the Management and Controls of the Hospital Deficits in the National Health Service* (in Greek). Athens: Ministry of Health, 1996.

36 Ministry of Development. *Report of the Committee on the Rationalisation of the Hospital Supplies System* (in Greek). Athens: Ministry of Development, 1996.

37 Ministry of Health and Social Security. *Report of the Committee on the Reform of Primary Health Care* (in Greek). Athens: Ministry of Health, 1995.

38 National Statistical Service of Greece. *Social Welfare and Health Statistics.* Athens: National Statistical Service of Greece, various years.

39 Liaropoulos L, Prezerakos P, Bila A. *Background Document on the National Program for the Hospital of 2010 and the 2nd EU Cohesion Framework* (in Greek). Athens:

Health Care and Cost Containment in Greece 399

IMOSY, 1996.

40 IKA. *Statistical Bulletin* (in Greek). Athens: IKA, 1996.

41 Pharmetrica. *Pharmaceutical Expenditure Trends* (unpublished paper). Athens: Pharmetrica, 1997.

42 Ranos C, Polyzos N. 1994. Pharmaceutical policy within the Greek NHS. In: Mossialos E, Ranos C, Abel-Smith B (eds). *Cost Containment, Pricing and Financing of Pharmaceuticals in the European Community: The Policy Makers' View.* Athens: LSE and Pharmetrica, 1994.

43 Vartholomeos J, Tinios P. The structure and reform of social security and the demand for pharmaceuticals in Greece. In: Mossialos E, Ranos C, Abel-Smith B (eds). *Cost Containment, Pricing and Financing of Pharmaceuticals in the European Community: The Policy Makers' View.* Athens: LSE and Pharmetrica, 1994.

44 Athanasopoulos G. *The Greek Pharmaceutical Market* (in Greek). Athens: Hellenic Association of the Pharmaceutical Industries, 1995.

45 Mossialos E, Ranos C, Abel-Smith B (eds). *Cost Containment, Pricing and Financing of Pharmaceuticals in the European Community: The Policy Makers' View.* Athens: LSE and Pharmetrica, 1994.

46 Government Accounting Office. *Trends in Public Capital Expenditures in Greece* (unpublished paper). Athens: GAO, 1990.

47 Kyriopoulos J, Niakas D. Economic and health policy issues in biomedical technology: the case of Greece. In: Malek M, *et al* (eds). *Strategic Issues in Health Care Management.* London: Wiley, 1993.

48 Liaropoulos L. *Private Health Insurance. Its role, problems and perspective in Greece* (in Greek). Athens: Financial Forum, 1993.

49 IMOSY. *Trends in Private Health Insurance Expenditure* (in Greek).Athens: IMOSY, 1996.

50 Abel-Smith B (chairman), Calltorp J, Dixon M, Dunning Ad, Evans R, Holland W, Jarman B, and Mossialos E. (coordinator). *Report of the Special Committee of Experts on the Greek Health Services.* Athens: Pharmetrica, 1994.

51 Ministry of Health and Social Security. *A Study on the Planning and Organisation of the Health Services.* (edited by Theodorou M, Karokis A, Polyzos N, Roupas T, Sissouras A, Yfantopoulos J) Athens: Ministry of Health and Social Security, 1994.

52 Sissouras A, Karokis A. The necessity for a unified health fund. In: Kyriopoulos J, Sissouras A (eds). *The Unified Health Fund.* Athens: Themelio, 1997.

53 Tountas J, Stefannson H, Frissiras S. Health reform in Greece: planning and implementation of a national health system. *International Journal of Health Planning and Management* 1995;10:283–304.

54 Kyriopoulos J. (ed.). 1995. Health Policy in Greece: Choices at the crossroad. Athens: Themelio (in Greek).

55 Ministry of Health and Social Security. *Report of the Committee on the Creation of a Unified Health Fund and the Decentralisation of the Health Care System* (in Greek). Athens: Ministry of Health, 1995.

56 Ministry of Health and Social Security. *Report of the Committee on the Reforms in the*

400 *Health Care and Cost Containment in the European Union*

Management of the Health Care Services in Greece (in Greek). Athens: Ministry of Health, 1995.

57 Abel-Smith B. *Cost Containment and Health Care in Europe.* London: Bedford Square Press, 1984.

58 Abel-Smith B, Mossialos E. Cost containment and health care reform: a study of the European Union. *Health Policy* 1994;28(2):89–134.

59 Mossialos E. Health policy in Greece. *Hellenic Medical Journal* 1996;1(1):33–5.

60 Ferrera M. *EC Citizens and Social Protection: Main Results from a Eurobarometer Survey.* Brussels: Commission of the European Communities, 1993.

61 Mossialos E. Citizens' views on health care systems in the 15 EU Member States. *Health Economics* 1997;6(2):109–16.

8 Health care and cost containment in Spain

GUILLEM LOPEZ I CASASNOVAS

8.1 Introduction

This chapter will focus on the following cost containment measures.

- Changes in the system of financing Spanish hospitals, entailing a move away from reimbursement methods to the purchasing of services based on activity, as evidenced by the evolution of the Catalan contracting-out method since 1986, the 1991 State Hospital Contracts Programme (*Contrato Programa*), and some other initiatives in the Basque Region.

- The creation in 1993 of a negative list of drugs which could no longer be reimbursed by social security (800 brand name products); some very recent experiments (for example in Valencia in 1997) on reference pricing (the maximum that the authority is willing to pay) for the most commonly prescribed drugs and proposals for pharmaceutical co-payment increases.

- Changes derived from the primary health care reform, begun in 1984 and still under way, involving the departure from a system based on capitation and hours of work to a system closely related to salaries and full-time employment in the new Health Centres.

- Efforts to create a basic package of publicly financed health care, best represented by the Guaranteed Health Care Entitlement of 1995.

- An analysis of the diversity in the way health services are managed across the decentralized Spanish autonomous communities.

I would like to thank A. Beith, P. Ibern, V. Ortún, J. Puig and D. Serra, from Centre de Recerca en Economia Salut-Universitat Pompeu Fabra, and E. Mossialos for their comments on an early version of this paper. Research support from the *Comisión Interministerial para la Ciencia y la Technologia* is also acknowledged (Spanish Department of Education, grant number PB94-0848).

402   *Health Care and Cost Containment in the European Union*

- Proposals to extend the MUFACE system (a publicly financed choice of public or private health insurer) currently restricted to civil servants, to the rest of the population.

The following overview of the Spanish health care system will attempt to set these cost containment measures in the relevant context.

8.2 Brief description of the Spanish health care system

8.2.1 General overview

Health care financing in Spain is a mixture of public (approximately 80 per cent of total health care spending) and private (20 per cent) financing. These figures remained fairly stable between 1980 and 1995 (Table 8.1). In 1995 total health expenditure amounted to PTE 5 billion, around 7.6 per cent of

Table 8.1 Main sources of health care financing in Spain

	Year	Source	Current PTE (billion)	Percentage
Public expenditure	1986	General taxation	270.0	23.8
		Social insurance contributions	843.7	74.3
		Other sources	22.3	1.9
		Total	1,136.0	
	1995	General taxation	2501.5	77.3
		Social insurance contributions	658.7	20.4
		Other sources	73.8	2.3
		Total	3,234.0	
Private expenditure	1986	Health insurance premiums (4.3 million enrollees)	71.1	23.7
		Out-of-pocket payments	228.9	76.3
		Total	300.0	
	1995	Health insurance premiums (5.7 million enrollees)	293.7	30.0
		Out-of-pocket payments	685.3	70.0
		Total	979.0	

Spanish Gross Domestic Product (GDP). In per capita terms, the figure was close to one thousand dollars in Purchasing Power Parities (PPPs) which is 10 per cent below the corresponding UK figure and 40 per cent below the average of western European OECD countries. However, when adjusted for income, the Spanish figure fits almost perfectly the standard OECD pattern.

The Spanish health care system is financed from public funds both through state transfers to the social security body (INSALUD)* and through social security contributions (payroll taxes) at a ratio (of the former to the latter) of 4 to 1. However, this ratio has been anything but stable between 1980 and 1996, varying from 1 to 4 at the beginning of the 1980s to a mid-1990s level of 4 to 1. This change is mainly due to the financial efforts to remove health care from the social security budget crisis.

8.2.2 Public health care expenditure

We can see from Figure 8.1 overleaf, that Spanish health care is founded largely upon a system of public financing, with public production also playing a relatively prominent role. The private expenditure share of the total is slightly below the OECD average, even after adjusting for GDP differences.

Despite this broad picture, some important variations exist among the different Spanish autonomous communities. For instance, in Catalonia, more than half of hospital expenditure is contracted out to non profit-making private producers and to public hospitals owned by organizations other than social security, such as local municipalities and the Red Cross. The amount of private expenditure in health care is also subject to relatively significant regional variations, being higher in richer regions. This is particularly true with regard to private insurance expenditure, although the same patterns that occur across regions can also be observed within a region.[1-3]

Given that the Spanish health care system was based on a National Health Service model, the reasons for establishing such a mix in funding sources in the past are unclear. These are not likely to be due to the potential impact of payroll taxes, as an earmarked tax to health expenditure, on individual behaviour or collective choice. In fact, current INSALUD fund-

---

* Since 1989 the amount of the transfer has been earmarked for health care spending (instead of being a non-defined part of the overall social security budget). This process was reinforced in the budgets for 1995 and 1996.

Figure 8.1 Main features of the Spanish health care system, 1995

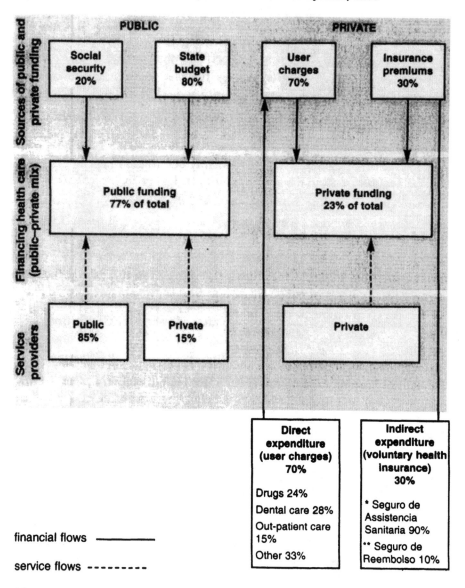

* Insurance companies arranging for the provision of health services via a network of office-based doctors and hospitals.
** Health care insurance companies reimbursing, fully or partially, out-of-pocket expenditure by the insuree.

Source: Author's own elaboration from different sources.

Health Care and Cost Containment in Spain 405

ing, which is financed from social security contributions, represents only a small proportion of nominal taxation, and is not believed to have any adverse effects on public perception. In any case, plans to reduce financial pressures on the social security budget by discontinuing these social security contributions and financing the Spanish health care system solely through general taxation, although started with the 1997 budget, have been postponed to the year 2000.* It could also be argued that the resistance to financing health services completely from taxes dates back to the beginning of the political decentralization process and the then desire of the Socialist Party not to generalize the transfer of powers to the autonomous communities. Thus, the provision of health care was retained within the auspices of social security (not transferable) rather than the state (transferable).

Public health expenditure in Spain is, in principle, limited to a budget. Nevertheless, this is frequently exceeded, and for this reason most of the actual expenditure figures included here refer to 1995, these being the latest available as data for 1996 and 1997 are not reliable (see section 8.2.5). The adjustment of public budgets over initial levels is mainly achieved by modifying certain budget items. This is particularly true of the figures for pharmaceutical expenditure which are usually underestimated, since these amounts can be modified without complex legal procedures (see Table 8.6).

As Table 8.2 shows, public health care expenditure increased from PTE 1,434,485 million in 1986 to PTE 2,677,551 million in 1995 at 1986 con-

Table 8. 2 Public health care expenditure (1986–95) at constant 1986 prices

Year	PTE million	Year	PTE million
1986	1,434,485	1991	2,346,687
1987	1,523,997	1992	2,340,686
1988	1,809,475	1993	2,466,688
1989	1,965,153	1994	2,620,286
1990	2,214,532	1995	2,677,551

Source: Ministerio de Sanidad y Consumo, 1997.[4]

---

* Indeed, the so-called *'Pacto de Toledo'* (a consensus agreement among all the political parties to reform the Spanish social security) removes social security contributions for health care and imposes finance by taxation, as was originally intended in the *Ley General de Sanidad* of 1986 (the law establishing the National Health Service in Spain).

406 *Health Care and Cost Containment in the European Union*

stant prices. However, the increase between 1986 and 1990 was 54.4 per cent, whereas that between 1991 and 1996 was only 14.1 per cent.

In brief, total health expenditure, according to OECD data for 1995, amounts to 7.6 per cent of Spanish GDP, with per capita health expenditure being just below one thousand dollars (in PPPs). Around 80 per cent of this figure is public health care expenditure and about 20 per cent accounts for private health care expenditure. Total expenditure on health rose from 3.7 per cent of GDP in 1970 to 5.7 per cent in 1985 and 7.6 per cent in 1995 (Table 8.3).*

Table 8.3 Evolution of (1) the total health care expenditure to GDP ratio and (2) the percentage of total public expenditure on total health expenditure (1970–95)

	Spain		European Union average*	
	(1)	(2)	(1)	(2)
1970	3.7	65.4	5.0	75.5
1980	5.7	79.9	6.9	80.6
1985	5.7	81.1	7.1	78.2
1990	6.9	78.7	7.3	78.6
1995	7.6	78.2	8.3	74.5

* non-weighted

Source: Ministerio de Sanidad y Consumo, 1996.[5]

Within INSALUD, the distribution of the budget in 1994 was as follows: primary care, 14.5 per cent; pharmaceuticals, 18.1 per cent; in-patient and out-patient hospital care, 63.2 per cent; research and training, 2.2 per cent and administration costs, 2.0 per cent. However, no explicit mechanisms exist for allocating resources between these spending catagories, either for

---

* However, there are considerable differences in spending between automonous communities (of which there are 17 in Spain). For 1994, the difference between the 15 per cent higher per capita regional health expenditure and the remaining 85 per cent was PTE 19,130, with an average per capita value of PTE 80,100 and a mean of PTE 78,877. Between 1986 and 1994, the annual average rate of increase was 13.17 per cent and its rank increased by 11.69 per cent.

Health Care and Cost Containment in Spain   407

INSALUD or for the Regional Health Authorities with health service management responsibilities. The majority of the latter are annually allocated a lump-sum payment based roughly on a per capita calculation and each year conflicts arise regarding the regional distribution of the total public health budget (see section 8.4.4).

8.2.3 Private health care expenditure

Private health care expenditure, which constitutes around one-fifth of the total health care expenditure, can be broken down into payments for voluntary health insurance (around 10 per cent of the total), direct payments, which are mostly for extra-hospital care (around 14 per cent), medicines (22 per cent) and other pharmaceutical supplies (10 per cent), dentistry (25 per cent), prostheses (9 per cent) and other expenses (10 per cent).* Table 8.4 shows that the total number of insured with voluntary health insurance increased by 20.5 per cent between 1990 and 1997. Over the same period the average premium increased by 105.7 per cent.

Table 8.4 Evolution of average voluntary insurance premiums and number of insured, 1990–97

Year	1990	1991	1992	1993	1994	1995	1996	1997
Total insured (000s)	5,420	5,489	5,709	5,644	5,710	5,733	6,294	6,505
Average premium (PTE, current prices)	23,670	30,987	35,340	40,143	43,196	46,196	46,129	48,691
Increase of average premiums over previous year	n.a.	+30.9	+14.0	+13.6	+7.6	+6.9	-0.1	+5.5

Source: Author's elaboration from MSD, 1996[6]; Dirección General de Seguros, Ministerio de Economia y Hacienda, Información Trimestral, several years.

---

* Data from the Encuesta de Presupuestos Familiares (1991 Household Expenditure Survey).[2]

408 *Health Care and Cost Containment in the European Union*

Between 1980 and 1990, the annual average increase of private expenditure in real terms was 2.6 per cent.* This also meant an enlarged share for private expenditure in family budgets (2.65 per cent in 1980 and 3 per cent in 1990).[2] Expenditure on dental care and drugs saw the highest increases in nominal terms, at 18.8 per cent and 24.4 per cent respectively. Despite these increases, the share of private to total health expenditure stayed constant or decreased slightly during the 1980s, owing to a higher increase in public expenditure (15.3 per cent in average annual nominal rate, versus 13.5 per cent for private health expenditure).

Private health expenditure is subject to an income tax deduction of 15 per cent.

8.2.4 Regulation of public provision of health care

The Spanish Constitution of 1978 provided for the decentralization of some responsibilities to the 17 Spanish autonomous communities (CCAAs). Seven of these (the Basque Country, Navarra, Catalonia, Galicia, Andalucía, Valencia and the Canary Islands) now have responsibility for health care services, managing approximately 55 per cent of total health care spending. With the exception of the Basque Country and Navarra (which have their own special system of financing),** the tendency for resource allocation to the regions has been to use capitation criteria, however, this process has varied from region to region.

The current Spanish health care system has evolved from a health service that was largely fragmented, characterized by scattered competencies and involving a multitude of bodies. Recently there have been moves towards an increased integration of services, made possible by the *Ley General de Sanidad* (LGS) of 1986. Efforts to improve the system include

---

* This was the last year covered by the General Household Expenditure Survey. The complete survey is conducted every five years.

** Under the *Concierto* (general agreement) the Basque Country and Navarra collect their own taxes and then pay for those services remaining under central control. These payments (*cupos*) relate to income. Whenever a public service is decentralized, the region no longer pays the central state for this service, and it can keep all the revenues collected. If the state was financing less than the corresponding amount of the share in the regional income in total (as usually happens in rich regions with regard to capitation), the transfer of a service implies additional money to the region.

Health Care and Cost Containment in Spain   409

moves to universalize public health care coverage, decentralize the management of health services and increasing public financing for health care by almost 1.5 percentage points in terms of GDP between 1982 and 1996. Despite these efforts, however, many groups remain dissatisfied with the current system of health care, notably:

- consumers, as regards the perceived quality of certain services, mainly in primary care;

- health professionals, who have continually pressed for higher wages and whose strikes of 1987 and 1995 resulted in significant INSALUD salary increases (20 per cent and 10 per cent, respectively). However, the 1997 budget again froze wage in the public health care sector; and

- the autonomous communities (excluding the Basque Country and Navarra), because of present resource allocation and budgetary mechanisms. Some claim to be receiving insufficient health care resources, while others argue that the present method for resource allocation is far from equitable, as it does not sufficiently allow for regional differences.

Without a doubt, the resource allocation dilemma is one of the main reasons behind the push for health sector reform in Spain. It is significant both to the current political debate questioning the legitimacy of the present model and to the question of how to control the public deficit. Despite the fact that macro health indicators in Spain are for the most part higher,* and health care spending lower, than the OECD average, the question of how to reform resource allocation will remain a key element of future reforms.

In fact, the feature of the Spanish health care system that probably stands out the most is the fact that Spain is one of the western nations in which the correlation between the apparent effectiveness of the health care system, the cost of health services and the level of satisfaction among citizens is lowest.** The reason for this low correlation may be found in the excessive regulation exerted by health authorities over the utilization of

---

* In 1994, life expectancy at birth was 81.0 years for women and 73.3 for men, perinatal mortality per 100 live births was 0.66 per cent and the infant mortality rate was 0.6 per cent.[7]

** See for example, the Blendon Report, commissioned by the *Comision de Analysis y Evaluacion del Sistema Nacional de Salud*, which allows for comparisons between different countries regarding satisfaction with health care services.[8] See Mossialos, 1997,[9] for the Eurobarometer Survey.

410 *Health Care and Cost Containment in the European Union*

health care services. In other words, the supply and demand for health care, with controls supposedly directed towards the improvement of the population's health status, today are highly bureaucratic. Direct production and financing of services, inspection of health care services through the regulation of patient flows, the assigning of population quotas (despite the measures introduced in 1994 and 1995 instituting a patient's free choice of specialist), fixed referral centres, administrative regulations regarding manpower policies and retribution schemes to health care personnel, the use of equipment – including amortization – by health care producers, are all examples of this bureaucratization.

Despite having been established in order to safeguard the welfare of Spanish citizens, it is not necessarily the case that all this regulation always benefits the consumer. It is more likely that, in reality, those who decide upon and finance the production of health care services are more concerned with ensuring the viability of the centres they administer and keeping their professionals satisfied than with meeting the wishes and requirements of citizens.

8.2.5 Recent evolution of health care spending and levels of financial sustainability

The Spanish health service has been financed via general taxation and social security contributions since 1978, when revenues and payments were first linked.* In 1988, resources transferred to INSALUD by the state represented 28 per cent of total resources. The 1989 Budget Bill (*Ley de Presupuestos Generales del Estado*) established a new system which contained a specific contribution by the state to INSALUD. Thus, at 80 per cent for general taxation and 18 per cent for social security contributions, the financing figures for 1995, broken down, completely reverse the 1988 figures.**

The percentage of per capita health care spending in total expenditure

---

* In fact, until the introduction of a single contribution in 1979, there were specific contributions for each Social Security Service. As of 1979, the contribution from the state was dedicated to financing the deficit of the entire system. From 1989 on, the state decided to increase its contributions to social security, thus ending its responsibility for the social security budgets.

** The remaining 2 per cent is mostly made up of revenues from third parties, for instance traffic accidents.

Table 8.5 Public national health system expenditure, 1982–96 (current prices, in million pesetas)

Year	Planned budget expenditure	% increase	Recorded* expenditure	% increase	Actual** expenditure	% increase	GDP annual % increase
1981	605,401		654,313				12.37
1982	695,447	14.8	762,498	16.5	–	–	15.70
1983	800,436	15.1	843,590	10.6	–	–	14.24
1984	875,214	9.3	900,756	6.8	–	–	13.26
1985	970,354	10.9	1,015,666	12.8	–	–	10.51
1986	1,049,032	8.1	1,154,811	13.7	–	–	14.66
1987	1,155,019	10.1	1,307,647	13.2	–	–	11.78
1988	1,350,682	16.9	1,497,547	14.5	1,640,000	–	11.11
1989	1,574,005	16.5	1,795,841	19.9	1,892,000	15.4	12.17
1990	1,851,144	17.6	2,065,984	15.0	2,171,000	14.7	11.32
1991	2,108,863	13.9	2,259,351	9.4	2,474,869	14.0	9.48
1992	2,389,141	13.3	2,564,707	25.9	2,755,858	11.4	7.47
1993	2,671,321	11.8	2,988,417	5.1	2,933,240	6.4	3.23
1994	2,845,480	6.5	3,225,516	7.8	2,982,301	1.7	6.23
1995	3,224,068	14.0	3,314,456	3.2	3,228,734	8.9	7.85
1996	3,484,068	8.1	3,526,045	6.4	n.a.	n.a.	6.40

* planned expenditure plus additional credit given during the financial year (includes repayment of debts from previous years).

** planned expenditure plus additional exenditure allocated to the year in which it was incurred.

Note: The recorded expenditure for 1992 and 1993 does not include expenditure incurred before 1991. The adjustment for 1992 and 1993 amounts to PTE 280,558 and PTE 140,282 million, respectively.

Sources: Ministerio de Sanidad y Consumo, 1998[10] and Ministerio de Economía y Hacienda, 1994.[11]

412   *Health Care and Cost Containment in the European Union*

in Spain reveals an average annual increase of 2.63 per cent from 1981 to 1991. For total INSALUD public expenditure, this figure was 14.45 per cent between 1986 and 1993. This translates to an absolute average spending per capita of 13.12 per cent, a figure much higher than the nominal GDP growth rate.

These figures are calculated by taking into account the accumulated debts of previous years and adding the excess spending to that initially budgeted.*

Table 8.6 Recent evolution of the deviations in public health expenditure for the national health system (%), 1981–96

	Recorded expenditure over planned budget	% actual versus planned budget expenditure
1981	8.08	n.a.
1982	9.64	n.a.
1983	5.39	n.a.
1984	2.92	n.a.
1985	4.67	n.a.
1986	10.08	n.a.
1987	13.21	n.a.
1988	10.87	n.a.
1989	14.09	20.2
1990	11.61	17.3
1991	7.14	17.4
1992	19.09	15.3
1993	11.97	9.8
1994	13.38	4.8
1995	2.80	0.1
1996	1.20	n.a.

Source: Author's own elaboration from Ministerio de Trabajo y Seguridad Social, 1992, 1994, 1997.[12–14]

---

* In order to understand some key aspects of the budgeting process in health care before 1994, see Sanfrutos.[15]

Health Care and Cost Containment in Spain 413

Without considering outstanding credit, in 1994, a deficit of PTE 68 billion was recorded for 1992, and PTE 56.5 billion for 1993. Tables 8.5 and 8.6 show the importance of comparing planned expenditure with recorded and actual expenditure, in order to understand the real evolution of health expenditure in Spain. The Working Group for Health Finance, which was created with a mandate to evaluate the shortfall in health care funding, established a programme of measures to close this gap. This was to be met partly through additional resources and partly through credit supplementation over the following four years. However, all of this greatly complicates knowledge about real health care expenditure. For example, after hearing the results of the above-mentioned Working Group, the September 1994 agreement of the Financial and Fiscal Committee (*Consejo de Política Fiscal y Financiera*) ended in recognizing a general debt of PTE 290 billion between 1992 and 1993, which had not been included in any previous health care calculations and had not initially been included in their own. For 1996, PTE 152 billion were added (PTE 90 billion in 1995). Some estimates show an overall deficit for the entire system of between one hundred and two hundred thousand pesetas a year, and an already accumulated debt of around half a billion pesetas.

Consequently, figures on public health expenditure must be analysed very cautiously. Table 8.6 shows the complexity of analysing public health care expenditure using existing records.

8.2.6 Public health care expenditure by components

As mentioned in previous sections, in 1994 hospital expenditure accounted for 63.2 per cent of total public health expenditure, having risen from 59.6 per cent in 1988, and 61.6 per cent in 1991.

The large size of pharmaceutical expenditure as a share of total public health expenditure is one of the ways in which Spain is different from other OECD countries (see Table 8.7 overleaf). Since the Medicines Act of 1990, there has been a concerted attempt to control these costs, but this has met with little success. Recent measures, discussed below, try to reduce both unit costs, by acting on the pharmaceutical industry and privately-owned pharmacies, and the prescription rates of Spanish physicians. Since 1980, the number of prescriptions has increased by 12 per cent, and consumption at current prices has multiplied sixfold. The evolution of pharmaceutical expenditure in recent years is included in Table 8.7.

Table 8.7 Recent trends in public health care expenditure and expenditure on pharmaceuticals (PTE billion, current prices), 1990–95

	Public health care expenditure	Pharmaceutical expenditure*	%
1990	2,171.0	419.9	19.3
1991	2,475.0	491.6	19.8
1992	2,756.0	565.0	20.5
1993	2,933.0	609.4	20.7
1994	2,982.0	643.7	21.5
1995	3,164.0	718.0	22.7

* This figure excludes co-payments and pharmacy profit margins.
Source: INSALUD, 1997.[16]

Lopez and Mossialos[17] have shown that it is the real increase in the type of prescriptions, rather than price variations in drugs, that explains this pattern of growth. While real drug expenditure increased by 264 per cent between 1980 and 1996, the relative price of drugs fell by 39 per cent and the number of prescribed items rose by only 10 per cent. Most of the increase can be attributed to new products, whose impact on health expenditure trends increased by 442 per cent between 1980 and 1996.

Primary health care represents around 15 per cent of total public health expenditure. Nowadays, primary care tends to be organized as an integrated system of production at the territorial level of the health area. However, this 'new' model still coexists with a traditional quota system based on part-time single-person practices, paid on a per capita basis. In contrast, the new primary health care teams are essentially group practices, mainly paid salaries. At present, two-thirds of the population are covered by these teams, but again regional differences exist, particularly in Catalonia, where the difficulty in persuading GPs to voluntarily change their status has led to lower levels of coverage.

In the field of primary care, Spain occupies an average position in terms of direct referrals per one thousand inhabitants, at 54.6 (80.5 for Norway, 24.4 for France).[18] Moreover, the ratio of successive to first visits illustrates the relevant role of specialists in hospital health care. The average time between initial referral and the actual medical visit is 12 days, again an average position in the European context.[18] Workload ratios show an extremely low percentage of home visits, just 6 per cent (15 per cent in the UK, 39 per

Health Care and Cost Containment in Spain 415

cent in France)[18] and a low number of visits per capita per year, 4.0 (11.5 for Germany, 11 for Italy, 7.5 for Belgium and 4.5 for the UK).[18]

The only part of dental care covered by the public system is tooth extraction, and thus this forms an important component of private expenditure on health. According to the Spanish Household Expenditure Survey, inequality in utilization of dental services is very high (the ratio of dental expenditure between the highest and the lowest income deciles was 4 in 1990, which has decreased from around 7 in 1980).

8.2.7 The hospital sector

The latest available data on the Spanish hospital system as regards the number of hospitals, sizes and bed numbers[19] reveal that, in 1995, the national health service (*Sistema Nacional de Salud*) comprised 198 hospitals (out of a total of 787 in Spain) which provided 86 thousand beds (out of a total of 169 thousand), concentrated for the most part in hospitals with more than 200 beds (which differs considerably from private non profit-making hospitals which generally have fewer than 200 beds) and, most importantly, with a high concentration of acute care patients (and fewer geriatrics and long-term care cases).* In 1980, the number of hospital beds per thousand inhabitants was 5.4 (5.8 for the EU unweighted average) which had decreased to 4.1 by 1994 (4.4 for the EU). Despite the fact that, for the same period, hospital admissions per thousand inhabitants increased from 9.3 to 10.4 and bed occupancy rate rose from 70 to 77.8, the average length of stay, measured in days, decreased from 14.8 in 1980 to 11.0 in 1994.

Data contained in the *Catálogo Nacional de Hospitales* reveal that 68 per cent of beds are publicly owned.** Of this sub-total, 83 per cent are for

---

* The beneficiary private sector (Red Cross and Church) totals about 135 centres, covering all sizes and types of assistance (including maternal, infant and psychiatric care and oncology).

** The distribution of public beds is less homogeneous in the autonomous communities with health care responsibility, both in terms of the status of hospitals (that is whether dependent upon the social security, municipalities or profit-making organizations) and the number of beds per inhabitant. For example, there are 0.78 beds which depend on the social security per thousand inhabitants in Catalonia, compared with 2.55 in Aragon and an overall average of 1.68. As regards total numbers of beds, there are 4.95 in the Basque Country and 6.1 in Navarra, compared with 3.8 in Galicia and 3.2 in Castilla la Mancha while the average is 4.35. Analysis of the private sector reveals 3.04 beds per thousand inhabitants in Catalonia compared with 0.2 in Extremadura and an overall average of 1.4.

416 *Health Care and Cost Containment in the European Union*

acute care. Public hospitals account for 73 per cent of total days of hospital stays and 75 per cent of discharges. The majority (98 per cent) of people working in these centres work 36 hours or more, while, at 66 per cent, the percentage is significantly lower for the private sector. Hospital specialists are paid a basic salary. Further small increments may be added to this salary, in a similar way to that used for the rest of Spanish civil servants, along with some complementary allowances. These are determined by law and vary according to the particular level of responsibility a post entails (head of service, head of section, extra duties performed, and so on).

In brief, until recently acute care hospitals belonging to the social security financed their current expenditure from a baseline calculated from previous expenditure, without any formal evaluation process being carried out. This was accompanied by negotiation between the financing body INSALUD and the management authorities of the individual health centres. Until recently, the cost per day of stay and per admission were the only two economic criteria used as external references of activity, collected in the *Informe Economico Funcional* of INSALUD (the INSALUD Report). Financing was through a global budget, without any distinction between programmes, services or hospital departments. Within each centre expenditure was then disaggregated, separated into in-patient care, out-patient services, teaching and research, although not in such a way as to be particularly reliable for cost comparison purposes.

In 1993, the INSALUD hospitals set up the so-called '*contratos-programa*' in the ten regions that remain centrally controlled.[20] This programme establishes agreements which link activity to global budgets. These agreements are determined annually and outline:

- the objectives of health care production — measured in *Unidades Ponderadas de Asistencia**(UPAs) and other related procedures; and

- health care financing, based on actual (average) costs, as well as additional sources of revenue (from coverage of third parties, traffic accidents, and the private sector).

The weighted results are as follows: medical stay, 1 UPA; surgery, 1.5 UPAs; obstetrics, 1.2 UPAs; paediatrics, 1.3 UPAs; neonatology, 1.3 UPAs; intensive care, 5.8 UPAs; emergencies without admission 0.3 UPAs; first

---

* Resource weighted health care units.

consultations, 0.25 UPAs; successive consultations, 0.15 UPAs; and ambulatory surgery (minor procedures), 0.25 UPAs.

Some services are calculated separately from the total amount and have separate set fees; for example, teaching, haemodynamics, haemodialysis (patient/month), renal extractions, renal transplants, hepatitis, cardiac and some ambulatory surgery.

As mentioned above, 'notional' prices were determined using average costs, but owing to the absence of any common accounting plans, these include only running costs (as defined by chapters I and II of the budget). Prices for some activities, such as those for laboratory services, dental extractions and transplants, were tentatively fixed centrally. In 1993, some decentralization occurred involving the contracting out of some services (dialysis, lithotripters, CAT-scans) to hospitals which then received the corresponding credits. These measures affected the activity of professionals through the development of incentive systems. In the past few years it appears that they may have resulted in an increase in day surgery and day hospitalization, thus reducing existing waiting lists.[21]* The Catalonian, Basque and Andalucian health services have taken similar measures, although differing in specific measurement tools.

Additionals innovations have been attempted in the Basque Country and in Andalucía, the former pursuing Patient Management Categories while the latter has opted to employ Diagnosis Related Groups (DRGs), although in both cases the application cannot be considered definitive since they are still at the experimental stage. A new payment system for the Catalonian hospitals is expected to be implemented in 1997. Real incentives for developing alternatives to in-patient care can only be found in this Catalan proposal, since this is not exclusively based on a system of reference payments. For the moment, case-mix adjustments in Catalonia are mostly based on DRGs, although their importance in calculating hospital finance is still low.

In summary, while hospital financing claims to be prospective, the lack of evaluation of actual spending results in its being retrospective. In reality, and despite the creation of the *contratos programas*, budgets are still not

---

* INSALUD surgery waiting lists contained 53,828 patients in June 1996, with an average wait of 207 days. In order to halve these figures, in July 1997 the Conservative Government put forward extraordinary measures to increase the health care budget. The results, however, have to be adjusted by case mix to take into account not only the number of patients but also the type of service involved.

418 *Health Care and Cost Containment in the European Union*

linked closely enough to activity. In the majority of cases, resources are simply related to expected activity, while variations in activity are only slightly compensated for by variations in resources. Undoubtedly, this step represents a gradual advance, but real risk decentralization to managers and professionals has not yet occurred.

As regards hospital decentralization, it should be pointed out that, within the margins of approved budgets, health care centre managers have control over variable personnel costs (that is, for extra hours and possible replacements), although there are restrictions on levels of payment. Personnel modifications are determined centrally, although it is possible to substitute among categories at the hospital level. Hospitals are also responsible for initiating disciplinary procedures, yet not for their resolution. Trade unions are still very strong as concerns manpower policies and with regard to decisions as to how variable productivity should be distributed. Regarding the contracting of goods and services, there are certain expenditure restrictions on the quantity of direct purchases allowed by health centres. In INSALUD this is set at PTE 50 million, while in Andalucía the figure is PTE 250 million. As a result, many centres seek to disperse direct small contracts in order to elude the fixed limits in the law of public contracting.[21] Moreover, Spanish health centres cannot autonomously decide how much to invest, as such decisions are planned and authorized centrally. Owing to the lack of any real inventories of fixed assets, there are also no plans for adequate relocation.

Of the 135,000 personnel having *estatutario* status ('estatuto' implies a sort of self-protecting law), hospital doctors are paid a salary, with the majority of them having a contract of 36 hours or more per week. There is also a *numerus clausus* university policy which has, since the beginning of the 1990s, decreased the number of medical graduates to around 5,000 a year (4,914 for 1997). This represents somewhere between a half and one-third of the respective figure in the 1980s.[22]

Moreover, certain incompatibilities exist within the system. Personnel wishing to maintain more than one post within the public sector must submit to a process of authorizations. However, work schedules in the public sector do permit further practice within the private sector, although those people taking up outside private practice lose a specific supplement received by those who choose voluntarily to dedicate themselves to the public sector. A system of partial dedication does exist which goes some way to making this essential incompatibility more flexible. Currently, this is only the case in Catalonia, although there are at present proposals to extend it to the rest of Spain.

Whether related to the cost of living index or to GDP, it is clear that over the past two decades there has been a significant decrease in the salaries of hospital doctors, although this has not followed a consistent pattern. If the evolution of salaries is divided into two periods, a better relative salary in real terms is observed for the period 1986–91, and a loss is recorded for the years from 1991 to the present. Joining these periods results in a practically neutral effect, except for the least qualified health care personnel who have experienced consistent salary losses.

The above data, which are analysed in more detail by López and Garcia Cestona,[23] seems to reveal that, between 1970 and 1986, hospital personnel policy regarding salary control was fairly rigorous, while employment policy could be considered bland, resulting in important manpower increases in hospitals. However, this combination seems to have been eroded over the past five years, during which time salaries have caught up incrementally – the result today probably being a relatively low productivity on the part of health professionals.

8.2.8 Health technology assessment

The Spanish National Office of Technology Assessment was formed in 1994. This coexists with several regional agencies: in Catalonia since 1991 (it became an independent agency in 1994), in the Basque country since 1992, in the Valencia Community since 1994 and in Andalucía since 1996. These offices assess the effectiveness of innovative medical treatments and disseminate the available evidence. The need for health technology assessment can be illustrated by the high variation in clinical practice (among regions, and between Spain and other countries of the European Union), for instance, in home oxigenotherapy for chronic patients.[24,25]

8.3 Some cost containment measures in the Spanish health sector

Reforms over the past decade have skirted the idea of introducing strong cost containment measures in Spain. In particular, in 1991 under the socialist government, the Abril Martorell Report[26] (named after the man who

420   *Health Care and Cost Containment in the European Union*

headed the Commission set up to evaluate and offer suggestions to the health sector) raised several recommendations to improve efficiency within the National Health Service, including (i) introducing a purchaser/provider split; (ii) creating a basic package of publicly provided health care; (iii) increasing funding from taxation yet maintaining social security contributions at around 30 per cent of total funding in order to increase cost consciousness among consumers; and (iv) searching for the introduction of nominal fees for some services such as pharmaceuticals (to include pensioners who currently pay nothing, but offsetting this measure with an increase in pensions), more as a cost consciousness measure than to generate further resources.

However, the central health organization, INSALUD, which has responsibility for the ten remaining regions, has encountered serious difficulties in its attempts to change the status quo. In consequence, with contracting out still only in the initial stages of development, the purchaser/provider split has so far failed to materialize and health care provider budgets still follow incremental routines. A basic package of health care measures to be provided publicly (*Catálogo de Prestaciones Sanitarias*) was approved in 1995.[27] However, the effectiveness of this basic package is debatable, since, far from narrowing services provided, the package in fact adds services to the care currently available. Moreover, social security contributions have been maintained at around 20 per cent of total health care financing. Finally, the planned introduction of nominal fees for some services (including those for pensioners), has yet to be implemented.

These and other more recent reform proposals are analysed below.

8.3.1 Types of expenditure effects derived from health care reform

A systematic analysis of the following set of fiscal effects, derived from health care reforms, will now be attempted:

(a) changes that generate a slope effect: a change between the pre- and post-reform growth rates;

(b) one-off changes in the level of expenditure: a one-off step drop followed by (starting from this lower level) a trend similar to that which existed prior to the reform;

(c) perverse changes: that is, an initial expenditure decline followed by a

Health Care and Cost Containment in Spain   421

rate of increase higher than that which was the case before reform, causing final expenditure levels to be higher than those forecast had reform not taken place; and

(e) successful changes: an initial downward shift followed by a lower slope in the rate of increase.

In this analysis, the policy measures on which we will focus, are:

(a) changes in the system of financing Spanish hospitals, moving from reimbursement methods to purchasing services based on activity, as measured by the UPA (*Unidad Ponderada de Asistencia*) in INSALUD's *Contratos-Programa*, which started around 1991;

(b) the 1993 Drug Bill, which created a negative list of 800 speciality group drugs no longer to be reimbursed by social security;

(c) the effects of past policies on drug consumption by the Spanish population at large (excluding those drugs dispensed in hospitals), looking at co-payment increases over time. These rose from 10 per cent in 1978 to 30 per cent in 1979 and 40 per cent in 1980;

(d) changes in pharmaceutical costs per capita between those covered by the MUFACE system* and the rest of the population;

(e) per capita costs under the new Primary Health Care Reform, instituted in 1984. This saw a departure from a system based on capitation and hours of work to a salary-based system and full-time employment in the new health centres;

(f) diversity in the way health services are managed among the decentralized regions in Spain;

(g) the Valencian experiment on reference pricing for the most prescribed drugs; and

(h) creation of a basic package of publicly provided health care, known as the Guaranteed Health Care Entitlement of 1995.

---

* At present civil servants in Spain are covered by special schemes. One such scheme, MUFACE, allows insured civil servants the option of choosing between either being publicly insured (through INSALUD) or being privately insured at no extra cost.

422 Health Care and Cost Containment in the European Union

8.3.2 Proposals and facts

The Spanish health care reforms and proposals most relevant to cost containment are the following.

8.3.2.1 Policy reforms for setting overall financial constraints Since September 1994, within The Commission for Financial and Fiscal Policy (*Consejo de Política Fiscal y Financiera*), there has been an agreement linking overall growth in public health care expenditure to nominal GDP increases. However, up to the present time, including both 1995 and 1996, this has rarely been the case, with health spending often rising above this level. For this policy to achieve greater credibility, it has been agreed that all savings achieved by cost containment in the health sector will be added to the GDP nominal increase for the 1997 budget. Nevertheless, Spanish public health budgets have not benefited from the reduction in pharmaceutical prices.

Linking public health spending and GDP is not a constitutional budgetary rule, but a political commitment that can change at any time. Indeed, the amount devoted to financing health care is the result of a political discussion process at the highest political level, involving initially the vice-secretaries of the different departments and then the Council of Ministers. Moreover, doubts currently exist as to how these ceilings may be enforced and respected in the near future. Per capita health expenditure is well below the European average and in almost no country, including the UK, have ceilings been able to reverse the growth trend. However, in support of the present proposal, we should point to the fact that the Budget Law for 1997 changes the budgetary legislation. It makes spending overruns more difficult, since, in principle, the amended legislation does not allow any additional – other than planned – finance in such situations.

8.3.2.2 Policy reforms on pharmaceuticals As mentioned above, co-payments are only available for drugs not dispensed in hospitals. Co-payments have now been maintained at a rate of 40 per cent since 1980, having previously stood at 10 per cent in 1978 and 30 per cent in 1979. Individual co-payments for pharmaceuticals are not usually covered by supplementary private insurance. Chronic patients are liable for only marginal co-payments*

---

* There is a range of medications for chronic diseases for which only 10 per cent of the cost is paid, with a ceiling of PTE 439 per prescription, updated annually. This reduced contribution was recently extended to drugs used in the treatment of AIDS.

Health Care and Cost Containment in Spain 423

while pensioners are entirely exempt. Evidence that co-payments reduce demand has only been shown by using the 'natural test' (other tests related to expenditure or number of prescriptions per capita are ambiguous because of the observed consumption flow from the non-exempt to the exempt population*) that is given by the increase over time of the consumer share in costs for non-pensioners and by the MUFACE system.** For the 1967-85 period, for which co-payments were raised from PTE 50 up to the current rate of 40 per cent of the retail price, Puig[28] estimated a demand price elasticity of between -0.13 and -0.15. This rather low figure is probably due to the significant transfer of prescriptions to the exempted elderly population and the potentially high income effects which occurred particularly during the early years of the period being analysed. The transfer of prescriptions was estimated by Puig to represent between 30 and 40 per cent of the elderly population (that is, 15 or 20 per cent of the total). For those covered by the MUFACE scheme, there is a flat-rate co-payment of 30 per cent which applies to everyone including pensioners. As a result, pharmaceutical per capita costs for MUFACE are 8 per cent lower than the average.[29]

A more recent policy is that which created a negative list of drugs. New regulations were put into place in 1994 establishing a negative list of drugs no longer to be reimbursed by social security. This list excludes specific groups of medications for minor symptoms: in particular, anabolic drugs, dermatological products, nutritional and anti-obesity drugs. In addition, 1,692 pharmaceutical specialities were also excluded, amounting to 19.8 per cent of the market total, with an average price of PTE 291 (the total average price was PTE 1,247). These measures created a 'shift', or short-term, effect in the rate of increase of expenditure followed, in 1995, by a rise to levels higher than those before the policy was implemented. Other effects recorded were an increase in the number of prescriptions transferred to pensioners and a higher utilization of substitute and more expensive drugs. In any event, the reduction partially affected some drugs already out of use.

An agreement establishing a system of profit reduction also exists between the government and the pharmaceutical industry; this has set annu-

---

* This is shown by the apparent increase of retiree drug consumption due to others using them to gain access to free prescriptions. As a result the per capita cost ratio (retirees versus non-retirees) is 9 to 1.

** As mentioned earlier, for those covered by the MUFACE system, there is a general co-payment of 30 per cent for everyone, including pensioners. As a result, pharmaceutical per capita costs for the MUFACE system are 8 per cent lower than the average.

424 *Health Care and Cost Containment in the European Union*

al growth ceilings for public expenditure on drugs at 7 per cent for 1996 and 4 per cent for 1997. In addition, pharmacies have been asked to offer discounts to the public payer of around 2 per cent.

The Valencian policy establishing a reference list for some drugs includes an exemption from this 2 per cent discount in return for agreeing to supply 38 specified drugs according to a set reference price. These 38 drugs account for 45 per cent of overall Valencian pharmaceutical expenditure.* Currently, supplying 'copies' of the original brands of pharmaceuticals is the only policy possible and accounts for 30 per cent of all prescriptions. This is because the present Spanish generic market constitutes only 3 per cent of all prescriptions, and the late adoption of the European legislation on patents does not allow for a rapid increase of the generic market in the near future.

In short, the Valencian experiment of reference pricing for the most frequently prescribed drugs, the cost of which amounts to over PTE 40 billion, is still in too early a stage to evaluate its effectiveness. Nevertheless, Valencian managers argue that the experiment has resulted in an average increase in pharmaceutical expenditure 40 per cent lower than the national figure.

8.3.2.3 The Guaranteed Health Care Entitlement Lack of scientific evidence on a treatment's safety or clinical effectiveness, the redundancy of other more cost-effective treatments, or debatable added therapeutic value (being simply for comfort or leisure), are some of the reasons for the creation of the basic package of publicly provided health care, the so-called Guaranteed Health Care Entitlement.[19]

As a result, explicitly excluded from public financing are psychoanalysis, sex change surgery (with some exceptions), spa treatments, and plastic surgery not related to accidents, disease or congenital malformation. Ironically, in comparison to services previously provided under public financing, this package actually implies a slight enlargement of services.[30] In particular, dental care has been extended to children (not only prevention and extraction), although the exact definition of this is difficult to determine, given its likely financial impact. Moreover, the basic package does not take into account waiting times and, in general, its conditions of provision (including geographical access) are rather ill-defined.

As far as we know, no health researcher has put any faith in the viabil-

---

* Valencia has a per capita pharmaceutical cost almost 35 per cent above the national average.

Health Care and Cost Containment in Spain 425

ity of the existing list of services and interventions (*Catálogo*) as a cost containment measure.

8.3.2.4 Investment and capital financing There have been no new developments in the financing of capital investment in Spanish health care. Amortization expenditure, the opportunity costs of investment and new investments are the key factors in understanding the process. No charge has been established on the utilization of public capital. New investments have for the most part been sacrificed in order to avoid budget overruns by INSALUD during the last two years. This has meant that capital financing problems have simply been deferred. In this context, the significance of capital and amortization expenditure is questionable, since these are little more than fictions of budget accountability, given the spending possibilities of centres in this field. The sum of the notional amortization costs for all centres is the spending of the central management body, but is treated as an accounting item that is registered simultaneously as spending and revenue, and the receiving body has no autonomy regarding its application. Its significance for the national budget is low, as it does not necessarily respond to capital stock, valued with a predetermined coefficient. Neither does any relationship exist between amortizations at hospital level and capital expenditure. The annual increase between 1988 and 1993 on capital expenditure has been 13.21 per cent for INSALUD, 24.9 per cent for Andalucía, 22.6 per cent for Catalonia and 21 per cent in total. There has been some criticism of the fact that INSALUD's cost containment efforts may have focused on short-term reduction of capital expenditure.

8.3.2.5 Hospital activity In recent years the number of acute hospital beds in Spain has declined slightly (in fact, to the levels of 1973) as the average length of stay has decreased. In general, chronic patients have filled empty acute beds. Despite the fact that the present Conservative government put forward some money for a drastic reduction in hospital waiting lists for surgery (no more than six months is the target), it has not empowered citizens with a charter of rights which would allow patients to be treated in another hospital or even in the private sector if they have to wait over a predetermined period. No public beds are available for private use. This favours the development of private investment, making the rationalization of existing facilities more difficult. Not only does duplication exist between public and private facilities, but also amongst Regional Health Authorities, partic-

426 Health Care and Cost Containment in the European Union

ularly when they have full powers to run health services and from a political view are tempted to become 'self-contained NHS providers'. Several Offices for Health Assessment, working under slightly different auspices, in Catalonia, the Basque Country, Madrid and Seville, illustrate this case. However, this may be taken as a political restriction resulting from the Spanish Constitution and not, strictly speaking, as an efficiency issue.

As mentioned earlier in this chapter, Spain has seen some innovation in its system of hospital finance. Probably the most important innovations in hospital activity have been the development of day care and out-patient clinics. The experiments of Catalonia and Galicia illustrate the strength of these innovations. However, because of the way hospitals are financed, the extension of these policies has not yet materialized. Administration costs may have increased. And although no data are available, these increases seem to have mainly been concentrated in the intermediate levels of care (Districts or Health Areas) rather than in sophisticated institutional management.

8.3.2.6 Analysis of the relationship between health care activity and hospital financing González and Villalobos[31] analysed the extent to which public hospital finance is sensitive to activity. The results* reveal a positive relationship between hospital size and case mix of the centre, using a method which incorporates nine principle factors and which links heterogeneity in the 'mix' of patients with average length of stay. The efficiency of beds by services is estimated using indicators based on the rates of global occupation of services. The conclusion reveals that average length of stay (the utilization component) varies more owing to the behaviour of doctors than to any lack of flexibility in shifting resources between hospital services.

For the most part, the complexity and severity of cases treated, the specialization and organizational efficiency of different centres explain average cost variations.** However, it should be pointed out that budgetary alloca-

---

* To this end, they applied diverse approximation methods to a broad case mix of activities and costs for 68 INSALUD hospitals. It is thus a proposal of methods for studying variations observed in cost and activity found in complexity – methods of concentration and relative severity – and allocative efficiency. This analysis is alternatively based on information theory, on factoral analysis and on multiple regression.

** However, the authors call attention to the fact that, even in 1991, financing of medium–large INSALUD hopitals was not really 'service-specialized', especially as the variable of inter-hospital average length of stay tended to follow general, organizational factors that affected the hospital as a whole.

tions do not seem to respond at all to the intensity of health care activities.

The weak relationship between financing and activity (using in this case an index based on the Theory of Information, and related to complexity and speciality factors) was shown for the case of Catalonia by López and Valor[32] using 64 basic illnesses from the 1987 *Encuesta de Salud* of Barcelona, and by López and Wagstaff[33] from a relatively homogeneous sample.*

Systematic influences can explain differences in observed costs between the distinct centres which make up the sample. These should be taken into account when considering the correlation between financing and activity.

With the estimation of the frontier cost model, and using panel or longitudinal data, it becomes possible to distinguish the distinct determinants of hospital costs for the sample of INSALUD hospitals between 1986 and 1989. The systematic influences are considered using a hospital cost function which expresses the cost per case as a function of the supply of beds, complexity of case mix, average duration of stay and so on. The uncertain influences are considered using the temporal and transversal dimension for the panel data: the idea being that while the uncertain 'shocks' can adversely affect the activity of the hospital in any given year, these uncertain influences should cancel each other out. In contrast, however, inefficiency is assumed to vary between hospitals, yet not in the long run. The resulting residual can be defined as 'inefficiency' only once both the systematic and uncertain effects which influence hospital costs are included. Such inefficiency should be penalized, rather that protected, when considering policies of hospital financing.

Their estimation reveals that a longer average length of stay, a high level of complex activity and proximity to the campus of a university hospital are clearly associated with some of the highest costs per case.[32,33] It was also found that, in practice, the fixed costs of hospitals are a function which increases with the number of beds, although this relationship between total fixed costs and supply of beds was not linear.

The results show that the average inefficiency in the Spanish hospital sector is quite high, equivalent to about 45.2 per cent of the average cost per case, with a substantial variation in inefficiency between distinct centres.

---

* Hospitals owned and managed by INSALUD, with more than 100 beds and a hospital supply that is not distorted by the proximity of large regional hospitals.

428 *Health Care and Cost Containment in the European Union*

These findings also confirm the point of view that, in order to evaluate inefficiencies in hospital spending, it is not possible to only address costs per case; factors which exert systematic (in particular those which look at the complexity of hospital activity) and uncertain influences on costs also need to be taken into account.

In a more recent study of INSALUD as a whole, González and Barber[34] found a positive correlation between the implementation of *contratos programa* and the reduction in the level of average inefficiency of the sample analysed. They carried out their analysis using temporal variations in efficiency (assessing the periods immediately prior to and following 1993) through the estimation of frontier cost functions and data envelope analysis. It should be pointed out that these decreases in inefficiency are around 13.5 per cent, which is considerably below the results of López and Wagstaff,[33] who find it to be around 30 to 35 per cent of the best practice observed. However, these results might be due to the use of prices as one of the explanatory variables in the cost function, calculated through average spending incurred in the inputs.

Quintana[35] linked the impact of territorial decentralization to hospital efficiency. He concludes that the diversification of management has not led to a wide spread improvement in efficiency. In particular, it was found that the Catalan management body yields similar grades of inefficiency (these being quite low) within its own centres, while those centres that are directly managed by INSALUD and those run by the *Servicio Andaluz de Salud* reveal greater levels of inefficiency. Nor was an improvement in management detected after 1987, when the reforms following the *Ley General de Sanidad* of 1986 were introduced.

A more recent study, by López and Wagstaff[36] on the efficiency (cost frontier) of the entire health network of the *Servei Catala de la Salut* (Catalan health care purchasing body), reveals a higher level of inefficiency in public centres than in private centres (one-third higher). Despite this, a significant correlation between inefficiency and size or status (basically teaching) of the centre is not proven. Both are factors which relate more to the public centres and are used to justify their higher relative cost.

When compared with results currently achieved using the UBA pricing mechanism based on lengths of stay, the results of the above study, outlining efficiency costs and 'prices' for lines of activity, indicate a much higher relative cost for emergencies. The opposite was concluded for ambulatory activity (although this was without any adjustment for case mix). The estimations practically favour the identification of emergency care on one (average) in-patient stay, the third part of these values not reaching the average of ambulatory activity in terms of cost. In conclusion, López and Wagstaff argue that a regulation which bases finance (both for public hospital centres owned by the social security and for contracted centres) on the rate currently established for publicly financed non-public hospitals would save around 17 per cent of current expenditure.

Finally, Prior and Solà, in a data envelopment analysis for hospitals in the Catalan network between the years 1987 and 1991,[37] also reveal high levels of inefficiency of around 30 per cent. This inefficiency is particularly associated with an excess of health care personnel, specifically doctors. They point out that a reduction in inefficiency could be achieved, not so much by reducing the size of hospitals (through bed reduction), but by significantly increasing consultations and applying a growth rate for discharges above that of stays. This would lead to a reduction in average length of stay, which would in turn reduce waiting lists without increasing a centre's maximum available capacity.

8.3.2.7 Health centres and the change in doctors' remuneration in primary care In an attempt to establish a more prevention-focused primary care service, teams of GPs, nurses and paediatricians (called *Equipos de Atención Primaria*) were created following the primary care reform in 1984 to increase consultation times, promote team working among professionals and to eliminate ambulatory specialist care. In 1996, these teams covered about 60 per cent of the Spanish population, although with significant regional variations. The reform succeeded in providing better working facilities for doctors in the new health centres, promoting team-working conditions (allowing centres to open for seven hours a day instead of two and a half) and providing a salary component with some incentives for following special programmes (such as smoking and breast cancer prevention). Although reform of the primary care sector has been achieved, significant regional differences remain in its application. This is particularly the case for Catalonia, where the opportunity costs to physicians accepting the new model are higher, and no extra billing is allowed.

It is not easy to evaluate the success of the reform in terms of cost containment, since the target is not quite the same as that pursued under the former system.[38] Costs of primary care have increased, emergency activity in hospitals has not decreased, and pharmaceutical costs seem to be lower but

430 *Health Care and Cost Containment in the European Union*

not significantly so if we adjust for the characteristics (such as age) of the prescribers (young health professionals seem to prescribe less). Users do seem to be more satisfied with the level of primary care service they receive; this is largely due to longer consultation times, averaging 6 minutes (having risen from 3.5 per visit), resulting from the extension of doctors' hours of work. However, this is not always regarded as having a positive medical effect since the extra consultation time may result from increased bureaucratic work and a lower productivity rate (that is, a lower number of patients being visited).

8.3.2.8 Patient choice A patient's right to choose has been extended from general practitioner to specialist care in obstetrics and gynaecology. Because this potentially affects the number of patients on a physician's list, it can affect the capitation component of a physician's remuneration. For the moment, no restriction has been imposed on these changes. However, according to information currently available, little use has so far been made of this right to choose.

For other areas of specialist care, a referral system exists that requires a certificate from the practitioner in order to gain access to hospital care. This takes time and usually delays health care treatments, resulting in the perception of a low quality service. However, the MUFACE system, which gives civil servants the right to choose between public and private insurers, has not been extended to the rest of the population.[39]

8.3.2.9 The effects of co-payments and excluding certain health services from public financing With regard to private premiums for complementary health insurance, Murillo and González[40] show that for the period 1972–89, the price elasticity was 0.44. This is to say that a 10 per cent increase in premiums reduced private demand for health insurance by around 5 per cent. Despite a significant reduction in those opting for private insurance, over the last decade private expenditure in health insurance has increased (to 0.90), largely as a result of the rising cost of premiums.

Aggregation here hides the fact that demand for private insurance is highly concentrated; although the Spanish average is just 8 per cent, in Catalonia one-fourth of the population is covered. The level of private insurance also has a strong, positive correlation with the head of the family's status (in terms of education), income and age.[1] This notwithstanding, complementary insurance is too diverse to allow for a refined estimation of its

Health Care and Cost Containment in Spain   431

sensitiveness to incomes and prices, and since insurance premiums are currently subsidized from income tax (a 15 per cent deduction on the tax bill), its full cost is not passed on to the insured. In addition, some policies are financially supported collectively by corporations as a component of fringe benefits.

There is a strong link between those dental services exempt from public coverage, constituting approximately 16.8 per cent of private health expenditure, and income. In terms of per capita expenditure, consumption of highly educated groups was between seven and eight times higher than that of the least educated group.

8.4 The short-term future of health care in Spain: the Conservative Party's (*Partido Popular*) health care policies

The *Partido Popular* (PP), in its 1996 political platform, stressed the need to improve quality in public health services, to increase consumer choice and satisfaction, to decrease waiting lists and to improve the overall efficiency of what has traditionally been a very bureaucratic service. The party addressed the need to continue with the following ongoing reforms:*

- adjustment of the purchaser/provider split;

- the more equitable distribution of resources to correct regional inequities;

- greater autonomy for health centres and hospitals, with more efficient management at all levels of the health system;

- increased participation and responsibility of health care professionals; and

- larger freedom of choice of citizens of health providers (either public or private producers).

---

* An early version of this section can be found in Lopez and Beith, 1996.[41]

432　*Health Care and Cost Containment in the European Union*

8.4.1 The proposals

Stressing the need to maintain the principles of universality, a service free at the point of use and solidarity, specific PP platform proposals included: (a) a financial audit of the Spanish national health system in order to calculate the pending debt of the system (budgets have consistently been overrun over the past decade) and to eliminate this debt and formulate a realistic and sufficient method of financing public health care in Spain; in addition to this, a financial audit of infrastructure, technology and personnel within the health sector would also be carried out; (b) the control of cost escalation through (i) reinserting ambulatory care more closely into hospital services, (ii) the establishment of a policy of generics in the pharmaceutical industry and (iii) the more efficient use of resources by health care professionals; (c) maintaining the system of public financing with both public and private provision; proposals here include breaking the traditional monopoly by introducing competition into the provision of health services (via the generalization of the so-called MUFACE model, although specifics to this end were not outlined in the PP platform); (d) the further decentralization of health care to the remaining ten regions which still do not have responsibility for the health care of their populations (although only after remaining regional debt has been calculated and paid off, as failure to take this step has caused many difficulties for the seven autonomous regions which at present have responsibility for health care); (e) improving information systems within the Spanish national health service and concluding the replacement of family cards for primary care with individual cards (spreading the policy of one card per individual instead of one card per family as was traditionally the case); (f) creating nationwide consumer choice for both primary care doctor and health centre and the creation of ambulatory surgery units and day hospitals; (g) completing the development of primary health care teams, which began in 1984 and by 1995 covered almost 90 per cent of the Spanish population; and finally (h) reducing waiting lists and depoliticizing health care management.

One other proposal outlined by the *Partido Popular* in its political platform has the potential to radically transform the Spanish health sector. In practice, however, this policy would be very difficult to implement. At present, civil servants in Spain are covered by special schemes. One such scheme, MUFACE, is exceptional as it allows insured civil servants the option of choosing between being either publicly (through INSALUD) or

Health Care and Cost Containment in Spain   433

privately insured. The *Partido Popular's* proposal consisted of expanding this scheme to around 3 million more self-employed workers, with the intention of later extending it to the entire Spanish population. At the time of writing, however, it is uncertain whether the PP will seek to move forward with this measure.

8.4.2 From proposals to actions

The *Partido Popular* has been in power since March 1996 and has to date implemented the following measures in the health sector:

- as outlined in its platform, the PP has established an Audit (a *ponencia*) within the Commission of Health and Consumption of the Congress of Deputies, with the mandate of analysing the national health system and advancing its consolidation by studying the measures necessary for guaranteeing a stable financing mechanism and the modernization of the system;

- the government has recently approved a decree, accepted by an absolute majority in the Congress, which modifies the management of public health centres and social service centres by allowing centres to be run according to rules other than those of public social security;

- a specific budget has been approved to finance the reduction of the existing hospital waiting lists to a maximum of six months;

- a policy designed to squeeze the profits of the pharmaceutical industry by restricting their revenue figures to a predetermined amount has been put forward. In addition, the legal authorization to open new pharmacies has been relaxed (lowering conditions up to now based on population and distance criteria); and

- more recently, the financial universalization of health care, by suppressing the payroll contribution as a source of health care financing, and the introduction of an equivalent transfer from general taxation, has been almost unanimously accepted.

In summary, in its first year in office, the *Partido Popular* has demonstrated (a) the difficulty of implementing radical changes within health care, whether or not these changes were part of the pre-election manifesto – that

434 *Health Care and Cost Containment in the European Union*

the MUFACE system has been neither abolished nor extended is excellent proof of this; (b) the relevance of arguments from the literature on health care reforms, as regards the purchasing–provision split, the allocation of budgets and greater accountability of clinicians; (c) some initial success in countering the relatively high pharmaceutical costs: the present minister, formerly an adviser of the drug industry, appears to be doing a better job in this respect than certain strong socialist cabinet members have in the past; and (d) a failure to depoliticize the management of public hospitals, since almost all the managers are being changed. The actions of the PP have at times contradicted the idea of a right wing party. There has been nothing new concerning health service limitations (the *Catálogo*) with regard either to private production (*concertacion*) or to the management of health care centres, or the suppression of the contributory source of finance of public health expenditure. Moreover, the government's reforms have met with more opposition from drug suppliers than from public professionals. The lack of revolutionary zeal with regard to health care reforms is best illustrated by the government's use of the term 'consolidation' in place of 'reform' when referring to its health care policies.

8.4.3 The actions: the parliamentary 'audit' for a 'modern and consolidated' Spanish national health system

Far from reaching a national consensus on the future of the Spanish health care sector, the Parliamentary Commission has finished its work with an open social debate on the future of the financing and regulation of the Spanish health system. This new disagreement among the conservative and socialist parties complicates the already confused Spanish health policy. In addition to the lack of consensus on how to deal with the system's shortage of finance, doubts about the role of private insurers in health care delivery have now emerged, with the communist and socialist speakers on health affairs accusing the popular and regional parties of 'destroying' the National Health Service. This accusation arises largely from the willingness of the present conservative and regionalist ruling parties to allow private insurers to take on a larger role in the delivery of health care to the population.

In fact, health policy in Spain is at present a complex puzzle with crossfire resulting from two different main themes. In the first place there exist different views on the extent of private production under public

Health Care and Cost Containment in Spain 435

provision. Secondly, there are differences of opinion concerning how best to finance health services and distribute resources, particularly with regard to the regions. Taking both factors together, we can see how political (and not only regional) financing problems are at the root of the current health care controversy. Spanish health policy is today a political tool in the fight for electoral support, and under these circumstances even minor and logical changes become impossible to implement and the status quo prevails.

The existing problems have in part emerged from the manner in which-health care services have been decentralized in Spain. Since the Spanish Constitution of 1978, 17 Spanish autonomous communities (CCAAs) have been created, some of them with important cultural and historical backgrounds and others as simple administrative groupings of provinces. Several CCAAs pushed for the devolution of important powers and currently seven of these CCAAs (the Basque Country, Navarra, Catalonia, Galicia, Andalucía, Valencia and the Canary Islands) have responsibility for health care services. As mentioned earlier, these regions now manage approximately 55 per cent of total Spanish health care spending. Most of the remaining CCAAs now also demand the devolution of health care responsibility.

With the exception of the Basque Country and Navarra (which have their own special financing systems), the allocation of resources to the regions has followed a capitation criterion, although the actual application of this measure has hardly been homogeneous. At present, no explicit adjustment is made for population age differences, cross-boundary flows, teaching and research costs for regional hospitals, nor any weightings for regional differences in the cost of living. This creates a large forum for debate, with each region favouring the solution that best suits its needs. In fact, each autonomous community has sought out a particular interpretation of 'health need' which, using some appropriately measured, weighted and aggregated empirical variables to approximate this, offers a solution for the regional financial deficit. However, since the starting point in regional health expenditure is far from being equal, once the health services were transferred, a shortage of money appeared in some regions. With this lesson in mind, the transfer of health care services to the Autonomous Community of Madrid is proving to be an almost impossible task under such a simplistic formula. In addition, in the past the government has followed a common practice of under-budgeting health expenditure for budget-setting proposals

436 *Health Care and Cost Containment in the European Union*

which have artificially lowered the distribution basis, and the pressures on public deficits now make it much more difficult to solve past problems. The 1998 budget proposal increases health finance by 8.5 per cent, well above the GDP nominal increase, but the revenue sources for this are still undecided. Current contenders are higher taxes on alcohol and tobacco and the introduction of new pharmaceutical co-payments for pensioners.*

8.4.4 Finance of the national health care sector and the regional allocation of resources

An agreement of the *Consejo de Política Fiscal y Financiera* was reached in November 1997. This established a General Fund for Territorial Distribution (accounting for 98.5 per cent of total resources), a Compensatory Fund (PTE 20 billion) and a Fund for the Cross-Boundary Flow of patients (PTE 48 billion).

The distribution of the first fund is purely on a capitation basis, with no adjustment made for age. This has necessitated the establishment of the second and third funds, designed to compensate those Communities which could argue that a purely capitation-based financing system would discriminate against them. The amounts allocated to different communities have not been estimated on the basis of empirical evidence regarding utilization of sources.

The solution is a political rather than a technical one, and basically favours Andalucía, Galicia and INSALUD. However, in order to avoid financial losses for Catalonia, some political 'amendments' have had to be made. Altogether this strategy has increased the cost of the 'solution' and, unfortunately, has not resolved once and for all the existing allocation problems. For no consensus exists on the distribution finally adopted.

Table 8.8 shows: (1) actual population for 1996 without adjustment for age differences, cross-boundary flows and teaching and research programmes; (2) the share of resources per region after the three funds come into operation; and (3) the 1997 actual increases in total finance over the previous allocation.

Finally, of the additional PTE 315 billion needed for the regional dis-

---

* The forecast expenditure for the National Health Service in 1998 amounts to PTE 3,835 billion (current) while the figure for 1997 was PTE 3,520 billion.

Health Care and Cost Containment in Spain 437

Table 8.8 Resource allocation between Spanish regions in 1997

	Population in 1996 (unadjusted)	Share of finance under the new system	Finance increase over previous system (1996–97)
Andalucía	18.07%	18.07%	+10.3%
Catalonia	15.75%	16.27%	+9.2%
Galicia	6.91%	6.93%	+7.0%
Valencia	10.23%	10.13%	+9.0%
Canary Islands	4.07%	4.02%	+12.4%

tribution (the cost of the agreement), 200 will have to be raised from additional general budgetary funds, 75 from higher tax revenues and 40 by fighting fraud in working day losses due to sickness (the so-called *incapacidad laboral transitoria*, at present financed by the central social security but managed by the regional health authorities). An extra PTE 65 billion is expected to be saved in 1998 from a new profit reduction agreement with the pharmaceutical sector, although as yet it is unclear what the powerful pharmaceutical lobby expects in return for its cooperation in this.

This all makes for a very complex strategy, particularly since, in the absence of any real reform, plans for additional health expenditure in the future are largely based on the current rate of budgetary expansion, which will be extremely difficult to maintain.

8.4.5 How these actions affect health policy problems

Following the regional devolution process, and despite past efforts to maintain a cohesive national health care system, results so far are not promising. Maintaining a uniform central policy on health care in Spain today no longer seems possible, or even, for that matter, entirely desirable. The latter point is illustrated by the Basque Country which, with a separate system of regional finance well rooted in its history, is able to finance health services at a rate almost 20 per cent above the per capita state average. The capitation system that initially benefited Galicia and Canary Islands, greatly

438   *Health Care and Cost Containment in the European Union*

improving their regional health infrastructure, is today obscured by current expenditure needs, arguably due to the lack of budgeting. The pure capitation-based system has always made life very difficult for Andalucía and Catalonia, causing annual budget overruns. The main effects of this are different waiting times for access to similar services, varying standards of quality in hospital health care, wage disparities among health professionals, different utilization rates for equal episodes, and even the provision of entirely different services. Recent examples of this are vaccination for meningitis C, rates in hip and knee replacement and services offered with some public education campaigns (breast cancer detection, for example).

However, it is perhaps difficult to expect any outcome other than regional disparities from any real process of devolution in health care. There are several reasons for this. First, existing territorial inequalities may be highlighted by devolution, though not necessarily caused by it. Secondly, generally speaking, fiscal federalism implies a level of disparity – different menus improve community welfare as opposed to the imposition of a bland central pattern of health care. In this sense, cultural and social differences among Spanish regions are very large. Thirdly, the relevant health inequalities in Spain still relate to individual social classes rather than specifically to regions – even a continuous redistribution of resources might never close the gap in regional health indicators. Some studies show that inequality reduction as a whole can be explained 90 per cent by personal rather than by territorial income redistribution.[42]

Thus any country seeking to decentralize responsibility for health care should heed the lesson of Spain and proceed differently. A more modest and suitable approach is, first, to define a basic policy, that is, what the public package of health care must include in any region for any citizen, based on consideration of the effectiveness criteria. A 'uniform average' in a decentralized context is in fact a 'moving average' and hence politically unenforceable. Second, in any decentralization process it is crucial that regional differences are financed by different regional fiscal efforts, and that equalization policies are well defined and their implementation well monitored. In the case of Spain, 'free lunches' for the autonomous communities in the delivery of health care do not make for sensible management and value-for-money health expenditure. Unfortunately, none of these factors is adequately addressed in Spain today and this makes the definition of any health policy at a general level extremely problematic.

References

1 González Y. La demanda de seguros sanitarios. *Revista de Economía Aplicada* 1995;III (autumn):111–43.

2 Rodriguez M, Murillo C, Calonge S. Evolución de la cuantía y la naturaleza del gasto sanitario privado en la década de los ochenta. *Hacienda Pública Española* 1993;monografico. Madrid. Instituto de Estudios Fiscales, 143–53.

3 Ibern P, López G, Ortún V. Informe per a la Comissió de Distribució de Recursos del Sistema sanitari de Catalunya (Report for the Advisory Comission on the Distribution of Resources in the Regional Health Service of Catalonia). *Fulls Econòmics* 1994;18:14–17.

4 Ministerio de Sanidad y Consumo. *Descripción y estado de situación del Sistema Nacional de Salud.* (Mimeo para la Ponencia de Sanidad del Congreso de Diputados), Madrid, 1997.

5 Ministerio de Sanidad y Consumo. *Descripción y estado de situación del Sistema Nacional de Salud.* 1996 (unpublished).

6 Merck, Sharp and Dohme (MSD). *Sistema gráfico de Información Sanitaria.* Madrid: MSD, 1996.

7 OECD. *Eco-Santé.* Paris: OECD, 1996.

8 Blendon R *et al.* Spain's citizens assess their health care system. *Health Affairs* 1991;10 (Spring):216–28.

9 Mossialos E. Citizens' views on health care systems in the 15 member states of the European Union. *Health Economics* 1997;6:109–16.

10 Ministerio de Sanidad y Consumo. *Presupuesto del Insalud 1997.* Datos y cifras, 1998.

11 Ministerio de Economía y Hacienda. *1990 Dirección General de Programación Económica.* Madrid: Informe de Ejecución, 1994.

12 Ministerio de Trabajo y Seguridad Social. *Cuentas y Balances de la Seguridad Social.* Madrid, 1992, 1994, 1997.

13 Ministerio de Trabajo y Seguridad Social. *Presupuestos de la Seguridad Social.* Madrid, 1992, 1994, 1997.

14 Ministerio de Trabajo y Seguridad Social. *Acuerdos de Liquidación del Presupuesto del INSALUD.* Madrid, 1992, 1994, 1997.

15 Sanfrutos N. El presupuesto sanitario en el contexto de la Seguridad Social. *Presupuesto y Gasto Público* 1993;10:101–12.

16 INSALUD. *Indicadores de la Prestación Farmacéutica del Sistema Nacional de Salud.* Madrid, 1997.

17 Lopez-Bastida J, Mossialos E. Spanish drug policy at the crossroads. *The Lancet* 1997;350(9079):679–80.

18 Lopez G, Ortun V, Murillo C. *El Sistema Sanitario Español: Informe de una década.* Madrid: Fundación BBV, 1998.

19 Ministerio de Sanidad y Consumo. *El Catálogo de prestaciones sanitarias públicas.* Madrid: Publicaciones del MSyC, 1995.

440 Health Care and Cost Containment in the European Union

20 Gavilanes E. La financiación de los hospitales en el ejercicio 1993: Los contrato programa. *Presupuesto y Gasto Público* 1993;10:159–62.

21 Cabasés J, Martín J. Diseño y evaluación de estrategias de desregulación en el sector sanitario público en España. In: López G, Rodríguez D (eds). *La Regulación de los Servicios Sanitarios en España*. FEDEA, Civitas, 1997, pp. 481–536.

22 González B. El mercado laboral sanitario y sus consecuencias en la formación: Numerus clausus. In: *La Formación de los Profesionales de la Salud. Escenarios y Factores Determinantes*. Madrid: Fundación BBV, 1997.

23 López G, Garcia Cestona MA. *Bases para una reforma de las políticas salariales y de empleo en el sector público: Una aproximación al sistema sanitario público*. Documentos de Trabajo de la Fundación BBV, Centro de Economía Pública, 1995.

24 Conde J. Evaluación de las tecnologías sanitarias y su relación con la calidad de asistencia. In: *La Formación de los Profesionales de la Salud. Escenarios y factores determinantes*. Madrid: Fundación BBV, 1997.

25 Borrás J, *et al*. Complex decisions about an uncomplicated therapy: reimbursement for long-term oxygen therapy in Catalunya (Spain). *Health Policy* 1996;35:53–9.

26 Ministerio de Sanidad y Consumo. *Informe Abril Martorell de la Comisión para la Reforma del Sistema Sanitario Español*. Madrid, 1991.

27 Ministerio de Sanidad y Consumo. *El Catálogo Nacional de Hospitales 1995*. Madrid: Publicaciones del MSyC, 1997.

28 Puig J. El gasto farmacéutico en España: efectos de la participación del usuario en el coste. *Investigaciones Económicas* 1988;12(1):45–68.

29 Ibern P. Gasto farmacéutico, responsabilidad individual y social. *Cinco Días* 1996;2(XII):17–18.

30 Cabases J. Priority-setting and guaranteed health care entitlement in Spain. *Eurohealth* 1996;2(4): 26–28.

31 González B, Villalobos J. Indicadores de actividades y costes en hospitales españoles. *Hacienda Pública Española* 1993;No.1 monográfico, IEF Madrid.

32 López G, Valor J. Algunas medidas para el seguimiento de la utilización de lo recursos hospitalarios. Aspectos teóricos y aplicación a los hospitales catalanes. Institut d'Estudis de la Salut; *Catalunya-Salut* 1987 (Sep–Dec):62–73.

33 López G, Wagstaff A. Competencia en Sanidad. *Moneda y Crédito* 1993;196:181–229.

34 González B, Barber P. Changes in public Spanish hospital efficiency after the program contracts. *Investigaciones Económicas* 1996;XX(3):377–402.

35 Quintana J. *Eficiencia relativa en la red de hospitales públicos españoles*. Documentos de Trabajo de la Fundación BBV, Centro de Economía Pública, 1995.

36 López G, Wagstaff A. La financiación hospitalaria basada en la actividad en sistemas sanitarios públicos, regulación de tarifas y eficiencia: el caso de la concertación hospitalaria en Cataluña. In: López G, Rodríguez D (eds). *La Regulación de los Servicios Sanitarios en España*. FEDEA, Civitas, 1997.

37 Prior D, Solà M. Planificación estratégica pública y eficiencia hospitalaria. *Hacienda Pública Española* 1995;136(1):93–108.

38 Gervas J, Ortún V. Regulación y eficiencia de la atención primaria en España. In: López

G, Rodríguez D (eds). *La Regulación de los Servicios Sanitarios en España*. FEDEA, Civitas, 1997.

39   Pellisé L. *Regulating Managed Competition in the Spanish Health Insurance Market. Capitation and Risk Selection in MUFACE.* (Unpublished doctoral thesis) mimeo, Univ. Pompeu Fabra, Barcelona, 1996.

40   Murillo C, González B. El sector sanitario en España. Situación actual y perspectivas de futuro. *Hacienda Pública Española* 1993;119:41–58.

41   López G, Beith A. The Spanish Partido Popular health reform proposals. *Eurohealth* 1996;2(3).

42   Ruiz-Huerta J, López Laborda J, Alaya I, Martínez López R. Relaciones y contradicciones entre la distribución personal y la distribución espacial de la renta. *Hacienda Pública Española* 1995;134:153–90.

9 Twenty years of cures for the French health care system

PIERRE-JEAN LANCRY AND SIMONE SANDIER

This chapter provides a brief summary of the main changes in the financing and delivery of health care in France over the past twenty years. Particular emphasis is given to the Juppé Plan, an ambitious reform plan which has been gradually implemented since 1996. The chapter also gives a brief overview of the main features of the French health care system, which allows a better understanding of the reforms' aims and contents, followed by an assessment of their potential impact.

9.1 The French health care system: social welfare and the delivery of health care until 1995[1]

On the whole, the French declare themselves satisfied with their health care system.[2] The population is almost universally covered by statutory health insurance (*Assurance-maladie*), a branch of the social security system which lifts the financial barriers to access to medical care provided by health professionals and the health care industry.

Affiliation to the *Assurance-maladie* is through different schemes, determined by an individual's socio-professional category. The main scheme, the *Regime General*, covers employees and pensioners from trade and industry sectors, as well as their families: that is, 80 per cent of the population. The *Regime General* is financed mainly by payroll contributions paid by both employees and their employers (respectively 6.8 per cent and 12.8 per cent of gross salaries).

Within the scheme of the *Assurance-maladie*, patients have freedom of choice in using health care services, but they contribute a significant proportion to covering the cost of care. Initially, patients pay the provider

443

444 Health Care and Cost Containment in the European Union

directly, being reimbursed later, but in most cases only partially. The difference is expressed through a patient cost-sharing scheme ('*ticket modérateur*'), which charges patients different amounts depending on the type of care and treatment necessary. However, there are exceptions to these general rules for certain patient groups, or types of diseases and treatments.

Eighty-seven per cent of the population are members of voluntary, supplementary sickness funds (*Mutuelles*), or purchase private insurance which complements the compulsory insurance, and covers to a varying degree of the charges that the *Assurance-maladie* does not reimburse. Due to the combined effects of the compulsory and the complementary coverage, different payers contribute differently to financing health care expenditure according to the type of services provided. Where direct payments (by the patient) only cover 13.9 per cent of the overall expenditure, the amount rises to 22 per cent in the case of physician services, to 20 per cent for pharmaceutical products, and reaches 40 per cent for dental treatment. Only 6 per cent of hospital charges are covered by direct payments.

The services and goods covered by the *Assurance-maladie* must be provided by registered health *providers* to come under the list of professional acts and reimbursable medicines. Moreover, these services and goods must also be prescribed by a doctor. In certain cases, such as eye-glasses and physiotherapy, prior approval is needed for reimbursement. Under these circumstances there is no limit to the number of services covered.

Services provided vary across a wide range. As far as ambulatory care is concerned, health professionals and health care facilities are mainly in the private sector. In contrast, the public sector dominates the field of hospital care.

The relationship between private doctors, their patients, and the *Assurance-maladie*, is regulated by contracts (*Conventions*), the last of which was signed by two doctors' trade unions in 1993, later joined by a third in 1995. Patients may consult a specialist without a referral by their general practitioner. Private doctors can prescribe any treatments or diagnostic tests for their patients. They are paid on a fee-for-service basis, according to a negotiated fee schedule. About 30 per cent of doctors ('*Secteur 2*') can exceed these fees (see section 9.3).

Three-quarters of all hospital beds are in the public sector, with the remaining quarter in the private sector. Changes in the number of beds or hospital equipment must abide by the '*Carte Sanitaire*'. Public hospitals are financed according to a global budget, whereas private hospitals are still paid on a per diem basis within a framework where expenditure targets are set.

Reimbursable drugs (which represent about 90 per cent of the pharmaceutical market) appear in a list that indicates their price and reimbursement rate, as set at ministerial level. Expenses coverage by the *Assurance-maladie* range from 35 per cent for non-essential drugs to 100 per cent for essential or expensive drugs.

According to comparative statistics from the OECD,[3] in 1997 France was classified third among the OECD countries, in terms of the share of GDP it devotes to health. In 1995, according to the figures of the French National Accounts (DNCS),[4] total health care expenditure amounted to 7,814 billion FRF, i.e. 10.2 per cent of GDP. Expenditure for medical goods and services represents 87.2 per cent of the total, the remainder consisting of research, training, preventive care and administrative costs. This rose to an average of 11,728 FRF per person, with an average growth of 3.2 per cent per year at constant 1995 prices, between 1980 and 1995.

In the long run, a reduction of the growth rate of health care expenditure per person at constant FRF has been observed. Over the five years between 1990 and 1995, the growth rate was +2.4 per cent per year (Tables 9.1 and 9.2 and Figure 9.1).

Table 9.1 Expenditure for medical goods and services: different types of care, 1975–95 (research, training, preventive care and administrative costs not included)

	1975	1980	1985	1990	1995
Expenditure for medical goods and services					
Total value, current prices (million FRF)	91,126	192,327	363,454	528,401	681,959
Value per person, constant prices* (FRF 1995)	5,828	7,370	8,758	10,422	11,728
Percentage of GDP	6.2	6.8	7.7	8.1	8.9
Share of different types of health care (per cent)					
Hospital care	46.7	53.0	51.4	48.4	49.3
Ambulatory care	27.9	26.3	27.4	29.4	27.8
– medical services	13.2	11.9	12.5	13.3	13.1
– dental services	6.6	6.9	6.4	6.6	6.1
Pharmaceuticals	22.2	17.5	17.7	18.2	18.5

* Value in current prices deflated by the General Consumer Price Index.
Sources: National Health Accounts[4] and ECO-SANTE.[5]

Table 9.2 Per capita expenditure for medical goods and services in 1995 and growth rates for certain types of care, 1975–95

Types of medical care	Value in 1995 (FRF)	Average annual growth rate (per cent) in constant 1995 prices			
		1975–80	1980–85	1985–90	1990–95
Hospital care	5,794	7.5	2.5	2.7	2.7
Ambulatory care	3,248	3.6	4.0	5.4	1.2
– Medical services	1,572	2.5	4.1	5.4	1.8
– Dental services	731	5.6	1.7	4.4	0.8
– Other	513	–	–	–	–
Pharmaceuticals	2,173	-0.1	3.3	4.6	2.6
Total expenditure for medical goods and services	11,728	4.8	3.1	4.0	2.4

Source: National Health Accounts.[4]

Figure 9.1 Evolution of health insurance expenditure in constant prices, 1970–95

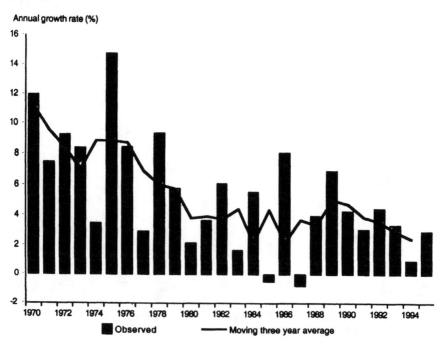

Since 1980, the modification of the reimbursement scheme has led to an overall decrease in the contribution of compulsory health insurance towards health care expenditure, from 76.5 per cent in 1980 to 73.9 per cent in 1995 (Table 9.3). In 1995 health insurance still contributed up to 90 per cent of hospital expenditure, but only about 60 per cent towards doctors' fees. An equal percentage was attributed to pharmaceutical expenditure, and less than a third to dental care expenditure.

On the other hand, supplementary health insurance (*Mutuelles*) and the private sector (families and private insurers) play a more important role in financing ambulatory care expenditure and pharmaceutical consumption.

Table 9.3 Sources of financing different types of health care in percentages, 1975–95 (research, training, preventive care and administrative costs not included)

Percentages	1975	1980	1985	1990	1995
Expenditure for medical goods and services					
Health insurance	73.2	76.5	75.5	74.0	73.9
General and local taxes	4.1	2.9	2.3	1.0	0.8
Supplementary health insurance (mutual funds)	3.8	5.0	5.1	6.1	6.8
Private expenditure*	18.9	15.6	17.1	18.8	18.5
of which direct payments	–	–	–	–	13.9
Total financing	100.0	100.0	100.0	100.0	100.0
Hospital care					
Health insurance	83.0	87.0	87.6	89.3	89.4
General and local taxes	7.0	4.6	3.5	1.4	1.0
Supplementary health insurance (mutual funds)	1.1	1.7	1.9	1.9	2.1
Private expenditure*	9.3	7.0	8.5	7.4	7.5
of which direct payments	–	–	–	–	6.1
Total financing	100.0	100.0	100.0	100.0	100.0
Total ambulatory care					
Health insurance	67.6	66.7	63.9	59.0	57.1
General and local taxes	1.4	0.9	0.9	0.7	0.6
Supplementary health insurance (mutual funds)	6.2	8.9	7.5	9.1	10.8
Private expenditure*	24.7	23.5	27.7	31.3	31.5
of which direct payments	–	–	–	–	23
Total financing	100.0	100.0	100.0	100.0	100.0

448   *Health Care and Cost Containment in the European Union*

Table 9.3 (continued) Sources of financing different types of health care in percentages, 1975–95

Percentages	1975	1980	1985	1990	1995
Services provided by office-based doctors					
Health insurance	75.1	74.3	69.3	61.6	58.7
General and local taxes	1.9	1.3	1.5	1.0	0.9
Supplementary health insurance (mutual funds)	7.4	9.4	7.4	8.6	10.5
Private expenditure*	15.7	14.9	21.8	28.8	29.9
of which direct payments	–	–	–	–	22.4
Total financing	100.0	100.0	100.0	100.0	100.0
Dental services					
Health insurance	50.7	48.5	43.8	36.0	31.5
General and local taxes	0.4	0.4	0.3	0.2	0.2
Supplementary health insurance (mutual funds)	5.2	9.4	7.9	10.4	13.6
Private expenditure*	43.7	41.7	48.0	53.4	54.8
of which direct payments	–	–	–	–	40.1
Total financing	100.0	100.0	100.0	100.0	100.0
Pharmaceuticals					
Health insurance	62.8	63.6	65.0	60.2	60.4
General and local taxes	1.9	1.1	1.1	0.8	0.6
Voluntary health insurance (mutual funds)	6.4	8.5	10.6	12.0	12.4
Private expenditure*	28.9	26.8	23.4	27.0	26.6
of which direct payments	–	–	–	–	19.8
Total financing	100.0	100.0	100.0	100.0	100.0

Source: National Health Accounts.[4]

* includes other voluntary health insurance.

9.2 Controlling health care expenditure: twenty years of efforts, 1975–95

Since the mid-1970s, the reduced rate of growth in economic activity and increasing unemployment have led to a fall in social security revenue, particularly that of the *Assurance-maladie*. Faced by new financing difficulties and the recurrent deficit in public accounts, the government and the

Assurance-maladie took measures that went beyond the ordinary management of the *Assurance-maladie*, which has evolved according to social, economic and technological change.*

New measures, aimed at 'controlling health care expenditure' (in fact slowing down the rate of growth in the expenses of the *Assurance-maladie*), were often introduced in plans labelled with an emphasis on 'rationalization', 'rebalancing', 'reappraisal' and 'rescue' plans. Other measures, decided on within the framework of the *Conventions* or by the Ministry of Health, are described in this chapter because they show a break with past tendencies and practices or because their effect is considerable and long-term.

When presented to the public, these measures are often accompanied by considerations of public health, quality of care, and equity; however, their aims are essentially economic. Most often, these measures attempt a short-term balancing of the social welfare accounts through a rise in revenues, or a reduction in expenditure. Other objectives are directed at reducing public deficits, and limiting the medium-term growth of the health sector, which is considered responsible for diverting resources from other social sectors, or from more productive activities.

In this section, the changes that took place during the last 20 years will be analysed by looking at the different areas concerned. Other means of analysing these changes, such as taking into account time-frames, instruments, objectives, impact and the nature of interventions, also enable us to draw some lessons. In fact, during the last 20 years, rationalization plans (often named after the ministers who proposed them), have been issued (on average) every 18 months. This shows that such measures were often of limited and short-term effectiveness.

The nature of these plans is primarily dependent on the instruments available to public institutions to guide the health care system within the existing regulatory framework. Table 9.4 gives a list of the main measures introduced between 1975 and 1995, prior to the Juppé Plan, aimed at improving the finances of the *Assurance-maladie*. This list which will be discussed below, can be read both chronologically and according to the nature of the measures, but is not exhaustive and does not enumerate the successive adjustments to prices, fees, lists of goods and reimbursable services.

---

* The extension of social welfare benefits to cover certain population groups, fee changes, and marginal changes in lists of reimbursable services.

450 *Health Care and Cost Containment in the European Union*

Table 9.4 Summary of main cost-containment measures introduced between 1975 and 1995

	Revenues of the Sécurité Sociale	*Benefits of the* Assurance-maladie: *reimbursement mechanisms*
Durafour Plan December 1975	Removal of ceiling on payroll contributions.	
Barre Plan September 1975	Supplementary source of finance: road tax.	Reduction of reimbursement rates for non-essential drugs. Increase of co-payment rates (ancillary services and transport).
Veil Plans April 1977– December 1978	Rise in contributions (salaried agriculture workers and active workforce). Contributions charged on pensions.	Reduction of reimbursement rate for some non-essential drugs (from 60% to 30%).
Barrot Plan July 1979	One-off contribution of pharmacists.	
1980 *Convention*		
Questiaux Plan November 1981	Twofold rise in car insurance. Partial removal of ceiling on payroll contributions.	
Beregovoy Plans July–September 1982	Contributions from the unemployed.	Introduction of a hospital co-payment fee (20 FF).
March 1983	Tax on pharmaceutical advertising (5%). Taxes on tobacco and alcohol.	Reduction of reimbursement rates from 70% to 40% for 1,258 drugs.
Delors Plan March–June 1983	One-off 1% levy on taxable income and subsequently on capital.	

Mechanisms for paying providers of care	Fees and charges for medical care	Other forms of management and control
	Reduction of VAT on drugs from 20% to 7%.	
		Constitution of an audit commission for the *Sécurité Sociale*.
	Freeze of doctors' fees and hospital daily rates. Ceilings on hospital expenditure increases.	
Doctors: introduction of the *secteur 2* with unregulated fees. (see section 9.3)		

452 *Health Care and Cost Containment in the European Union*

	Revenues of the Sécurité Sociale	Benefits of the Assurance-maladie: reimbursement mechanisms
1984		
Dufoix Plan May - June 1985		Increase of co-payment rates for some services. Reclassification of 379 drugs.
Seguin Plan November 1986 - 1987	One-off 0.5 % levy on 1985-1986 incomes. Supplementary 2 % tax on tobacco.	Extension and revision of the list of the 254 diseases exempted from co-payment. Limited co-payment exemption. Abolition of reimbursement for vitamins.
Evin Plan September 1989	Modification of part of the restrictive measures of the Seguin Plan.	Re-establishment of some co-payment exemptions.
1990 *Convention*		
December 1990 - 1991	Introduction of the *Contribution Sociale Generalisée* (CSG) - fixed at 1.1% for 1991. Increase of the tax on pharmaceutical advertising.	Abolition of reimbursement for 'anti-fatigue' drugs.
Bianco Plan July 1991	Increase of payroll contribution to health insurance by +0.9%.	Hospital co-payment fee increased from 33 to 50 FRF. Abolition of reimbursement for drugs containing magnesium or oligo-elements.
1992		Regulation agreements with adjustment measures. (*Objectifs Quantifiés Nationaux*, OQN). Ceiling caps were introduced for three sectors: biology (+7%); nursing (+9.7%); private practices (+5.2%).

Mechanisms for paying providers of care	Fees and charges for medical care	Other forms of management and control
Gradual introduction of global budgets for public hospitals.		
	Reduction of VAT on drugs from 7% to 5.5%.	
	Reduction of VAT on drugs from 5.5% to 2.1%.	
Significant restrictions of the *secteur 2* of office-based doctors		Introduction of the concept of medical cost-containment.
		Global budgets for ambulatory care. Hospital reform law.
	Revision of nomenclature for radiological procedures.	The pharmaceutical industry asked to reduce sales. Reduction of wholesale margins. Changes in the therapeutic categories concerning the level of reimbursement.

454 *Health Care and Cost Containment in the European Union*

	Revenues of the Sécurité Sociale	Benefits of the Assurance-maladie: reimbursement mechanisms
1993		
1993 - Veil Plan and *Convention*	Increase of the CSG from 1.1% to 2.4%.	Reduction (5 points) of reimbursement rates. Increase of hospital co-payment fee (55 FRF).
1994	New expenditure targets: doctors +3.4%; physiotherapists +5% biologists +3.4 %; nurses +4.5%; pharmaceuticals +3.2%.	
Announcement of Juppé Plan November 1995	Introduction of a more comprehensive set of measures, including structural measures. (See text for details)	

The measures can be grouped as follows:

(1) During the past 20 years, governments have generally preferred to increase the amount of resources available to the *Assurance-maladie* in order to limit their deficit in the short-term. This strategy, which is politically less risky than reducing benefits, was put in place by enlarging the salary base of payroll contributions, as well as by progressively increasing contribution rates from both employees and employers. To complement payroll contributions, new resources from taxes and other levies on revenues have also been allocated to the *Sécurité Sociale*. These new resources (initially conceived as small and temporary provisions), have been gradually adopted on a wider scale as ordinary sources of financing. Salary contributions rose from 1.5 per cent to 6.8 per cent between 1975 and 1995. During the same period, employers' contributions increased from 2.5 per cent to 12.8 per cent.

(2) Measures which affect the degree of public financing of health care expenditure are often opposed by public opinion. An overall increase in co-payment rates in 1967 had to be reviewed the following year after public demonstrations of social discontent. After this experience, the government waited 25 years before proceeding with another measure of this kind, establishing a general increase in patients' financial contribution to their health care expenses in the summer of 1993. Prior to this reform, the *Assurance-maladie* reduced its obligations to finance cer-

Mechanisms for paying providers of care	Fees and charges for medical care	Other forms of management and control
		Establishment of a pharmaceuticals agency.
		Introduction of treatment guidelines (*RMOs*) and patient medical records. Setting of a prospective expenditure target.

tain expenses through partial measures with direct or indirect effects. Those having a direct effect include the limitation of exemptions from co-payment (*Plan Seguin*, 1986); the introduction of patient charges to cover hospital hotel costs (*Plan Beregovoy*, 1983); and successive adjustments of pharmaceutical reimbursement rates to a level as low as zero, varying according to types of drugs. One measure having an indirect effect on the share of health care expenditure financed by the *Assurance-maladie*, was the creation of a sector of doctors with unregulated fees in 1980, which shall be discussed below.

Beyond their short-term effects, the restrictive measures taken in the field of social welfare have led to a fall in the participation of the *Sécurité Sociale* in financing health expenses. As a result, a growing number of people have resorted to complementary insurance. Between 1980 and 1995, for instance, the component of health care expenditure financed by the *Mutuelles* increased: from 5.0 per cent to 6.8 per cent of overall health care expenditure; and from 8.5 per cent to 12.4 per cent for pharmaceutical expenditure.

The declining role of the *Sécurité Sociale /Assurance-maladie* has certainly affected the equity of access to health care.*

---

* When the compulsory social welfare benefits and complimentary benefits do not cover the difference, inequalities in the use of health care tend to increase.[6]

456　*Health Care and Cost Containment in the European Union*

In the early 1970s, measures regulating the relationship between the state and the *Assurance-maladie* on one side, and private providers of care on the other, were generally concerned with the supply of health care. Firstly, a *numerus clausus* was introduced in medical schools, in order to reduce the number of doctors in the medium- and long-terms. Secondly, a fixed number of training posts for specialists was set for hospitals, which was expected to influence the distribution of doctors between general practice and specialist care. Finally, the *Carte sanitaire* was introduced to ensure that the demand for health care was met with appropriate hospital services, as well as to control the diffusion of high technology (see section 9.4).

During the 1980s new measures were introduced, initially targeting the methods of payment of providers of care either directly, or through more general cost containment measures. Subsequent steps have focused on professional practices.

9.3 Private doctors*

In 1995, expenditure on private office-based doctors accounted for approximately 14 per cent of spending on medical goods and services. However, their prescriptions for treatments and diagnostic procedures provided by other professionals affect virtually all health care expenditure.

As a deferred effect of the reduction of the *numerus clausus*, the growth rate of the medical workforce has declined in recent years, falling from +5 per cent in 1988 to +0.7 per cent in 1995. Currently, the number of private doctors is stagnant, whereas the proportion of specialists is growing (44 per cent in 1975 and 47 per cent in 1995). Overall, the medical workforce is ageing and the proportion of women is increasing.

The reforms which have affected private doctors during the last 20 years have had no effect on the three distinctive features of the French health care system appreciated in particular by patients and doctors, namely: the patient's free choice of doctor; free access to specialists; and the direct payment of doctors' services by patients.

One of the main reforms was the introduction of the '*secteur 2*' which was introduced with the 1980 *Convention*. This gave doctors the opportu-

---

* Self-employed doctors.

nity of exceeding negotiated fees, in exchange for reduced benefits (sickness benefits, pensions), and made patients or their private insurers liable to pay the difference between actual and negotiated fees. The advantages to the *Assurance-maladie* were twofold: on the one hand, it contributed to creating divisions amongst doctors, making them less aggressive during fee negotiations, since those belonging to the *secteur 2* would be able to increase their prices beyond negotiated fees; on the other hand, the expenses of the *Assurance-maladie* would only be partially affected by real price increases. In 1980 the *Assurance-maladie* defended itself from the critics of a 'two-tier health care system', by arguing that in a context of excess supply, market mechanisms would limit the number of doctors in the *secteur 2*, as well as the price increases.

It is true that, since it was introduced, *secteur 2* has contributed to containing the increase in doctors' fees, keeping growth rates between 1980 and 1995 at an average of +0.24 per cent per year in constant 1995 FRF. However, the development of *secteur 2* throughout the 1980s has posed a threat to the principle of equal access to care. The proportion of doctors billing fees has decreased, from 81.6 per cent in 1980 to 68.2 per cent in 1990 (general practitioners from 89.9 to 77.7 per cent and specialists from 70.0 to 57.0 per cent). The difference between actual and negotiated fees has also widened from 5 to 10 per cent of negotiated fees over the same period. Hence, the 1990 *Convention* attempted to limit the development of *secteur 2*, which had proven not only undesirable from an equity viewpoint, but also ineffective in decreasing the amount of services provided and in improving their quality. As a result, restrictive measures were introduced, regulating access to *secteur 2*. In 1994 the proportion of doctors in this sector had dropped to 28.5 per cent (19 per cent of general practitioners and 39.5 per cent of specialists).

Subsequent *Conventions*, especially from 1980 onwards, made explicit reference to the activity of doctors and a number of new concepts were introduced. The years in the following examples refer to the first time the term was used rather than to the actual introduction of a measure:

Tableaux statistiques d'activité (statistical tables of doctors' activities, including average prescription patterns) 1971;

Maîtrise des dépenses (cost containment) 1980, later abandoned;

Bon usage des soins (appropriate use of services) 1985;

Maîtrise médicalisée des dépenses (clinical cost containment) 1990; and

458 *Health Care and Cost Containment in the European Union*

Enveloppe globale (global budget for the health sector) 1990.
However, these measures, given their vague nature and absence of sanctions, had only a limited impact on regulating the volume of medical activities.

In 1993, three measures to rationalize the provision of health care were introduced. They also had the effect of challenging doctors' professional autonomy by introducing controls:

- The possibility of forcing doctors to prescribe the most appropriate services, without duplication, according to treatment guidelines (*Références Médicales Opposables – RMOs*) produced with reference to treatments and interventions. Sixty-five *RMOs* were produced in 1994, and 147 in 1995. These are expected to cover, progressively, all sectors of medical care. Doctors who do not abide by the guidelines are, in principle, subject to financial sanctions varying according to the frequency and gravity of negligence. However, controls by the *Assurance-maladie* are still limited, and there are several ways of appealing against a sanction.

- The introduction of '*carnet de santé*'(medical records in the form of a small booklet carried by patients) aimed at limiting the access to multiple doctors and avoiding conflicting and redundant prescriptions.

- The setting of a prospective target growth rate (+3.4 per cent in 1994) for private doctors' fees and prescriptions expenses.

During the first few months following their introduction, *RMOs* appeared to be an effective measure in curbing the expenditure of the *Assurance-maladie*. However, a subsequent acceleration in the rate of growth of health care expenditure proved its effectiveness was only temporary. A more detailed analysis has shown that *RMOs* have indeed influenced pharmaceutical prescriptions (see section 9.5).

Medical records have also had only a limited effect. During the first phase of their introduction they were to be targeted at 4 million people aged over 70 who sufferred from more than one disease. In fact, medical records were given to only 45,000 people before this measure was suspended with the introduction of the Juppé Plan in November 1995. There is no evaluation of the impact of medical records on health outcomes or medical practices.

9.4 Hospitals

Hospital care accounts for approximately half of total health care expenditure. A planning instrument, the *Carte Sanitaire*, was introduced by a law approved on 31 December 1970, based on the assumption that the availability of hospital beds induces greater demand given that beds must be filled. As a consequence, the step taken for containing hospital expenditure was the rationalization of hospital capacity. The *Carte Sanitaire* defines the regions and sectors into which the health care system is divided, as well as the nature and role of the facilities available to the population. It also defines standard ratios of hospital beds and equipment *per capita* for both the private and public hospital sectors.

On the one hand, the *Carte Sanitaire* has effectively contributed to limiting the growth of hospital beds. However, beds are only one of the factors in hospital supply. Thus, it did not prevent the rapid increase of hospital expenditure which took place before the early 1980s, due to staff and salary increases. Approximately 70 per cent of hospital costs are in fact devoted to staff costs, salaries, and related social charges.

In 1991, a new law introduced a complementary planning instrument called the *Schéma Régional d'Organisation Sanitaire* (SROS), which regulates the geographical distribution of equipment and activities at a regional level. The SROS tasks include reorganization of the emergency services, networking health care facilities, and reducing or converting the use of hospital beds. A law, approved in July 1994, allowed for the closure of hospitals services with limited activity. This measure, however, is regularly opposed by local political interests, firstly because it touches upon people's sensitivity about the issue of access to health care; and secondly, it affects local economic and employment levels.

Public hospitals were the first sector in which global budgets were introduced in 1984. Since 1985, all publicly financed hospitals are no longer paid on a *per diem* basis (a method deemed to generate inflation), but are allocated a global budget aimed at covering most of their costs. The budget is calculated on the basis of past expenditure, allowing for a rate of growth set at the start of the financial year (11.8 per cent in 1980, 5.7 per cent in 1985, 4.2 per cent in 1990 and 2.1 per cent in 1996). The possibility of introducing a complementary budget for those expenses which cannot be predicted at the start of the financial year (such as salary rises or new treatments), has yet to be explored. It seems that while global budgets played a

460 *Health Care and Cost Containment in the European Union*

significant role in the decrease of hospital expenses, since the growth rate had already slowed prior to their introduction, other factors must also have had an effect. The annual rate of growth in the volume of care provided by public hospitals dropped from 7.4 per cent (on average) between 1975 and 1980, to 2.2 per cent between 1980 and 1982. Other factors also influenced this trend, but the most important was the reduction in general inflation rates. Certain technical advances and new pharmaceutical treatments, as well as the high number of private doctors, contributed to the practice of shortened hospital stays, strengthening primary and home care.

Between 1982 and 1995, the hospital share of expenditure for medical goods and services diminished sharply (from 53 per cent to 48 per cent).

Nonetheless, after ten years of experience, global budgets were judged unsatisfactory. Hospital expenditure and its contribution to total expenditure decreased, but the allocation of resources according to a uniform rate of growth did not reduce the disparities between hospitals. This measure failed to take into account the volume and quality of the output produced. Combined with this, a low allocation of resources can act as a brake on the introduction of new technologies, and constitute an incentive to the selection of patients. A new system (*Programme de Medicalisation de Systemes d"Infomation* – PMSI), aimed at enhancing the medical component of information systems and outcomes, based on the US DRGs (Diagnosis Related Groups), was set up in order to measure hospital outputs. The information collected is used as a basis for hospital planning, where the notion of output replaces the administrative notion of the hospital bed. This new system is expected to contribute to the harmonization of methods of payment between private and public hospitals.

9.5 The pharmaceutical sector

Pharmaceutical expenditure for both prescription and over the counter drugs, represents 18.4 per cent of the total expenditure for medical goods and services in France. This percentage is clearly higher than in most European countries and North America. Although comparisons are difficult to make, it seems that doctors in France, and general practitioners in particular, prescribe more drugs per visit (3.2 items) than their counterparts in other countries. It also seems that the consumption of certain types of drugs (anti-depressives, vasodilators, antibiotics) is also higher in France than in other countries. Additionally, though drug prices are usually lower in France, the frequent use of new products and the virtual absence of generics, makes the average cost of drugs consumed rather high when compared with other countries.

Until recently, the control of expenditure has meant acting on two components of pharmaceutical costs for the *Assurance-maladie*: prices, and reimbursement rates.

In addition to setting a specific pricing method at the production level, there have also been several reductions of VAT on drugs (1976, 1987, 1990) as well as reductions in wholesale and pharmacy distribution margins.

Since 1976, reimbursement rates have fallen from 70 per cent to 40 per cent for certain drugs treating 'non-serious diseases'. The reduction of reimbursement rates, and in some cases exclusion from any reimbursement at all, for specific categories of products has been one of the most frequently used measures (1978, 1982, 1985, 1987, 1991). In addition, all products were affected by a general rise in patient contributions to pharmaceutical expenditure in 1993 (Veil Plan).[7]

The reduction of reimbursement rates automatically led to a decline in the role of the *Sécurité Sociale* in financing pharmaceutical expenditure. This occurred without there being a long-term decline in the consumption of drugs. A study based on consumption surveys[6] showed that the consumption of only two categories of drugs (digestives and vitamins) were affected by the decline of the reimbursement rate – both decreased slightly between 1980 and 1991. However, consumption had increased in all the other categories. The new measures appear to have had an effect, in this particular case, because they went in the same direction as changes which were taking place in medical practice.[8]

In 1994, the combination of prices and volumes became the subject of an agreement between pharmaceutical companies and the state. According to the agreement, from 1995 onwards companies must commit themselves to promoting an appropriate use of drugs, within the framework of a national expenditure target. Sanctions in the form of price reductions can be applied when consumption exceeds targets. In 1994, the growth rate was much lower than the target, set at +3.2 per cent (+0.7 per cent for the expenditure financed by the *Sécurité Sociale* and +2.1 per cent for total pharmaceutical expenditure). However, in 1995 the share of pharmaceutical consumption financed by the *Sécurité Sociale* increased by 6.9 per cent. It

462   *Health Care and Cost Containment in the European Union*

appears that until now there have been no price reductions as provided for in the above agreement.

RMOs (treatment guidelines) concerning prescriptions also represent an indirect mechanism for controlling pharmaceutical expenditure. A study[9] on their implementation showed that some of them were effective, for example, the decline in the use of second- and third-generation cephalosporines for common respiratory infections. The same study estimated that in 1994, the application of *RMOs* led to overall savings of FRF 337 million. Nevertheless, this represented only 0.5 per cent of the total cost of medical prescriptions, due to the limited application of *RMOs*. In 1995, the effect of the previous years' guidelines continued, although at a slower pace, and new guidelines induced further changes in prescribing behaviour.

9.6 Other health care sectors: biology, auxiliary services and private hospitals

Since 1976, auxiliary services (nursing staff and physiotherapists) have been subjected to decreases in coverage rates. Regulatory agreements with biologists, private nurses and hospitals in 1992, and with physiotherapists in 1994, followed a different logic. These agreements are all based on the concept of budgeting, with different adjustment mechanisms according to different types of profession. These include: application by professional category or individual; re-payment of all expenditure exceeding budgets; activity ceilings; and the absence of fee upgrades in the case of budgetary noncompliance.

On the whole, these measures allowed for a downturn in expenditure trends. This is particularly evident in the case of private nurses and biologists, to the extent that one wonders how an economic agreement with laboratories could have such consequences (i.e. reduction) on the volume of doctors' prescriptions. The annual growth in expenditure on laboratory services at constant prices was 10.6 per cent between 1980 and 1985, and only 1.0 per cent between 1990 and 1995.

9.7 The Juppé Plan

In 1995, the growth rate of *Assurance-maladie* expenditure was relatively high (+3.2 per cent in constant FRF). This occurred not only because growth had been moderate in the previous year,* but also because of the upgrading of doctors' fees at the beginning of 1995, which took place in a pre-election context unfavourable to restrictive measures.

On 15 November 1995, the Prime Minister Alain Juppé, aware of the expected deficit, presented the *Assemblée Nationale* with a programme of reforms of the *Sécurité sociale*, which would affect the three branches of: sickness, family benefits and pensions. On the one hand, the '*Plan Juppé*' (which differed slightly from programmes announced in the electoral campaign six months earlier by the President of the Republic) announced emergency measures aimed at covering previous deficits, while on the other, it set down the guidelines for a financial and operational revision of the health care system in the medium term.[10] The *Juppé Plan* gathered together different ideas gleaned from earlier reports on the future of the French health care system.[11,12]

The *Juppé Plan* proved extremely controversial, provoking social turmoil at the end of 1995. Its central proposals were nevertheless preserved, and are currently being implemented.** This section will only deal with the parts of the reform affecting the *Assurance-maladie* and the health care system.

The Juppé Plan offered some standard, short-term measures which were aimed at increasing social security revenues or curbing the progression of expenditure in a number of ways:

- increasing contributions by pensioners, the unemployed and private doctors;

---

* In 1993 and 1994, the expenditure of the *Assurance-Maladie* grew at a relatively slower rate (+2.9% in 1993, and +0.4% in 1994). This was partly due to a generalized increase of co-payment rates implemented on 1 August 1993, and to the psychological or economic effect of the introduction of *RMOs* in 1994.

** The implementation of the measures set out in the Juppé Plan entailed a complex process of legislative reform: first a constitutional reform, then a law authorising the government to pass legislation through decrees, and finally the adoption of 5 decrees between January and April 1996. Decrees specifying the details of the implementation process will follow.

464 Health Care and Cost Containment in the European Union

- reducing coverage rates with an increase of the hospitalisation co-payment rate from FRF 55 to 70;

- imposing an exceptional tax of FRF 2.5 billion on the pharmaceutical industry;

- targeting the growth rate of hospital and general medicine expenditure for 1996–97 to equal general inflation (+2.1 per cent).

There were also further plans to introduce reinforced control mechanisms. These measures started to be implemented at the beginning of 1996. In 1997 Parliament voted for a cap of +1.7 per cent on health care expenditure increases.

As a long-term measure, the Plan instuituted an 'exceptional' income tax for a period of 13 years aimed at discharging the debt of the *Sécurité Sociale* (FRF 250 billion). The tax of 0.5 per cent of total income was introduced in 1996.

The Plan also aimed to introduce universal coverage by the *Assurance-maladie*, a progressive widening of its sources of finance (including a switch from payroll contributions to general tax revenue) as well as the control of its expenditure. To these ends, a number of structural measures (more innovative but requiring more time to be implemented) related to different areas of the health and social security system: the health care system's general management, the financing and management of the *Assurance-maladie* and the organisation of health care delivery. New supervisory and management bodies were set up, operating above and below existing bodies: councils supervising the finances of the *Sécurité sociale*, the *Agence nationale d'accréditation et d'évaluation en santé* (ANAES), the *Unions regionales des caisses d'Assurance-maladie*, and the regional hospital agencies *(Agences Regionales de L'hopitalisation)*.

In addition, the French Parliament now participates in the general management of the health care system. It deliberates on the revenue and expenditure trends of compulsory social security regimes by voting laws on the financing of the system. The role of the state has also been strengthened by new measures regulating the management of the *Assurance-maladie*. Trade union representation within the new management boards has been modified in favour of employers' representatives. Mandatory targets have also been set for the activities of the *Assurance-maladie*.

Long-term agreements on objectives and management have been

signed between the state and the funds of the *Sécurité sociale*, accompanied by annual amendments after the publication of the *Sécurité Sociale* finance law. These agreements and their amendments concern first, the instruments and expected results of the internal management of funds; second, long-term government strategies in the field of public health, medical workforce and pharmaceuticals; and finally, the compliance to the cost objectives for general practice. The conditions of implementation of these agreements are examined by the *Conseil de Surveillance.*

The decree referring to the 'medically driven control of health expenditure' presented a long list of measures concerning different aspects of care: access, supply, quality, prices, and expenditure. Some measures are ready for implementation while others require further action by the government, the managers of the *Assurance-maladie*, and those who represent the medical profession.

The most important innovation in the field of access to care is the introduction of the *carnet de santé* (medical records in the form of a small booklet) which patients must present when seeking medical attention, and in which doctors should record the information relevant to any follow-up. The introduction of patients' records started in autumn 1996. It is anticipated that this will effectively limit the number of visits and redundant prescriptions.

In an effort to reduce medical staff in the short-term, private doctors are being encouraged to retire early, starting from the age of 56. Another measure with a similar aim is the six month extension of general practitioner training. Continued medical training has now been made compulsory.

Several measures have set criteria for the reimbursement of services provided by private doctors under the *Assurance-maladie*. These include:

- inclusion in a list of reimbursable services;

- electronic transmission of information;

- compliance to treatment guidelines (*RMOs*); and

- reference to the contractual agreements on the expenditure of the *Assurance-maladie* for determining the volume of activities and prescriptions.

Though the application of global or individual sanctions for non-compliance with the above criteria has been established, the exact nature and details of how these sanctions should be applied have yet to be fixed. Decisions on the

466 *Health Care and Cost Containment in the European Union*

application of sanctions will be determined by instruments which will contribute towards enhancing the information available on medical activities, such as the coding of services, prescriptions and diseases.

The Juppé Plan allows for experimental projects on new ways of delivering health care. These projects must be accepted by the sickness funds and, although they may cover a wide variety of plans, only volunteers (doctors and patients) may participate.

In the field of hospital care, the issues of quality and cost containment are similar to those in ambulatory care, but the role played by the funds of the *Assurance-maladie* is less important and the state's supervision is more direct. Regional hospital agencies are responsible for the planning of facilities, and the allocation of resources to both private and public hospitals under the direct supervision of the ministries in charge for health and social security. The accreditation of hospitals and services, as well as the production of guidelines for good medical practice, are ensured by the ANAES, whose president and director are nominated by the health minister. The plan emphasizes the cooperation between public and private facilities, and encourages hospitals to promote alternatives to hospitalization, as well as to develop health care networks with private doctors.

The plan also touches upon pharmaceutical products. A drug can only be prescribed for the therapeutic purposes for which it was registered in the list of reimbursable products. Prescriptions must comply to *RMOs*. However, despite the encouraged use of generics, there are no clearly defined guidelines as to how this should be achieved.

9.8 Conclusions

During the last 20 years, cost-containment measures have targeted the *Assurance-maladie* rather than considering health care expenditure as a whole. Some of these measures, such as the increase in payroll contributions or the reduction in services provided, have achieved their objective of improving the *Assurance-maladie*'s finances in the short-term. On several occasions, the growth of expenditure related to services covered by the *Assurance-maladie* and overall health care has slowed significantly. This phenomenon, which sometimes occurs in the interval between the announcement and the implementation of new measures, is more the result of psychological influences on people's behaviour, rather than a sign of the measures' effectiveness.

This does not mean that cost-containment measures only have a short-term effect. Over a long period of time, a slow but certain deceleration in the growth rate of health care expenditure increases can be observed. Several social and economic developments as well as cost containment measures have had an impact on this growth rate.

Some of the factors affecting decision-making are contradictory, often in conflict with the decision-makers' objective of balancing finances at the national level. By affecting positively the sector at which it is aimed, while having negative repercussions on other sectors, the overall impact of a measure can be diminished or even nullified. This effect occurs, for example, when constraints imposed on hospitals create a higher demand for primary and community care, or when the reduction of reimbursement rates for some drugs causes their substitution with more expensive products.

Some measures might also prove contradictory because their medium-term effects differ from their initial objectives, which were decided upon in a different context. This is best illustrated by the regulations concerning the medical workforce (see section 9.3).

Between 1975 and 1995, the most frequently used cost-containment-measure was increases in cost-sharing. Another aim of these increases was to increase the revenue of the *Assurance-maladie*. This is may be very effective in the short-term. However, the reduction of reimbursement rates, widely used for pharmaceuticals, seems to have been abandoned due to its unpopularity, its discretionary application and its minimal long-term effectiveness. The resulting increase in prices to the consumer did not contribute to reducing consumption, but on the contrary, led to the development of complementary insurance (*Mutuelles*). The subsequent introduction of global budgets has proved more effective in controlling the expenditure of the *Assurance-maladie*, but has had no influence on the delivery of care or equity. This measure was maintained by the Juppé Plan and is now accompanied by other measures aimed at improving the quality of care.

1996 saw the commencement of the implementation of the Juppé Plan. Emergency financial measures came into force and most of the administrative framework was set up. In December 1996, the *'Loi de Financement de la Sécurité Sociale'* was passed and 1997 saw, for the first time, a cap on the growth of health expenses.

In June 1997, a new left-wing administration unseated the right-wing

468 *Health Care and Cost Containment in the European Union*

government. In spite of this major political change, there has been no significant alteration in health policy so far. Even though the Plan Juppé contributed to the fall of the previous administration, the newly elected government has continued to implement most of the measures based on the existing legislation.

In early 1998 the situation was as follows:

For the second year of the reform, the deficit of the *Sécurité Sociale* as a whole (health, family benefits, pensions) exceeded the target envisaged when Prime Minister Juppé presented his plan (1996 forecast: FRF 17 billion deficit, actual: FRF 52 billion deficit; 1997 forecast: FRF 12 billion surplus, actual: estimated at FRF 47 billion deficit). The gap between forecast and actual deficit is due mainly to a lack of revenue rather than to an increase in expenditure. To address this issue, the Jospin government has decided to extend the period of the 'exceptional' 0.5 per cent income tax from 13 to 18 years.

The second *'Loi de Financement de la Sécurité Sociale'* was more generous than the first. The rate of increase allowed in 1998 was higher than in 1997: +2.2 per cent (+1.7 in 1997) for total reimbursed expenses. The breakdown by type of care was +2.1 per cent for ambulatory care (+2.0 in 1997) and +2.2 per cent for hospital care (+1.4 in 1997).

The rates, which have legal force at national level, are divided at regional level according to rules based on the age of population for ambulatory care. The allocation formula for the hospital sector adjusts for discrepancies in the cost of provision of care. For instance, the rates of growth for hospital expenses vary from +0.35 per cent (Paris region) to +2.55 per cent (Poitiers region).

As far as health care expenditure is concerned, it is unlikely that the targets for 1997 will be met fully for all catagories of care. For example, the increase in expenditure for GPs is likely to fall within the +2.4 per cent target, but that of specialists is expected to exceed the +1.4 per cent cap.

A two-tier *Convention* between the doctors' union and the sickness funds was signed in March 1997. The agreement includes provisions applicable to GPs and specialists both jointly and separately. The GPs *Convention* allows doctors to become *'médicin référent'*, a kind of gatekeeper to the system. This is voluntary for both doctors and patients. Under this system GPs must keep a detailed record for their patients and 10 per cent of their prescriptions must be for generic drugs. There are financial incentives to join the scheme for both patients and doctors. Normally the patient has to pay the provider directly and then has to wait for reimbursement. Under the *'médecin référent'* scheme the direct payment is only 30 per cent and if the patient has a complementary insurance (such as a *Mutuelle* or private insurance) it is possible that no charges are asked of the patient. Doctors receive an extra annual payment of FRF 150 per registered patient. By the end of 1997, only 12.5 per cent of GPs had joined the scheme as many are concerned about the risk of increased control by sickness funds.

The above points illustrate the continuity of French health policy under, first Juppé and now Jospin. Similar economic constraints have driven the health policy decisions of both governments, and this may be why such an important popular measure as universal coverage based on residence, announced by Juppé, has not yet been implemented.

However, it is likely that the present government will be more inclined to negotiate with the stakeholders in the health care system. Prime Minister, Jospin announced as early as July 1997 (within weeks of his appointment), that a major consultation of all stakeholders, *'Etats Généraux de la Santé'*, would take place. This meeting proved very difficult to organize and has already been postponed twice. It is now due to take place in 1998. Measures to enhance public health can be expected, but it is unlikely that major changes will be recommended regarding the financing and delivery of health services.

References

1   Duriez M, Lancry P-J, Lequet-Slama D, Sandier S. Le système de santé, Paris: CREDES, PUF, *Que sais-je?* 1996;3066.

2   Mossialos E. Citizens' views on health care systems in the 15 EU Member States. *Health Economics* 1997;6(2):109-16.

3   OECD. *Health Data 1997.* Paris: OECD, 1997.

4   MSSPS, SESI. *Les Comptes Nationaux de la Santé: 1993–1994–1995.* Paris: SESI, 1996.

5   Logiciel ECO-SANTE FRANCE 4.0, Paris: CREDES. 1996/07.6

6   Mizrahi A and A. *Etat de Santé, Vieillesse Relatif et Variable Sociodémographiques.* Paris: CREDES. 1994 no. 999.

7   Lecomte T, Tonnelier F. *Prescription et Diminution Du Taux de Remboursement.* Paris: CREDES 667, June 1985.

8   Lecomte Th. *La Consommation Pharmaceutique en 1991: Evolution 1970–1980–1991.* Paris: CREDES. 1994/12.

9 Le Fur Ph, Sermet C. *Les Références Médicales Opposables: Impact sur la Prescription Pharmaceutique.* Paris: CREDES. 1996/03.

10 Le Plan Juppé. In: numéro spécial *Droit Social* 3, 1996/03.

11 Rochaix L, Khélifa A, Pouvourville G de. *Santé 2010: Équité et Efficacité du Systéme de Santé: Les Enjeux.* Paris: CGP, 1993/06.

12 Soubie R, Portos JL, Prieur C. *Livre Blanc sur le Système de Santé et D'assurance Maladie.* Paris: La Documentation Française, 1994.

10 Health expenditure and cost containment in Ireland

JENNY HUGHES

10.1 Introduction

Health expenditure in Ireland is heavily influenced by Government budgetary considerations. During the 1970s, health spending as a percentage of gross domestic product (GDP) increased rapidly; however, as the economy went through a difficult period in the 1980s this trend was reversed. With the easing of the budgetary crisis, and the recovery in the economy in the late 1980s, expenditure on health once again increased.

In the 1980s, to restrain the growth in health spending, various cost containment strategies were adopted. Major reforms included: the introduction of capitation payments in place of fee-for-service payments to general practitioners for the treatment of people with medical cards; the introduction of charges for out-patient visits and for in-patient care in public beds by non-medical card-holders; and the introduction of various mandatory and voluntary price and volume control measures to curtail the growth in pharmaceutical expenditure. Measures adopted more recently to contain costs include the use of case-mix analysis in the setting of hospital budgets and the introduction of drug budgeting.

Before examining these and other measures introduced to contain health care costs the chapter begins with a description of the Irish health care system.

10.2 The Irish health care system

The Irish health care system is a unique mixture of public and private financing. The principal source of finance is general taxation; however, voluntary insurance also plays an important role, with over 35 per cent of

472   *Health Care and Cost Containment in the European Union*

the population covered by schemes operated by the Voluntary Health Insurance (VHI) Board. The two principal payers in the system are the Department of Health and the VHI.* However, on behalf of the Department of Health (DoH), eight health boards fund and manage public services locally and the General Medical Services (Payments) Board (GMS), established jointly by the health boards, fund general practitioners (GPs) and pharmacists who provide services to medical card-holders.

The mixed financing arrangements in place in the Irish health care system has resulted in a mixture of publicly and privately delivered health services. The providers of health care services include independent pharmacists (retail chemists) and GPs, voluntary general hospitals (some of whose beds are private), public general hospitals (some of whose beds are private), public special hospitals (for geriatric, mentally handicapped and psychiatric patients), community health services (including home nursing, dental, aural and ophthalmic services), and private general and psychiatric hospitals.

Figure 10.1 depicts the main features of the Irish health care system.

10.3 Health care expenditure

Health care expenditure is composed of public and private spending.

Public health expenditure, as defined by the Commission on Health Funding, includes:

* non-capital expenditure on statutory health services by the Department of Health, excluding charges for private accommodation in public hospitals and other income such as emoluments and superannuation, retensions from pensions, other receipts such as payments for agency services and investment income;

* expenditure (by agencies other than the Department of Health) of grants from the European Social Fund towards the training of disabled persons.

* expenditure from the National Lottery allocated to community health services and the Health Education Bureau;

---

* On 1 January 1997, the British United Provident Association Limited (BUPA) commenced trading in the Irish health insurance market.

Health Expenditure and Cost Containment in Ireland 473

Figure 10.1 The system of health care in Ireland

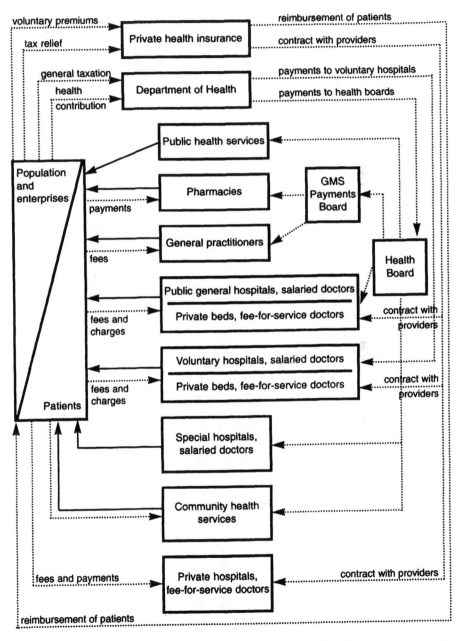

Source: OECD, 1992.[1]   Financial flows ·······▶   Service flows ⎯⎯▶

Table 10.1 Public expenditure on health, 1960–93

£ million	1960	1970	1975	1980	1985	1986	1987	1988	1989	1990	1991	1992	1993
Net non-capital expenditure	19.5	72.8	242.6	701.0	1169.3	1219.0	1221.5	1231.5	1318.0	1463.9	1631.0	1829.7	2016.6
European Social Fund	-	-	0.6	8.2	18.9	17.1	18.3	17.8	22.9	23.6	24.9	26.6	27.6
National Lottery	-	-	-	-	-	-	3.5	4.5	4.9	8.6	21.5	30.3	18.4
Treatment benefits	0.4	1.0	2.8	6.3	15.3	16.6	16.7	18.2	16.1	15.5	17.0	17.4	23.8
Total non-capital expenditure	19.9	73.8	246.0	715.5	1203.5	1252.7	1260.0	1272.0	1361.9	1511.6	1694.4	1904.0	2086.4
Capital expenditure	0.8	3.7	10.0	35.0	57.0	58.7	57.6	42.3	45.0	44.2	35.9	33.0	33.4
National Lottery capital expenditure	-	-	-	-	-	-	-	2.0	3.0	2.0	6.6	11.0	11.0
Total capital expenditure	0.8	3.7	10.0	35.0	57.0	58.7	57.6	44.3	48.0	46.2	42.5	44.0	44.4
Total public expenditure	20.7	77.5	256.0	750.5	1260.5	1311.4	1317.6	1316.3	1409.9	1557.8	1736.9	1948.0	2130.8
Total public expenditure as % of GDP	3.3	4.8	6.8	8.0	7.1	6.7	6.3	5.9	5.6	5.7	6.1	6.5	6.6

Source: Department of Health, various years.[2]

Health Expenditure and Cost Containment in Ireland 475

- expenditure on medical benefits available under the Social Insurance Fund, from the Department of Social Welfare; and

- capital expenditure (e.g. spending on long-term assets such as buildings and equipment) by the Department of Health.

In Table 10.1 public expenditure on health in nominal terms and as a percentage of GDP are shown for selected years from 1960 to 1993. During the 1960s and the early part of the 1970s public expenditure on health increased. Following the first oil crisis and the budget imbalances associated with them, there was a slowdown in growth. However, towards the end of the 1970s, expenditure picked up and by 1980 public spending on health had increased by over 160 per cent in real terms on the 1970 level. During the budgetary crisis of the 1980s the growth in expenditure was curtailed once again. Following the 1987 and 1988 public expenditure cuts and the recovery in the economy, growth in expenditure resumed. This trend has continued into the 1990s, with public health expenditure increasing to 6.6 per cent of GDP in 1993.

Capital expenditure by programme is presented in Table 10.2. During the budgetary crisis of the late 1980s capital expenditure was cut. With the recovery in the economy in the early 1990s, expenditure on all programmes has picked up.

Non-capital expenditure accounts for about 95 per cent of all public health spending. It is divided into three major programme areas (Table 10.3, overleaf): community care; special hospitals; and the general hospital programmes. These programmes are subdivided. The community care pro-

Table 10.2 Estimated capital expenditure by programme, IEP million (current prices), 1987–93

	1987	1989	1991	1993
Community health services	1868	808	837	1127
Community welfare	952	364	223	105
Psychiatric	4,939	988	360	2,902
Services for the handicapped	4,279	495	1,004	2,026
General hospitals	45,577	41,345	27,576	32,130
Total	57,615	44,000	30,000	38,290

Source: Department of Health, various years.[2]

Table 10.3 Estimated non-capital expenditure by programmes and services, IEP million (current prices). 1987–96

	1987	1989	1991	1994	1996
Community Protection Programme	**19700**	**23160**	**26210**	**40232**	**54738**
Prevention of infectious diseases	5670	8140	9249	14745	19277
Child health examinations	6840	6866	7831	8766	9824
Food hygiene and standards	3490	3554	4057	7583	8805
Drugs Advisory Service	790	1000	1058	1450	-
Health promotion	290	1040	1131	2270	3399
Other preventive services	2620	2560	2884	5418	13433
Community Health Services Programme	**186300**	**229180**	**260780**	**371626**	**433948**
GP services (including prescribed drugs)	125900	160000	176688	250026	271661
Subsidy for drugs purchased by non-medical card-holders	10500	16700	19963	39057	60999
Refund of cost of drugs for long-term illness	8500	10500	11132	17159	21384
Home nursing services	21155	21810	26888	30569	32288
Domiciliary maternity services	1960	1810	2102	2390	2524
Family planning	145	150	165	175	2385
Dental services	13290	13350	18353	25799	34740
Ophthalmic services	4000	4000	4512	5368	6834
Aural services	850	860	977	1083	1133
Community Welfare Programme	**102575**	**108500**	**140500**	**200729**	**133377**
Cash payments and grants for disabled persons	57680	62410	74200	96176	—
Mobility allowances for handicapped persons	380	410	469	646	1040
Cash payments to persons with certain infectious diseases	545	570	657	759	840
Maternity cash grants	70	50	30	34	27
Domiciliary care allowances for handicapped children	5490	5830	6645	7785	8729
Cash payments to blind persons	1050	1130	1293	1515	1837
Home help services	6500	6660	9379	10703	11458
Meals-on-wheels services	1620	1630	1751	1903	1949
Grants to voluntary welfare agencies	9900	9850	22443	30860	34036
Supply of milk to expectant and nursing mothers and children <5 years covered by medical cards	950	910	968	1072	1097

Pre-school support services	540	550	587	1554	1691
Boarding out of children	2700	2920	3131	9634	10490
Payment for children in residential homes	6750	6940	8395	26032	46777
Welfare homes for the aged	7840	8080	9884	11312	12623
Adoption services	560	560	668	744	783
Psychiatric Programme	**158200**	**158110**	**183390**	**215850**	**233199**
Service for the diagnosis, care and prevention of psychiatric ailments	158200	158110	183390	215850	233199
Programme for the Handicapped	**132800**	**141000**	**164920**	**222756**	**267519**
Care in special homes for the mentally handicapped	77300	83930	107034	144859	167747
Care of mentally handicapped persons in psychiatric hospitals	28560	29080	24821	31298	32633
Care in day centres for the mentally handicapped	7620	8280	10643	17143	20871
Assessment and care of the blind	1920	1940	2070	2552	3514
Assessment and care of the deaf	590	600	639	767	1006
Assessment and care of persons otherwise handicapped	13550	13710	15699	22060	26151
Rehabilitation service	3260	3460	4014	4077	15597
General Hospital Programme	**655775**	**697490**	**897060**	**1146609**	**1276548**
Services in regional hospitals	151750	167010	222156	294214	337360
Services in public voluntary hospitals	259700	274730	367544	475383	518024
Services in health board general hospitals	125155	132710	166009	200320	226309
Contributions to patients in private hospitals	15000	15300	16698	27326	30380
Services in district hospitals	25990	26750	31166	37350	40046
Services in health board long-stay hospitals	60680	62840	73151	87398	93536
Ambulance services	17500	18150	20336	24618	28893
General Support Programme	**64650**	**67560**	**79140**	**92856**	**107586**
Central administration	7400	9630	12385	13233	16024
Local administration	35000	36280	40693	44997	47566
Research	2300	1300	1631	2769	3411
Superannuation	14250	16650	19465	23026	31142
Finance charges	5700	3700	4966	8831	9443
Gross non-capital total	**1320000**	**1425000**	**1752000**	**2290658**	**2506915**

Source: Department of Health, various years.[2]

478   *Health Care and Cost Containment in the European Union*

gramme includes community protection; community health and community welfare. The special hospitals programme is concerned with the provision of services to the mentally ill and handicapped, and the general hospital programme involves service provision in regional, general and district hospitals. There are overlaps between programmes so care must be taken in interpreting the breakdown. However, expenditure on all programmes (in nominal terms) has increased over the past ten years.

An alternative series on public health spending is given in the National Accounts (Table 10.4). The levels and trends in the data are similar to those in Table 10.1, however there are two differences between the series. First, the National Accounts data represent gross expenditures, whereas the data from the Health Statistics are net of income from charges for maintenance in private and semi-private accommodation in public hospitals, and deductions from pay for emoluments and superannuation, retentions from pensions, investment income and other receipts such as payments for agency services. Second, the National Accounts data excludes income support programmes administered by the Department of Social Welfare. For the purposes of international comparisons, the National Accounts series on health expenditure is preferable.[3] However, this series is only available up to 1988.

The bulk of resources devoted to health care come from public sources, however, private expenditure accounts for a small proportion of total expenditure.* Private health expenditure includes:

- VHI expenditure comprising the claims and administration expenses of the VHI;

- other non-household expenditure, made up of small employment-based schemes which also offer health insurance;

- household expenditure based on Central Statistics Office (CSO) estimates of private spending on medical goods and services net of refunds under health insurance and drug subsidy schemes; and

- expenditure on private hospitals etc.

In Table 10.5 private health expenditure at current prices and as a percentage of GDP are shown for selected years from 1960 to 1993. Private expenditure as a percentage of GDP has remained relatively constant during the

---

* Data on private expenditure is limited and often based on estimates.

Table 10. 4 Public expenditure on health, 1976–88 (National Accounts Basis)

	1980	1981	1982	1983	1984	1985	1986	1987	1988
Total current expenditure (IEPm)	695.6	812.7	959.5	1047.7	1091.2	1192.5	1237.6	1249.5	1247.3
Total capital expenditure (IEPm)	52.1	60.0	49.3	53.3	56.1	57.5	63.7	61.4	48.0
Total public expenditure (IEPm)	747.7	872.7	1008.8	1101.0	1147.3	1250.0	1301.3	1310.9	1295.3
Total public expenditure as % of GDP	8.0	7.7	7.5	7.4	7.0	7.1	6.9	6.5	6.0

Source: Central Statistics Office, various years.[4]

Table 10.5 Total private expenditure on health, 1960–93

	1960	1970	1975	1980	1985	1986	1987	1988	1989	1990	1991	1992	1993
VHI expenditure (IEPm)	0.3	2.8	8.7	30.9	103.6	117.4	150.1	164.9	158.0	171.1	184.9	203.6	203.1
Other non-household expenditure (IEPm)	0.1	0.3	1.0	2.9	4.9	5.0	5.0	5.1	5.5	6.1	6.7	7.6	8.0
Household expenditure(IEPm)	10.1	25.6	34.4	125.1	211.8	227.5	231.1	246.9	260.1	277.0	307.2	331.7	382.4
Private capital expenditure(IEPm)	–	–	–	–	32.6	21.3	37.5	41.5	50.0	42.0	32.7	32.7	25.0
Private expenditure (IEPm)	10.5	28.7	44.1	158.9	352.9	371.2	423.7	458.4	473.6	496.2	531.5	575.6	618.5
Private expenditure as % of GDP	1.7	1.8	1.2	1.7	2.0	1.9	2.0	2.0	1.9	1.9	1.9	1.9	1.9

Source: Central Statistics Office, various years.[4]

480 *Health Care and Cost Containment in the European Union*

period of analysis. However, it is interesting to note the substitution between public and private expenditure. Between 1970 and 1975 private expenditure declined as public expenditure increased, and in the late 1980s when public expenditure was cut private expenditure increased slightly.

10.4 Financing of expenditure on health

The Irish health service is financed from public and private sources. Public financing accounts for approximately 75 per cent of total funding. Over the past twenty years publicly funded health care services have been financed predominantly from general taxation. A specific pay-related health contribution of 1.25 per cent on the incomes of non-medical card holders (up to a limit of IEP 23,200), charges for public hospital services by non-medical card-holders, and receipts under European Union (EU) regulations in respect of health services provided to EU nationals, are the other sources of financing.

Exchequer spending on health services is determined by the Department of Health and the Department of Finance. With the exception of public voluntary hospitals whose budgets are negotiated individually with the Department of Health, funding for the provision of public health services is provided on the basis of annual budgets to the eight health boards. Each health board has the responsibility of allocating funds across the different health care programmes (i.e. community care, special hospital and general hospital programmes) as well as ensuring that the budgets are respected. The Department of Health also monitors events to ensure budgets and activity targets are met.

Table 10.6 Sources of funds for public non-capital health services, 1987–96

	1987	1989	1991	1993	1995	1996
Exchequer	89.4%	87.0%	88.4%	87.6%	88.4%	88.3%
Health contributions	8.2%	9.8%	9.0%	9.6%	9.4%	9.2%
Receipts under EU regulations	2.4%	3.2%	2.6%	2.8%	2.2%	2.5%
Total	100%	100%	100%	100%	100%	100%

Source: Department of Health, various years.[2]

The remaining 25 per cent of health funding comes from private sources – health insurance companies and households. A large proportion of private expenditure on health care is covered by the VHI, and household expenditure on health services accounts for about 15 per cent of total current health spending[5] (Table 10.5). Household expenditure, except for those with medical cards, includes GPs' fees, the costs of drugs, the fees of dentists and opticians not covered under the Pay Related Social Insurance Treatments Benefits Scheme, and public hospital charges. It is worth noting that some private spending is also supported from public funds through tax relief on health insurance premiums and the availability of income tax relief for certain unreimbursed medical expenses exceeding IEP 100 in one year for an individual or IEP 200 a year for a family. In 1988–89 the Revenue Commissioners estimated that the cost of income tax relief on medical insurance was IEP 41.8 million and the cost of relief on unreimbursed medical expenses was IEP 2.4 million for 1987.[6]

10.5 Commission on health funding

During the 1980s the reduction in public expenditure and concern over the financing and delivery of health care resulted in the establishment of the Commission on Health Funding. Its task was to examine the financing of the health services and to make recommendations on the extent and source of the future funding required to provide an equitable, comprehensive and cost-effective public health service and on any changes in administration which seem desirable for that purpose. The Commission reported to the Minister for Health in September 1989.[6] A number of recommendations were made in the Report.

The main recommendations with regard to funding and eligibility were as follows:

- The health services should continue to be primarily tax-funded through general taxation, but there should be a supplementary role for private financing.

- There should be only two categories of eligibility, with the lowest income group remaining eligible for all health services and the remainder of the population eligible for core services (including all hospital care, a range of health services in the community excluding GP care,

482 *Health Care and Cost Containment in the European Union*

and prescribed drugs over a certain value) free of charge.

- Patients using public hospitals should choose between public and private in-patient care and those choosing private care should bear the full cost.

- The Commission believed that user-charges had a useful role to play in a public funding system provided they were regulatory in nature.

- Income tax relief on health insurance and on unreimbursed medical expenses should be phased out.

The principle recommendations made by the Commission in relation to administration and management were:

- The establishment of an administrative structure which would separate political and executive functions. The Minister and the Department for Health would concentrate on policy formulation while the Health Services Executive Authority (HSEA), a new national body, would be responsible for the management of the health services and for the allocation of funds to health agencies. Health boards would be transformed into health councils with responsibility for service delivery in each region.

- A Performance Audit Unit should be established to assist the Minister for Health in assessing the overall effectiveness of the services.

With regard to information and evaluation, the Commission suggested that better management information systems should be developed for health and social services. In particular, they called for more cost-benefit analyses and more health technology assessment.

With respect to the various health services, it was recommended that:

- general practitioner care should continue to be paid for by those who can afford to do so;

- there should be a common admission policy including a common waiting lists for public and private patients in public hospitals; maximum waiting times should also be published;

- regulatory charges are a useful deterrent to unnecessary utilization of out-patient services; any in-patient charges for public services should be aimed at cost-sharing; and should be subject to a yearly maximum;

- specific roles and catchment areas should be designated for all public hospitals;

- hospitals should be funded according to an agreed level of service based on activities and the case-mix based cost of meeting this service;

- public voluntary and private hospitals should be required to obtain a licence in order to ensure the maintenance of standards;

- a mix of public and private consultant practice in public hospitals should continue; consultants should be free to engage in private practice in the hospital where they hold their main public appointment; private practice at another hospital should take place only with the agreement of the employing public hospital;

- there should be a comprehensive review of the medical manpower requirements of all public hospitals with a view to establishing a grading structure for consultant positions;

- health insurers should seek to negotiate maximum chargeable fees with consultants and to devise ways of reducing the risk of unnecessary private expenditure;

- a Drugs and Therapeutic Committee should be established for GPs and hospitals to assist in the evaluation of prescribing patterns and the development of therapeutic guidelines;

- a limited list of pharmaceutical products for use in the public system should be introduced, and the HSEA should negotiate the trade prices of these products; and

- prescription charges should not be imposed on medical card-holders.

A number of the recommendations made by the Commission were implemented. In the following sections these changes will be highlighted.

10.6 Eligibility for health services and the structure of health charges

Entitlement to health services depends on eligibility, calculated on the basis of personal income. There are two categories of eligibility, and the category to which a person belongs determines what services he should pay for

484 *Health Care and Cost Containment in the European Union*

Table 10.7 Access to health care: eligibility for public health services, 1996

Category One

General practitioner care

All prescribed medicines

All in-patient public hospital services in public wards (including consultant services)

All out-patient public hospital services (including consultant services)

Dental, ophthalmic and aural services and appliances

Maternity and infant care services

A maternity cash grant of IEP 8 for each child born.

Category Two

All in-patient public hospital services in public wards (including consultant services) subject to a daily charge of IEP 20 up to a maximum of IEP 200 in any consecutive 12 month period

All out-patient public hospital services (including consultant services)

Attendance at accident and emergency departments, subject to a charge of IEP 12 where the patient does not have a referral note from a GP

Maternity and infant care services

A refund of expenditure on prescribed drugs and medicines under the Drug Refund Scheme, Drug Cost Subsidisation Scheme, or Long-Term Illness Scheme

---

Source: Department of Health, 1996.[7]

and what services he is entitled to free of charge. In Table 10.7 the entitlements of those in *Category One* and *Category Two* are outlined.

Persons with *Category One* eligibility are individuals who are judged to be unable to arrange GP services for themselves and their dependents without undue hardship. Such persons and their dependents have full eligibility for all health services without charge. This includes free GP and pharmaceutical services; free maintenance and treatment in public wards of hospitals (including consultant services); free specialist out-patient services at public clinics; free dental, ophthalmic and aural services; and a free mater-

Table 10.8 Category One patients, 1977–94

	Numbers in Category One	As a % of the total population
1977	1,233,150	38.63
1980	1,199,599	35.62
1985	1,303,273	36.84
1986	1,323,035	37.40
1987	1,342,233	37.88
1988	1,324,849	37.45
1989	1,256,818	35.76
1990	1,221,284	34.86
1991	1,237,772	34.94
1992	1,263,001	35.60
1993	1,274,621	35.77
1994	1,286,632	36.49

Source: General Medical Services (Payments) Board, 1977–94.[8]

nity and infant care service (including the services of a GP during and for up to six weeks after pregnancy). Fully eligible persons are issued with medical cards by their health board. Entitlement to a medical card depends upon personal income and circumstances. Income guidelines are revised each year. About a third of the population are in this category (see Table 10.8).

The remainder of the population (those that do not qualify for a medical card) have *Category Two* eligibility. These persons are entitled to all in-patient public hospital services in public wards (including consultant services) subject to certain charges; all out-patient public hospital services (excluding dental and routine ophthalmic and aural services); attendance at accident and emergency departments subject to a charge where the patient does not have a referral note from his or her doctor; a maternity and infant care service (including the service of a GP during pregnancy and up to six weeks after the birth); and a refund of expenditure on prescribed drugs and medicines in excess of a specified amount under either the Drug Refund Scheme, the Drug Cost Subsidisation Scheme, or the Long-Term Illness

486 *Health Care and Cost Containment in the European Union*

Scheme.

Under the Drug Refund Scheme, all persons with *Category Two* eligibility who incur expenditure of more than IEP 90 per quarter on prescribed drugs and medicines, are entitled to a refund from the health board in excess of IEP 90. The Drug Cost Subsidisation Scheme (introduced in 1990) is also available to persons who do not have a medical card but who are certified as having a regular and ongoing requirement for prescribed medicines in excess of IEP 32 per month. Those who qualify under this scheme apply to the health boards for authorization which entitles them to pay only up IEP 32 each month. The GMS Board, on behalf of the health boards, makes payments for the balance due to pharmacists. The Long-Term Illness Scheme provides without charge drugs, medicines and other medical requisites for the treatment of *Category Two* patients with certain long-term illnesses and disabilities (e.g. mental handicap, cystic fibrosis, epilepsy, haemophilia).

It should noted that a three-category entitlement system was in operation until 1991, with those without medical cards being divided into *Categories Two and Three* on the basis of an income ceiling. *Category Three* persons were entitled to free maintenance in a public hospital ward but were liable for consultant's fees. In addition they were liable for maternity and infant care services in the community. *Categories Two and Three* were then combined to produce the two-category system which is currently in existence.

In 1987 charges were introduced for the utilization of public hospital services by those in *Category Two (and Category Three)*, almost two-thirds of the population.* Initially patients were required to pay IEP 10 for the first visit to a hospital out-patient or accident and emergency department. Currently, the charge is IEP 12. This applies only to the first visit of any episode of care. It does not apply to attendances at out-patient clinics. A charge of IEP 10 per day was also introduced for in-patient care up to a limit of IEP 100 in a year. A daily charge of IEP 20 now applies to stays in public wards of public hospitals, up to a maximum of IEP 200 in any consecutive 12 month period. This limit applies regardless of the number of hospitals to which a patient is admitted. Public hospitals also have semi-private

---

* Women receiving maternity services, children up to six weeks of age, children receiving treatment for mental handicap, mental illness, cystic fibrosis, spina bifida, hydrocephalus, haemophilia or cerebral palsy, children referred from child health clinics, and persons receiving services in respect of infectious diseases are exempt from public hospital charges.

and private accommodation and persons occupying semi-private or private beds must pay for that accommodation, irrespective of their category of eligibility. These charges, set by the Department of Health and applied across all public hospitals, have always been imposed on users of the services. However, the levels have increased substantially since 1980 when the charges for a semi-private and private bed were IEP 9 and IEP 12 respectively. At present these charges are IEP 104 per night for a semi-private bed and IEP 132 per night for a private bed in major public hospitals, with lower charges for smaller hospitals. These public hospital in-patient charges are covered by the VHI. Out-patient charges in public hospitals are also covered, but only when total expenditure in the year exceeds a fixed amount. The health insurance package offered by BUPA also covers in-patient and out-patient charges.

Since the introduction of health charges, no study has formally examined the impact of charges on the utilization of services. However, according to Nolan,[5] the utilization of hospital services was unlikely to change given that the charges for out-patient care were lower than the cost of seeing a GP and the charges for hospital in-patient care in a public ward were not applicable to medical card-holders and were covered by the VHI for those with health insurance.

10.7 The Irish hospital system

The Irish hospital system is made up of a mix of public and privately owned and funded hospitals (Table 10.9 overleaf). The public hospital system comprises two distinct sub-groups; Health Board hospitals and public voluntary hospitals, differentiated primarily by the degree of state funding attributable to each. The private hospitals meanwhile, are owned and managed privately and receive no direct funding from the state.

Health Board hospitals (regional, county and district hospitals), as their title indicates, are managed by the country's regional health boards, as established in 1970 by the Department of Health. Each health board receives an annual budget from the Department of Health, from which all health services are funded. Within the Health Board services, any hospital's allocation is at the discretion of the relevant regional board. Typically, the budget of each hospital is determined on a historic expenditure basis, and adjusted for inflation, pay awards, projected changes in service provision and govern-

488 *Health Care and Cost Containment in the European Union*

Table 10.9 Number of hospitals in Ireland, selected years

	1977	Number of hospitals 1986	1993
Health Board hospitals*	97	87	78
Voluntary public hospitals	47	40	27
Private hospitals	16	23	22
Total	160	150	127

Source: Department of Health, various years.[2]

* Health Board hospitals include district, regional, county, fever and orthopaedic hospitals.

ment policy on overall public expenditure. Recently, case-mix analysis has been used in a small number of Health Board hospitals to determine budgetary allocation.

Voluntary public hospitals (general teaching, non-teaching and special hospitals) have traditionally been owned and operated by religious orders. However, the dwindling number of people in religious orders has in some cases led to the incorporation of hospitals by charter or statute, working under lay boards of governors often selected by the Minister for Health. Voluntary public hospitals receive annual funding directly from the Department of Health. This accounts for most of the hospitals' funding. In the past, budgets to voluntary public hospitals were determined solely on the basis of their previous year's spending. In 1991 the Department of Health established a National Case-Mix Project to examine the potential uses of case-mix analysis for both resource allocation and hospital level applications. The decision to use case-mix measures in setting part of hospital budgets was taken in 1993. Data on hospital activity and on hospital costs were combined to adjust the funding allocation to 14 acute hospitals in 1993 and 23 in 1995. The principal is now established and has been used increasingly in the allocation of budgets. In 1995, 12.5 per cent of hospital budgets were allocated using case-mix analysis. The Department of Health plans to increase this percentage annually, in addition to expanding the case-mix analysis to out-patient and day-care services.

The case-mix measure adopted by the Department of Health are

Diagnosis Related Groups (DRGs).[9] Every case treated by an acute hospital is assigned to one DRG. The grouping system currently in use in Ireland contains 492 DRGs. Assignment is based on primary diagnosis, secondary diagnosis, procedures performed, discharge status, age, and sex. These details are gathered from the Hospital In-Patient Enquiry (HIPE). By grouping the in-patient cases of each hospital into a set of DRGs, each hospital's workload can be analysed and compared in case-mix terms. The cost information needed to calculate the cost of each DRG comes directly from each hospital through the Specialty Costings programme run by the Department of Health. This programme gathers costs for each specialty area within hospitals, and data for ten cost centres are extracted. The cost centres include the intensive care unit, theatre, drugs, radiology, hotel costs, supplies, laboratory, physician, administration and other miscellaneous costs. These cost centres are allocated to DRGs, some on the basis of daily costs, others using a set of service weights (i.e. a set of relativities that express the expected use of services between DRGs). The activity and cost data are combined to calculate a case-mix index (CMI) for each hospital. The CMI represents a measurement of the costliness/complexity of each hospital relative to any other hospital in the sample. For example, a hospital with a CMI of 1.15 has a caseload which would be expected to cost 15 per cent more than the national average. Using the CMI, hospital budgets taking account of case-mix measurement are calculated. Adjustments are made using a blend of the hospital's own cost per case (85 per cent) and the average cost per case of all hospitals in the sample (15 per cent). For a review of the case-mix adjustment approach adopted by the Department of Health see Wiley, 1995.[10]

Currently, the private hospital sector consists of 22 hospitals owned and managed privately, either on a non-profit or profit basis. These hospitals receive no direct state funding. Approximately 90 per cent of private hospital patients are insured with the VHI. Given that the VHI has traditionally been the principal provider of private medical insurance, it has considerable control over the private hospital sector. For example, the VHI introduced capping of expenditures by hospitals as a part of an emergency measure to contain expenditure following the sudden deterioration in its financial position in the late 1980s. What was initially a temporary measure is now a control mechanism and has been extended from hospitals to consultants.[11] Capping works by limiting the amount the VHI pays each hospital during the year. Once a hospital has reached its limit in pure capping terms, then it cannot attract private insured patients, or if it does, it cannot reclaim costs.

490   *Health Care and Cost Containment in the European Union*

However, the VHI has introduced some flexibility into this system using a variant of marginal cost pricing (i.e. treatment costs for patients above the baseline quota could be recovered at between 25 per cent and 40 per cent of actual cost).

Approximately 16 per cent of in-patient beds are privately owned. In addition, about 20 per cent of the beds in the public hospitals are used by the private sector. In total, therefore, over 30 per cent of hospital beds are used for privately financed health care.[12] Since the late 1970s however, the number of in-patient beds in public hospitals has declined quite significantly[11] (Tables 10.10 and 10.11). Most of the decline in public hospital beds occurred between 1986 and 1988, when the bed complement fell from 16,876 to 13,632. This was primarily due to the closure of county and district hospitals as a result of rationalization and expenditure cutbacks associated with the fiscal crisis. Consequently, the increase in private hospital beds, particularly after 1986, was due to the reduced availability of beds in publicly funded hospitals. During this period there was also an increase in the number of day-beds, as many surgical procedures previously requiring overnight stays were performed on a day-case basis. Day-case activity is an area of growing importance in Irish hospitals. In 1993 day cases represented almost one-third of total hospital activity[2] (Table 10.12).

Since the early 1980s community-based services for the mentally ill and the handicapped have been developed as alternatives to institutional care. For example, the number of people residing in psychiatric hospitals

Table 10.10 Distribution of hospital beds between the public and private sectors, selected years

	Number of hospital beds		
	1977	*1986*	*1993*
Health Board hospitals*	9,044	9,507	8,193
Voluntary public hospitals	8,332	7,369	5,451
Private hospitals	1,502	n/a	2,500 **

Source: Department of Health, 1980 and 1993.[2]

* Health Board hospitals include district, regional, county, fever and orthopaedic hospitals.

** Estimate.

Health Expenditure and Cost Containment in Ireland   491

Table 10.11 Health Board, district and public voluntary hospitals: main features of activity, 1986 and 1994

	Number of hospitals		Average number of in-patient beds available	
	_1986_	_1994_	_1986_	_1994_
Health Board hospitals *	39	36	6,584	6,392
District hospitals **	48	42	2,923	1,835
Public voluntary hospitals	40	27	7,369	5,461

	Patients discharged		Average length of stay (days)	
	_1986_	_1994_	_1986_	_1994_
Health Board hospitals *	273,411	300,876	7.3	6.3
District hospitals **	16,641	11,093	n/a	n/a
Public voluntary hospitals	276,053	222,011	7.7	7.0

Source: Department of Health, various years.[2]

* Health Board hospitals include regional, county, fever and orthopaedic hospitals.

** District hospitals are general practitioner staffed hospitals with units for medicine, minor surgery, and frequently for obstetrics and paediatrics. Many of these hospitals cater for longer-stay patients, hence the high average length of stay.

n/a Not available.

Table 10.12 Health Board, district and public voluntary hospitals: day-case activity*, 1987 and 1993

	Number of day beds available		Number of day cases	
	_1987_	_1994_	_1987_	_1994_
Health Board hospitals	n/a	208	23,613	52,394
District hospitals	n/a	0	3,233	863
Public voluntary hospitals	n/a	313	61,559	130,624

Source: Department of Health, various years.[2]

* A day case is defined as a patient who is admitted to hospital on an elective basis for care and/or treatment which does not require the use of a hospital bed overnight and who is discharged as scheduled.

492   *Health Care and Cost Containment in the European Union*

and special units in general hospitals has fallen from 12,484 in 1984 to 6,657 in 1993. In the same year, over 2,000 patients resided in community-based hostels compared with just 791 in 1984, and the number of day-care facilities increased from 32 to 145 over the same period. In the Four Year Action Plan, included in the strategy document *Shaping a Healthier Future*,[13] the expansion of community-based services for mentally ill and handicapped people remains a key policy objective.

10.7.1 Manpower and manpower controls

The number of persons employed by publicly funded hospitals and health boards has fluctuated significantly over the past 20 years. In 1977 just over 50,000 people were employed in the public health sector, this increased to 66,060 by 1981. However, during the budgetary crisis of the late 1980s and the embargo on public sector employment, the numbers employed in the health sector declined to 56,357 by 1988. During the embargo, temporary posts were discontinued and those who retired were not replaced. Since then, however, the numbers employed have increased, and in 1993 there were almost 62,000 employed in the public health sector. Almost 65 per cent of those working in the public health sector are employed by health boards. Voluntary and joint board hospitals accounted for a further 27 per cent, and mental handicap and specialist agencies employed the remainder. Health board recruitment decisions are taken at board level but in accordance with the Minister for Health.[14] Voluntary hospitals and other agencies are responsible for the selection of their own staff.

The number of hospital consultants has remained relatively constant since the early 1980s. In January 1995 there were 1,064 consultants practicing in public hospitals, compared with 1,085 in 1984. The number and type of consultant appointments in hospitals is regulated by *Comhairle na n-Ospideal* (Hospital Council). Since 1991, consultants can commit themselves to different categories of hospital appointment. These appointments vary in salary levels and the facility to work in private practice, in association with the service commitment in public hospitals.[15] Consultants are paid by salary for their work with public patients, and on a fee-for-service basis for private patients. Non-consultant hospital doctors working in the public sector increased from 1,824 in 1984 to 2,430 in 1993. Like the consultants, these doctors are paid by salary.

Health Expenditure and Cost Containment in Ireland 493

No data is available on private sector employment.

10.8 General Practitioner services

The General Practitioner (GP) service is also a mixture of public and private provision. The General Medical Services (GMS) is the public scheme which covers about 1.28 million people. Under the GMS scheme, those who are unable to arrange GP medical and surgical services for themselves or their family receive a medical card entitling them to free medical services. All patients in Ireland can choose their own GP, but whereas private patients may switch doctors at will, medical card-holders must register with a GP who participates in the GMS scheme (in 1995 1,652 GPs registered in the scheme). GMS patients who wish to change their GP must apply to the health board to do so, and the health board arranges the transfer to another participating GP. On transferring, the new doctor receives payment for any services provided to the patient.

The operation of the public scheme has been the subject of repeated discussions with the medical organizations since 1972. The principal features modified over the years have been the method of payment to doctors (from a fee-for-service to capitation system in 1989), and the establishment of a GP unit in the Department of Health and in each health board.

In February 1989, the government introduced capitation payments in place of fee-for-service payments for the care provided by GPs to GMS patients. Capitation payments were introduced because of concerns that the fee-for-service method of paying GPs encouraged over visiting, over prescribing and the medicalization of minor illnesses.[6] The rate of capitation per patient is determined by the age and gender of the patient, and the distance between the patient's home and the doctor's practice. The 1997 capitation fees payable under the GMS scheme are shown in Table 10.13 overleaf. These are annual payments for each patient on the doctor's list. There are also a number of special services which attract a fee in addition to capitation (for example, excisions, recognised vein treatment, ECG tests and their interpretation). The scheme allows for superannuation and various forms of leave payments.

It was expected that the change to the capitation system would curb visiting by medical card patients and that this in turn, would result in a decrease

494 *Health Care and Cost Containment in the European Union*

Table 10.13 Capitation fees per patient per annum as at 1 January 1997

Ages	Up to 3 miles		3–5 miles		5–7 miles		7–10 miles		Over 10 miles	
	M	F	M	F	M	F	M	F	M	F
0–4	35.69	34.83	37.60	36.74	40.41	39.55	43.17	42.32	46.61	45.76
5–15	20.73	20.98	21.53	21.75	22.68	22.92	23.80	24.03	25.22	25.43
16–44	26.48	43.26	27.50	44.29	29.00	45.79	30.47	47.26	32.31	49.10
45–64	52.83	58.05	55.30	60.52	58.91	64.12	62.46	67.71	66.90	72.11
65+	55.66	62.12	62.47	68.92	72.59	79.03	82.53	88.96	94.85	101.29

Source: General Medical Services (Payments) Board.[8]

in prescribing and drug costs. The impact of the change from fee-for-service to capitation is difficult to establish as there is no longer detailed administrative data on GP visits. However, anecdotal evidence suggests that the number of consultations has declined by up to 20 per cent on the pre-1989 level.[16] Both the GMS drugs bill and the number of prescriptions issued have continued to increase since the introduction of capitation payments (Table 10.14). It is difficult to determine what factors have contributed to these trends, hence a much more detailed analysis of visiting and prescribing rates is required before the impact of capitation can be fully assessed.

In 1992 a major review of the GMS Scheme was undertaken by the Department of Health. During that process the blueprint document *The Future of General Practice in Ireland* [17] was developed and became an integral feature of an agreement between the Minister for Health and the Irish Medical Organisation (IMO) on the arrangements for the provision of primary health care services and the development of general practice.

In the document, a number of key problems preventing the development of general practice were highlighted. For example, general practice was overly fragmented, with 59 per cent of GPs operating from single-handed practices and only 13 per cent operating from practices with three or more doctors. Moreover, many GPs were isolated both from one another

Health Expenditure and Cost Containment in Ireland 495

Table 10.14 Summary of statistical information relating to the GMS Scheme, 1988–94

Doctors	1988	1989	1990	1991	1992	1993	1994
Total payments (IEP)	44,601	51,580	56,369	59,618	73,698	86,234	89,446
Doctors' payment per person (IEP)	33.19	40.02	73.86	46.38	55.35	65.99	67.48

Pharmacies	1988	1989	1990	1991	1992	1993	1994
Total cost of prescriptions (IEP)	87,245	100,885	107,208	113,730	128,894	133,274	141,012
Number of forms (000s)	7,055	7,132	7,136	7,546	8,016	8,65	8,740
Number of items (000s)	13,818	14,282	14,636	15,478	16,534	17,252	17,906
Cost per form (IEP)	12.37	14.15	15.02	15.07	16.08	15.74	16.13
Cost per item (IEP)	6.31	7.06	7.32	7.35	7.80	7.72	7.88
Total cost of stock orders (IEP)	5,486	6,499	6,651	6,621	7,176	6,328	6,446
Overall cost of medicines (IEP)	92,731	107,384	113,859	120,350	136,070	139,602	147,458
Pharmacy payment per person (IEP)	69.01	83.32	92.24	97.78	108.32	110.47	115.01
Overall payments (IEP)	137,332	158,964	170,228	179,968	209,768	225,836	236,904
Overall payment per person (IEP)	102.20	123.34	136.10	144.16	163.67	176.46	182.49

Source: General Medical Services Board Financial and Statistical Analysis of Claims and Payments, 1992–94.[8]

and from hospitals. It was felt that these features of the organizational structure led to the duplication of costs, inefficiencies in the use of resources and increased workloads for doctors. The lack of a private patient list also meant that many GPs were not aware of the size of their total practice population in terms of either named patients or numbers. Other problems highlighted were the dearth of epidemiological data relating to disease and morbidity in the community and variations in practice styles.

A number of suggestions were made as to how to reorganize and aid the development of general practice. For example, proposals for reorganizing general practice at a national and regional level called for the establishment of a general practice unit in the Department of Health and within each health board. The national unit was to coordinate the work and functioning of the regional units. The regional units, on the other hand, were to provide support for work within general practice, to identify areas where additional services could be provided more cost-effectively (and to enter into arrangements with individual practices to provide these services), to improve the interface between general practice and hospital and other health services, to allocate resources for the funding of the service, and finally to assist GPs to prescribe appropriately and cost-effectively. In 1993, the Department of Health, in conjunction with the IMO, established a national general practice unit and general practice units within each health board.

At a practice level the aim was to organize general practice in such a way as to preclude the necessity for patients to attend hospitals as a first point of contact. The way in which this could be achieved was to provide a comprehensive range of general practice services at all times, which meant satisfactory out-of-hours cover. The fact that the majority of GPs were single-handed prevented the achievement of this objective. However, it was proposed that group practices would be set up in urban areas or towns with a minimum of three doctors in full partnership. Cross cover for nights and weekends could be provided within this group, and the doctors would work from an appropriately equipped medical centre. The centres could be provided and equipped by the health boards or on a joint venture approach. In addition, it was suggested that multi-centred group practices could be established. These would involve at least three doctors working in full partnership from different locations and providing cross-cover for one another. They would have their own centres of practice and also a central medical centre with equipment and facilities available to the entire group. A further way in which these centres could be established would be doctors working in the vicinity of a general hospital entering into cooperation with one another by continuing to work from their own centres of practice but pooling all resources such as staffing and equipment, and agreeing to provide full cross-cover. Single- and two-handed practices would be supported and recognized where group or multi-centred practices were unworkable. The provision would be that adequate weekend and night cover would be made available. Access to equipment in group practices by these doctors would be encouraged.

It was recognized that in the short- to medium-term, practice arrangements as they existed would continue. However, it was proposed that pilot practices would be established along the lines of the models discussed above. Any future contracts for the GMS, particularly in major urban areas, would be expected to provide continuous care on a 24-hour/7 day-a-week basis. Incentives would be provided for a number of different night and weekend arrangements.

In the case of the individual GP, a number of measures were needed to enable the GP to better carry out his or her role in the community. These measures included closer contact between GPs and other health and social services. It was envisaged that the general practice units in the health boards could have a significant role in this area. Other areas included establishing agreed protocols for investigation, treatment and care in the community, looking at the area of prescribing, the collection of information, and register of patients.

In 1993 the Government established a fund of IEP 12.5m out of which specific payments were made for developments in line with the document *The Future of General Practice in Ireland*. Annual payments were regarded as investments to be recouped as savings materialized. The fund was invested in four ways: IEP 4.5m was paid as an additional allowance for realistic rostering and out-of-hours arrangements; IEP 3m was paid towards practice maintenance equipment and development; IEP 1.5m was paid as a supplementary grant to those employing nurses and/or secretaries; and IEP 3.5m was paid for specific developments outlined in the document, including the establishment of national and regional general practice units.

The duration of the agreement between the IMO and the Department of Health was two years beginning on 1 January 1993, after which time the agreement was due to be reviewed. The review agreement came into effect on 1 January 1995. In the review, it was agreed that accountability arrangements were to be put in place so that any service changes arising from the

498   *Health Care and Cost Containment in the European Union*

provision of the General Practice Development fund could be analysed. In particular it was accepted that the General Practice Unit of each health board would discuss with individual GPs the manner in which investments were being used to improve facilities and services for patients. On the basis of the review, the fund was increased by 2.4 per cent from 1 January 1995.

Almost 85 per cent of all GPs in the country participate in the GMS scheme, though for the bulk of these, receipts under the GMS will not be their only source of income. They will also have private patients (those not covered by medical cards) who pay on a fee-for-service basis. GP's fees for private patients are set by the market, although there is no competition over price. The private GP system is diffuse, and there is little information published along the lines of the GMS system.

10.9 Pharmaceuticals*

In Ireland expenditure on pharmaceuticals accounts for approximately 10 per cent of total health care expenditure. Figures relating to private expenditure on pharmaceuticals are not available. However, on the basis of the Schemes operated by the Department of Health, pharmaceuticals account for an increasing proportion of health care resources. Figures published recently indicate that the drugs bill for 1994 was IEP 194.22 million, for 1995 it was IEP 215.89 million and for 1996 it amounted to IEP 235 million.

To control the growth in expenditure, various mandatory and voluntary price and volume control measures have been introduced by the Department of Health. For example, since the introduction of the General Medical Service Scheme in 1972, agreements for the supply of drugs to the health care services have existed between the Department of Health and the Irish Pharmaceutical Health Care Association (formerly the Federation of Irish Chemical Industries) which represents a large proportion of pharmaceutical manufacturers and distributors. The first agreement provided for price uniformity, volume discounts to hospitals, and rebates to the GMS for all products supplied under the Scheme. But it did not govern the level of pharma-

---

* For a more detailed analysis of the pharmaceutical industry in Ireland, see Nolan A, 1994.[16]

Health Expenditure and Cost Containment in Ireland 499

ceutical prices. However, in 1980 when Trident Management Consultants recommended that trade prices for drugs should be related to those in the UK, following a review of the supply arrangements, a new agreement was formed which provided for hospital discounts and rebates to the GMS together with limits on the amount by which the Irish trade price of drugs could exceed those obtained in the UK. The principal terms of the second agreement were as follows:

- trade prices of individual medicines limited to 115 per cent of the UK trade price;
- average trade prices limited to 107.5 per cent of the average UK trade prices;
- price increases permitted for the duration of the Agreement;
- manufacturers rebate equivalent to 4 per cent of GMS sales;
- hospital discount of 15 per cent on orders over IEP 100;
- freedom of the doctor to prescribe the medicines of his or her choice;
- freedom of access for new medicines to the GMS scheme; and
- Department of Health reserved the right to influence the general prescribing habits of doctors.

This agreement between the Department of Health and the Irish Pharmaceutical Health Care Association was revised in 1986, 1987, 1990, 1993 and 1997. The principal terms of the current agreement, which came into effect on 1 August 1997 for a five-year period, are as follows:

- prices of existing products are frozen for 5 years;
- doctors are free to prescribe the medicines of their choice, although the DoH is permitted to influence the prescribing habits of doctors;
- pharmacists must dispense the medicines prescribed by doctors;
- new products granted a product authorisation are reimbursable in the GMS and other community drug schemes, while existing products reimbursable in the GMS scheme remain so;
- the DoH reserves the right to seek cost benefit studies for any new product;

500 *Health Care and Cost Containment in the European Union*

- the pricing of new medicines are limited to the lesser of the currency adjusted UK wholesale price and the average of the currency adjusted wholesale prices in Denmark, France, Germany, the Netherlands and the UK;

- price modulation is permitted on the basis that such modulation is cost neutral;

- the rebate paid by the industry for medicines dispensed under the GMS scheme is reduced from 5 per cent to 4 per cent, and a further reduction to 3 per cent will apply from 1 August 1998 to 31 July 2002; and

- supplies to hospitals and health boards are now invoiced at trade price less 15 per cent on orders over IEP 500. Previously the discount was on orders over IEP 100.

Although the Department of Health has predominantly used the supply agreements with the pharmaceutical industry to control prices, it has also attempted to control the volume of medicines supplied to patients. In October 1982, about 900 over-the-counter (OTC) medicines were deleted from the list of drugs and medicines which could be prescribed under the GMS scheme. The objective of the exclusions was to restrict expenditure under the GMS to preparations of significant therapeutic value, and to discourage individuals from visiting their GPs to obtain prescriptions for OTC medicines. However, the exclusion of certain items from the list of reimbursable products resulted in the prescription of newer and more expensive alternatives, because they were free. Consequently, in 1989 the Department of Health restored two of the de-listed categories – mild pain-killers and anti acids – to the list of reimbursable products.

During this period attempts were also made to increase the awareness among prescribers of the price differentials between products with the same formulation. For example, the GMS Payments Board distributed to doctors, free of charge, a bulletin providing information on prices and the alternative preparations available. In 1990, the Department of Health introduced a National Drugs Formulary which had as its stated objective 'the rational use of medicines through safe, cost-effective prescribing'. The Formulary was prepared by a joint working group of the Department of Health and the Irish Medical Organisation. The failure of the Formulary to achieve its stated objectives resulted in the introduction of an agreement between the Department of Health and the Irish Medical Organisation relating to the set-

Health Expenditure and Cost Containment in Ireland 501

ting of prescribing targets and cost-effective prescribing for general practitioners participating in the GMS scheme. In the years prior to the agreement, the cost of prescribing to the GMS had been rising at approximately 11 per cent per year.[16] As the price of drugs had not risen, the reasons for this increase were attributed to volume increases and the substitution of more expensive drugs. To encourage GPs to pursue the objective of responsible and cost-effective prescribing, indicative prescribing targets were established for each GP and it was agreed that a proportion of any savings generated were to be invested in the development of general practice. The General Practice Units within each health board, set up under the same agreement, were to encourage appropriate prescribing by ensuring that appropriate information was issued to GPs at regular intervals showing how savings could be made as regards prescribing. In addition, members of the Units were expected to visit GPs periodically to discuss prescribing patterns, to target high-cost/volume prescribers, and to encourage all practices to review repeat prescriptions regularly.

The overall impact of indicative drug targeting and the effectiveness of the General Practice Units on prescribing patterns and total drug expenditure are difficult to quantify, given that both measures have only been in existence a few years. However, in a recent survey of GPs undertaken by the Centre for Health Economics (University of Dublin), preliminary results indicate that drug budgeting has altered the prescribing habits of GPs in relation to GMS and private patients. A review of the drug budgeting scheme, commissioned by the Department of Health, has just been published.[18] The objective of the review was to 'determine the effects of the Indicative Drug Target Savings Scheme on the quality of patient care in the GMS with particular reference to changes in prescribing patterns'. Two hundred GPs, 250 pharmacists, 50 hospital physicians and 1000 patients were surveyed to obtain their views on the scheme.

Unfortunately there is no information available on whether the quality of patient care has been affected by the introduction of drug budgeting. However, the majority of GPs surveyed believed that the scheme had resulted in an improvement in patient care. From the survey of GPs, a small number claimed that vulnerable groups in society, such as the elderly and chronically ill patients, were being denied optimum care. This finding was supported by hospital physicians and pharmacists. It is also of concern that hospital discharge prescriptions were being changed more frequently by GPs. Hospital physicians surveyed encountered a number of patients who had

502   *Health Care and Cost Containment in the European Union*

experienced adverse clinical effects as a result of drug substitution. The unreliability and poor quality of certain generic products were also points raised by GPs and pharmacists.

The patient survey revealed that a large number of people were unaware of the drug budgeting scheme. Many were confused and unhappy about changes in their prescribed medication to a generic brand. Complaints to doctors and pharmacists have increased as a consequence. While the majority of patients claimed that they would be willing to consume less expensive versions of drugs, there was an unwillingness to take more frequent doses of shorter acting drugs.

The report concluded with a list of recommendations, including a call for the establishment of a national pharmacoepidemiology database and a linked prescribing and morbidity database, the introduction of quality assurance instruments, the use of pharmacoeconomic evaluations, the development of local area formularies, and more patient participation in the scheme.

The effect of government controls on the growth in prices of pharmaceuticals, the level of prices in Ireland in comparison with those in other countries, the penetration of the market by generics, and the growth in expenditure on pharmaceuticals in the public sector, were analysed by Nolan.[16] She concluded that while price increases may have contributed to an increase in expenditure in the past, since 1990 the Agreements between the IPHA and the Department of Health have resulted in downward pressure on prices. In comparing the prices of the top-twenty branded products across 12 European countries, she found that Ireland had moved from ninth to seventh position between 1988 and 1992. The penetration of the market by generics was low. She found that the generic medicines share of the market had remained at 6–7 per cent since the mid 1980s. This is attributable to a number of causes: the fact that doctors are free to prescribe the medicines of their choice; their belief that patients are less likely to be compliant in taking their medication if the physical appearance changes with each issue; the pressure to prescribe generically has not been strong, as pharmacists are not permitted to substitute and must by law dispense what appears on the patient's prescription; and that generic manufacturers in Ireland have chosen to market branded generics as opposed to unbranded generics. Finally,

---

* For a more detailed analysis of the private health insurance market in Ireland see Kinsella and O Healai, 1997.[19]

Health Expenditure and Cost Containment in Ireland 503

in analysing the growth in expenditure, Nolan found that expenditure on medicines in the GMS scheme, the Long-Term Illness Scheme, and the Drug Refund Scheme, had almost doubled between 1982 and 1992.

10.10 Private Health Insurance*

The Voluntary Health Insurance (VHI) Board was established in 1957 as a non-profit state sponsored body, under the Voluntary Health Insurance Act. Its primary role at that time was to provide cover for hospital charges to those on high incomes who fell outside the scope of the public sector services. A secondary role was to attract subscribers from among those eligible for free services, with a view to encouraging the notion of self-reliance and reducing some of the financial burden on the Exchequer.

Private health insurance in Ireland is supplementary to public entitlement. However, over 1.3 million people subscribe to the VHI in order to gain more rapid access to certain medical procedures as well as a higher standard of non-medical facilities (Table 10.15 overleaf). Since its establishment, VHI membership has grown steadily throughout the 1960s and 1970s. After a substantial rise between 1980 and 1982, membership as a percentage of the population remained static until 1987 when significant growth resumed. In more recent years membership of the VHI has levelled off.

Health insurance premiums are typically paid for by the individual or the individual's employer as part of their salary package. Group schemes exist in many companies, thus enabling members to avail themselves of reduced premiums of approximately 10 per cent. Until recently, health insurance premiums qualified for tax relief at the member's highest rate of tax. In the Finance Act of 1994, however, tax relief on health insurance premiums was reduced to the standard rate of tax, currently 27 per cent. It is likely that this tax concession will be eroded in the coming years.

The VHI monopoly of private health care insurance has enabled it to adopt community rating from the outset. Under this system, premiums for a given level of benefits are set at the same rate for all subscribers irrespective of age, sex and health status. The Health Insurance Act, which came into effect on 1 July 1994, opened the way for competition in the health insurance market. However, the Act requires insurers operating in the market to comply with the principles of community rating; that is to provide open

504 *Health Care and Cost Containment in the European Union*

Table 10.15 VHI Membership and percentage of the population covered, 1958–93

	Membership	Percentage of population
1958	23,238	0.8
1960	78,778	2.8
1967	288,496	10.0
1968	321,777	11.0
1969	357,051	12.2
1970	386,726	13.1
1975	524,525	16.5
1978	645,165	19.5
1979	697,346	20.7
1980	843,309	24.8
1981	935,804	27.2
1982	995,284	28.6
1983	1,013,745	28.9
1984	1,028,194	29.1
1985	1,033,261	29.2
1986	1,032,709	29.2
1987	1,037,780	29.3
1988	1,078,423	30.5
1989	1,107,954	31.5
1990	1,129,543	32.2
1991	1,165,624	33.1
1992	1,193,965	33.6
1993	1,222,205	34.3

Source: Department of Health, Voluntary health Insurance Board, various years.[2,20]

enrolment (i.e. no individual who wishes to enroll may be turned away); and to offer life-time cover (i.e. an insurer will not be allowed to refuse to renew a contract on the basis of excessive claims). In order to support community rating/open enrolment all insurers are obliged to provide a minimum level of benefits relating to hospital in-patient services. The existing legislation, and in particular the establishment of a risk equalization fund, prevents insurers from using product design and selective marketing techniques to obtain low-risk individuals. The risk equalization scheme involves an insurer with a majority of low-risk individuals contributing to a fund, and one with high-risk profiles receiving compensation from a jointly funded pool in order to balance the impact of open enrolment. To date, BUPA is the only company of this type to begin trading on the Irish market.

The transition to the new market structure has not been without difficulty. BUPA Ireland's products, a low-cost community-rated medical care plan and a risk-rated cash plan, were opposed by Government and the VHI just days before BUPA was to begin trading. Essentially, they believed that the strategy of separating products adopted by BUPA Ireland undermined the principle of community rating, and feared a reduction in the numbers covered by the VHI and an overloading of the public medical care system. BUPA, on the other hand, argued that its strategy was consistent with the Health Insurance Act which excluded cash plans from the Regulations. However, following intensive government pressure, including the threat of de-registration, BUPA Ireland agreed to introduce a new range of community-rated products and to replace existing cash plans with a range focused on the established cash plan market.[19]

These difficulties in the private health insurance market highlighted a number of ambiguities and distortions in the legislation. They may also explain why only one company to date has entered the private health insurance market. It is generally believed that other possible entrants want to observe the functioning of the risk equalization fund, and are waiting for the scheduled evaluation of the Regulations in 1998 before committing themselves to the Irish market. Future developments in this market are difficult to predict given recent events.

10.11 Technology assessment

The Department of Health has control over expenditure on new medical

506 *Health Care and Cost Containment in the European Union*

equipment which cannot be financed from the current budget of the health board or hospital. Health boards or hospitals requiring new equipment apply directly to the Department for funding. However, in recent years many hospitals have organized voluntary fundraising activities to assist with the purchase of expensive medical equipment and have only approached the Department for financial support to operate or maintain this equipment. The Department has no control over the purchase of equipment in the private sector.

Technology assessment is undertaken on an ongoing basis by medical, engineering and administrative staff at the Department of Health. No independent technology assessment unit exists in Ireland, despite the recommendation of the Commission on Health Funding for the establishment of a multi-disciplinary department within an Irish university to undertake joint epidemiological, clinical and economic research. However, with the publication of the health strategy document, *Shaping a Healthier Future*, calls for the introduction of formal systems of appraisal have once again been made.

10.12 Dental services

For persons with *Category One* eligibility and their dependents and preschool and national school children referred from child health examinations, dental treatment and appliances are available without charge from over 300 dentists employed by the health boards. Other individuals (paying the full rate of Pay Related Social Insurance) are entitled to free dental services such as dental examinations, diagnosis and scaling, and subsidized treatment such as fillings, extractions, dentures and root canal therapy, under the Pay Related Social Insurance Scheme administered by the Department of Social Welfare. For the remainder of the population not covered by the Health Board, Social Welfare or employer funded schemes, the full cost of dental services provided by private practitioners must be met from their own resources. Routine treatment is not covered by the VHI. Similarly, the scheme of tax relief for unreimbursed medical expenses excludes routine dental treatment.

Public expenditure on dental treatment under Health Board schemes amounted to just over IEP 20 million pounds in 1993 compared with IEP 13 million in 1987. Expenditure under the Social Welfare scheme amounted to

Health Expenditure and Cost Containment in Ireland 507

just over IEP 19 million in 1995 compared with a little over IEP 12 million in 1987. Expenditure data on private dental treatment is not available. However, a study undertaken in 1987 estimated that private expenditure amounted to IEP 52 million, or two-thirds of all expenditure on dental treatment.[21]

In May 1994 the Dental Health Action Plan which focused on ways of improving oral health and the public dental services was published. The objectives outlined in the Plan and in the health strategy document *Shaping a Healthier Future* included the phased extension of eligibility for public dental services to children under 16 years; the phased improvement of primary and secondary orthodontic care for all children; the expansion of hospital oral surgery services to provide adequately for those who require specialized treatment; the phased introduction of new arrangements for the provision of dental care for eligible adults; and improvements in school dental services to ensure the systematic screening of children in three designated classes in primary and post-primary schools.

10.13 Shaping a Healthier Future: A Strategy for Effective Health Care in the 1990s[13]

In April 1994, *Shaping a Healthier Future* was published. The principal theme of the Strategy was the reorganization of the system to ensure greater effectiveness and efficiency in the planning and delivery of health services. Three key principles underpin the Strategy: equity, quality of service, and accountability.

Uniformity in the eligibility and charges for services, reductions in waiting times for public services, and special attention to disadvantaged groups were specified as essential steps in the pursuit of an equitable health service. The identification of health development sectors (i.e. geographic areas or population groups with low health status) and ways of improving the health status of these sectors through the establishment of pilot schemes, were policy objectives outlined in the Strategy. Since the publication of the Strategy, some pilot projects have been established to consider access to health care for travellers. Issues being addressed include the processing of medical cards and a peer-led health promotion intervention programme. A policy document on travellers' health is to be published.

508   *Health Care and Cost Containment in the European Union*

In the pursuit of quality, both technical and service quality were highlighted as being essential attributes. Hence, providers of services should ensure that the best outcome is achieved given the resources expended (technical quality), and that the consumer is satisfied (service quality). To guarantee technical quality, the development of information systems, the evaluation of technology (a formal system of technology assessment is to be introduced) and the promotion of clinical audit were recommended. Measuring consumer preferences and the levels of consumer satisfaction were deemed important in the Strategy. Since the publication of the Strategy, each health board has appointed new Directors of Public Health. These Directors have begun to evaluate the health needs of their areas and to identify health outcome measures so that improvements can be made in the planning and delivery of services.

Finally, formal legal and financial accountability arrangements were recommended, and those providing services were asked to take responsibility for the achievement of agreed objectives. To assist with these objectives, a major reorganization of the health services was set out in the Strategy. Some of the changes outlined in the Strategy include the replacement of the Eastern Health Board with a new authority which would have full responsibility for health and social services in the Eastern region while the remaining health boards (to be re-named health authorities) would be responsible for all services within their regions. Further, the Department of Health would no longer be involved in the detailed management or direct funding of individual services. Instead the Department would be responsible for advising and supporting the Minister in determining national policy and the annual health estimates, determining the financial allocation of the regional authorities, determining the overall personnel policies within which health authorities function, monitoring and evaluating the service and financial performance of the authorities against national objectives and standards, and identifying and supporting the introduction of more effective management practices. Since the publication of the Strategy, each health board and voluntary agency has been required to draw up a detailed service plan at the beginning of each financial year, and proposals for the re-structuring of the Eastern Health Board have commenced.

A Four Year Action Plan was an integral part of the Health Strategy. The Plan includes national targets for reductions in risk factors associated with premature mortality, targets for improvements in other indicators of health status, and objectives for service development. Areas addressed in the

Plan include health promotion, general practitioner services, dental services, women's health, family planning, children's health, child care and family support services, travellers' health, drug misuse, food and medicine control, acute hospital services, HIV/AIDS, ill and dependent elderly, palliative care, mental illness, and disability. For each service area deficiencies and ways of improving the existing system were outlined.

All of the areas identified in the Four Year Action Plan are currently being addressed. For example, problems with GP services included the fragmentation of general practice and the isolation of GPs, the lack of epidemiological data relating to morbidity in the community, the lack of defined practice population, and the high proportion of the population who do not closely identify with one GP. Plans to improve the service included the establishment of single-centre or multi-centre group practices which would provide a comprehensive range of primary health care services, the development of a detailed information network for GPs, the introduction of a system of patient registration and the development of protocols of combined care for specific conditions between consultants and GPs. Since the publication of the Strategy document, changes which have occurred include better rota arrangements for out-of-hours cover in rural areas, more practice support staff, the establishment of a National Medicines Information Centre, and health board general practice units are encouraging the development of referral, discharge and therapeutic protocols by GPs and hospital consultants.

10.14 Conclusions

The Irish health care system combines public and private financing with public and private provision. Over the past 10–15 years a number of reforms have been introduced to improve the financing and delivery of health services. To assess the effectiveness of these policies some key indicators may be examined – health expenditure, hospital data and health outcomes.[1,12]

The trends in nominal health expenditure have previously been discussed. However, key findings from the latest OECD survey of the Irish economy suggest that Ireland has experienced a reduction in the share of GDP devoted to health compared with many other OECD countries. In their view this reduction is attributable to the control of public health expenditure.

510 *Health Care and Cost Containment in the European Union*

Hospital productivity has also improved over the past decade due to better management of hospital facilities.[12] For example, the admission rate to Irish hospitals for in-patient care has fallen, the use of day-care treatment has increased, the average length of stay fell by 29 per cent between 1980 and 1993, the average bed occupancy rate has increased to nearly 85 per cent, and the number of hospital beds has declined by 40 per cent. Further improvements in productivity are likely with the extension of case-mix analysis for hospital budgeting.

The health of the population has also improved in recent years. Life expectancy at birth has increased substantially, while loss of life among the young has declined.[1,12] However, it is difficult to attribute these changes solely to the provision of improved health services.

Over the coming years, significant changes in the financing and delivery of health care services are unlikely. However, some policy changes are necessary as a number of pressures on the health care system emerge.[12] Areas which need to be addressed include: the rise in the pay of health service personnel and in the overall cost of medicines paid for by the Government; the existence of a bureaucratic hospital management system with little devolution of budgetary authority and lack of communication between management and medical staff; the divide between public and private provision of medical care, whereby patients use hospitals rather than GP services because charges are lower; and competition within the private health insurance market.

References

1 OECD. *The Reform of Health Care: A Comparative Analysis of Seven OECD Countries.* OECD, 1992.

2 Department of Health. *Health Statistics.* Dublin: Stationery Office, various years.

3 Nolan B. *Health Service Utilisation and Financing in Ireland.* Dublin: The Economic and Social Research Institute, General Research Series Paper No. 155, 1991.

4 Central Statistics Office. *National Income and Expenditure.* Dublin: Stationery Office, various years.

5 Nolan B. *Charging for Public Health Services in Ireland: Why and How?* Dublin: The Economic and Social Research Institute, Policy Research Series Paper No. 19, 1993.

6 Stationery Office. *Report of the Commission on Health Funding.* Dublin, September 1989.

Health Expenditure and Cost Containment in Ireland 511

7   Department of Health. *Information Guide to Our Health Services*. Dublin, 1996.

8   General Medical Services (Payments) Board. *Annual Report*. Dublin, various years.

9   Wiley MM, Fetter RB. *Measuring Activity and Costs in Irish Hospitals: a Study of Hospital Case-Mix*. Dublin: The Economic and Social Research Institute, Paper 147, 1990.

10 Wiley MM. Budgeting for acute hospital services in Ireland: the case-mix adjustment. *Journal of the Irish Colleges of Physicians and Surgeons* 1995;24(4):283–90.

11 Durkan J. *Health Care Expenditure in Ireland – A Comparative Analysis and Policy Issues, Centre for Health Economics*. Dublin: University College Dublin, Working Paper 94–4, 1994.

12 OECD. *OECD Economic Surveys 1996–1997*. OECD, 1997.

13 Stationery Office. *Shaping a Healthier Future: A Strategy for Effective Health Care in the 1990s*. Dublin: Department of Health, 1994.

14 Hensey B. *The Health Services of Ireland*. Dublin: Institute of Public Administration, 1988.

15 Comhairle na n-Ospideal. *Annual Report, 1992*.

16 Nolan A. *Medicine Costs in the Context of Overall Health Care Costs in Ireland*. Dublin: University College Dublin, Centre for Health Economics, Working Paper 94-2, 1994.

17 Department of Health. *The Future of General Practice in Ireland* (not available publicly).

18 Murphy M. *Review of Indicative Drugs Target Saving Scheme*. July 1997. (commissioned by the Department of Health from the University of Cork, not available publicly).

19 Kinsella R, O Healai R. *Private Medical Insurance in Ireland: Issues and Challenges*. Dublin (unpublished paper).

20 Voluntary Health Insurance Board. *Annual Report and Accounts*. Dublin, various years.

21 Coopers and Lybrand. *Oral Health Care Manpower 1986–2000*. Dublin, 1987.

11 Cost containment and reforms in the Italian National Health Service

GIOVANNI FATTORE

11.1 Introduction

This chapter focuses on the Italian health care system in the early 1990s and discusses the two main issues which have dominated policy action: the reform of the NHS (established in 1978) and the reduction of public health care expenditure. The first section briefly describes the structure of the Italian National Health Service (NHS). The two subsequent sections review the NHS during the 1980s. Section 11.5 discusses the main cost containment measures adopted in the 1990s, while section 11.6 examines the content of the health care reform approved in 1992 and provides a critical interpretation of this reform. A brief description of the expanding private health care market follows, and some final remarks close the chapter.

11.2 The Italian National Health Service

In 1978, a radical reform re-shaped the Italian health care system. The old system based on compulsory social insurance was replaced with a National Health Service. This transformation had few precedents in the history of the Italian social policy[1] and constituted one of the most radical health care reforms in Western Europe since the end of the Second World War.*

---

* For a global description of the evolution of the Italian health care system see OECD, 1994[2] and Whitaker, 1994.[3] For detailed descriptions of the 1978 reform see also Citoni and Di Biase, 1990[4] and Garattini, 1992.[5]

Such a grand reform was made possible by the exceptional political momentum of that time. The legislation that created the Italian NHS was approved by a National Solidarity coalition including the Communist Party. This coalition, which lasted just one year, was the political expression of the *'Compromesso Storico'*, a search for agreement on basic democratic and social issues between the two dominant social and ideological movements in Italian society at the time: the Communists and the Christian Democrats.

Consequently, the principles of solidarity, statism and social participation largely inspired the health care reform. Expressed by both the Communist and Christian Democrat parties, albeit with significant differences, these principles shaped a vision of the new health care system that has been labelled 'full democratic universalism'.[1] The fundamental ideas underlying the Italian NHS are that health services have to be made available to everyone on the basis of need, with no differentiation or discrimination among citizens and no barriers at the point of use, and that the system should be subject to popular democratic control at national, regional and local level. Also, the institutional and organizational structure of the Italian NHS was strongly influenced by the idea that barriers between levels of care had to be suppressed and that all the different types of services (preventive, curative, rehabilitative, related to the environment) had to be provided to a specific population by a single organization.

Most of the features of the system which emerged from the 1978 reform reflected these principles. Coverage was made universal by offering entitlement to NHS services to all Italian citizens and permanent residents. Sickness funds were abolished and all the financial resources which were fuelling the previous system were channelled into the government's budget. Legislative and procedural disparities among the beneficiaries of the sickness funds were cancelled, while most health care workers were made civil servants under national contracts.

The NHS is financed through the National Health Fund, annually determined in the government budget (*legge finanziaria*). Although the 1978 reform advocated the use of general taxation revenues to fund the NHS, payroll taxes have always been the most important source of financing. In 1996, they accounted for 53 per cent of the Italian NHS current expenditure, while general national taxation covered about 39 per cent (Figure 11.1).

From an organizational point of view, the reform allocated political and administrative responsibilities on health matters to the three main levels of public authority: the State, the regions and the communes. At the national

Figure 11.1 Funding sources of the Italian NHS in 1996

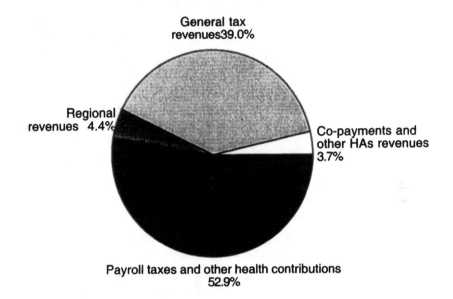

Source: Ministero del Bilancio, 1996.[6]

level, the Ministry of Health is responsible for comprehensive planning, the allocation of resources among regions, the negotiation of contracts with the NHS personnel and with private providers, and most of the regulatory functions concerning drugs and medical equipment. Regions provide the intermediate tier of the NHS, between the Ministry of Health and the local health units. Italian Regions were established in the early 1970s and are provided with legislative power. In the health care field, their main functions were to plan health services in the region consistently with national priorities, to allocate financial resources among local health units, and to monitor and evaluate their performance.

Lastly, until 1990, communes were the third institutional tier of the NHS, as they had to give strategic guidance to local health units and appointed their management boards. Local health units, which numbered 659 before the 1992 reform, were the key elements of the Italian NHS. They were designed to achieve a complete integration of the whole range of health care activities to promote the health conditions of the population, thus

516   *Health Care and Cost Containment in the European Union*

ending the former fragmentation of the health care system. As a consequence, their tasks included: primary care, sanitation, out-patient specialist services, family planning services, acute and long-term hospital care, mental health, provision of medicines, occupational health, rehabilitation, veterinary medicine and, until recently, several activities related to environmental hazards.

11.3 The 1980s: institutional weaknesses and implementation problems

The health care system which emerged from the 1978 reform had various shortcomings. These had three main sources: the weaknesses of the institutional framework designed by the legislators, the ambiguous role of the private sector and the social and political climate of the 1980s which, in turn, influenced the implementation of the reform.

Seen almost twenty years later, the institutional arrangement chosen for the Italian NHS looks 'baroque'. In theory, democratic control of the system was assured by the political accountability of public authorities to voters at three levels: national, regional and local. In practice, this kind of accountability was very difficult to achieve for two reasons: (a) voters could not relate their judgements about the NHS to a particular political tier; and (b) the accountability chain was weakened by the proportional representation system which tends to generate multiparty and unstable coalition governments. Rather than being democratically controlled, the system was over-politicized, especially at local level.[7] In fact, management board members were part-time politicians with little or no previous experience in health care administration.[8]

Health policy-making reflected the NHS structure based on three institutional tiers. Calls for greater autonomy and responsibility at regional and local level were countered with national attempts to keep the system under financial control and to assure the geographical equity goals of the 1978 reform. As a result, relationships between the three tiers were often based on conflicts, decision-making processes were slow and cumbersome, and the scope of accountability at each tier was unclear.[9, 10]

Unlike some other countries with a National Health Service, such as the UK, a significant share of the Italian NHS budget is spent on private for-

Cost Containment and Reforms in the Italian National Health Service 517

profit and non-profit-making organizations. In 1982, 9.7 per cent of the NHS budget was used to fund private hospitals and a further 5.8 per cent to fund private specialists. In 1995, the corresponding figures were 10.5 per cent and 2.5 per cent.[6] The public-private mix in the provision of health services is thus a structural feature of the Italian NHS, particularly in the central and southern regions of the country.

While the private hospital sector may have played a relevant role in improving access to care for populations residing in areas lacking public facilities, the contribution of contracted providers to the development of the Italian NHS has been questioned.[11] In many circumstances private providers used their competitive advantages in terms of flexibility and autonomy to improve ancillary services, to introduce new expensive technologies and, presumably, to secure themselves the most remunerative patients. The relationship between private providers and the NHS was neither complementary nor competitive. It was not complementary because Local Hospital Units (LHUs) and regions could not manage a strategic control over these providers. And it was not competitive because, *de facto*, the market shares of private providers were in political hands and were independent of their performance.

With the 1978 reform all hospital doctors became public employees. However, public employment and private practice were not made legally incompatible.[11] Doctors opting for reduced-time status (28 hours instead of 38 per week) within the public service were allowed to practice privately. In 1987, more than one-third of public hospital doctors opted for this status. In addition, there is large anecdotal evidence that private practice is very common among doctors opting for a full-time status.

Dual practice poses two main problems. The first concerns equity: despite principles established by the 1978 reform, the presence of dual practice can make access to medical services dependent on private payments. Results of a national survey conducted in 1990 show that more than 10 million specialist visits were privately funded by patients.[12]

The second problem is related to perverse incentives at work: attracted by additional income, privately practising doctors have strong incentives to expand (or at least to preserve) their private market and, consequently, to leave unmet demand in the public sector. It is therefore clear that dual practice may discourage doctors from pressing for more efficiency in the public system.

There was little evidence of any strong political commitment to fix the

518 *Health Care and Cost Containment in the European Union*

problem of dual practice in the 1980s. However, there was, and remains, no easy solution to this problem once the basic framework of the NHS was established. The NHS reform was 'naive' in its attempt to control the medical profession. It formally attributed to doctors a civil servant status, along with the consequences, such as lack of financial incentives, career progression mainly based on age, and job security. However, doctors *de facto* enjoyed a wide degree of freedom to achieve professional and economic satisfaction outside the public sector.

The weaknesses of the structure envisaged for the NHS were amplified by inadequate policy-making and implementation during the 1980s. Since the beginning of the decade, a shift in the ideological and political climate changed the attitude towards the Italian welfare state. As in many other Western societies, popular enthusiasm for welfare programmes decreased and cost containment issues started to dominate the political agenda. In 1979, the influence of the Communist Party on Italian politics at national level started to decline and a moderate alliance replaced the coalition which had approved the reform bill. The new government included the Liberals, a minor party that opposed legislation in 1978, but provided three Ministers of Health between 1985 and 1995.

As a result of this political shift, health policy never ranked very high in the national political agenda during the 1980s. Presumably, the ruling coalition felt that the principles behind the NHS were not aligned with their political ideas, but at the same time felt that radical health policy action was a dangerous ground for political confrontation. Two consequences derived from this lack of political commitment to legislative and policy action. First, the national government was very slow in amending the reform bill, although it was clear from the beginning that corrections were needed.

Second, there was a very weak commitment to implementation issues. Such a radical reform would have required a massive investment to support health planning and financing at central and regional level, to build new information systems, to provide clear guidance to the local health units, to promote large educational programmes aimed at training health and administrative personnel. Instead, very little attention was paid to these issues so that implementation proceeded slowly and without clear and effective guidance from the Ministry of Health. Moreover, the planning system envisaged by the 1978 reform was never implemented: in the 1980s no National Health Plan was made operational and only a few regions produced regional plans.

Cost Containment and Reforms in the Italian National Health Service 519

11.4 The 1980s: first attempts to cost containment

In a decentralized system such as the Italian NHS, scope for keeping the system under financial control is influenced by the way power is distributed among the three tiers of government. To a certain extent, the national tier can be considered a third payer with only limited control over the expenditure processes. Indeed, while the national government perceived the political costs of funding the system and hence tried to keep expenditure under control, the LHUs did not have strong incentives to do so as high expenditure benefited local politicians and their voters.

It is likely that only the devolution of strong financial responsibility to the regions and LHUs could have protected the national tier from overspending. But this was not possible, mainly because the centralized nature of the Italian fiscal system prevented any attempt to enforce Regions' and Local Authorities' financial accountability. Also, the unspecified right to health care enshrined in the 1978 reform provided ample room for local and regional claims that funding was inadequate and that overspending was unavoidable in order to provide essential care to the population. Predictably, as Mapelli had already suggested in the early 1980s, this situation produced a vicious circle.[13] Total funding was determined on the basis of macroeconomic compatibility, with little regard for expected expenditure and no account taken of future deficits. During the fiscal year, the regions and LHUs ran short of resources and claimed that without additional funds adequate care could not be provided. As a result, the central government conceded supplementary funding and, often, promised to cover deficits. Finally, confident that any deficit would be met by the State, regions and LHUs planned to overspend, *de facto* acting without an actual financial constraint. The impact of this *modus operandi* had three main consequences:

(a) health care expenditure during the 1980s and the early 1990s always exceeded planned budgets; *ex-ante* funding differed from *ex-post* expenditure with regional and local tiers being the real decision-makers on the levels of expenditure;

(b) the NHS was dominated by a climate of acute uncertainty over financial resources, creating a tendency to day-to-day management;[11] and

(c) this situation favoured the introduction of various cost containment measures that interfered with the LHUs' autonomy and further delegit-

520 *Health Care and Cost Containment in the European Union*

imized the determination of the national NHS budget as a way to keep the expenditure under control.[14]

Since the late 1970s Italian governments have adopted two main types of cost containment measures: co-payments on pharmaceutical and out-patient care, and regulations aimed at limiting specific LHUs expenditure.[15] As far as the former are concerned, they have been very erratic over time as it is shown in Table 11.1.

The first (very modest) co-payment system was introduced in 1978 on 'non-essential' drugs. It was then substantially revised in 1983, when a proportional charge (15 per cent) was introduced. However, co-payments were effectively capped since patients were only required to pay up to a certain amount.

Co-payments, as well as the maximum amount due per prescription, were increased several times during the 1980s and the early 1990s. With the 1994 re-classification of the positive list (see below), the co-payment system was radically revised. At present, patients pay 50 per cent of the price of drugs classified in class B (a relatively short list of products) and ITL 3,000 (ECU 1.5) per item prescribed (up to ITL 6,000) for drugs covered by the NHS.

In 1982, specialist visits, laboratory tests and other diagnostic procedures were also subjected to co-payment. Being very unpopular, regulation on this co-payment has been changed several times and was even abolished between 1986 and 1989. In 1994, patients were required to pay the full cost of out-patient care up to ITL 100,000 per visit. Despite the fact that this amount was lowered to ITL 70,000 in 1995, the amount of co-payment for out-patient care appears substantial. At present, patients' revenue as a share of gross cost is probably higher for out-patient care than for pharmaceuticals.

The introduction of co-payments has been accompanied by a long list of rules establishing exemption criteria. Initially, these criteria were mainly based on personal income. The system was then gradually refined by taking into consideration family size, age and occupation. At the same time, full exemption was also granted to the disabled, to individuals affected by certain chronic illnesses, and to pregnant women.

These measures contributed to raising additional funds and, presumably, to reduce consumption. Unfortunately, however, the reduction in consumption caused by co-payments is unknown as there are no recent studies

Cost Containment and Reforms in the Italian National Health Service 521

Table 11.1 Major changes in patient charges regulations for pharmaceutical and out-patient care between 1978 and 1995

Year	Pharmaceuticals	Out-patient care
1978	A moderate fixed-charge system is introduced on drugs classified "not essential".	
1982		A charge system is introduced on specialist visits and diagnostic procedures (15% of cost subjected to a maximum amount).
1983	Drugs are classified into three classes: A no charge; B and C are subject to co-payment (15% + flat rate).	
1987		The charge system is abolished.
1989	Proportional co-payment is increased and differentiated according to two classes of drugs (30% and 40%); a ceiling on the amount due on each prescription (ITL 30,000) is introduced. Exemption criteria are substantially enlarged.	The charge system is reintroduced at a higher rate (30%).
1992	Co-payment percentages and the ceiling per prescription are increased (30% and 50%; ITL 50,000).	
1993	Exemption criteria are radically changed: pensioners can get a bonus of 16 free prescriptions per year.	Criteria for exemption from charges on out-patient care are made more similar to those for drugs.
1994	The positive list is radically revised (see section 11.3.1). The bonus system is abolished; income selectivity is replaced by age selectivity.	Non-exempted patients pay for out-patient care up to ITL 100,000.
1995	Income criteria added to age selectivity for exemption to co-payment.	The ITL 100,000 deductible is lowered to ITL 70,000.

Sources: Mapelli, 1995;[15] Farmindustria, 1997.[16]

522   *Health Care and Cost Containment in the European Union*

attempting to estimate the charge/volume elasticity.

Whatever the potential impact, in practice the effect of co-payment regulation was weakened by the large number of exemptions. In 1991, the number of exempted people was almost a quarter of the population, while this segment of the population was responsible for three-quarters of total public pharmaceutical expenditure.[17]

Measures aimed at limiting specific types of LHU expenditure, the second set of measures mentioned above, were very popular during the 1980s. They included freezes on staff hiring, ceilings on the purchase of goods and services, and the introduction of standards in the provision of hospital care (in terms of personnel per bed ratios, minimum occupancy rates, minimum beds per hospital). Although these measures seemed to be sensible in a situation where large savings were supposed to be achievable by just improving the efficiency in the provision of services, they were based on the assumption that production processes could be regulated from central government. Instead, not only did most of these measures not produce the expected results, but they also tended to increase the degree of bureaucratic control over the LHUs, limiting further the scope for the development of managerial control and accountability in public health care organizations.[9]

Overall, the cost containment measures undertaken during the 1980s were not very effective: the proportion of GDP spent on the NHS increased from 5.6 per cent at the launch of the reform to 6.3 per cent in 1990 (Table 11.2). The budget for the NHS was always overshot so that NHS expenditure has never been known in advance, and the NHS has accumulated a deficit of ITL 67,000 billion from its inception to 1995.[15] However, NHS expenditure did not explode during the 1980s: the rate of growth was lower than that forecast at the launch of the reform, and part of the increase is attributable to the fact that access to health services was made universal and that differences in per capita expenditure among regions were reduced.

11.5 The 1990s: reducing public expenditure becomes a must

The cost containment imperative gained political momentum in the early 1990s. After having accumulated an impressive public debt during the 1980s, Italy was forced to take decisive action to reduce its public deficit. A growing awareness of the need to improve the public financial performance finally pervaded the political agenda, under pressure from the requirements

Cost Containment and Reforms in the Italian National Health Service 523

Table 11.2 Public health care expenditure in the European Union, 1980–95

	Public health care expenditure as % of GDP				Public health care expenditure as % of total health care expenditure			
	1980	1985	1990	1995	1980	1985	1990	1995
Austria	5.4	5.2	5.3	5.9	68.8	77.6	75.0	75.6
Belgium	5.5	6.0	6.7	7.0	83.4	81.8	88.9	87.8
Denmark	5.8	5.3	5.3	5.3	85.2	84.4	82.3	82.7
Finland	5.1	5.7	6.5	5.8	79.0	78.6	80.9	74.7
France	6.0	6.5	6.6	8.0	78.8	76.9	74.5	80.6
Germany	6.3	6.6	6.3	8.2	79.2	77.9	76.8	78.4
Greece	2.9	3.3	3.5	4.4	82.2	81.0	82.3	75.8
Ireland	7.2	6.1	4.9	5.1	82.2	77.4	74.7	80.8
Italy	5.6	5.5	6.3	5.4	80.5	77.2	78.1	69.6
Luxembourg	5.7	5.5	6.1	6.5	92.8	89.2	93.1	92.8
Netherlands	5.9	5.9	6.1	6.8	74.7	75.1	72.7	77.1
Portugal	3.7	3.4	4.3	5.0	64.3	54.6	65.5	60.5
Spain	4.5	4.6	5.4	6.0	79.9	81.1	78.7	78.2
Sweden	8.7	8.1	7.9	5.9	92.5	90.4	89.9	81.6
United Kingdom	5.0	5.0	5.1	5.9	89.4	85.8	84.1	84.3
EU	5.6	5.5	5.8	6.1	80.9	79.3	79.8	78.7

Source: OECD Database 1997.[18]

of the Maastricht Treaty. As a result, various ways to cut public expenditure have been explored: from reducing funding for local governments, to putting ceilings on public-sector wage increases, from delaying major infrastructure investments, to reforming the pension system.

As a major component of public expenditure, NHS expenditure has been the target of many measures. Indeed, because of constraints in other sectors, special attention has been focused on health expenditure, an area in

524 *Health Care and Cost Containment in the European Union*

which the government has a greater degree of freedom.[19] Within health care expenditure, the preferred target of cost containment policy during the 1990s was the pharmaceutical sector.

11.5.1 Reducing the drug bill

In 1992 an impressive series of scandals made Italian people aware that hundreds of politicians, senior civil servants, 'experts' and businessmen systematically handled bribes, using public money for political and personal purposes. To most Italians, the corruption of the old regime is symbolized by what happened with pharmaceuticals. The Minister of Health (a prominent medicine professor), the head of the Pharmaceutical Division of the Department of Health, the President and most of the members of the committee in charge determining prices, the President of the Italian Pharmaceutical Industry Association, and many company executives were charged with systematically giving and receiving bribes for drug registrations and pricing.

With the pressure mounting to contain expenditure, this situation favoured the most radical change in Italian pharmaceutical policy ever. The first step of the new area was to re-define the positive list. In 1994, a renewed Committee for Drugs (CUF - *Commissione Unica per il Farmaco*) re-classified products into three categories: drugs for severe and chronic illness (class A, no proportional co-payment), drugs of therapeutic importance (class B, 50 per cent co-payment) and other drugs (class C, not available under the NHS). A fixed charge of ITL 3,000 (ECU 1.5) per item was introduced on all NHS prescriptions (classes A and B). The fixed rate is paid by almost all citizens, while large population groups (elderly, low income individuals, pregnant women etc.) are exempted from the proportional co-payment due on drugs in class B.

The CUF was mandated by the Government to make decisions consistent with an annual budget for 1994 of no more than ITL 10,000 billion, ITL 2,400 billion less than the expenditure in 1993. In three months it prepared the new positive list according to four criteria: (a) demonstration of clinical efficacy, documented by controlled clinical trials; (b) the risk-benefit balance of the therapy; (c) acceptability of the therapy to patients; and (d) cost of the therapy. The new list was radically different from the previous one, since government funding for several hundred active ingredients was

Cost Containment and Reforms in the Italian National Health Service   525

Table 11.3 Pharmaceuticals covered by the NHS and public pharmaceutical expenditure, 1992–95 (ITL billion)

Year	Number of active principles (class A: fully reimbursed)	(class B: 50% reimbursed)	Net public expenditure (a)	Co-payment on products covered by the NHS (b)	Total (a)+(b)
1992	115	1,404	14,491	2,833	17,324
1993	115	1,380	12,616	2,433	15,049
1994	652	119	10,379	1,339	11,718
1995	687	120	9,782	1,557	11,339

Source: Garattini *et al.*, 1995;[20] Bozzini and Martini, 1996.[21]

eliminated (Table 11.3).

Almost simultaneously, price regulation was radically modified. In 1993 the Committee on Pharmaceuticals (*CIP Farmaci*), the body charged with determining drug prices was abolished, and a year later the Interdepartmental Committee on Economic Planning (CIPE) announced a new method of regulating prices that replaced the previous one based on cost estimates derived mainly from information provided by companies.

The basic principle of the new system is that prices are free but cannot exceed Average European Prices (AEP). For the sake of simplicity only France, Germany, Spain and the United Kingdom are taken into consideration in deriving the AEP. For each of these four countries, national prices are converted into Italian lira using Purchasing-Power-Parities (PPPs), a well-known price index widely used for international comparative studies. The Government required that prices above AEP were lowered immediately, while prices below were allowed to increase only by 20 per cent per year.

Not surprisingly, the pharmaceutical industry considered various elements of the new pricing system as a subterfuge to depress prices. In particular, it was the use of PPPs instead of exchange rates that was most fiercely criticized. It has been argued that using PPPs to convert national currencies artificially imposes differences in the prices of pharmaceuticals across Europe, and can penalize companies that purchase licenses, raw material or unfinished products abroad since their prices reflect exchange rates instead

526   *Health Care and Cost Containment in the European Union*

of PPPs.[22] *

In 1995 the pharmaceutical sector was once again the target for NHS savings: a generalized price cut of either 2.5 or 5 per cent was mandated by the government and the annual increase for products with price below the European Average was not granted. Concurrently, the Government announced, in very general terms, its interest in introducing a reference price system.

One year later an Italian version of reference pricing was introduced. The new pricing system can be summarized under the statement 'same prices for same drugs'. The basic idea is that prices of products made of the same active principle, with the same method of administration and having the same or comparable pharmaceutical form, must have the same price per unit of compound. For example, suppose an active ingredient (AI) is marketed in four different products. For each of the four products the price per unit of the AI (i.e. the cost per mg) is calculated by dividing the price of each product by the total amount of AI that it contains. The lowest value among the four unit prices is then multiplied by the amount of AI contained in each product. The results of these calculations are the new prices (obviously, for one product the price remains unchanged).

This methodology looks like 'phase 1' of the German reference price system. However, despite the very basic idea of this 'pricing' methodology, prices were not freed – if the company does not accept the new price the product is delisted. As expected, many pharmaceutical companies reduced prices to maintain their products under NHS coverage. Some other companies decided not to reduce prices and their drugs were consequently delisted. As a result, more than 400 products were delisted and over 150 had their prices reduced by an average of 7 per cent**

The Budget Law for 1997 includes measures to curb further public pharmaceutical expenditure, but this time targeting pharmacists rather than producers. It turns the pharmacist's margin, previously set at a fixed 26 per cent proportional rate, into a system where pharmacists are forced to provide a

---

* The *'Consiglio di Stato'* has recently found that the way the AEP is calculated is illegitimate. Consequently, new legislation modifying various aspects of the system is awaited.

** A new deliberation of CIPE concerning innovative products registered through the centralized European procedure has been recently announced. The deliberation contains innovative elements such as that prices will be set by means of a negotiation, and that economic arguments are fully part of the material to be processed and discussed between the government and companies.[23]

discount to products covered by the NHS. Different discount rates apply to different price ranges in order to make the pharmacist's margin regressive (the higher the price, the lower the pharmacist's margin rate). This change is expected to reduce substantially the remuneration of pharmacists.

As a consequence of all these measures, Italy has been very effective in cutting public pharmaceutical expenditure. In just three years, expenditure was reduced by 32 per cent, that is ITL 4,600 billion (ECU 2.3 million). In 1992 public pharmaceutical expenditure was about 0.9 per cent of GDP. By 1996 this percentage has fallen to about 0.6 per cent.

The reduction in public pharmaceutical expenditure has been achieved without strong opposition from political parties, consumer associations or trade unions. Nor, with some exceptions, have doctors and patients shown any great dissatisfaction with the present list of drugs covered by the NHS. There are, however, situations where delisting has increased private expenditure as GPs and specialists have not modified their prescribing behaviour. Possibly this is because, at the individual patient level, the expectation is that delisted products are more beneficial. In fact, there has been a shifting effect from public to private expenditure (Figure 11.2). It is not yet clear

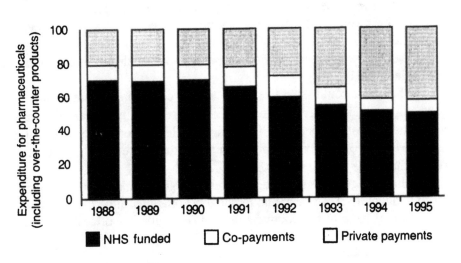

Figure 11.2 Public and private expenditure as percentage of pharmaceutical expenditure, 1988–95

Note: Private expenditure includes over-the-counter products.
Source: Farmindustria, 1996.[16]

528   *Health Care and Cost Containment in the European Union*

whether private pharmaceutical expenditure is a serious burden on low income groups.

Before 1993, pharmaceutical policy was legally and illegally driven by industrial interests. Since then, the health policy point of view has dominated the scene, completely neglecting the industrial policy perspective. In recent years the Italian government has fully used regulatory and monopsonistic power to get the best deals for the NHS. One attitude has been common to four different government coalitions: they all looked for savings from the pharmaceutical bill. It is evident that cutting pharmaceutical expenditure was more technically feasible and politically viable than implementing other cost containment measures.

11.5.2 Other cost containment measures

Accounting for more than 40 per cent of total public health care expenditure, the cost of personnel directly employed by the NHS is a key determinant for keeping expenditure under control (Table 11.4). Obviously, two elements constitute personnel costs: the number of employees and their unitary cost. As far as the volume of the NHS workforce is concerned, the central government has tried for many years to impose limitations on regions and local health units, mainly freezing staff hiring or turnover. Table 11.5 reports the recent trend in the number of NHS employees: during the entire period 1987–94 the number of NHS employees has constantly increased. However, while the number of nurses and especially doctors has increased substantially over the whole period, the number of non-health professionals has fallen since 1991.*

Although it could have been effective in containing personnel costs, controlling manpower actually resulted in greater rigidity in managing services and in costly procedures to circumvent legislation. Also, regulating manpower was considered at odds with attributing more managerial autonomy to hospitals and local health units.

In Italy wage and salary negotiations for NHS workers are underwritten at national level. There are no regional negotiations, although the implementation of parts of the contracts depend on regional and local decisions

---

* Interestingly, despite similar expenditure (both in absolute terms and as a percentage of GDP) Italy employes almost 500,000 less people in the NHS compared with the UK.

Cost Containment and Reforms in the Italian National Health Service 529

Table 11.4 Public expenditure in 1995 and the rate of increase between 1983 and 1995

	ITL billion 1995 (%)	Rate of increase (%) 1983–88	1988–91	1991–95	1983–95
Personnel	39,900 (41.3)	48.6	75.6	7.9	181.4
Goods and services	18,500 (19.2)	69.5	74.2	15.1	239.6
Primary Care (GPs)	5,550 (5.8)	37.5	63.6	-0.4	124.2
Pharmaceuticals*	9,800 (10.1)	80.7	62.3	-34.9	90.8
Private hospital care	10,500 (10.9)	64.0	66.4	16.9	219.0
Private specialist care	2,480 (2.6)	110.0	10.3	-33.7	53.6
Other	9,840 (10.2)	77.7	131.8	31.8	654.6
Total NHS Expenditure	96,570 (100)	61.7	65.8	2.9	188.7

* dispensed through pharmacies
Source: Ministero del Bilancio, various years.[6]

Table11.5 NHS employees at 1st January 1987, 1991 and 1994

	1987 Units	%	1991 Units	%	1994 Units	%
Medical and Dental Doctors	79,820	13.3	91,661	14.1	100,372	14.8
Nurses	224,697	37.4	239,729	36.9	254,726	37.7
Other Health professionals	56,184	9.3	66,715	10.3	76,576	11.4
Total Health professionals	360,701	60.0	398,105	61.4	431,674	63.9
Administration personnel	66,742	11.1	73,858	11.4	72,686	10.8
Other personnel	173,934	28.9	176,936	27.3	171,559	25.4
Total NHS personnel	601,377		648,899		675,919	

Source: Ministero del Bilancio, various years;[6] Ministero della Sanità, 1994.[17]

530 *Health Care and Cost Containment in the European Union*

and circumstances. For example, while national contracts envisage 'productivity premiums', their actual level depends on financial viability at regional level.

In the period 1991–95 three main factors contributed to keep labour costs at a relatively modest rate of increase (less than 2 per cent per year in nominal terms; see Table 11.4). First, renewal of national contracts was postponed several times.* Second, increases in wages and salaries agreed between the government and trade unions were less generous than in the past so that they were aligned with the actual inflation rate. Third, 'productivity premiums' and the use of overtime were cut as required by national legislation and, in some regions, were further reduced. These two components of labour costs are an easy target of cost containment because, by definition, they are flexible. It should be noted, however, that where these premiums were correctly used to stimulate productivity or where overtime was used to cope with increasing unmet demand, the curtailment of the flexible part of the salary may have caused a decrease in output and, in some circumstances where additional health services are contracted out to meet demand, an increase in expenditure.

As mentioned earlier, private provision is another important source of NHS spending. Private hospital care and out-patient care absorb 10.5 per cent and 2.5 per cent of NHS expenditure (Table 11.4) respectively. Given the size and the scope for flexibility in contracting with private providers, this component of health care expenditure is another potential easy target for cost containment policies. In fact, after a rapid increase during the 1980s, expenditure for private out-patient care has substantially decreased, partly because high co-payments have diverted part of the demand to the private sector.

The situation concerning private provision of hospital care is slightly different since NHS reimbursement was stabilized in real terms. Hospitals have been the only private health service suppliers of the NHS not seriously hit by cost containment measures during the early 1990s. There are three reasons for this. First, the amount of hospital care contracted from the private sector is decided at regional level. Despite attempts to make the regions more financially responsible, it is clear that the pressure to contain costs is

---

* It should be noted that postponement of the renewal of labour contracts only postpones higher expenditure, it does not contain costs. In fact, the new contract includes a compensation for the period not covered by the previous contract.

much stronger at national than at regional level. Second, private hospitals form a relatively powerful lobby and benefited, until recently, from the support of a large number of physicians who used to supplement their NHS salaries with work in the private hospital sector. Third, containing private hospital care funded by the NHS clearly conflicts with the mixed market envisaged by the 1992 reform. Despite the fact that implementation is still in the early stages, the reform envisages a more active role of private hospitals in the NHS. As a consequence, the position of the private hospitals in the health care arena has already been strengthened.

A major cost containment measure which has always been adopted in Italy, as in other countries, is underfunding capital expenditure. As explicitly admitted by the Ministry of Budget and Economic Planning, funding for capital investments is very marginal.[6] In 1994 it amounted to ITL 300 billion, approximately 0.3 per cent of current expenditure. Large investments in physical infrastructures are rarely implemented and the age of NHS buildings is rapidly increasing. Maintenance works and medical equipment are generally purchased using current expenditure funds as well. Although the need of nursing homes and other forms of long-term institutions has explicitly been recognized for many years, investments in this field are proceeding very slowly.

In order to renew the capital assets of the NHS, an extraordinarily large programme of funding for new capital investments was decided in 1988. However, out of the ITL 30,000 billion (ECU 15 billion) envisaged by the Parliament in 1988, by 1995, only ITL 3,000 billion (ECU 1.5 billion) had been allocated to specific projects.

11.6 The 1992 reform of the NHS

Cost containment has dominated the health policy agenda in the early 1990s. However, parallel to legislation aimed at reducing public expenditure, a radical reform of the NHS was approved in 1992 and amended in 1993. Although it will take time to understand the consequences of this reform, it is clear that it will probably influence expenditure trends and cost containment policies in the next decade. In this section the main elements of the reform are presented and some implications for cost containment discussed.

The need for a substantial revision of the structure of the NHS became

532   *Health Care and Cost Containment in the European Union*

evident in the mid-1980s. However, during the 1980s only minor corrections were introduced. It was only in 1989 that the first broad plan aimed at revising the NHS was presented to Parliament. The first legislative measure was approved two years later. This dramatically reduced local political interference: management boards became supervisory committees (with no day-to-day management responsibilities) and were later abolished altogether, and a new cadre of administrators (supposed to have experience in health administration) were appointed and overseen by the regions. In 1991 a comprehensive reform plan was finally approved by the Senate, but not by the Chamber of Deputies because of the early conclusion of the legislature.

Finally, in 1992, the new Parliament approved a 'framework' Bill, including some general principles on the basis of which the government was delegated to reform the NHS. Both the general principles (L. 421/1992) and the specific legislation (Dec Leg.vo 502/92) included the changes envisaged by previous plans, but at the same time they introduced radical new elements. Four themes characterize the 1992 reform: decentralization, managerialism, a quasi-market in health service provision, and opting out of the NHS.

11.6.1 Decentralization

Under the reform, the national government maintains a central role in financing the system and in defining criteria to guarantee uniform availability of health services across the country. Collection of financial resources for the NHS remains a national responsibility and each region continues to receive funding calculated in accordance with its resident population with adjustments for cross-boundary flows. Funding for capital expenditure is to be distributed to overcome the disparities in the availability of public facilities (still lacking in some southern regions).

The national tier also defines a set of basic services to be equitably provided across the country. Regions are accountable to the national tier to provide this minimum range of services. Regions are also financially accountable; that is, they have to cover any deficit incurred with their own revenues to guarantee the set of basic services or to provide services above this level. In theory, regions can increase local taxes and compulsory health care contributions, and can introduce regional co-payments. In practice, it is unlikely that regions would use this option given the present centralization

Cost Containment and Reforms in the Italian National Health Service   533

of the fiscal system. Only a substantial decentralization of the fiscal system can guarantee strong financial accountability at regional level. In fact, even after the implementation of the 1992 reform, regional deficits have continued to be the rule and only a few regions have used their own resources to reduce their deficits.

In addition, it should be noted that the set of basic services envisaged by legislation has never been specified. Indeed, there is no explicit link between the resources made available by central government and the services that regions are expected to provide.[24] Accordingly, it remains unclear what the NHS is mandated to provide.

Regions are also responsible for increasing the size of LHUs and for setting up new regulation concerning their organizational structure, accounting systems and managerial development. The 659 local health units, instituted by legislation approved prior to 1992, have now been merged and regrouped to form 228 health authorities (*Aziende Sanitarie Locali*).[25] By the end of 1986, 84 hospitals were also given 'self-governing' status.

The 1992 reform almost completely eliminated the local tier of the NHS, putting LHUs and 'self-governing' hospitals under regional control. Accordingly, both these types of organizations are now 'public enterprises' accountable to the regions. In addition, the role of the regions has been strengthened by the nature of the 1992 reform as it provided a framework, rather than a precise set of new rules. By requiring substantial regional legislation, the 1992 reform attributes to regions a central role in re-shaping the system.

11.6.2 Managerialism

One of the main criticisms of the Italian NHS has focused on managerial issues.[7,9,11,26,27] Critics have pointed to the lack of accountability of LHU administrators, the poor performance of consensus management, the burden imposed on the LHUs by unnecessary bureaucratic constraints, the lack of management systems (i.e. information systems, managerial accounting, planning procedures), and the various constraints limiting the scope of human resource management. It is thus not surprising that the 1992 reform tried to deal with managerial issues in the NHS.

First of all, it eliminated consensus management by replacing the 'directing office' (a body composed of senior managers of LHUs) with a

534 *Health Care and Cost Containment in the European Union*

general manager appointed by the region for a five-year term. As a consequence, a clear accountability line between regions and the newly established health authorities was introduced and formal power (and responsibility) was attributed to a single person. To limit patronage and to guarantee their management skills, general managers now have to be chosen from a regional list of candidates possessing relevant managerial experience and a university degree.

The reform also strengthened the accountability chain within HAs and self-governing hospitals by attributing to general managers the appointment (through private contracts) of the two senior managers, one for health matters and the other for administrative affairs. In order to increase the accountability of consultants and other senior managers, a new regime regulating access to and dismissal from consultant posts was also introduced. However, this measure is expected to produce effects only in the long run, as those who held a consultant post when the reform was approved retain the right to opt for the old and more protective rules. In addition to these changes, a broader reform of the Italian Public Administration and the national contracts for NHS employees signed in 1996 are gradually introducing more flexibility in the management of human resources and more scope for articulated carrier paths and reward systems.

The 1992 reform also introduced a new body in the health authorities: the Council of Health Professionals. This body represents medical doctors (the majority of the elected representatives) and other health professionals. It has to be consulted by the general manager for major decisions concerning health issues, but it is not provided with binding power. It is too early to know whether the Council will be an effective way to provide top management with technical advice, or whether it will become the medical counterpart of general management. Nevertheless, the risk of increasing resistance to change and of slowing down decision-making processes is evident.

Other reform measures that were aimed at improving management effectiveness included: the abolition of various bureaucratic controls over the decisions of general managers, the gradual introduction of new accounting systems replacing those based exclusively on financial information, the attribution to HAs and self-governing hospitals of a certain (limited) degree of freedom in borrowing, the requirement that public hospitals have between 6 and 12 per cent of their beds reserved for paying patients, and, more generally, encouragement to adopt new management systems. Most of these measures were almost universally welcomed. But behind the long-awaited recognition of the importance of management issues, a substantial improvement in the way public health care organizations are managed seems to depend on at least two conditions.

The first condition concerns the incentives at work in the system. Organizations tend to align management systems, and more generally, managerial culture to the social and institutional environment in which they operate. Therefore, actual managerial changes will mainly depend on institutional changes, rather than on legislation requiring them to do so.

The second condition relates to the facilitating role that the state and regions can play. Changes are built upon significant investments in human and capital assets. Changes are thus unlikely to happen if they are not supported by adequate funding, training programmes, benchmarking activities, investment in IT equipment and so on.

Despite the fact that self-governing hospitals may be an essential element of a quasi-market, the decision to make some hospitals independent of the HAs was originally motivated by management considerations. While in 1978 the idea of strong integration between different sectors of care prevailed, and consequently HAs were conceived as large multi-purpose organizations (managing everything from highly specialized hospital units to veterinary care), during 1980s it was gradually realised that this kind of integration created inefficiency and lack of flexibility. In addition, real coordination between hospital care and other sectors proved to be difficult, and large hospitals tended to have a dominant position in many HAs.

The 1992 reform dealt with this issue in two ways. First, it allowed hospitals which have national relevance and are highly specialized to become independent of the LHUs, to obtain organizational, managerial, accounting and patrimonial autonomy. The criteria required to obtain self-governing status were defined in the reform and are related to the provision of highly specialized services, medical training and emergency services. University hospitals were automatically given this status. Despite uniform national criteria, the regions played a major role in deciding how many and which hospitals could become self-governing. As a result, the number and the characteristics of these hospitals vary greatly from one region to another.

The second type of measures included in the reform refers to hospitals that remain under HA control (the vast majority): they are provided with a certain degree of autonomy and a separate accounting system, and, when run by the same HA, they are encouraged to merge or to form networks.

536 *Health Care and Cost Containment in the European Union*

11.6.3 The Italian 'quasi-market'

As noted by Citoni and Di Biase in 1992,[4] the first reform plan put to the Parliament made no provision for competition among health care providers. The measures expected to stimulate competition within the NHS appeared for the first time in the 'framework' bill in 1992 and did not derive from any previous document or consultative paper. Nor were they the result of the work of a formally established advisory body. It should also be noted that legislators never used words such as 'competition' and 'market'. However, the new funding rules for hospital and specialist care suggest, at least potentially, the activation of a new institutional environment where public and private providers will compete for patients and resources.

Since January 1995 regions have been required to fund public and private hospitals according to a prospective per-case-payment system. A phase-in period of three years was planned. In the first year, 80 per cent of funding for hospital care was allocated on an historical basis and the new payment system played only a marginal role. However, from 1998 regions are expected to fully implement the new system.

Regions are free to establish their own prospective per-case-payment systems, but they cannot set up fees exceeding those defined by the national government. The DRG classification forms the basis of the reimbursement system for in-patient hospital care. In addition to the 489 diagnostic categories, reimbursements per admission are differentiated between ordinary and day-hospital admissions and between acute, long-term and rehabilitative care. A first official document (*Decreto del Ministero della Sanita' del 15 Aprile 1994*) borrowed US Medicare weights, but the monetary values reported in a later decree (*Decreto del Ministero della Sanita' del 14 Dicembre 1984*) did not reflect these weights.[28] The details of the methodology that was followed to derive these values sometimes appear unclear. Furthermore, the information on costs was derived from a sample of only eight hospitals, mainly located in the northern regions. Not surprisingly, in many quarters it was argued that these values do not reflect actual average costs and that new cost exercises should be carried out to improve the system. According to the reform, a prospective system for ambulatory care is also to be introduced. However, the shift towards fee-for-service funding of ambulatory care is still on the drawing board in many regions.

With the 1978 reform the private sector was attributed a complementary role, supplementing public provision for certain services and in geographic

Cost Containment and Reforms in the Italian National Health Service   537

areas where public provision was underdeveloped. However by the 1980s, the presence of the private sector was already more than complementary and this tended to produce duplication of services by public and private providers and, therefore, excess capacity.[11] The 1992 reform shows a new attitude towards the private sector: private institutions were fully legitimized as a component of the provision side of the NHS, as patients are now free to choose between public and private organizations and the same prospective system should apply to both the types of providers.

The reform contains no real device to regulate the role of the private sector, the only exception being the requirement for private (but also public facilities) to be accredited. It is too soon to know whether the accreditation system will be used to limit the growth of the private sector. However, the few words contained in the reform bill regarding accreditation suggest that its role should be limited to guaranteeing minimal organizational and structural requirements.

To understand the logic of the 'quasi-market' system (implicitly) envisaged by the 1992 reform, it is useful to try to define a classification of the way market elements can be introduced in a publicly-funded system. Comparing the British and the Swedish reforms, Saltman and von Otter, 1989[29] made a distinction between the *mixed market* model, where the purchasing function is attributed to public authorities allowed to choose among public and private providers (the British model), and the *public competition* model where competition is restricted to public providers and funding reflects patients' freedom of choice (the model tried out in some Swedish counties). In a more recent paper, this basic distinction was elaborated into the bi-dimensional classification summarized in Table 11.6.[30,31] The horizontal dimension denotes the provider function; it distinguishes an arrangement in which providers are publicly-owned, and those in which both pub-

Table 11.6 A typology of quasi market in secondary health care

Purchasing Arrangement	Provider institution capital ownership	
	Public	*Mixed*
Consumer-led	Some Swedish counties	Italy
Agent-led	British NHS (in practice)	British NHS (in theory)

Source: Adapted from Saltman *et al.*, 1991[30] and Harrison and Pollit, 1994.[31]

538 *Health Care and Cost Containment in the European Union*

lic and private organizations are in the same competitive arena. At least in theory, the reformed British NHS has the features of a mixed market model since private providers are permitted to bid for Health Authority and GP fundholder contracts. The vertical dimension of Table 11.6 represents the purchasing function. It distinguishes between an arrangement in which patients are free to choose among providers (who are then reimbursed by a third party), and an agent-led arrangement in which purchasing decisions are taken by entities acting on behalf of patients. Along this dimension the British reform is clearly positioned on the agent-led quadrant: patients cannot exercise choice of provider because Health Authorities and GP fundholders have control of the purchasing function. In contrast, the Italian reform locates the NHS in the mixed patient-led quadrant.

In order to understand the potential effects of the Italian version of the 'quasi-market' model, it is thus crucial to consider together the new prospective per-case-payment system, the mixed market on the provider side and the patients' freedom of choice on the demand side. These three elements create a model in which providers compete on quality (at least as perceived by patients) and the NHS (either through regions or LHUs) acts as a third payer.

It is difficult to make predictions about the consequences of this model. However, at least three potential risks can be identified.

(a) Per-case-payment systems coupled with patient choice create incentives and pressures to carry out more cases and hence may lead to loss of control over total costs.

(b) Regions may have limited strategic control over providers (especially those that are privately owned).

(c) Unless the payment system is differentiated between public and private providers, publicly-owned institutions might lose their market share and hence incur large deficits. In fact, public hospitals are subjected to many constraints that limit their flexibility and hence their market responsiveness.

There is a growing awareness of these risks among policy-makers, as witnessed by the introduction of variants of the prospective system in which the reimbursement is gradually reduced if the actual volume of care exceeds the targeted one (for example, legislation in the Emilia Romagna and Veneto Regions),[32] and the proposal to use contractual arrangements between

Cost Containment and Reforms in the Italian National Health Service 539

LHUs and independent hospitals to keep the volume of care under control.[28] The implementation of the model designed by the reform, may not be sustainable because it provides regions and LHUs with little power to 'manage' the competitive arena and to keep public expenditure under control. Obviously, measures like those just mentioned above introduce corrections that may alleviate some of the expected shortcomings. Nevertheless, it is doubtful that such corrections can solve the fundamental inconsistencies of the model. The concomitant presence of patient choice, public-private mix on the provision side, and the prospective per-case-payment form seems incompatible with controlling public health care expenditure and providing guidance to the supply side of the system.

11.6.4 The short life of 'opting-out' of the NHS

Another, yet more radical measure was introduced in the first version of the 1992 reform: one article of the reform bill gave regions the possibility of allowing individuals or categories of individuals to opt out of the NHS, provided that they had purchased an insurance policy covering at least the benefit package provided by the NHS. Opting-out citizens would have continued to pay their share of taxes and compulsory contributions, but they would have been provided with a voucher to be spent on the private market. Both for-profit insurance companies and non-profit mutual societies would have been allowed to cash these vouchers and, eventually, to ask for additional contributions for supplementary coverage. As Ferrera[1] argued, the opt-out clause touched the very heart of the NHS. It would have introduced market mechanisms on the funding side, probably inducing competitions among insurers based on differentiation of benefits and premiums, selection of 'good' risks and other devices that are generally found in insurance markets. To mitigate the effects of patient selection, sophisticated formulae to risk-adjust these vouchers should have been developed, although incentives for residual 'cream-skimming' would have undoubtedly remained. In the long run the Italian health care system would have dramatically changed. Probably, it would have moved towards a two-tier system, with the majority of the population covered by private plans and the residual part (mainly the elderly, the disabled and the chronically ill) covered by a deprived NHS.

The opt-out clause represented a strong attack on the universalist principles underlying the NHS. Not surprisingly, the left and part of the centre

540   *Health Care and Cost Containment in the European Union*

spoke out strongly against it. But despite this opposition, the 'opt-out' clause was part of the legislation approved in 1992. A few months later, however, the new Minister of Health, a leftist Christian Democrat, reformulated the article of the reform bill concerning the opt-out clause so to eliminate it (Dec Leg.vo 517/93).

11.7 The private market

In the early 1980s approximately 80 per cent of health care needs were financed publicly (Table 11.2). According to the OECD database, by 1995 this had fallen to 70 per cent, almost 9 points less than the EU average. Only in Portugal does public spending account for a lower fraction of the total. It is possible that in the OECD database Italian private health care expenditure is overestimated. However, these figures do suggest that private health care expenditure is growing very fast and that the NHS is losing its market share.

The most updated information about public expenditure concerns expenditure on drugs. In 1988 the NHS covered about 70 per cent of the value of the drug market, including over-the-counter products (see Figure 11.2). In 1995 this percentage was just over 50 per cent. As mentioned earlier, the new positive list prepared in 1994 excluded hundreds of active compounds from NHS reimbursement. The reduction of public expenditure was only partly attributable to a decrease in the use of drugs. Most of the savings from the drug bill corresponded to increases in private expenditure.

The scope of the private market is probably even larger in the specialist ambulatory care sector. According to a 1990 national survey involving 24,000 families, 55.7 per cent of out-patient visits were fully paid by patients (or by their private insurers).[12] This figure includes visits to dental clinics. If these services are excluded, privately paid specialist visits account for 46 per cent of the total. It is difficult to estimate the value of this part of the private market because there is no data on prices charged for specialist visits. Assuming that the average price is ITL 70,000, the value of private specialist ambulatory care can be estimated at about ITL 2,600 billion. Since this value is based on data from a survey conducted in 1990–91, a period where co-payments for public specialist care was lower than it subsequently became, it is likely that it underestimates the actual value of the private market for specialist ambulatory care.

The extent of the private hospital market is largely unknown. According

Cost Containment and Reforms in the Italian National Health Service 541

to the Ministry of Health census,[33] there were 1114 public hospitals and 664 private hospitals operating in Italy in 1991. Of the private institutions, on average much smaller than the public ones, 102 did not have contractual agreements with the NHS. Assuming that the average patient turnover of privately-funded and NHS-funded private hospitals are equal, hospital care privately paid for by Italians would be about ITL 1,500 billion (ECU 750 million). This figure probably underestimates the value of the market since most of the hospitals with contractual arrangements with the NHS also admit privately-paying patients.

The vast majority of private funding is not mediated by insurance providers. It is estimated that in 1993 the insurance market accounted for ITL 3,000 billion (ECU 1,500 million).[34] Several types of carriers provide health insurance products: open, company-based and industry-based mutual funds, as well as commercial insurance companies. The latter cover approximately 50 per cent of the market and have been very active recently. In the period 1989–93 they had an average annual increase of almost 13 per cent.

It is estimated that in the early 1990s the private insurance market (including funds) covered 3 million people,[33] a little more than 5 per cent of the Italian population. This figure is low when compared with the extent of the private market for health services. In the United Kingdom, a country with a smaller private sector, it is estimated that 11 per cent of the population held an insurance policy in 1995.[35]

According to the estimates provided above, the average cost per insured person is about ITL 1 million (ECU 500). In 1995 public per capita expenditure was ITL 1.7 million. Therefore, it is likely that most of the people privately insured hold complementary policies and/or that policy-holders have low health risk profiles. Both these hypotheses are confirmed by qualitative research.[33, 36]

11.8 Conclusions

Cost containment has always been on the NHS agenda. However, while during the 1980s it was more nominal than factual, since the early 1990s there has been decisive action to stabilize public health care expenditure. The most radical measures have involved pharmaceutical expenditure. Nevertheless, less dramatic but still very effective measures contained

Figure 11.3 Trends in Italian public health care expenditure at current and 1995 prices, 1983–95

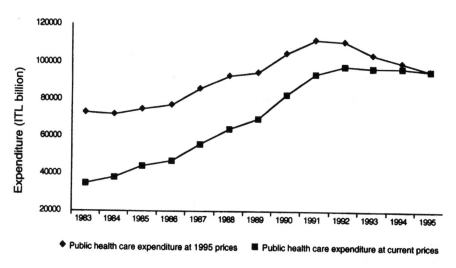

♦ Public health care expenditure at 1995 prices   ■ Public health care expenditure at current prices

Source: OECD database, 1997.[18]

expenditure on personnel and private 'contracted-out' ambulatory care.

Overall, cost containment measures have been very successful: public expenditure has been reduced in nominal terms (from ITL 96,300 billion in 1992 to ITL 93,400 billion in 1995, see Table 11.2 and Figure 11.3) so that it decreased as a percentage of GDP from 6.3 per cent in 1992 to 5.4 per cent in 1995. As a result, Italy is among those EU members devoting the lowest share of their GDP to public health care.

It is difficult to identify which measures contributed most to the exceptional cost containing results achieved during the period 1992–95. Probably, the main determinant was the low increase of expenditure for personnel. Through postponing national negotiations, the reduction of the flexible part of labour costs ('productivity premiums' and remuneration of overtime) and freezing staff hiring and turnover the main component of public health care expenditure was kept at a very low rate of increase. Also, the new positive list and the new pricing system for pharmaceuticals played relevant roles. However, pharmaceutical expenditure is a minor component of public health care expenditure and was successfully managed by central government, while control of the remaining NHS resources is mainly in regional

Cost Containment and Reforms in the Italian National Health Service 543

hands. In fact, it is the regional level that one should also look at to understand why expenditure has been controlled in recent years. The key issue to understanding the change of attitude towards health care expenditure may be found in the new institutional arrangements introduced by the 1992 reform. While during the 1980s local political control rendered the financial accountability of provider organizations very weak, the 1992 reform uncoupled providers from local community control and made easier the establishment of more rigid financial discipline.

Although successful in improving the Italian public deficit, these measures have put the NHS under strong financial pressure: in the last few years, LHUs and self-governing hospitals have had to be managed with declining resources in real terms. There is no systematic collection of data on private health care expenditure in Italy. However, evidence in the previous section suggests that the private sector is growing fast and, consequently, that a decreasing fraction of demand for health services is met by the NHS.

Some radical health care reforms in Europe have been promoted for cost containment reasons (for example in Germany and France). The Italian 1992 reform, however, was mainly motivated by other reasons, that is, to revitalize a system lacking incentives for efficiency, managerial accountability, strategic control over providers and public satisfaction.* Although the regionalization of the system is expected to increase financial accountability at decentralized levels, even this part of the reform appears to be driven by a general trend towards decentralization of the Italian State rather than by cost containment considerations.

The reform may have a strong impact on public expenditure. The main reason for this is related to the feature of the Italian quasi-market. As suggested above, moving from global budgets to fees-per-case and fee-for-services for secondary care may weaken the control over this important component of public expenditure, especially in the regions where private providers are well established.

Whether or not the 1992 reform will re-shape the Italian NHS, and in

---

* See for example Ferrera, 1993 [37] who shows the results of a European public opinion survey on health services conducted in 1992. According to these results only 34 per cent of the Italian sample thought that the quality of health care was good, while 82 per cent felt that health services were inefficient. See also Blendon et al. 1990 [38] and Mossialos, 1997 [39] for striking results concerning the high level of public dissatisfaction with the NHS.

544   *Health Care and Cost Containment in the European Union*

what way, is still difficult to forecast, despite the fact that three years have already passed since its inception (in fact, implementation of the reform started in 1994). It is likely, however, that the Italian NHS of the future will be dominated by two strategic issues: the balance of power between the State and the regions, and the attitude of the NHS towards private providers.

References

1   Ferrera M. The rise and fall of democratic universalism: health care reform in Italy, 1978–1994. *Journal of Health Politics, Policy and Law* 1995;20(2):275–302.

2   OECD. *The Reform of Health care Systems: A Review of Seventeen OECD Countries.* Paris: OECD, 1994.

3   Whitaker D. The health care system in Italy. In: Hoffmeyer UK, McCarthy TR (eds). *Financing Health Care.* Dordrecht: Kluwer Academic Press, 1994 pp 513–84.

4   Citoni G, Di Biase R. *Il Sistema Sanitario Italiano: Prospettive di Riforma.* Rome: ISPE, 1992.

5   Garattini L. *Italian Health Care Reform.* York: CHE Occasional Papers, 1992.

6   Ministero del Bilancio e della Programmazione Economica. *Relazione Generale sulla Situazione Economica del Paese. Anni 1987–1995.* Roma: Poligrafico dello Stato, various years.

7   Freddi G (ed.). *Rapporto Perkoff.* Bologna: Il Mulino, 1984.

8   Ferrera M. La composizione partitica e socioprofessionale dei comitati di gestione nella legislatura 1980–1985. In: Ferrera M, Zincone G. *La salute che noi Pensiamo. Domanda Sanitaria e Politiche Pubbliche in Italia.* Bologna: Il Mulino, 1986.

9   Borgonovi E. Il servizio sanitario nazionale: caratteristiche strutturali e funzionali. In: Centro Studi Confindustria (ed). *Stato ed Economia: Lo Stato Come Spende.* Roma: Il Sole 24 Ore, 1988 pp 469–90.

10   Buratti C. Successi e fallimenti del servizio sanitario nazionale: un bilancio dei primi dieci anni. *Economia Pubblica* 1990;20(3):145–54.

11   France G. Cost containment in a public-private health care system. *Public Budgeting and Finance* 1991;11(4):63–74.

12   Istat. Indagine multiscopo sulle famiglie. *Condizioni di Salute e Ricorso ai Servizi Sanitari (volume 10).* Roma: Istat, 1994.

13   Mapelli V. Il fondo sanitario nazionale e la sua ripartizione. In: Brenna A (ed). *Il Governo della Spesa Sanitaria.* Roma: Sipi, 1984.

14   Fattore G, Garattini L. L'allocazione delle risorse finanziarie nel Servizio Sanitario Nazionale: il quadro teorico e una soluzione pratica. *Economia Pubblica* 1989;19(12):541–56.

15   Mapelli V. Cost-containment measures in the Italian health care system. *Pharmacoeconomics* 1995;8(2):85–90.

Cost Containment and Reforms in the Italian National Health Service 545

16 Farmindustria. *Indicatori Farmaceutici.* Roma: Farmindustria, 1997.

17 Ministero della Sanita' Dipartimento della Programmazione. *Attivita' Gestionali ed Economiche delle U.S.L. Anno 1994.* Roma: Ministero della Sanita', 1994.

18 OECD. *OECD Health Data 1996.* Paris: OECD, 1997.

19 Fausto D. Italy, advances in health economics and health services research. *Comparative Health Systems* (Supplement 1) 1990 pp 211–40.

20 Garattini S. Cultural shift in Italy's drug policy. *The Lancet* 1995;346:5–6.

21 Bozzini L, Martini N. Drug policy – from chaos toward cost-effectiveness. *The Lancet* 1996;348:170–1.

22 Zammit-Lucia J, Dasgputa R. Reference pricing: the European experience. *Health Policy Review* (paper no. 10). London, 1995.

23 Fattore G, Jommi C. Il prezzo dei farmaci innovativi tra regolazione e mercato. *Mecosan* 1997;22:103–11.

24 Del Vecchio M. *Guaranteed Entitlement to Health Care: An Italian Point of View*, Paper presented at the "Hard Choices in Health Care' conference held in London, 21 November 1995.

25 Tannozzini T. Sistema contabile, solo 9 regioni adottano il provvedimento. *ASI* 1997;4 (27 Geannio).

26 Borgonovi E. Dalla sanita' di Stato allo Stato per la salute dei cittadini. *Mecosan* 1992;3:6–12.

27 Mapelli V. L'intervento pubblico nel settore sanitario: il caso dell'Italia. In: Ghetti V (ed.). *Deregulation Versus Regulation nei Sistemi Sanitari in Cambiamento.* Milano: F Angeli, 1987.

28 Taroni F. *DRG/ROD e Nuovo Sistema di Finanziamento degli Ospedali.* Roma: Il Pensiero Scientifico Editore, 1996.

29 Saltman RB, von Otter C. Public competition vs mixed markets: an analytical comparison. *Health Policy* 1989;11:43–55.

30 Saltman RB, Harrison S, von Otter C. Designing competition for publicly funded health systems. In: Hunter D (ed.). *Paradoxes of Competition for Health.* Leeds: Nuffield Institute for Health Studies, 1991.

31 Harrison A, Pollit C. *Controlling Health Professionals. The Future of Work and Organization in the NHS.* Buckingham: Open University Press, 1994.

32 Artico P. Il sistema degli incentivi finanziari nel nuovo assetto della sanità veneta: aspetti teorici e scelte operative. *Mecosan* 1995;14:59–77.

33 Garattini L, Mantovani L, Salvioni F, Sangalli F, Scopelliti D. *L'intervento Privato in Sanità.* Milano: Kailash, 1995.

34 Piperno A. Il sistema sanitario in Europa e negli USA. *Banca e Lavoro* 1994;20(supplement):24–37.

35 Laing W. *Laing's Review of Private Health Care.* London: Laing and Buisson Publications, 1996.

36 Battaglia G. Il Mercato Assicurativo in sanità: il quadro italiano e le prospettive di sviluppo. *Mecosan* 1993;7:18–25.

546 *Health Care and Cost Containment in the European Union*

37 Ferrera M. EC *Citizens and Social Protection: Main Results from a Eurobarometer Survey.* Brussels. Commission of the European Communities, 1993.

38 Blendon RJ, Leitman R, Morrison I, Donelan K. Satisfaction with health systems in 10 countries. *Health Affairs* 1990;9(2):185–92.

39 Mossialos E. Citizens' views on health care systems in the 15 Member States of the European Union. *Health Economics* 1997;6(2):109–16.

12 Health care and cost containment in Luxembourg

ELIAS MOSSIALOS

12.1 Introduction

Luxembourg remains committed to universal health insurance, which currently covers 99 per cent of the population. Those excluded can have their contributions paid for them if their incomes are sufficiently low as to entitle them to social assistance.[1] Health insurance was extended to people receiving the 'minimum income guarantee', itself a provision introduced in 1986 (see Section 12.5.5). The system is publicly funded and services are mainly privately provided by contracted-out providers. All reforms have respected the fundamental principles of Luxembourg's health care system, namely the free choice of provider by the patient, as well as the compulsory contracting out of all providers who must strictly respect the negotiated fixed fees. Providers cannot opt out of the agreements, neither can they negotiate individually with the health insurance system. This has to be done by their associations. There is no referral system and office-based doctors (both general practitioners and specialists), dentists and other health professionals are paid on a fee-for-service basis.

The government fixes the rates of contribution for health insurance through regulation. What can be reimbursed or paid for under health insurance is defined by law, and by the Union of Sickness Funds' statutes amendments. These may be adopted at the Union's delegates' meeting, and must be approved by the Ministry of Social Security. The Government has the authority to approve new hospital construction or additions and the installation of heavy equipment in accordance with the national hospital plan. It has

---

I am grateful to Mr Gérard Scholl and Ms Marianne Scholl of the Inspection Générale de la Sécurité Sociale, Luxembourg, for providing useful material and for making very useful comments on earlier drafts of this chapter.

548   *Health Care and Cost Containment in the European Union*

no power to regulate pharmaceutical prices but approves products sold in the country. Health services are covered by health insurance on the basis of medical authorization preceding their delivery. A different medical authorization is necessary for prescriptions administered by different providers and suppliers. If this condition is not fulfilled, the prescription is not reimbursed by health insurance. Moreover, the benefits delivered must correspond to those stated in the prescription, and repeat prescriptions cannot be issued.

According to the statutes, when a medical service is submitted to the medical board for authorization, the board may refuse payment by the health insurance organizations if the treatment/supply exceeds the ceiling of what it considers useful and necessary.

In 1992, major reforms focusing on four central themes were introduced:[2]

- the reorganization of the health insurance system with the establishment of a Unified Health Insurance Fund (the Union of Sickness Funds) with the parallel retention of the nine professionally-based health insurance funds;

- changes in the financing of the health sector including a projected fixed budget for health insurance;

- a new financing system for hospitals with the introduction of individual projected hospital budgets;

- new regulations for the negotiations between the health insurance funds and the providers.

Figure 12.1 presents the financing and delivery of health services in Luxembourg following the 1992 reforms.

The measures taken as a consequence of these reforms are too recent to be fully evaluated. The lack of both primary sources of data and adequate secondary sources, also makes this task difficult. Given this, it was necessary to conduct in-depth interviews with key policy-makers in order to obtain an understanding of how the financing of the health system in Luxembourg operates, with particular emphasis on cost-containment measures. However, the views expressed in this chapter are those of the author and do not necessarily reflect the views of those who provided information and commented on policy developments. This chapter analyses health care expenditure trends during the last 10 years, examines the 1992 reforms, and

Figure 12.1 Financing and delivery of health care in Luxembourg (1997)

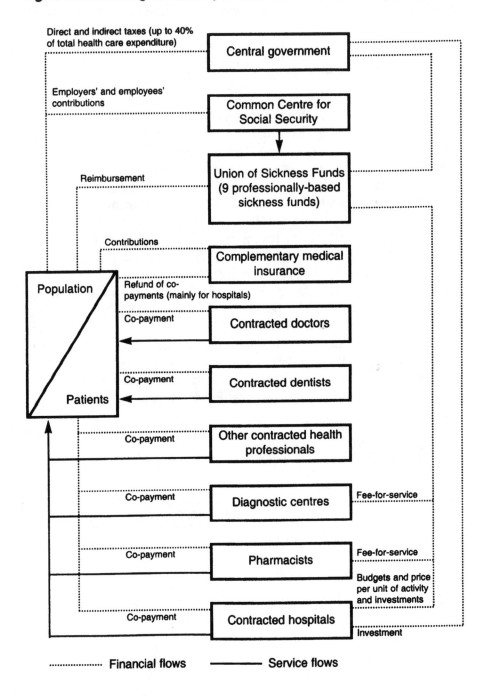

550 *Health Care and Cost Containment in the European Union*

describes the various cost-containment measures that have been introduced. Drawing on this information, the policy options for the future are discussed.

12.2 Health care expenditure

Although per capita health care expenditure in US$ Purchasing Power Parities is one of the highest in the EU, health care expenditure as a percentage of Gross Domestic Product (GDP) is relatively low. This is because Luxembourg's per capita GDP is the highest in the EU. As Table 12.1 shows, health expenditure has been relatively stable during the last ten years. The table presents data included in the OECD databank as well as data provided by the Inspection Générale de la Sécurité Sociale (IGSS) in Luxembourg. The IGSS data covers only public expenditure on health. There are some divergences from the OECD data concerning the size of public expenditure. According to the OECD data, private expenditure on health is negligible. In fact, for 1993 the OECD gives the same figure for public and total expenditure on health (6.2 per cent of GDP). In 1992, it was estimated that direct payments accounted for 10 per cent of total health care consumption.[3] This figure did not include expenditure for OTC pharmaceutical products. In addition, in 1994 the benefits provided by CMCM (voluntary health insurance) were estimated to account for 2.2 per cent of the benefits provided by the Union of Sickness Funds. If these estimates are cor-

Table 12.1 Health care expenditure in Luxembourg as a percentage of GDP, 1985–94

	1985	1990	1991	1992	1994
Public expenditure on health (OECD)	5.5	6.1	6.0	6.2	n.a.
Total expenditure on health (OECD)	6.1	6.2	6.2	6.3	5.8
Public expenditure on health (IGSS)	5.5	5.7	5.8	6.0	5.84*

Notes: n.a. not available.
   * estimate.
Sources: OECD Health Data, 1996,[4] Ministère de la Sécurité Sociale, 1997.[5]

Health Care and Cost Containment in Luxembourg 551

rect, and the data provided by the IGSS represents the actual level of public expenditure on health, then the total health expenditure in Luxembourg must be higher than that reported in the OECD database.

An analysis of public health care expenditure trends between 1975 and 1994 is shown in Table 12.2 overleaf. Total public health care expenditure increased by 172.4 per cent between 1975 and 1994 (in constant 1975 prices). The highest growth rate was that of cash benefits for maternity care (1656.5 per cent), followed by transport expenses (766.1 per cent) and surgical and anaesthetic expenses (631.7 per cent). During the same period, revenue from the contributions of active persons rose by 134 per cent and subsidies from government by 407.5 per cent. The Union of Sickness Funds currently runs a surplus, resulting mainly from the increased subsidies from government.

12.3 The health insurance reforms

A series of measures to contain costs were introduced in the period 1981–83. These mainly included increases in co-payments, a negative list for drugs, a special measure for 1983 when doctors were asked by law to concede a reduction of total remuneration, and the adjustment of the pay of hospital employees with the cost of living. These led to a one-off reduction in expenditure. Following this, the increase in costs resumed. As a result, the income of the Sickness Funds was not covering their expenditure. In July 1992, the government took new measures. They established a new central body (the Union of Sickness Funds) with wide responsibilities for the nine health insurance funds. Since the 1992 reforms, the management of health insurance has been the responsibility of the Union of Sickness Funds on the one hand, and the nine funds organized on the basis of socio-professional structures on the other. Since 1994, the new body annually produces a balanced budget for the combined funds which retains a reserve of between 10 and 20 per cent of annual turnover, which is subject to governmental approval. The law provides for indicators on several levels, which would activate redressing mechanisms in case of budgetary imbalance. A four-party committee comprising representatives of the employers, employees, the government and health professionals, has been appointed to suggest proposals on the specific measures to be introduced. It can make any recom-

552 *Health Care and Cost Containment in the European Union*

Table12. 2 Expenditure of Sickness Funds in 1975 prices, 1975–94

	1975	1980	1985	1990	1991
Benefits in kind					
Medical	780.0	1108.2	1223.2	1669.8	1771.2
Dental	156.0	221.0	248.5	304.9	313.2
Transport	9.0	15.5	21.0	50.6	57.2
Pharmaceuticals	693.0	828.0	984.9	1477.9	1518.7
Surgical and anaesthetic expenses (excluding doctors' fees)	75.0	177.4	238.9	377.1	402.7
Other curative and therapeutic	337.0	212.2	941.2	1713.7	1759.3
Dental prostheses	118.0	163.4	167.9	214.1	227.2
Examination and treatment by radiology and imaging	90.0	134.6	163.4	314.2	321.6
Hospital hotel costs	686.0	1150.3	1286.7	1722.4	1783.2
Maternity care	0.0	107.2	100.4	129.0	123.8
Total benefits in kind	2944.0	4117.9	5376.1	7973.6	8278.0
Benefits in cash					
Sickness	1202.0	1024.7	1131.8	1424.3	1501.3
Maternity care	25.0	127.2	171.9	299.7	343.5
Total benefits in cash	1227.0	1151.8	1303.8	1724.0	1844.8
Administrative cost	159.0	334.2	369.9	476.7	481.7
Total expenditure	4330.0	5603.9	7049.8	10174.2	10604.5

Source: Ministère de la Sécurité Sociale, 1996.[5]

1992	1993	1994	Growth rate 1975–94	Growth rate 1990–94	Annual growthrate 1975–94	Annual growth rate 1990–94
1982.0	2228.8	2140.8	174.5%	28.2%	5.5%	6.4%
331.1	377.2	310.9	99.3%	2.0%	3.7%	0.5%
72.3	89.7	77.9	765.0%	54.2%	12.0%	11.4%
1689.9	1892.3	1774.7	156.1%	20.1%	5.1%	4.7%
458.4	507.6	548.8	631.7%	45.5%	11.0%	9.8%
1955.5	2127.0	1981.3	487.9%	15.6%	9.8%	3.7%
234.3	242.6	227.0	92.4%	6.1%	3.5%	1.5%
352.8	413.1	305.9	239.9%	-2.6%	6.7%	-0.7%
1775.2	2127.9	1756.1	156.0%	2.0%	5.1%	0.5%
131.1	136.5	97.9	–	-24.1%	–	-6.7%
8982.6	10142.7	9221.4	213.2%	15.6%	6.2%	3.7%
1645.1	1713.8	1616.5	34.5%	13.5%	1.6%	3.2%
385.1	429.5	439.1	1656.5%	46.5%	16.3%	10.0%
2030.2	2143.3	2055.6	67.5%	19.2%	2.8%	4.5%
496.5	536.5	518.4	226.1%	8.8%	6.4%	2.1%
1509.2	12822.5	11795.5	172.4%	15.9%	5.4%	3.8%

554 *Health Care and Cost Containment in the European Union*

mendation concerning the financing of the system. Meanwhile, from August 1992 the combined contributions falling equally on employers and employees for financing health care, were raised from 4.7 per cent of the payroll to 5.0 per cent. There is a maximum contribution which is 5.0 per cent of five times the social minimum reference wage. The minimum contribution is fixed at 5.0 per cent of the social minimum reference wage for the active insured, whereas for pensioners the minimum contribution is 30 per cent higher.[3] The contributions are collected centrally for all branches of social security by the Common Centre of Social Security and are allocated to the Union of Sickness Funds. This Union is responsible for paying for hospitals' expenditure and for all the benefits directly provided on a fee-for-service basis in Luxembourg and abroad, but sickness funds continue to reimburse the recipient for certified expenditure on goods and services.

Table 12.3 Government's contribution to total public health care income between 1985 and 1995

Year	Government's contribution (%)
1985	33.8
1990	38.8
1991	37.9
1992	38.1
1993	36.6
1994	37.3
1995	34.5

Source: Author's estimates based on Ministère de la Sécurité Sociale, 1996.[5]

Instead of paying for specific items of expenditure as in the past, it was laid down that in future, the calculation of government subsidies would be mainly based on the amounts contributed by employers and employees or by pensioners. The government subsidizes the care of pensioners, who consume more health care compared with the active population, and whose contributions to health care are lower. The subsidy is equivalent to 250 per cent of the contributions of the pensioners, whereas the subsidy for the active population is 10 per cent of their contributions. In addition, the expenses due to maternity care are entirely borne by the government. Table 12.3 shows the evolution of the government's contribution to total health income over the last 10 years. The government's contribution increased from 33.8 per cent of total health care income in 1985 to 34.5 per cent in 1995. However, the figure for 1995 includes an one-off subsidy in order to cover expenses for outstanding invoices for past expenditure. The government covers part of the hospital investments as well as normal maternity insurance benefits (98 per cent of expenditure) or expensive treatments.

12.4 Voluntary health insurance

The mutual aid societies and the mutual medico-surgical fund (Caisse Médico-chirurgicale Mutualiste – CMCM) have a long tradition in sickness insurance. In order to join CMCM the contributor has to belong to a sickness fund in Luxembourg and to a mutual aid fund. The latter counted 297,000 members in 1995 (approximately 75 per cent of the population). CMCM's financing is based on the contributions of its members which vary according to their age and when they join, and which should be sufficient to cover all expenses and maintain a reserve fund which cannot exceed half of the annual benefits.

The tax system encourages membership of mutual aid societies on two levels:

1. by exempting them from revenue and property tax; and,

2. by making contributions paid to them deductible from the income tax of the head of the household.

The government also subsidises these organizations.

The benefits reimbursed by the CMCM are mainly co-payments for medical treatments in hospitals in Luxembourg or abroad and dental treatments (mainly dentures), but are very limited compared with the benefits reimbursed by the Union of Sickness Funds (corresponding to only 2.2 per cent of those benefits in 1994). The CMCM does not reimburse co-payments for pharmaceuticals.

556 *Health Care and Cost Containment in the European Union*

12.5 Cost-sharing

12.5.1 Pharmaceuticals

Pharmaceuticals included in the official list and which are not excluded from reimbursement (negative list) are classified in three categories. For each one there is a specific reimbursement rate. Pharmaceuticals needed by in-patients are totally reimbursed. In the case of drugs dispensed in hospitals, there is no need for prior authorization by the medical board.

The usual reimbursement rate for pharmaceuticals prescribed at primary health care level is 80 per cent (20 per cent co-payment) and was introduced in 1983. The special reimbursement rate of 100 per cent is applied to pharmaceuticals which do not normally contain more than one active substance and treat long-lasting diseases or special diseases. There is an official list of these medicines. This special rate is also used in the case of particularly serious medical conditions which are indicated in another list. It is estimated that there is no co-payment for 29 per cent of pharmaceuticals.[2]

The reduced 40 per cent reimbursement rate refers to pharmaceuticals with a more limited therapeutic value, which are included in an extensive list (for instance, painkillers, anti-flu drugs, and energizers). Non-essential medicines are not reimbursed.

12.5.2 Office-based doctors

Office-based doctors may work in practices within the hospital or at an out-patient setting. A co-payment of 5 per cent for consultations and home visits has been retained with the extra co-payment of another 20 per cent for the first home visit within a period of 28 days.

There is no reimbursement without prior authorization or justification by the medical board in case of:

1. more than one regular consultation or visit to a general practitioner or a specialist of the same specialty within 24 hours, unless it involves emergency services;

2. more than two regular consultations or visits to a general practitioner or a specialist of the same specialty within a period of seven days; and

Health Care and Cost Containment in Luxembourg 557

3. more than ten regular consultations or visits to the general practitioner or a specialist of the same specialty within a period of five months, unless there are consultations or visits offered during a long stay at a geriatric institution or a hospital.

12.5.3 Hospitals

For second-class hospital beds the co-payment is currently LUF 214 per day. This is not linked with the cost of hospitalization. The flat rate daily charge for in-patients, other than maternity cases and those for occupational accidents and diseases, is still increased in line with the cost-of-living index. An increase of 2.5 per cent in the index triggers an increase. There is no co-payment for second-class maternity care.

Supplementary expenses aimed at improving the patient's personal convenience, including additional charges for first-class hospitalization, are not reimbursed.

Consultations and visits by doctors have to be paid separately by health insurance. They are fully reimbursed for patients occupying second-class beds. For first-class hospitalization, an additional fee (66 per cent on top of the fixed fee) is charged by the doctors.

12.5.4 Dental care

All dental services on the list of medical and dental services that exceed the annual amount of LUF 1200 – which is covered by health insurance – are reimbursed at 80 per cent of the fixed prices.

The cost of dentures is covered at 80 per cent of the fixed prices, except for maxilla-facial prostheses which are fully covered. Dentures, other than those made from precious metals, are free to patients providing they have had their teeth examined in each of the two preceding years. Otherwise 20 per cent of the cost must be paid.

Dental descaling is covered only once for a period of 365 days. A prior estimate is required in the case of certain dentures and orthodontic treatment. The CMCM also provides a fixed sum for dental treatments authorized by the health insurance funds.

558   *Health Care and Cost Containment in the European Union*

12.5.5 Other

Certain co-payments depend on conditions whose form may vary with age: i.e. replacement of visual aids, orthodontic treatment, and prostheses.

With regard to visual aids, health insurance covers a fixed amount (LUF 1600) and a pair of eye-glasses every two years. There are restrictions for children under the age of 14. Orthodontic treatment is only covered once, following authorization. Different types of prosthesis are covered following the authorization of the Social Security Medical board, unless their price is lower than LUF 5000.

The social assistance scheme or the local social services office covers the co-payment of those with insufficient income, defined by a 1986 law. The law established a minimum income level for each household depending on the age and number of its members. Medical examinations of pregnant women are also fully reimbursed. According to a law of 1977 a pregnant woman has to be examined six times by a doctor. One of these examinations has to be made by a dentist. Following confinement, a further examination must take place at the earliest date after a period of two weeks.

12.6 Health benefits and rationing

The insurance scheme does not cover all those benefits which are not included on the different lists and exceed the principle of the useful and the necessary. This has led to a real inventory of the useful and the necessary which are precise in the provision of care on the basis of the needs of each patient according to his/her state of health. Treatment cannot exceed what is useful and necessary, and must be done in the most economical way possible; thus conforming to the principle of efficiency of treatment and to scientific data and medical ethics. Annex C of the statutes of the Union of Sickness Funds indicates explicitly the diseases, treatments and diagnostic means which are excluded from reimbursement (Table 12.4), and list 1 of Annex D enumerates the medicines which are not covered by health insurance.[6]

The Union of Sickness Funds statutes impose sanctions on individuals who are considered to have abused the system.

A user is seen to have abused the benefit system of health insurance when:

Health Care and Cost Containment in Luxembourg 559

Table 12.4 Services and interventions excluded from reimbursement

1. The health insurance funds do not cover the antenatal diagnosis of any chromosomal anomalies and foetal malformations through amniocentesis, choriocentesis or sample of foetal blood, with the exception of the following cases:
- women over 35 years of age;
- mothers who have already given birth to a child-carrier of a chromosomal abnormality;
- fathers and mothers who are carriers of an anomaly in the structure of their chromosomes;
- any foetal malformations, delay in the intra-uterine development or anomalies in the quantity of the amniotic liquid discovered during an ultrasound; and
- families with a history of genetic diseases.

2. Health insurance does not cover any maternal serum tracers in the antenatal detection of the trisomy of chromosome 21.

3. Health insurance covers the infertility treatment of the couple after its diagnosis has been reported to the Social Security Medical Council through a detailed certificate produced by the insured person or his/her doctor. Moreover, prior authorization is required for the following treatments:
- in vitro fertilization; and
- intra-cytoplasmic injection of sperm.

Both the above treatments are limited to a maximum of four attempts.

Cases which infertility treatment does not cover include:
- following a tying of the fallopian tubes or a vasectomy; and
- when a woman is over forty years of age.

4. Osteodensiometry.

5. Surgical or laser treatments of refraction.

6. Surgical treatment of obesity is not covered unless there is a detailed medical report stating that all previous non-surgical treatments have failed. Prior authorization from the Social Security Medical Council is required for the coverage which is reserved to persons with a BMI (Body Mass Index) higher than 40.

7. The replacement of breast implants for which no express authorization was given by the health insurance in the first place.

560 *Health Care and Cost Containment in the European Union*

- the user consults more than two different doctors of the same specialty within six consecutive months without prior authorization by the medical board; and/or

- services of more than three doctors of any specialty are provided without authorization by the medical board within a period of three months. This rule exempts the services of dentists, radiologists, ophthalmologists and anaesthetists.

Decisions of the medical board certifying abuse are notified to the insured person in the form of a decision subject to objection or appeal according to common law. Insofar as the decisions are not appealed against or are not challenged in court, and within the time limits set by the law, they are effective immediately and compulsory penalties are implemented by the relevant authorities.

Sanctions are implemented in a similar way in the case of a judgement based on a prior final decision confirming abuse.

Those benefits which health insurance organisations refuse to cover are communicated to the insured person as well as to the doctors and providers in question.

12.7 Paying the doctor and the dentist

The establishment of practices by doctors and dentists are not planned or controlled.[7] Doctors' and dentists' fees are subject to annual negotiations between the health insurance system and the representatives of the providers' associations. In practice, the level of fees tends to increase roughly in line with the cost of living. The fixed fees apply to both office-based and hospital doctors.

The 1992 health insurance reforms have changed the methods of negotiating and fixing the fees of doctors, dentists and other health professions. A nomenclature was established that defines all medical and nursing procedures and determines their relative value on a more rational basis. An extended list of acts defines every act by a fixed price (key) and a weighting coefficient which creates a hierarchy. The value of the key expressed in monetary units is fixed by contract. When the act or the service involves the use of medical equipment/technology, the list can fix a specific coefficient

Health Care and Cost Containment in Luxembourg 561

to cover its cost. The key for medical acts in 1997 was fixed at LUF 113.46.[8] The key for dental acts is LUF 120.95 and that for nursing acts is LUF 67.66.[9] There are separate keys for physiotherapists, pathology and clinical biology, opticians and speech therapy specialists. Table 12.5 presents some examples of medical acts where a different coefficient applies.

Table 12.5 Medical acts and weighting coefficients in 1997

Act	Coefficient	Fee*
Consultation with general practitioner	6.75	765
Consultation with specialist**	7.00	795
Consultation with cardiologist	5.65	640
Consultation with ophthalmologist	9.00	1,020
Emergency visit by paediatrician	17.70	2,010
Regular visit by paediatrician	12.00	1,360
Cervical biopsy	7.05	800
Mastectomy for malignant tumour	107.55	12,205
EEG	13.05	1,480

Notes: * The key for 1997 was fixed at 113.46 LUF.
** Internal medicine doctors, endocrinologists, haematologists, and nephrologists.
Source: Union des Caisses de Maladie, 1997.[8]

The adjustment of the value of the key letter is negotiated annually by the signatory parties of the agreement before 1 August, and should not exceed the growth of the average amount of contributions to health insurance of the active contributors. With respect to medical tests and clinical biology laboratories, it should not exceed the growth of the cost of living index.

A binding calendar is laid down for fixing fee levels either by agreement or arbitration. The increase in the total volume of medical procedures provided may be taken into account in the negotiation. The acts and services and prostheses reimbursed by health insurance are included in different official lists.

Finally, the acts and services are jointly fixed by the Ministers of Health

562   *Health Care and Cost Containment in the European Union*

and Social Security on the basis of detailed recommendations by the Commission of the Nomenclature, the Medical College and the Supreme Council of Health Professionals which are each invited to give an opinion.

As to the collective agreements, the Minister for Social Security controls the legality of the adjustment of the key-letter value and in case of dispute can refer it to the arbitral Social Security Council.

12.8 Pharmaceuticals

There is no positive list and there have been no further exclusions from payment under health insurance since 1979 when certain vitamins, tonics and comfort medicines were excluded. Now that hospitals have their own pharmacies, some of them are introducing limited lists for use within the hospital. Lists of the prices of a limited range of comparable products are sent to doctors. There is some evidence of a greater willingness on the part of doctors to prescribe generics.

Luxembourg imports all pharmaceutical products. Prices are normally calculated on the basis of the retail price in the country of origin or the retail price in Belgium taking into account an adjustment of the different tax rates on the value added applied in the country of origin.

The retail margins of pharmacists are controlled and, since 1983, pharmacists are required to pay social security 5 per cent of the official price of each product. Pharmaceuticals dispensed to patients on presentation of their insurance card are reimbursed directly to the pharmacists by the health insurance funds, and the pharmacists have to pass on the statement to the Union of Sickness Funds in a standard form. In return, the Union reimburses the equivalent of 80 per cent of the average monthly sum before the 18th day of each month.

Pharmaceutical expenditure reimbursed by health insurance increased by 14.4 per cent between 1994 and 1995.[5] A breakdown of expenditure according to the reimbursement level is provided in Table 12.6. The data presented exclude hospital consumption and non-reimbursed pharmaceuticals.

Out-of-pocket expenditure for pharmaceuticals which are partly reimbursed by health insurance amounted to LUF 730,025 million in 1995. This corresponds to 25.19 per cent of reimbursed expenditure. This amount does

Health Care and Cost Containment in Luxembourg 563

Table 12.6 Pharmaceutical expenditure (in million LUF) in Luxembourg according to the reimbursement level, 1994–95

Reimbursement Level	1994	1995	Percentage Difference 1994-95
40 per cent	106.3	173.8	63.5%
80 per cent	1,713.1	1,877.3	9.6%
100 per cent	713.2	847.0	18.8%
Total reimbursed expenditure	2,532.6	2,898.2	14.4%
Out-of-pocket expenditure	587.7	730.0	24.2%
Total expenditure	3,120.3	3,628.2	16.3%
Out-of-pocket expenditure as a percentage of total pharmaceutical expenditure	18.8%	20.1%	—

Note: Estimates exclude OTC products and pharmaceuticals excluded from reimbursement.
Source: Ministère de la Sécurité Sociale, 1996.[5]

not include out-of-pocket expenditure for OTC and non-reimbursed products. The out-of-pocket expenditure increased by 19.49 per cent between 1994 and 1995.

12.9 The hospital system

The aim of the 1992 hospital reform was to achieve greater efficiency and cost control, increase transparency in hospital activity, and to treat hospitals in a fair way, independently of their status and according to specific tasks and their individual activities.[10]

In order to achieve these goals the government had to introduce a number of complementary legislative measures. The system of financing hospitals, which involved 'chasing the act', had led to a surplus of short-stay beds and a shortage of long-stay beds. Reclassifying beds as long-stay since 1992 has been achieved in some cases. But the procedure for requiring hospitals to transfer long-stay cases to nursing homes is slow and cumbersome. There is no problem of waiting for admission for acute hospital care, but those in

564 *Health Care and Cost Containment in the European Union*

need of long term care (which is not covered by health insurance) have to wait for about 18 months. In 1993, Luxembourg's acute hospital system (not including psychiatric and rehabilitation units) comprised 18 hospitals. About half the hospitals belong to private non-profit or religious organizations. The remainder are run by local authorities or are public and semi-public. The government would like to reduce the number of hospital beds from 2,629 (or 6.8 beds per 1,000 inhabitants) to 2,342 (or 6.03 beds per 1,000 inhabitants) by transferring acute beds for the use of the chronic sick. Implementation of this proposal will be contentious.[2] A small reduction in the number of beds was achieved through the closing down of the small local hospital units. More than half of the hospitals are private non-profit institutions. The rest are owned by the local communities. There is only one private for-profit hospital in the country.

There are plans to extend day hospital care as well as home care programmes with both home nurses and home helps. In 1989 an inter-ministerial commission was established to coordinate arrangements for the care of the aged at home wherever possible. Table 12.7 shows the evolution of the average length of stay between 1984 and 1994. Despite its decline the average length of stay in Luxembourg is still high compared with other EU Member States.

Table 12.7 Hospitals – average length of stay

Population	1988	1994
Active	9.07	8.95
Retired	23.32	16.27
Total	14.52	12.02

Source: Ministère de la Sécurité Sociale, 1996.[5]

A 1994 regulation introduced the National Hospital Plan (Plan Hospitalier National).

This plan deals with:

- the allocation of acute beds according to real needs;

- the concentration of beds in larger units in order to provide continuity and medical audit, and to optimize the allocation of health professionals according to the volume of activity;

Health Care and Cost Containment in Luxembourg   565

- the importance of research into the quality of care and patient safety; and
- the consideration of increasing rehabilitation needs, especially of the elderly.

The hospital plan favours the grouping of hospitals to create synergies. The Plan also defines the number of beds in different regions as follows:

Centre	1221 beds	(52.2% of total beds)
North	324 beds	(13.8%)
South	797 beds	(34.0%)

The aim is to achieve a more equitable allocation of hospital beds and equipment on the basis of the geographical distribution of the population.

Four follow-up hospitals (with 151 beds) were also established in order to save room in the acute hospitals and play the role of units for a medium length of stay. This is also undertaken by the psychological rehabilitation centres (257 beds) and the aftercare and functional rehabilitation centre (217 beds).

Hospitals which offer emergency services are obliged to reserve some beds for the immediate admission of patients. With regard to non-urgent treatments, admission of patients for stationary treatment is completed within a reasonable period of time. In 1995 almost 25 per cent of hospital admissions were limited to one-day stays.

12.10 Hospital budgets

Before the health insurance reform in 1992, sickness funds covered the cost of hospital care by means of three principal mechanisms, namely the daily fee, the payment of certain acts and supplies, and the surgical fees. The system of payment for hospital treatment has become considerably more complicated over the last ten years. Although the system of fixing a price scale was successful in conferring to the hospital sector an overall balance of some sort, it did not allow the revenue to be balanced with the expenditure of each hospital. The volume of medical acts increased significantly and the unbalanced method of fixing a price scale was no longer providing an incen-

566 *Health Care and Cost Containment in the European Union*

tive for the provision of quality medical care at a low cost. At the same time the invoicing system was very complex and did not provide the information necessary to assess the quality of services or estimate the cost per service.

All hospitals (public and private) which are part of the hospital plan have been paid on a global budget basis since 1 January 1995. The budgets are negotiated between the new central body (Union of Sickness Funds) and each hospital separately. These budgets continue to exclude payments to doctors which are reimbursed on a fee-for-service basis.

The Union of Sickness Funds covers the payments of the hospital sector within the budgets fixed separately for each hospital on the basis of its projected activity during the next one or two budgetary years. Budgets include the reimbursement of movable and real-estate investments, provided that they have not been subsidized by the government. To the extent that the investment is subject to prior authorization by virtue of a legal or statutory clause, the reimbursement is only granted if authorization has been given.

Exempted from budgeting are: foreign health insurance benefits, those made on the grounds of personal convenience of the insured person, as well as benefits provided to people not entitled to the protection of Luxembourg's law, or any bi- or multilateral social security agreement.

Methods of reimbursement are regulated by a written agreement concluded between the Union of Sickness Funds and the Hospital Association. The representativeness of the Hospital Association is estimated by the number of their members and their seniority. The same agreement deals with the appointment of a Hospital Budget Commission.

12.11 Hospital Budgeting Process

Before 1 April of each year, the Ministry of Social Security prepares a circular with an assessment of the foreseeable development of the exogenous economic factors which could affect hospital budgeting. Until 1 May the signatory parties of the agreement negotiate the terms of budgeting.

Each hospital submits its budget by 1 June to the Union of Sickness Funds which verifies whether it conforms to the provisions of the law, the regulations and the agreements, as well as to the Ministry's circular.

By 1 September, the Union of Sickness Funds submits any final disagreement to a Hospital Budget Commission.

Hospitals are financed via three different routes:

1. The first route is non-activity related and mainly concerns funding for hospital maintenance. The Union of Sickness Funds pays each hospital at the beginning of each month a sum equal to one-twelfth of the non-activity-related expenses, provided for by the projected budget.

2. The second route finances the expenses which are directly proportional to hospital activity. These are paid according to the accomplished units of activity in different departments of the hospital on the basis of an account comprising the number of units of activity which were realised in each patient case. The activity is not linked with a specific diagnosis. The activity is defined by a number of units such as normal hospitalised days, intensive care hospitalised days, surgical operations, laboratory tests, X-Rays, MRIs, lithotripsies, haemodialysis, physiotherapies and polyclinical activities. Prices are calculated by dividing the total budget allocated for a specific activity by the estimated volume of this activity. The hospital has to provide health insurance with an individual invoice for every patient which shows the number of units consumed for each type of activity.

3. The third route concerns lump-sum payments for specific treatments. This is the case for maternity care (without pathological complications).

The pay of hospital employees is indexed to the cost of living, with an increase of 2.5 per cent triggering an increase in pay. This is the case with all employment contracts in Luxembourg. Increases above this level are subject to negotiation between the association of hospitals and the trade unions. In practice, pay increases may be delayed if hospitals are unable to afford increases.

The budget can be amended at the request of the hospitals or the Union of Sickness Funds in the event of projected economic conditions being overtaken by real events.

The average daily hospitalization fees fixed within each hospital budget are different even within the same hospital category. This occurs without any possibility of creating competition between the different hospitals, since such a step would require quite a large number of offers which could not be the case in Luxembourg.

There is no competition between the public and the private sector insofar as the latter is subsidized by the State according to the same criteria

568 *Health Care and Cost Containment in the European Union*

as the former. Finally, each hospital board is required to produce an annual activity report.

12.12 Control of medical equipment and investments

The list of reimbursed acts and the regulation of doctors' and dentists' fees define precisely the providers' acts which can be reimbursed by health insurance. In practice this policy restricts private medical practice investments to technologies and equipment which are approved by health insurance.

The National Hospital Plan defines the criteria for the organization of the hospital system. As described above, the Plan determines the hospital regions and defines the evolution of the hospital system per region; sets the criteria for the classification of services and hospitals, and assesses the need for equipment and appliances which are either expensive or have particular conditions of use. Legal and statutory provisions allow for the establishment of norms governing the allocation of staff in different hospitals and their equipment in the area of leading technology.

Nineteen categories of medical equipment are controlled. These can only be installed if permission is granted by the Ministry of Health. An inventory lays down the need for equipment and appliances which are either particularly expensive or require a very specialized environment. This inventory is updated every three years. There are no special arrangements for evaluating new technologies.

Under a Law of 1990, the government pays 50 per cent, and in some cases 80 per cent, of the cost of any capital schemes it approves. The hospitals have to find the remaining funds from their accumulated surpluses or from borrowing. This gives the government tight control over capital schemes.

The government subsidizes both the movable and real-estate investments of hospitals. Nevertheless, this assistance is reserved only for those investments which respond to a certain health need. The law regulating investments distinguishes between the creation of beds, the creation or modernization of a service and the purchase or replacement of equipment.

Ordinary replacement of equipment is not subsidized by government. Subsidies are given when the equipment is a new technology or improves the provision of services, provided that there is coordination between hospitals to avoid duplication of purchases.

Health Care and Cost Containment in Luxembourg 569

Moreover, the government defines both the steps of applying for and the procedure of granting this aid, on the advice of a permanent Committee for the Health Sector.

A second source of financing hospital investments is provided by the blueprint agreement concluded between the Union of Sickness Funds and the Association of Hospitals in compliance with the 1992 health insurance reform law. Duly authorized investments according to hospital legislation, are opposable to health insurance, provided that they meet the criterion of useful and necessary. In principle, individual hospital budgets comprise the paying off of investments insofar as they have not been financed by the government within the context of the law The hospital expenditure budget, which is also opposable to health insurance, does not comprise in any way those investments which were subsidized by the government.

12.13 Manpower control

During the period 1980–95, the number of doctors almost doubled. In 1995 there were 648 doctors in Luxembourg compared with 348 in 1980. The number of dentists also increased considerably over the same period: from 85 in 1980 to 215 in 1995. Table 12.8 shows that the greatest increase was in the number of general practitioners and dentists, whose average rate of increase was 5.5 per cent and 6.4 per cent respectively. This is in comparison to that of specialists who showed a 3.7 per cent increase rate. Since 1993, however, the rate of increase of medical practioners seems to have slowed down.

Table 12.8 Evolution of the number of doctors and dentists between 1980 and 1995

	1980	1995	Annual growth rate 1980–95
General Practitioners	99	221	5.5%
Specialists	249	427	3.7%
Dentists, including stomatologists	85	215	6.4%
Total	433	863	4.7%

Source: Ministère de la Sécurité Sociale, 1996.[5]

570 *Health Care and Cost Containment in the European Union*

12.14 Medical profiles

Although, in early 1983 agreement was reached with the medical profession that a system of medical profiling should be introduced, it has not yet been implemented. There are doubts as to how effective such a scheme would be in view of the fact that doctors do not reveal diagnoses to the Sick Funds.

The Audit Commission is competent to certify a justified deviation of the professional activity of a care provider on the basis of activity reports drawn up by the Social Security Medical Board. It can summon the provider in question to a hearing, examine his or her explanations, and proceed to carry out an investigation. If the deviation is proved to be unjustified, the provider can be warned and this is notified to the signatory parties of the collective agreement.

In the case of an unjustified deviation of a provider's activity, each of the signatory parties of the agreement can call the on Lower Council for Social Insurance, which can arbitrate in disputes and suspend a provider from health insurance for up to six months. Other measures include issuing warnings, requesting doctors and other providers to return fees, asking doctors to pay back part or the total payment for the services prescribed and consumed, imposing a fine of up to LUF 500,000, and publishing the actions taken. Providers have the right to appeal to the Higher Council for Social Insurance for amounts higher than LUF 30,000. The appeal has a suspensive effect.

12.15 Control of administrative costs

Health insurance administrative costs are estimated to be 4.4 per cent of total public expenditure on health. The constant rise in the number of people who cross the border to work makes the procedures for reimbursement of expenses more complicated, and this fact makes it necessary for the insurance agents to become familiar with reimbursement conditions and fees both within the country and abroad. The increasing complexity of procedures, due to international developments and the implementation of new reforms, does not currently allow for a reduction in the administrative costs.

12.16 Alternatives to hospital care

Nursing homes are provided by the Ministry of Health, while homes and day centres for the mentally ill and mentally handicapped are either run by the Ministry of Health or the Ministry for the Family. The Ministry of Health has recently begun organizing services for the aged to prevent transfer to hospital for minor illnesses. Elderly people who need constant care are accepted in geriatric nursing homes; these are run by the public health services or by the private sector.[2]

Home care programmes are being developed by the Ministry of Health through local government and contracts with non-governmental organizations, but such services are poorly coordinated. Since 1989, a monthly cash allowance has been made available to those providing care at home; where the person requiring care has an income below a certain level. Consideration is being given to a scheme of insurance to cover the costs of social care for dependent persons. The main directions of this new scheme were outlined by the government in 1996 and are currently being discussed with all the relevant organizations and stakeholders.

12.17 Conclusions

Luxembourg has achieved the provision of a comprehensive health care system which is not very costly when measuring health care expenditure as a percentage of the country's GDP. Health care expenditure has been relatively stable over the last ten years, and the 1992 reform enhanced the unified and universal character of the system. Citizens have free access to primary care and hospitals since there is no gate-keeping system.

The 1992 reform strengthened the monopsony role of the central administration by introducing a central body for health insurance, by specifying the negotiation process between purchasers (health insurance) and providers, and by introducing a projected fixed budget for health insurance and individual budgets for hospitals. The 1994 National Hospital Plan is expected to link the allocation of hospital facilities to the needs of the population, and provide for alternatives to hospital care by increasing the number of rehabilitation centres and the units of medium length of stay.

There are still a number of unresolved issues. The parallel existence of the central body and the nine insurance funds may increase bureaucracy and administrative costs. The abolition of the nine funds is, however, politically contentious; although in the long-run it could contribute to the strengthening of the purchasing and monopsony powers of the system. The lack of a referral system and the fee-for-service payment of doctors, dentists and other care providers can also lead to cost escalation. On the other hand the introduction of relative value fees combined with a potential for fee reductions in the negotiation of the fee nomenclature (in case of high volume consumption) may prove to be an effective safeguard. The development of appropriate information systems and audit mechanisms could also contribute to an assessment of the quality of care, reduction of duplication of services and the development of more sophisticated payment systems for hospitals and doctors.

References

1 Abel-Smith B. *Cost Containment and New Priorities in Health Care*. Aldershot: Avebury, 1984.

2 Abel-Smith B, Mossialos E. Cost containment and health care reform: a study of the European Union. *Health Policy* 1994;28(2):89–134.

3 Wagener R. Luxembourg. In: *The Reform of Health Care Systems: A Review of Seventeen OECD Countries*. Paris: OECD, 1994.

4 OECD. *OECD Health Data*. Paris: OECD, 1996.

5 Ministère de la Sécurité Sociale. *Rapport Général sur la Sécurité Social 1996*. Luxembourg: Inspection Général de la Sécurité Sociale, 1996.

6 Ministère de la Sécurité Sociale. *Aperçu sur la Legislation de la Sécurité Social 1996*. Luxembourg: Inspection Général de la Sécurité Sociale, 1996.

7 Hemmer CA. The health care system in Luxembourg. In: Casparie AF, Hermans HEGM, Paelinck JHP. *Competitive Health Care in Europe*. Aldershot: Dartmouth, 1990.

8 Union des Caisses de Maladie. *Nomenclatures des Actes et Services des Médecins et Médecins-Dentistes: Tarifs 1997*. Luxembourg, 1997.

9 Union des Caisses de Maladie. *Nomenclatures des Actes et Services des Proféssions de Santé: Tarifs 1997*. Luxembourg, 1997.

10 Consbrück R. La nouvelle législation hospitalière Luxembourgeoise. In: Standing Committee of the Hospitals of the European Union. *European Citizens' Rights and Health*. Brussels: BelgoHope, 1996.

13 Developments in health care cost containment in the Netherlands

MIRJAM VAN HET LOO, JAMES P KAHAN AND KIEKE G H OKMA*

13.1 Introduction

Like other industrialized countries, the Netherlands has witnessed a rapid growth of health care expenditure in the last three decades. It has often been stated that the two major determinants of this growth are the ageing of the population[a] and the development of new medical technologies.[1,2] However, OECD studies point to other factors in explaining this growth: supply factors such as the number of medical professionals and the capacity of health care institutions, and demand factors such as rising income levels and consumer expectations.[3] Growing supply and demand have resulted in increasing absolute health care costs. This increase runs counter to a general policy that sees the need for health care costs to be controlled in order to keep health care affordable, accessible and of high quality. As with other countries, Dutch health policies are increasingly focused on cost control measures in an effort to contain the growth of public spending.

There are many actors influencing health care expenditure, including public and private insurers, general practitioners (*huisartsen*), alternative and other providers, and of course consumers. Other important players are the Parliament (approving budgets), the Ministry of Health, Welfare and Sport, and the Health Department (designing and implementing policies).

---

* We wish to thank Paul Belcher, Jonathan Cave, Erik Frinking, Elias Mossialos and an anonymous reviewer for their helpful comments and reviews of earlier drafts of this chapter.

(a) In 1980, 11.5 per cent of the population was over 65 years of age; by 1995 this was 13.1 per cent. Among the elderly, the proportion of 'very old' (over 80 years) is also growing.[4]

574 *Health Care and Cost Containment in the European Union*

Each year, the Health Department publishes a survey of current and future health care expenditure. Over time, this survey has gradually acquired the status of a spending ceiling rather than an expenditure estimate. The government influences prices and tariffs by providing central guidelines for charges for health care services.(b) When Dutch governments deemed these general measures inadequate, they introduced more direct cost control measures.[5]

There have been several recent attempts at reform and cost containment in the Netherlands. These include:

- shifting coverage for various services and pharmaceuticals between the various coverage categories ('delisting of services'), which shifts the burden of payment between the public and private sectors, as well as to the consumer;

- introduction of cost-sharing in the form of an out-of-pocket deductible for health care expenditure beyond primary care;

- setting function-based budgets for hospitals;

- substituting out-patient for in-patient care;

- implementing practice guidelines based on evidence-based cost-effectiveness;

- manpower control; and

- use of financial information systems.

Before considering these and other attempts at cost containment in detail, an overview of health care in the Netherlands is provided below.

13.2 An overview of the Dutch health care system

Health care in the Netherlands is largely provided by self-employed professionals and private organizations, guided by government policies and self-

---

(b) These guidelines are developed by the Central Council for Health Care Charges (*Centraal Orgaan Tarieven Gezondheidszorg*, or COTG) and are subject to approval by the Minister of Health.[5]

Developments in Health Care Cost Containment in the Netherlands 575

regulatory guidelines.[6] In-patient care is provided by general, single-speciality and university hospitals, psychiatric hospitals, institutes for mentally handicapped persons, retirement homes and nursing homes. Almost all hospitals (88 per cent) and other in-patient service providers are private institutions, working on a non-profit basis. There is a well-developed system of out-patient care, provided by general practitioners, district nurses, home helpers, midwives, physiotherapists, dentists, pharmacists and independent specialists. In addition, hospitals and clinics provide a wide range of day-care services; maternity clinics; centres for convalescence; centres for the disabled; abortion clinics; and ambulatory plastic surgery, dermatology and orthopaedics.[7] Most of the general practitioners, dentists, physiotherapists and other health care professionals working outside hospitals are self-employed.

General practitioners traditionally have had and continue to have a strong gatekeeper function. The general rule is that patients must visit their general practitioner for referral to specialist care. This procedure is mandatory under the sickness fund scheme, except in the case of emergency. Most private insurance companies stipulate that patients should first visit their general practitioner, but are, in practice, lenient in enforcing this rule. Specialists inform the general practitioner of diagnosis and treatment so that he or she can take over the treatment when the patient is referred back.[7] General practitioners receive payment for treatment by means of a capitation fee for those insured by a sickness fund, and by fee-for-service for the privately insured.[5]

In 1996, total health care expenditure amounted to NLG 60 billion.[2,(c)] The largest share is spent on hospitals and specialists,[(d)] followed by institutional care for the elderly, out-patient care, pharmaceuticals and medical aids, care for the disabled, mental health care, management and miscellaneous, and prevention. Table 13.1, overleaf, shows that the breakdown of health care expenditure is rather stable over time. Table 13.2, also overleaf, shows the breakdown of health care expenditure as provided by the Central Bureau of Statistics.[8]

The current government has agreed to a real growth of health care

---

(c) 2.18 Dutch guilders to one ECU.

(d) Specialist services are costed separately from other in-hospital expenditure. This aspect of expenditure is discussed below.

576 *Health Care and Cost Containment in the European Union*

Table 13.1 Total health care expenditure, 1990–96 (Ministry of Health)

	1996*	1995*	1993*	1990*
Hospitals and specialists	33%	31%	33%	33%
Institutional care for the elderly	18%	18%	18%	18%
Out-patient care	14%	17%	17%	17%
Pharmaceuticals and medical aids	9%	11%	10%	10%
Care for the disabled	9%	9%	8%	8%
Mental health care	7%	7%	7%	7%
Management and miscellaneous	7%	7%	5%	5%
Prevention	1%	1%	1%	1%

* Not all columns add up to 100% due to rounding.

Table 13.2 Total health care expenditure, 1980–94 (Central Bureau of Statistics)

	1994*	1990	1980
Intramural care	53%	55%	58%
Extramural care	42%	39%	37%
Miscellaneous**	5%	6%	5%

*   most recent data available.
** this category includes inspection services and management.

expenditure of 1.3 per cent per year. However, pressure from both demand and supply sides makes it difficult to remain within this boundary. In 1995 and 1996, actual expenditure substantially exceeded the spending ceiling, and for 1997, the government agreed to increase the budget by NLG 376 million.[e]

Absolute health care costs (HCC) are constantly rising, but the HCC

(e) The extra NLG 376 million will be mainly spent on the admission of new medicines (anti-AIDS and beta-interferon) and solving the bottlenecks in home care.

Developments in Health Care Cost Containment in the Netherlands 577

relative to the Gross Domestic Product (GDP) has been rather stable since the mid-1980s. This also holds for the HCC adjusted for inflation in the medical sector relative to the GDP adjusted for inflation in the economy as a whole. Table 13.3 shows the share of HCC in the GDP (Wildevuur, 1996) and the share of the adjusted HCC in the adjusted GDP, with 1989 as the year of reference.[9]

Table 13.3 Health care costs (HCC) compared to the Gross Domestic Product (GDP), 1981–95

Year	HCC (NLG billion)*	HCC/GDP (per cent)*	HCC/GDP (corrected for inflation in the medical sector)
1981	35,528	10.1	n.a.
1985	40,710	9.6	n.a.
1990	48,844	9.5	9.23
1991	52,560	9.7	9.23
1992	55,570	9.8	9.28
1993	57,781	10.0	9.38
1994	59,463	9.8	9.32
1995	60,005	n.a.	n.a.

* Based on current prices.

In 1996, there were 156 general, specialized and teaching hospitals in the Netherlands, with over 55,000 beds. Between 1980 and 1994 several changes occurred in general hospitals. These were not only due to new medical technology, but also to changes in the budgeting system. The average length of hospital stay declined by 28 per cent (from 14.0 to 10.1 days). In spite of a reduction of over 16 per cent in the number of beds (from 73,150 to 61,605 beds), occupancy rates declined from 83.3 per cent to 71.7 per cent. In 1994 the government reduced the standard for the number of general hospital beds from 3.4 to 2.8 per 1000 habitants. Furthermore there are about 150 specialized institutions for psychiatric care, 340 nursing homes, over 1200 retirement homes, and over 100 institutions for the mentally impaired.

578 *Health Care and Cost Containment in the European Union*

13.3 Dutch health insurance

The health insurance system in the Netherlands consists of both compulsory and voluntary insurance. The compulsory sickness fund scheme (ZFW) covers over 60 per cent of the Dutch population, with almost all of the remainder covered by some form of private health insurance, typically provided as an employment benefit.[f] The entire population has been covered by the compulsory exceptional medical expenses scheme (AWBZ) – which covers long-term care – since 1968. In addition to these compulsory schemes, private insurance agencies offer additional voluntary coverage.

Figure 13.1 Financial flows in the Dutch health care system

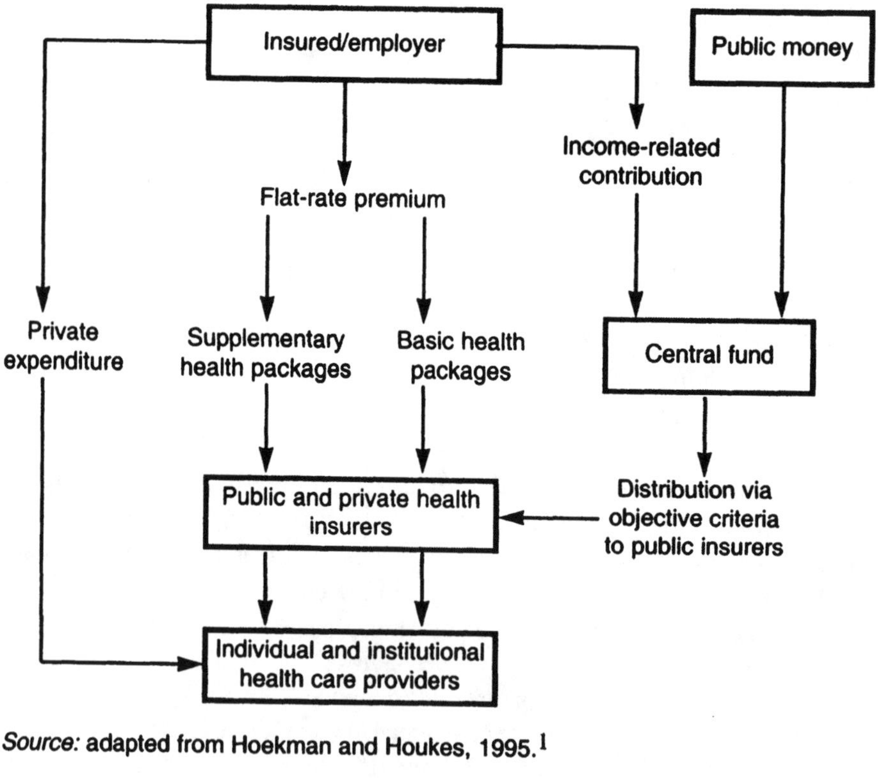

Source: adapted from Hoekman and Houkes, 1995.[1]

(f) This coverage is compulsory from the supply side. Everyone desiring coverage may obtain it at specified rates.

Developments in Health Care Cost Containment in the Netherlands 579

The financial flow of the Dutch health care system, pictured in Figure 13.1, is a complicated scheme that can bewilder a person unfamiliar with the Dutch political tradition of negotiation, compromise and consensus formation. Thus, the system is fed by both flat-rate and income-related contributions from the insured and their employers, as well as governmental contributions from general revenues. These monies are managed by private and public insurers, through two major categories of a basic health package plus supplementary packages for additional voluntary coverage.

Table 13.4 shows how health care has been financed in 1990, 1995 and 1996. Comparison of present patterns with ones before 1990 are not possible, because in 1989 the Ministry of Health combined the accounting of health and social care.[2] Table 13.5 shows the percentage of AWBZ and ZFW funded health care in 1980, 1990, and 1994.[8] As the Central Bureau of Statistics has not followed the lead of the Ministry of Health in combining health and social care in its statistical analysis, the 1980 percentages in Table 13.5 are comparable to other years. The higher AWBZ expenditure in Table 13.4 compared to Table 13.5 reflects social care for the long-term ill. The shifts in Table 13.4 and 13.5 between AWBZ and ZFW can be explained by the shifting of some provisions (e.g. pharmaceuticals) between health care packages (see below).

Table 13.4 Main sources of financing the system, 1990–96

	1996	1995	1990
AWBZ	33%	42%	32%
ZFW	35%	28%	33%
Private health insurances	15%	12%	16%
Government subsidy	10%	10%	10%
Miscellaneous (mainly private expenditure)	7%	8%	9%

Source: Ministry of Health, 1996.[2]

Table 13.5 AWBZ and ZFW, 1980–94

	1994	1990	1980
AWBZ	58%	46%	38%
ZFW	42%	54%	62%

Source: CBS, 1997.[8]

580 *Health Care and Cost Containment in the European Union*

In its health policy programme, the 1994 coalition government(g) distinguished between three funding categories of health care, with different degrees of government intervention.[10] The first category is the AWBZ, covering care in special institutions, nursing homes, hospital stays exceeding 365 days, and different categories of care for the elderly. The government maintains the primary responsibility for this insurance. The second category contains the different insurance schemes for regular medical care covering services such as general practitioners, medical specialists and hospital care. Like its predecessors, the present cabinet wants to shift responsibility for regular medical care to health insurers and health providers. The third category contains care that is not included in the other two funding categories, such as cosmetic surgery and dental care for people over 17. Which services fall into which category is subject to change, most notably in terms of the composition of health insurance packages. There is much debate about the coverage of mandatory health insurance. In particular, 'delisting' of services (i.e. moving services from the second to the third category) has proved to be very contentious.

The so-called Dunning Commitee[11] recommended criteria for including (or excluding) health care services in the mandatory insurance schemes. These criteria are:

- **necessity:** care is necessary when people cannot take care of themselves, when people cannot participate in society because their lives are threatened or when an illness results in a patient not being able to function normally in society;

- **effectiveness:** care must be effective;

- **efficiency:** efficient care must be given priority over inefficient care; and

- **individual responsibility:** one can set limits to solidarity, when the costs are high and the chance of an effect is very slight.

The Committee recommended that services failing to meet all four criteria be excluded from mandatory health insurance.

(g) The present government was formed in 1994 and is a coalition of the socialist party (PvdA), the 'liberal' conservative party (VVD), and a centre-left reformist party (D'66). The Minister of Health is the leader of D'66.

Developments in Health Care Cost Containment in the Netherlands   581

In recent decades, the Dutch health insurance system has undergone rapid transformation, with traditional relationships giving way to a more market-oriented health care system.[7] The reform proposals of the 1986 Dekker Committee sought to introduce a 'regulated market', aimed at increasing the efficiency of health care services while enhancing solidarity between different groups of insured.[12] After lengthy debate, the then Dutch government decided to implement the Committee's recommendations for a market-oriented reform of the health care system. One of the core elements of these recommendations was the introduction of a population-wide social health insurance based on regulated competition. In this system, regulated competition among insurers and health care providers would replace direct government control over prices and productive capacities. Services provided within the plan's policy would account for about 75 per cent of total expenditure on health care and social welfare. In a later stage, the Cabinet increased this percentage to 95 per cent in order to comply with European Union legislation and to increase popular support through policy consid-erations of income solidarity.[13]

Although the Dekker Plan was never fully implemented, and indeed some of its enacted changes were later rescinded, some important changes took place in the health insurance system.[12] Decision-making power over planning and contracting was shifted from the government to the health insurance agencies. Fifty years after its introduction, the mandatory contracting of services by the sickness funds was abolished. Maximum tariffs (as a ceiling under which the contracting parties might agree on lower tariffs) replaced fixed tariffs. The changes in the health insurance scheme led to increased business risks for private health insurers.

The three funding categories listed above saw changes to long-term care, regular medical care and private health insurance.

13.3.1 Long-term care: the exceptional medical expenses act (AWBZ)

Although the AWBZ was initially intended to fund long-term institutionalized care, it was extended to cover the financing of home nursing, home care, out-patient psychiatric care and some other services.[14] The scheme is financed by income-related contributions by employers levied out of wages, together with general taxation and other social insurance contributions.

One core element of the Dekker reforms entailed the introduction of a

582 *Health Care and Cost Containment in the European Union*

population-wide social insurance covering a wide range of health care and related social services. Following the Committee's proposal, the government decided to use the AWBZ as the vehicle for creating this insurance. It started to expand its coverage by gradually shifting entitlements from the mandatory sickness fund insurance and private insurance to AWBZ. Another measure attempted to change the balance between flat-rate and income-related premiums. Apart from the income-related AWBZ contributions, a flat-rate premium was introduced in 1991, but this was eliminated in 1995.

The 1994 coalition government decided to reverse some of the Dekker reform measures. In 1996, several entitlements shifted (back) from AWBZ to ZFW and private insurance. These included medical aids, pharmaceuticals, rehabilitation, and hearing aids. This was accompanied by a corresponding decrease in the income-related premium from 8.85 per cent in 1995 to 7.35 per cent in 1996. Further, the Cabinet proposed to introduce income-related cost-sharing for different health care services. To enable the administration of these charges, health care provision would be linked to patient social security ('SoFi') numbers. The first such cost-sharing schedule includes a deductible of NLG 50 as well as an income-related contribution for accessing home care. Further, the Cabinet introduced the option of cash payments for certain categories of patients rather than services in kind (the 'personalised budget'), and allowed institutions to seek customers and to provide out-patient services. For some services, the AWBZ may subsidize innovative experiments aimed at increasing efficiency, better collaboration between services or new organization of services geared to improve responsiveness to consumer demand.

13.3.2 Regular medical care

13.3.2.1 Sickness Funds Insurance (ZFW) In the nineteenth century, labour unions acting as organised consumer groups initiated voluntary health insurance for their members.[15] The 1941 *'Ziekenfondsbesluit'* was the first step towards social health insurance, introducing mandatory sickness fund membership for low-income wage earners.[12] The current Sickness Fund Act has been in force since 1966. The sickness funds insurance is a compulsory health insurance scheme for employees earning less than a certain income level (in 1995: NLG 59,100). The government policy is to keep the per-

Developments in Health Care Cost Containment in the Netherlands 583

centage of the population covered by the ZFW relatively stable. This stability is shown in Table 13.6, which illustrates that there has been very little fluctuation in ZFW coverage over time.

Table 13.6 Private Insurance vs. ZFW, 1985–94

	Private	*ZFW*
1985	33.6%	66.4%
1990	38.6%	61.4%
1991	38.6%	61.4%
1992	38.6%	61.4%
1993	38.4%	61.6%
1994	37.8%	62.2%

The ZFW expanded and now also accepts people over the age of 65 earning less than a certain income level who previously took out private insurance (in 1995: NLG 34,350), and certain groups of people entitled to unemployment or disability allowances. Today, over 60 per cent of the Dutch population carries sickness fund insurance. It is financed by income-related contributions from employers. As part of the Dekker reforms, in 1989 the government also introduced a flat-rate premium paid by the employee.

In recent years, some important changes in the ZFW have taken place.[13] The measures reveal a mix of policy considerations, including the desire to strengthen income solidarity, cost controls and the contracting flexibility of health care services. The main measures are as follows.

- ZFW membership expanded, and it now accepts people over 65 with pensions below a certain level (in 1995: NLG 34,350), and people entitled to unemployment and disability allowances. This expansion changed the character of ZFW from an employment-related social insurance to an income-related health insurance scheme.

- As of 1992, sickness funds may negotiate lower fees than the officially set maximum level. Further, the funds may now determine their own working area (instead of being limited to legally-defined regional catchment areas).

584 *Health Care and Cost Containment in the European Union*

- Private health insurance companies are allowed to establish a new sickness fund.

- As of 1992, sickness fund members have the option once every two years to register with the fund of their own choice. Funds must accept each eligible applicant.

- As of 1993, sickness funds receive a (partially) risk-adjusted per capita payment from the Central Fund.(h) From 1941 to 1991 all funds received full reimbursement of their expenditure. With this change, they are increasingly becoming risk-bearing enterprises.[12]

- As of 1994, the funds may selectively contract with self-employed doctors, such as general practitioners or physiotherapists. Before, the funds had to contract with each provider in their working area who wanted a contract.

- From 1991 onwards, there have been several changes in the composition of the type of care covered under the ZFW. Several health care services, such as cosmetic surgery (1991), spectacles and lenses (1993), non-prescription drugs (1995), dental care over the age of 18 (1995) and dental care over the age of 17 (1996) have been removed from ZFW coverage. In addition, the provision of other health care services, such as physiotherapy, Cesar therapy and Mensendieck therapy(i) was limited (1996). As of 1996, a medical examination for women between 30 and 60 years of age to screen for cervical cancer has been fully covered by ZFW insurance.

- As of 1996, the government shifted medical aids, pharmaceuticals, rehabilitation and hearing aids (back) from AWBZ to ZFW. It also abolished the flat-rate premium for the AWBZ. As a result, the flat-rate premium for the ZFW rose from NLG 16.50 per month in 1995 to NLG 27.10 per month in 1996. These steps resulted in a net premium rise of

---

(h) The Central Fund channels income-related contributions and tax subsidies to the sickness funds.

(i) As of 1996, only nine sessions of physiotherapy per year are compensated unless the problems are declared chronic, in which case all treatments will be covered. For both Mensendieck and Cesar therapy (which are both kinds of ergonomic therapy mainly focused on the way people walk, sit, lift things, etc.) nine sessions per year will be covered, with the possibility of another nine sessions.

Developments in Health Care Cost Containment in the Netherlands 585

NLG 1.25 per employee per month.[16]

- As of 1997, all those insured by ZFW face a co-insurance of 20 per cent of medical costs up to a maximum of NLG 200, or NLG 100 for people dependent on social security income.[j] This co-payment is waived for some kinds of health care, such as general practitioner visits,[k] basic dental care (when covered at all) and hospital costs of pregnancy. For in-patient hospital care, hospital day care and rehabilitation with hospitalization, there is a fixed co-payment of NLG 8.00 per day. The increase in patient out-of-pocket payments will be partially compensated by a decrease in the flat-rate premium. Existing cost-sharing for medical aids, ambulance services, prescription medications and maternity care will be maintained.[2]

13.3.2.2 Private Health Insurance Employees earning more than the ZFW ceiling and the self-employed are insured through voluntary private health insurance. Although voluntary, only very few do not insure at all.[17, (l)] Most of the companies offering private health insurance are non-profit. The services offered and the premiums that have to be paid differ per insurance company. A typical policy covers at least regular medical care, with the amount and nature of elective care highly variable. Generally, private health insurers tend to follow the guidelines of the ZFW in terms of what is considered regular medical care. The participant pays for this insurance, either directly or through an employment benefit package negotiated with the employer.

Recent changes in the private health insurance system are as follows.

- After the elimination of the voluntary sickness fund scheme for elderly people and for some other groups in 1986, the government introduced a separate insurance scheme for those privately insured with low incomes or with access problems.[18]

(j) It is important to mention that the income effects of certain measures often dominate the debate on social policies. This reflects the deep-rooted egalitarian tradition of Dutch society.[12]

(k) Visits to medical specialists must be preceded by a visit to the general practitioner. The cost containment dynamics of this form of co-payment are complicated, and the effects in terms of amount of care consumed are uncertain.

(l) The voluntary aspect of this health insurance opens up the possibilities of moral hazard and adverse selection. However, neither appears to be a problem at present.

586 *Health Care and Cost Containment in the European Union*

- As of 1992, private health insurers (like the sickness funds) are allowed to negotiate lower fees than the maximum rates.

- In 1994 several private health insurance companies established new sickness funds.[13]

- As of 1997, private health insurers introduced a deductible of about NLG 200 on all policies in order to keep pace with the sickness funds. This step was informally agreed upon with the Health Ministry, and is intended to correspond to the introduction of co-insurance in the ZFW.[2]

13.3.2.3 Regular Medical Care: Health Insurance Access Act (WTZ) The Health Insurance Access Act (*Wet op de Toegang tot Ziektekostenverzekeringen*, or WTZ) was enacted in 1986 to offer health insurance to specific groups of insured (mostly low-income, high-risk persons). The act was motivated by the (political) goal of safeguarding access to health insurance for all citizens, with a reasonable distribution of the financial burden over all population groups. The Cabinet introduced WTZ as a temporary measure, awaiting a more fundamental restructuring of health care. However, ten years on the 'temporary' WTZ is still there.[12]

Those aged over 65 with incomes above the ZFW coverage ceiling are eligible for a standard policy from private insurers, called the WTZ package. This standard package is comparable with the services offered under the ZFW and has a maximum allowable premium. There is also a WTZ package available for people who, because of exceptional medical circumstances, are not eligible for a private health insurance policy. The coverage provided by this package is the same as that of the standard package for the elderly, but the maximum premium amount is different.[17, 19] The premiums paid to the WTZ do not cover the expenses of the insurance companies, and private health insurers have to recover the shortfall via 'transfers' in the form of additions to the premiums charged to those insured through regular private health insurance.[2]

Recent changes in the WTZ are:

- In a major step taken in 1991, a WTZ package at a rate of NLG 178.60 per month (in 1995) was made available to everyone who was not able to obtain private insurance at this rate. This step in effect capped premium charges by private insurers. In this way, the government indirectly introduced a maximum premium for the basic benefits package available through the private health insurance market.[19]

Developments in Health Care Cost Containment in the Netherlands   587

- A slight modification in 1992 enabled all privately insured students who received state grants to obtain a basic benefits WTZ package for a special maximum premium which is somewhat less than half the amount paid by the other WTZ-insured.[19]

- The WTZ has always had a deductible of NLG 150 per person for non-clinical specialist care (e.g., physiotherapy, alternative medicine). As of 1997, this was changed to NLG 200 per policy (NLG 100 for single-person households).[2]

13.3.3 Voluntary supplementary health insurance

Supplementary health insurance is voluntary insurance which covers some of the third – or elective – category, i.e. those services that are not covered through AWBZ and ZFW/WTZ basic benefit packages. This insurance can be a supplementary plan purchased in addition to ZFW/WTZ insurance, or can be combined with regular medical care for private insurance. The premium for supplementary health care insurance varies according to the insured's financial status and the services covered. Examples of coverable elective care are: non-preventive dental care (for people over 17), alternative medicine treatments, medical expenses incurred in foreign countries, maternity care, non-physician-provided therapies, and medical aids.[16] The premiums for supplementary health care have risen as health services are removed from the second component and must therefore be insured through this type of coverage. The providers of supplementary health insurance compete in part on what care they will cover, deductibles, maximum amount, and how much they will charge for those services.[m] About 40 per cent of those insured through the ZFW purchase supplementary health care insurance. It is impossible to break down private insurance premiums into coverage for regular medical care and supplementary care. On balance, the charges have not led to any reduction in health care consumption. For example, after adult dental care was removed from the second category package, most ZFW subscribers purchased third category dental insurance.

(m) For example, one sickness fund offers one policy which covers 75 per cent of the costs of dental care with a maximum of NLG 300 per year. While another, more expensive policy, which covers 75 per cent of such costs, has a maximum of NLG 1000 per year.

588 *Health Care and Cost Containment in the European Union*

13.4 Policies to contain health care expenditure

Governments may consider a wide range of cost containment measures in health care, including global budgets for all or parts of health care expenditure; budgets for institutions or funding agencies; price controls; allocational mechanisms; consumer incentives; and changes in payment methods. Dutch governments have chosen a mix of different cost control approaches. This section provides an overview of these measures, broken down into the three major funding categories (long-term care, regular medical care and elective care). It should be added that rationing is not included as direct rationing is unknown in the Netherlands. However, many health care systems contain indirect rationing in the form of waiting lists or other methods. In most cases, admission to and position on waiting lists are based on explicit criteria, which include both medical and non-medical factors. In addition, there are guidelines for maximum waiting times.

13.4.1 Overall budgets for health care expenditure

As shown in Table 13.1, health care expenditure has shown a continuous growth in recent decades. The current Cabinet agreed on limiting the overall growth of health expenditure to 1.3 per cent per annum in the period 1994–98.[10] This entailed a spending ceiling of NLG 61 billion for 1996.[2] As this budget ceiling has no legal status, it cannot strictly be enforced. Within this overall 'budget', the government sets spending targets for different sub-sectors such as hospital care, mental care or ambulatory care.

13.4.2 Budgeting sickness funds

One of the measures proposed by the Dekker Committee was the introduction of prospective budgets for sickness funds. This shifts decision-making power as well as financial risks from the central administration to the individual funds. Although the current government decided not to continue the health reforms of its predecessors, it continued sickness fund budgets based on a capitation formula, including criteria such as age, sex, region and employment status. In order to allow for adjustments, the degree of financial risk for the funds is being gradually increased over a number of years.

13.4.3 Cost containment in regular medical care

Cost containment measures in regular health care services include budgets for hospitals, delisting of services, cost-sharing, changing payment methods, price controls for pharmaceuticals, controlling capital investments, and substituting in-patient with out-patient care. This sub-section briefly addresses each of these.

13.4.3.1 Budgets for hospitals Until 1983, the funding arrangement for hospital care was open-ended. Dutch hospitals received fixed payments for the number of nursing days and numbers of operations and diagnostic and therapeutic activities they performed. This payment method encouraged output maximization by providers.[1] In 1983, the government introduced a prospective budget financing system for in-patient care in general hospitals. The budgets were largely based on historical costs (1982 levels plus some adjustments). Within these budgets, hospitals had the freedom to allocate their funds. In general, budget financing creates incentives to control production. However, it also created incentives to spend all of the allocation as underspending might lead to lower budgets in following years.[1] In 1988 the government decided to replace the historical budgets by functional budgets, and gradually to shift to the new budgeting system as some hospitals saw a large difference between their historical budget and the functional budget. The essence of functional budgeting is that hospitals should be paid an equal budget for performing equal tasks. The transition from historical to functional budgets caused major budget shifts (positive or negative reallocations of more than 8 per cent occurred) between hospitals.[20] The functions on which the budgets are based are:[1]

- medical function: all activities of medical specialists (diagnosis and treatment);
- hotel function: facilities of the hospital which benefit the patients (food, cleaning, porter, etc.);
- specialized services: centralised services, such as burn centres and cardiac surgery, where care is provided for people who live outside the hospital catchment area; and
- settlement function: the availability of the facility; infrastructure (energy, maintenance, interest, etc.).

590   *Health Care and Cost Containment in the European Union*

The medical and hotel functions are part of the budget negotiated with the health insurance agencies. The compensation for special services and the settlement function is determined by the COTG. In 1992 the functional budgeting system was slightly revised. Major changes were the rise in the rate for day care visits[n] and weighting the rates for admissions and first outpatient visits.[20] Table 13.7 shows the budget for hospital care and the hospital expenses for selected years 1980-1992.

Table 13.7 Budget for hospital care and hospital expenses, 1980–92

	Budget for hospital care*	Hospital expenses*
1980	-	7639
1983**	8812	8874
1988***	9457	9439
1990	10434	10660
1992	11778	12148

*   Current prices.
**   Historical budgets.
*** Functional budgets.

13.4.3.2 Delisting of services In the early 1990s, the Dutch government delisted some services from AWBZ, ZFW, and WTZ insurance.[o] These include cosmetic surgery, alternative treatments, dental care for those over 17, eye-glasses and lenses (except for people whose visual impairment constitutes a major handicap). Further, on the advice of the Sickness Fund Council, some medical treatments were delisted as well.[p] There was a limit to the reimbursement for physiotherapy, and ergonomic therapies. Proposals to delist oral contraceptives for women over 18 years of age and long-term

---

(n) This change was made in order to stimulate substitution of patient care by day care.

(o) It should be mentioned that cost-shifting, not overall savings, was often the primary motive for delisting.

(p) The following treatments were delisted, following a health technology assessment: extensive surgery for stomach cancer, electrostimulation for loss of blood circulation in legs, excimer laser for coronary artery blockage, hormone growth treatment in neutropenia and fever, and regional-level care for attempted suicides.

Developments in Health Care Cost Containment in the Netherlands 591

psychotherapy were floated but dropped after meeting much public resistance. Some services such as artificial insemination, taking a taxi to treatment, speech therapy and household help after home birth are still under review.[q]

13.4.3.3 Cost-sharing Cost-sharing in health insurance requires the individual patient to pay part of the costs of medical care received. There are different forms of cost-sharing: deductibles, co-insurance, co-payments, or the delisting of services. Conversely, there may be hidden government subsidies when employers deduct their contributions from taxes, or when patients declare exceptional medical expenses as tax-deductible expenses.

Apart from co-payments for home care, nursing home care and residence in retirement homes, cost-sharing has historically not been a significant factor in Dutch health care. However, for home care and nursing homes co-payments have always been substantial. Other (early) examples of cost-sharing, since rescinded, include a co-payment by the ZFW-insured of NLG 25 for every first polyclinic visit (1987–90) and a NLG 2.50 co-payment for prescription drugs (1983–90).[21] The present system includes cost-sharing for medical aids, ambulance services, prescription medications and maternity care. In 1996, the Cabinet announced new cost-sharing measures. Briefly, these include a NLG 50 deductible for home care (replacing the membership due of a traditional home care organization), co-payments for regular medical services with a maximum of NLG 200 per policy per year for the ZFW and WTZ-insured, and an informal agreement for the corresponding deductible for other private insurance.[2]

13.4.3.4 Changing payment methods About half of all medical specialists in general hospitals work as independent consultants on a fee-for-service basis. Salaried specialists work mainly in teaching hospitals, psychiatric hospitals, and in some specific categories of specialities (in particular, paediatrics and rheumatology). The number of specialists working in their own practice or ambulatory health centres is limited. Until 1996, specialists' fees were not part of hospital budgets, and specialists would send a separate bill to the patient or insurance agency.[22]

(q) Speech given by Minister of Health E. Borst-Eilers at the European Health Policy Forum, Leuven, Belgium, 12 December 1996.

592 *Health Care and Cost Containment in the European Union*

The 1982 Health Tariff Act stipulated that health insurers have to offer contracts to all medical specialists, based on a fixed fee schedule set by the COTG. In contrast to budgets of hospitals, reimbursements of specialists remained open-ended. A degressive fee scheme (a physician is paid a lower fee per unit of service if the volume of his or her services exceeds a predetermined level) applies to sickness fund patients. In 1984, the scheme was extended to patients with private health insurance. Moreover, all private fees were cut by 5 per cent.[22]

In 1989, the representative organizations of medical specialists, hospitals, and insurance agencies agreed upon a 'Five Parties Agreement' or FPA. Although the government was not a formal party to the agreement, it ratified the results.[22] The FPA entailed the following:

- harmonization of descriptions of entitlements of sickness funds and private health insurance;

- harmonization of fees of the sickness funds and private health insurers;

- price adjustments of health services in terms of their relative resource utilization; and

- efforts to reduce existing income inequalities between different specialities.

Another important decision under the FPA was the acceptance of an expenditure target for specialist care. If expenditure exceeded this level, overruns would be offset by fee cuts in subsequent years. This way, medical specialists could no longer offset a loss of income by increasing their services.[22]

However, the introduction of an expenditure target has not led to reduced costs. On the contrary, specialist care grew by an average of 6.3 per cent over the period 1990–92 (compared to 2.6 per cent between 1980 and 1989), whereas the FPA aimed at zero growth. There were substantial cost overruns as the number of medical specialists and demand for health services continued to grow, and there was a lack of reliable and timely information.[22]

In 1995, the government agreed with medical specialists and hospitals to start experiments with integrated payment systems and participatory management models for hospitals and professionals. These experiments ('local initiatives'), heavily subsidized by the government, started in almost all general hospitals. The initiatives led to tripartite agreements among specialists, hospitals and insurance companies. As participation was higher

Developments in Health Care Cost Containment in the Netherlands 593

than expected, and as participants were exempted from budget cuts as a compensation for earlier cost overruns, the experiments resulted in higher expenses than expected. The experiments will continue in 1998.[2] Similar projects focus on increasing the quality of medical care.

13.4.3.5 Controlling expenditure for pharmaceuticals The Dunning Commission[11] stated that there are too many pharmaceuticals on the market and that their prices are too high. The Commission favoured the introduction of a national essential medicines list with pricing measures and lists of medicines that will not be paid for. The resulting government policy aimed at reducing the expenditure on medicines by means of: increasing price competition, reducing the prices of medicines and removing some medicines from the basic health insurance package.[r] Table 13.8 shows the expenditure on pharmaceuticals in recent years.[2, 9] Recall from Table 13.1 that these are between 9 and 11 per cent of total health care expenditure.

In 1993, the government excluded anthroposophic and homeopathic medicines from AWBZ coverage and in 1994, self-medication (with some exceptions) as well as some other medicines.[2] In addition, the pharmaceuti-

Table 13.8 Pharmaceutical expenditure, 1990–97

Year	Expenditure in NLG millions*
1990	4053
1991	4390
1992	4728
1993	5154
1994	5246
1995	5431
1996**	5261
1997**	5142

* current prices.
** estimated.

(r) The criteria for admission of medicines into the basic health insurance are: necessity, effectiveness and efficiency of care, and achieving a therapeutic value. Both existing and new medicines are judged according to these criteria.

594   *Health Care and Cost Containment in the European Union*

cal companies offered to reduce costs of medicines by 5 per cent.[9, 19] Despite these measures, expenditure on pharmaceuticals rose from NLG 4.1 billion in 1990 to NLG 5.4 billion in 1995.[23] In 1996, the government shifted pharmaceutical entitlements from AWBZ to ZFW and private health insurance.

An earlier attempt at cost control of pharmaceuticals is worth mentioning. In 1983 a co-payment of NLG 2.50 per prescription (*'medicijnknaak'*) was introduced. It resulted in a decrease of the number of prescriptions, but an increase of the number of items per prescription. The government withdrew the *'medicijnknaak'* in 1990.

13.4.3.6 Controlling capital investments[(s)] Capital investments are not part of regular hospital budgets and are under central government control. Since the late 1970s, consecutive Dutch governments have tried to reduce overcapacity of in-patient health care by limiting the number of beds, encouraging mergers and regional regrouping of hospital facilities. The level of capital investments increased substantially since 1980, and after some years of reduced growth, there was an increase in total capital investments; reflecting government policies to expand nursing home capacity and to contain the expansion of general hospitals (Table 13.9).[23, 24]

Table 13.9 Capital equipment investment, 1980–93 (expenditure in NLG millions)*

Year	General hospitals**	General hospitals**, mental hospitals, mental institutions and nursing homes
1980	818	1360
1985	617	1056
1990	1816	2476
1991	1473	2389
1992	1349	2298
1993	1344	2440

*   current prices
** excluding academic hospitals

(s) Including land and grounds, buildings, installations, stock, equipment, construction and external services.

Developments in Health Care Cost Containment in the Netherlands 595

13.4.3.7 Substituting out-patient for in-patient care As in other countries, Dutch health policies attempt to restrain hospital admittance. The Ministry of Health increased the funding for out-patient care and home care services. These efforts have borne fruit. In the last decade, in-patient care decreased, and hospital day care (including day surgery) expanded rapidly from 204,000 in 1984 to 592,000 in 1994. The number of rehabilitation treatment days increased from 539,000 in 1989 to 733,000 in 1994. The average length of stay in hospitals dropped in the same period from 12.5 to 10.1 days, reflecting changes in medical technology as well as effects of government policies.[23, 25, 26, 27]

13.4.4 Cost containment in long-term care

This sub-section addresses several cost containment measures in the long-term care insurance AWBZ, including nursing home care reforms, substituting in-patient with out-patient care, subsidies for innovation of care, and cash entitlements.

13.4.4.1 Nursing home care Compared to other countries, the Netherlands has a long tradition in publicly funded-nursing and retirement homes. In fact, its capacities are the highest in the world. The expansion of nursing home capacity was based on the assumption that the ageing of the Dutch population would lead to increased demand for institutionalized care. Further, smaller families and changing labour markets were anticipated to reduce the willingness and capacities of families to take care of ageing relatives. The introduction of the long-term care insurance into the AWBZ in 1968 encouraged the expansion of these institutions, so that there are now more people in nursing homes at any point in time than there are in hospitals.[21](t) In recent years, however, the government has taken different policy measures to slow down the growth, or even decrease the capacities of nursing and retirement homes. To reduce waiting lists, the institutions were allowed to expand their services by 4 per cent. This measure led to the provision of some extra beds, but also to substitution of in-patient with out-

---

(t) There are more hospital beds (about 61,600 in 1994) than nursing home beds (about 52.000). However, the occupancy rate of hospital beds is about 71.7 per cent, while the occupancy rate for nursing home beds approaches 100 per cent.

596 *Health Care and Cost Containment in the European Union*

patient care.[4] This also increased demand for home care. The government responded to this demand by expanding specialized district nursing, domestic help and medical appliances, and by providing subsidies for short-term home care (especially home care after hospitalization). Further, it proposed to increase competition in the provision of home care services, but these proposals met strong opposition from the home care organizations and in Parliament.

13.4.4.2 Innovation in long-term care Policies to substitute in-patient with out-patient care also applied to other areas of long-term care. In 1994, the government set up a separate fund (*'Zorgvernieuwingsfonds'*) for subsidizing innovations in mental health care.[9, (u)] The amounts channelled through this fund were NLG 31.7 million in 1994, NLG 55.2 million in 1995, NLG 74.9 million in 1996 and NLG 81.6 million in 1997.[(v)] The health insurance agencies are in charge of the administration of these funds, but the government has ultimate responsibility. Like other countries, Dutch policies for mental health care aim to reduce the volume of in-patient care, and to offer providers more possibilities to experiment with new kinds of care.

13.4.4.3 Cash benefits After experimenting for two years, the government introduced cash benefits enabling patients to decide what kind of care to purchase within these resources.[28] The resources allocated each patient are based on the number of hours he or she needs help. The aim of this system is to strengthen the responsibility of the care recipient and to stimulate individualized care. In 1995, the possibilities for patients to opt for cash benefits instead of entitlements in kind were introduced for home care, and in 1996 for care for the handicapped – two major areas of chronic care. In spite of initial administrative difficulties, most recipients of the cash benefits have

---

(u) As of 1993 there is also a *Zorgvernieuwingsfonds* for the elderly, and as of 1996 there is a *Zorgvernieuwingsfonds* for the handicapped.

(v) A part of the money in the *Zorgvernieuwingsfonds* is earmarked for special targets, such as social pensions for the homeless with psychiatric problems and care focused on specific problem groups in the four largest cities in the Netherlands (disabled persons, ethnic minorities, alcoholics, drug addicts, persons seeking asylum, etc.). The amounts involved were NLG 8.65 million in 1994, NLG 16.50 million in 1995, NLG 36.20 million in 1996 and a projected NLG 42.50 million in 1997. The remainder, the non-earmarked money, is mainly spent on psychiatric home care, rehabilitation in jobs and assisted living at home (*begeleid zelf-standig wonen*).

Developments in Health Care Cost Containment in the Netherlands   597

been enthusiastic about this option. After labour unions and the Social Affairs Ministry objected to the fact that a recipient could hire anyone on an informal base, thereby avoiding formal labour contracts, the government decided to require formal employers' status of the beneficiary. This has led to extensive administration, and to critical debates in Parliament about the management of the new programmes.

13.4.5 Cost containment by miscellaneous policies

Some policies are not primarily focused on cost containment, but still contribute to this goal. This sub-section reviews policies regarding manpower control, practice guidelines, new technologies, financial information systems, and quality assurance.

13.4.5.1 Manpower control Recent decades have seen a steady increase in the number of people entering the health care professions. However, there are policies to restrain medical school and nursing education enrolment. In addition, there is state control over the number of consultants working in hospitals. Following the general reduction of hospital capacity, there has been a decline in the number of consultants from 141,151 in 1992 to 137,105 in 1994. A similar trend occurred in academic hospitals, but the reverse happened in psychiatric hospitals, homes for the mentally handicapped, and nursing homes.[23, 25, 26, 27]

13.4.5.2 Controlling new technology While some medical technologies can save money, experience has shown that in general the introduction of new technology in the Netherlands, like in other countries, led to higher health care costs.[4] Among other factors, this is due to the lack of incentives for industry to develop cost-reducing technology, the lack of direct links between doctors and patients, and professional incentives to use technology.[29] Since 1985 the Netherlands has had a formal policy focused on health care technology assessment. Since 1988, the Investigative Medicine Committee of the Health Insurance Council made NLG 36 million a year available for the Investigative Medicine programme. This is a programme oriented to clinical research, emphasising technology assessment.[30] There is government control over the admission and dissemination of new and expensive technologies, such as heart surgery and radiotherapy.[11] The

598 *Health Care and Cost Containment in the European Union*

Medicines Evaluation Board registers new pharmaceuticals after assessing its efficacy, safety and pharmaceutical quality criteria. The Board is not allowed to refuse a product which is already registered in another EU country. Until recently, all approved medicinal products were available through the national health insurance system. However, some products have been delisted.[31] New medical devices have to be approved by the Netherlands Organization for Applied Scientific research (TNO) or the KEMA testing, research and consultancy organization; manufacturers may also certify their own products.[31]

Other new products require no formal approval, and innovation is left to the health care system itself. The application of technology is seen as the responsibility of health care professionals, and must assure adequate quality of care. At present, there is no policy to evaluate all innovative developments in terms of their (cost-)effectiveness before they enter the health care system. Within the present health care system, the major screening is the decision as to whether or not to include a new technology in the social health care insurance.

13.4.5.3 Practice guidelines Several studies established that there are great regional variations in practice, indicating frequent inefficient, unnecessary, or useless actions. The Dunning Committee proposed restrictions on provider autonomy.[11] These restrictions were based on the need to achieve:

- quality assurance through appropriate supervision of medical actions and the involvement of patients, insurers, and institutions in determining standards of quality;

- accountability of the physician to the broader society as well as to the individual patient, especially in regards to the costs of care; and

- an efficient and justifiable distribution of limited resources.

The Dunning Committee stated that the main responsibility for appropriate care rests with the professions and their organizations. In order to reach this goal, they must work with others in society to develop the standards for appropriate care. The Committee recommended that scientific associations, professional organizations, and health facilities themselves must take the initiative in setting up protocols, guidelines and lists of appropriate care. Also, the organizations of insurers and patients should be involved in the development of such standards.

Developments in Health Care Cost Containment in the Netherlands 599

The Ministry of Health recently announced a new programme to expand practice guidelines founded on medical technology assessment. This programme will perform technology assessments (including a major cost-effectiveness component) on frequently performed and expensive procedures, leading to the establishment of evidence-based guidelines for those procedures. This will be followed by efforts to change professional practice by implementing the guidelines. In this way, it is believed medical practice can be more cost-effective with no loss in the quality of care.

13.4.5.4 Financial information systems In health care, there are growing possibilities to use financial information systems.[2, 32] However, as decision-making in health care is highly decentralized, the collection of data for the information systems is difficult. The Ministry of Health does not track all financial transactions; indeed, most expenditure is made by insurance companies (public and private) and individuals (co-payments and deductibles). The most important sources of financial data are the Sickness Fund Council (*Ziekenfondsraad*), the COTG, the statistics bureau of private health insurance companies (Vektis), and the Central Bureau of Statistics (CBS). Thus the Ministry has to collect information from a large number of sources, which are dependent on individuals or insurance agencies. It sometimes takes a long time before all information is available, and not all information is reliable. In 1995, the Ministry of Health set up a Task Force on Health Care Information in order to improve the quality of financial data. The specific objectives of the task force are to:

- harmonize definitions of terms concerning health care financing;

- achieve consistency of the financial estimates produced by the Ministry of Health and the Health Insurance Funds Council;

- speed up data collection; and

- obtain better information regarding the payments of the Ministry of Health.

It is also expected that this will lead to improved control of costs.

13.4.5.5 Quality assurance The Dutch government considers quality assurance to be a major policy goal. The primary responsibility for quality of care rests with the providers. Also, the contracts between providers and insurance agencies should contain references to the quality of care. Further,

600 *Health Care and Cost Containment in the European Union*

the government supports certification activities of providers. In this system, government acts as controller of quality systems, and recorder of the certification. However, the development and implementation of quality assurance systems rests largely on self-regulation.[11]

13.5 Conclusion

During the last decades, Dutch health care underwent rapid transformation. In 1988, the Dekker Committee recommended the introduction of a population-wide social health insurance, merging the different funding sources for health care and related social services, and eliminating the difference between sickness fund insurance and private health insurance.[12] Based on this proposal, the Dutch government started to implement fundamental changes in the existing funding system of health care. The 1994 coalition government decided not to continue the health care reforms of its predecessors, but to opt for incremental adjustments of the existing system instead. However, in spite of this new course, Dutch health care witnessed major changes (van de Ven and Schut, 1994).[13] The debates on a market-oriented health care system themselves encouraged anticipatory behaviour.[12] Health insurance agencies, providers of care and consumers' organizations took new market positions and developed new roles. The major organizations of medical professionals and other providers initiated activities aimed to develop quality improvement and quality assurance systems. There was a marked increase in cost-accounting systems by health care institutions, and most institutes are in a process of gradual transition from input to output-pricing. The sickness funds and private health care insurance agencies have begun close collaboration.

The present health care policies aim at controlling the growth of health care expenditure and at increasing the efficiency and flexibility of care by encouraging innovations in health care.[2] The guiding principles of the present Cabinet are: (1) a new equilibrium of collective and individual responsibilities, (2) gradual convergence of sickness funds and private insurers, (3) cost containment, and (4) increased (financial) responsibilities for insurers, providers and the insured.[10] These general principles translate into measures for cost control and gradual improvements in the existing health insurance system. On the one hand, the present health policies con-

Developments in Health Care Cost Containment in the Netherlands 601

tinue the shift in decision-making power from the government to the consumers, insurance agencies and providers of care. On the other hand, the government resumed a dominant position in long-term care. Throughout all the changes to date, the percentage of health care expenditure within the private sector and the amount of out-of-pocket expenditure have remained stable. Although changes to the policy supporting this stability have been discussed, no concrete proposals have emerged to date.

The Dutch Minister of Health, Else Borst-Eilers, MD, still has some important subjects on her agenda for the second half of her cabinet period. These include reducing waiting lists in health care, the integration of specialists in hospitals, and completing the process of care renewal.[33] The main focus of the present health policy is on cost containment while maintaining quality and accessibility of care. So, not only policies focused on cost containment, but also policies aimed at improving care and enlarging the efficiency of care, are on the agenda for the future.

References

1 Hoekman PH, J Houkes. *Economie van de Zorgsector; Een Inleiding in de Economie van de Gezondheidszorg en de Maatschappelijke Dienstverlening.* Groningen: Wolters-Noordhoff, 1995.

2 Ministry of Health. *Jaaroverzicht Zorg 1997.* Rijswijk, September 1996.

3 Oxley H, MacFarlan M. Controlling spending and increasing efficiency. *Health Care Reform. The Will to Change.* Paris: Organisation for Economic Cooperation and Development, 1996.

4 Commissie Strategische Heroriëntatie Gezondheidszorg. *Gezondheidszorg in tel.* Utrecht: Nationaal Ziekenhuisinstituut, Publication No. 193.890, September 1993.

5 Grünwald CA, Mantel AF. Health systems in 12 Member States: The Netherlands. In: Leadbeater N. *European Health Services Handbook.* 1992. pp. 102–15.

6 Grinten TED, van der. Scope for policy: essence, operation and reform of the policy of Dutch health care. In: Gunning-Schepers LJ, Kronjee GJ, Spasoff RA (eds). *Fundamental Questions about the Future of Health Care.* Netherlands Scientific Council for Government Policy, The Hague: SDU Uitgevers, 1996.

7 Centraal Bureau voor de Statistiek (CBS). *Statistics Netherlands International Comparison of Health Care Data.* Voorburg/Heerlen, 1996.

8 Centraal Bureau voor de Statistiek (CBS). *Statistisch Jaarboek 1997.* Voorburg/Heerlen: SDU Uitgeverij, 1997.

9 Ministry of Health. *Financieel Overzicht Zorg 1995.* Rijswijk, September, 1994.

10 Tweede Kamer der Staten-Generaal. *Regeerakkoord 1994.* Kamerstukken II,

602 Health Care and Cost Containment in the European Union

1994–1995, 23715, No. 11. Den Haag: SDU Uitgeverij, 1994.

11 Government Committee on Choices in Health Care. *Choices in Health Care.* Zoetermeer: Ministry of Health, Welfare and Culture, 1992.

12 Okma GH. *Studies on Dutch Health Politics, Policies and Law.* PhD Thesis, University of Utrecht, 1997.

13 Ven WPMM van de, Schut FT. Should catastrophic risks be included in a regulated competitive health insurance market?, *Social Science and Medicine* 1994;39:1459–72.

14 Veen E van der, Limberger HHB. The assurance of appropriate care. In: Gunning-Schepers LJ, Kronjee GJ, Spasoff RA (eds). *Fundamental Questions about the Future of Health Care.* Netherlands Scientific Council for Government Policy, The Hague: SDU Uitgevers, 1996.

15 Abel-Smith B. The escalation of health care costs: how did we get there? *Health Care Reform. The Will to Change.* Paris: Organisation for Economic Co-operation and Development, 1996.

16 Zorg en Zekerheid. *Veranderingen in de Zorgverzekering.* Leiden, 1996.

17 OECD. *The Reform of Health Care; A Comparative Analysis of Seven OECD Countries.* Paris: Health Policy Studies No. 2. 1992.

18 Okma GH. De Wet op de toegang tot ziektekostenverzkeringen opnieuw voor het voetlicht. *Sociaal Maandblad Arbeid.* 1994(3):130–41.

19 Dijksterhuis WHK, Wever LJS. *Jaarboek gezondheidszorg; Overzicht van ontwikkelingen in beleid en regelgeving.* Houten: Bohn Stafleu van Loghum, 1995.

20 Maarse HAM. Fixed budgets in the in-patient sector: the Case of the Netherlands. In: Schwartz FW, Glennerster H, Saltman RB (eds). *Fixed Health Budgets: Experience from Europe and North America.* Chichester: John Wiley & Sons Ltd., 1996.

21 Abel-Smith B. *Cost Containment and New Priorities in Health Care: A Study of the European Community.* London: London School of Economics, 1992.

22 Lieverdink H, Maarse H. Negotiating fees for medical specialists in the Netherlands. *Health Policy* 1995;31:81–101.

23 Centraal Bureau voor de Statistiek (CBS). *Statistisch Jaarboek 1996.* Voorburg/Heerlen: SDU Uitgeverij, 1996.

24 Centraal Bureau voor de Statistiek (CBS). *Statistisch Jaarboek 1992.* Voorburg/Heerlen: SDU Uitgeverij, 1992.

25 Centraal Bureau voor de Statistiek (CBS). *Statistisch Jaarboek 1993.* Voorburg/Heerlen: SDU Uitgeverij, 1993.

26 Centraal Bureau voor de Statistiek (CBS). *Statistisch Jaarboek 1994.* Voorburg/Heerlen: SDU Uitgeverij, 1994.

27 Centraal Bureau voor de Statistiek (CBS). *Statistisch Jaarboek 1995.* Voorburg/Heerlen: SDU Uitgeverij, 1995.

28 Tweede Kamer der Staten-Generaal. *Het persoonsgebonden budget.* Tweede Kamer, vergaderjaar 1994–1995, 23904, No. 14, Den Haag: SDU Uitgeverij, 1995.

29 Gelijns AC, Rosenberg N. Making choices about medical technology. In: Gunning-Schepers LJ, Kronjee GJ, Spasoff RA (eds). *Fundamental Questions about the Future*

Developments in Health Care Cost Containment in the Netherlands   603

of Health Care. Netherlands Scientific Council for Government Policy, The Hague: SDU Uitgevers, 1996.

30 Banta HD, Oortwijn JW, van Beekum WT. *The Organization of Health Care Technology Assessment in The Netherlands*. TNO Prevention and Health (by order of Rathenau Institute), The Hague, November 1995.

31 Ministry of Health. *Medical Technology Assessment and Efficiency in Health Care*. Rijswijk, 1996.

32 Tweede Kamer der Staten-Generaal. *Informatiebeleid in een Veranderend Stelsel van zorg; InformatievoorZiening ten Behoeve van Rijksoverheid en Parlement in het Licht van Bestuurlijke Vernieuwing en de Stelselwijziging*. Tweede Kamer, vergaderjaar 1991–1992, 22540, Nos. 1-2, Den Haag: SDU Uitgeverij, 1992.

33 Wildevuur SE. Zorg moet doelmatiger: Jaaroverzicht Zorg 1997. *Medisch Contact*, Jaargang 51, 27 September 1996.

14 Health expenditure and cost control in Austria

ENGELBERT THEURL

14.1 Introduction

The Austrian health care system is organized along the principles of the Bismarck-model of social insurance.* It is therefore confronted with the specific advantages and obstacles of this model with respect to cost containment strategies. To illustrate and judge cost containment policy in Austria a short review of the institutional/constitutional framework of the Austrian health care system has to be given. Based on this background the specific policies of cost containment which were undertaken recently or are planned for the near future, are illustrated. Important cost containment strategies of the recent past are:

- the reorganization of the hospital financing system;

- the reorganization of long-term care;

- the introduction of a comprehensive plan for health care service capacities (especially in-patient capacities); and

- changes in cost-sharing and in the financing of pharmaceuticals.

These strategies will be discussed in more detail later in the chapter, which in turn ends with a short summary of selected recommendations for future reforms of the Austrian health care system.

---

* For a general view of the Austrian health care system see Beirat für Wirtschafts- und Sozialfragen, 1996;[1] Bundesministerium für Gesundheit, Sport und Konsumentenschutz, 1994;[2] OECD, 1994[3] and Österreichisches Bundesinstitut für Gesundheitswesen, 1994.[4]

606   *Health Care and Cost Containment in the European Union*

The chapter concentrates on the public part of the health care sector. The compulsory Austrian health insurance system is part of the social insurance system (Sozialversicherung) and covers, via its different funds (civil servants, workers in the private sector, self-employed and farmers, etc.), the health care costs of nearly all of the population. Although there are differences in the service packages of the different insurance funds, these funds offer almost universal basic coverage against health expenditure risks in a multi-tiered health care system.

The private health insurance companies act as a second stage and play quite an important role in the field of in-patient and out-patient health care. At the moment, the role of the private health insurance system has stagnated to some extent. Financial incentives to subscribe to private insurance plans have been reduced by income tax reforms in recent years. Currently the main advantages for people with private health insurance coverage are: reduced waiting times (especially for specialists outside the hospital), greater possibilities for the free choice of doctors, the free choice of doctors in hospitals, the provision of additional services not covered by the social health insurance system, and better 'hotel services' in hospitals. The quality of in-patient care provided by hospitals should be by law the same for all patients. Direct out-of-pocket expenditure plays an important role in dental care and pharmaceuticals.

14.2 The institutional framework of cost containment policy in Austria

Constitutionally Austria is a *federal state* with a three-tier system of government, divided into the central (federal government), regional (provinces) and local authorities (local communities). The assignment of functions and powers over spending and revenue are based partly on constitutional and partly on non-constitutional laws. The assignment of most functions and powers over spending can be described as moderately decentralized, even though decentralization is mainly characterized by 'a decentralization of law enforcement'. However, the distribution of revenue-raising powers is centralized to a very high degree. There exists practically no revenue-generating automony (in particular, tax sovereignty) at either state or community levels. Besides this, intergovernmental transfers play an important role. In the distribution of these responsibilities a distinction has to be made between an area of sovereignty and an area of private enterprise administration ('*Privatwirtschaftsverwaltung*'). In the first area, the state acts as an institution endowed with enforcement measures, whereas in the latter area, the state has to act like a private economic unit.

The distribution of powers and the assignment of functions according to the Austrian Federal Constitution, Articles 10–15, exclusively applies to the area of sovereignty. Within the area of private enterprise administration, however, each regional and local authority can within certain restrictions – territorial ones, for example – act independently of the assignment of authority in the area of sovereignty.

This rule also applies to activities in the health care sector. The preconditions for such activities are the *political will* to perform these activities and adequate *financing possibilities*. It is also basically accepted that all areas which are not regulated by the constitutional distribution of authority fall within the competence of the regional authorities (provinces). This is especially important for new public tasks such as environmental protection.

A prominent feature of the Austrian constitution with far-reaching consequences is the fact that while general health care matters predominately fall within the central state's authority, central government only has responsibility for hospitals insofar as it establishes the functional structure of the system, the mechanisms of finance, and sets minimal standards for the regional distribution of in-patient services. Regional governments have key competencies in this area, as they are responsible for implementing legislation, its execution, the administration of health financing and financial consequences.

Regarding the horizontal distribution of functions of the central state, the federal government's authority in health care is shared between the Ministry of Labour, Social Affairs and Health, and the Ministry of Science, Transport and Arts. The state's responsibility for health care basically covers regulatory functions. The financing of the health care system is, with some exceptions (such as medical research and education), not a task of the state. Medical care outside hospitals is organized and financed on a contract basis between the regional chambers of physicians and the social security funds.

This assignment of functions has several significant consequences for the Austrian health care system and for specific strategies of cost containment:

- At the level of the state, health care policy is largely characterized by

608 *Health Care and Cost Containment in the European Union*

regulatory control. Only matters of medical research and the education of doctors are financed directly by the state from the science-related budget. Medical care provided by registered doctors (outside hospitals) is financed by the social health insurance system alone, while in-patient treatment is financed from a number of sources: from social health insurance funds and funds from the state, provinces and the communities. The compulsory social health insurance system is based on individuals' occupations and is financed by income-based contributions of employers and employees. Coverage is also given to unemployed and retired people through this system. No extra contribution has to be paid for family insurance against health risks. The influence of economic interest groups in the social health insurance system is very high (the system of social partnership), because of Austria's corporatist political and economic tradition.

- The health care policy of the federal state in the past has been weakened by a largely dysfunctional distribution of authority between the Federal Ministry of Health and the Federal Ministry of Labour and Social Affairs. The main task of the latter was the regulation of the social insurance system. It was not until 1972 that a separate Federal Ministry of Health was established. However, this ministry has so far only been endowed with minimal authority. The task of regulating health care policy at an Austria-wide level cannot be performed on this basis. For this reason, there were also no overall budgets for the health care system as a whole and no clear policy strategies for national health priorities. Furthermore, no clear mechanism for the regional distribution of resources in the health care sector exists. The regional distribution is the result of various decisions to decentralize at the different levels of the health care system. Since the reorganization of the federal government in 1997 the Ministry of Health has been part of the Ministry of Labour and Social Affairs, thereby diminishing some of the federal level coordination problems in health policy which existed in the past.

- The relationship between the state, the provinces and local communities in health-related questions, is largely characterized by the fact that the responsibility for implementing hospital legislation falls within the competence of the provinces. Thus, an Austria-wide regulation of hos-

Health Expenditure and Cost Control in Austria   609

pital capacities (i.e. number of beds, large-scale medical equipment) is only possible to a limited extent. In order to lessen the numerous regulatory deficiencies resulting from this, a central fund (KRAZAF) was set up in 1978 with the aim, among other things, of regulating hospital investments, optimizing the geographical pattern of hospital care to prevent under-provision and the duplication of high-technology equipment, and introducing modern strategies of cost control. This fund was supervised by the central government. Members of the fund were the central government, the provinces, local governments and the social insurance funds. However, for a number of reasons, most particularly its composition, this hospital cooperation fund has not fulfilled expectations. The role of this fund changed fundamentally through the reform of hospital financing in 1996.

- This deficiency in the regulation of hospital capacities is aggravated by the fact that hospital capacities and out-patient capacities – supplied by registered doctors – are planned and regulated separately. The regulation of hospital capacities is essentially the duty of the provinces. However, the regulation of out-patient capacities (especially the regional distribution of doctors) is applied within the framework of long-term bilateral agreements between the Chamber of Physicians, which has regional competence at the level of the provinces, and the Main Association of Social Insurance Funds (a kind of coordinating body for social security funds at the level of the state), in cooperation with the regional social insurance funds. Given the high possibilities of substitution between in-patient and out-patient care, this arrangement hinders the optimal division of labour between the two institutions of health care.

- Important care organizations which may act as substitutes for health care institutions, such as social welfare facilities, nursing facilities, care for the aged, etc., fall within the competence of the provinces and the local communities. This leads to many coordination problems between these services at the regional level. These coordination problems between health care institutions and other care institutions are particularly aggravated by the increasing proportion of old people in the total population and the growing incidence of chronic diseases associated with this increase.

610 *Health Care and Cost Containment in the European Union*

Figure 14.1 The decision-making process in the Austrian health care system

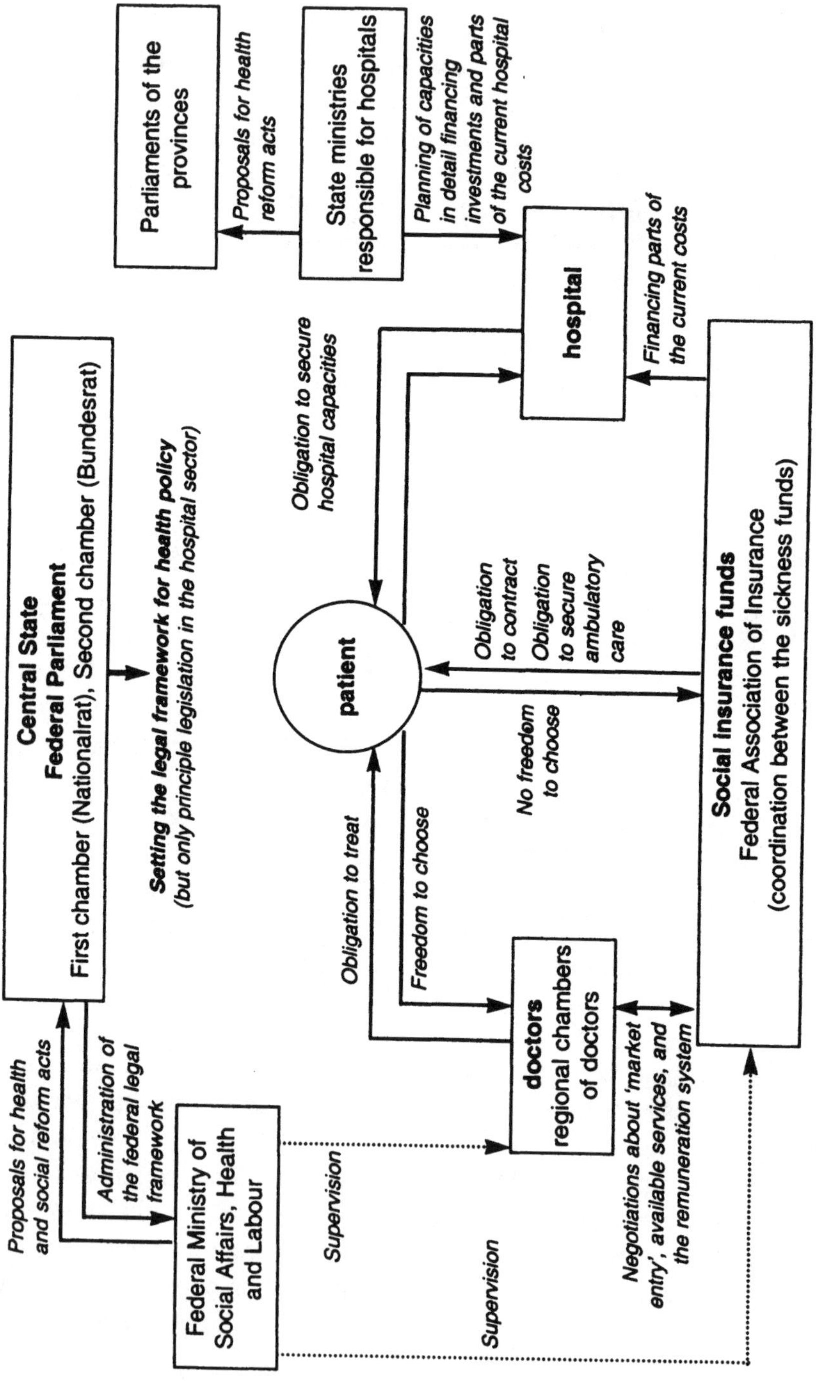

- Parliaments of the provinces
- Proposals for health reform acts
- State ministries responsible for hospitals
- Planning of capacities in detail financing investments and parts of the current hospital costs

- **Central State**
  Federal Parliament
  First chamber (Nationalrat), Second chamber (Bundesrat)
- *Setting the legal framework for health policy*
  (but only principle legislation in the hospital sector)

- Proposals for health and social reform acts
- Administration of the federal legal framework
- **Federal Ministry of Social Affairs, Health and Labour**
- Supervision
- Supervision

- **doctors**
  regional chambers of doctors
- Obligation to treat
- Freedom to choose
- No freedom to choose

- **patient**
- Obligation to secure hospital capacities
- **hospital**
- Financing parts of the current costs

- Obligation to contract
- Obligation to secure ambulatory care

- Negotiations about 'market entry', available services, and the remuneration system

- **Social insurance funds**
  Federal Association of Insurance
  (coordination between the sickness funds)

Figure 14.1 gives an overview of the basic structure of the decision-making process in the Austrian health care system and of the basic relations between the purchasers and providers of health services.

14.3 Some evidence on the development of health expenditure in Austria

Before the cost containment strategies in selected sectors of the Austrian health care system are presented, a short overview of the development of health expenditure in Austria will be given. Data from the OECD Health Data 96 were used for this comparison. Figure 14.2 shows the ratio of total expenditure on health to GDP in Austria for the period 1960–95.

As a percentage of GDP health expenditure increased from 4.4 per cent in 1960 to 9.6 per cent in 1995. We can see two noteworthy shifts in the development of the level of health care expenditure in this period. The first occurs during the first oil-price shock in 1974/75 and the second since 1992.

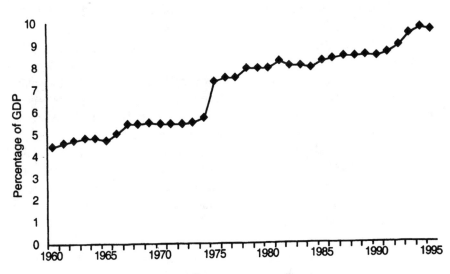

Figure 14.2 Total expenditure on health as a percentages of GDP in Austria, 1960–95

Source: OECD Health Data, 1996.[5]

612 *Health Care and Cost Containment in the European Union*

Table 14.1 Average annual growth rate of total health expenditure and GDP, 1960–95

Period	GDP	Total health expenditure	Elasticity of health expenditure to GDP
1960–65	8.6	10.0	1.16
1965–70	8.8	13.0	1.47
1970–75	11.8	18.1	1.54
1975–80	8.7	10.3	1.18
1980–85	6.3	6.9	1.09
1985–90	6.0	6.7	1.12
1990–95	5.5	9.4	1.71

Source: OECD Health Data, 1996.[5]

From a global perspective therefore, Austrian cost containment policies were not particularly successful in the recent past. This is especially true in comparison to the Scandinavian countries, which were able to stabilize or decrease health expenditure as a percentage of GDP. In Table 14.1 the increase of the health expenditure is separated into a five-year average growth rate of total health expenditure and GDP. The last column shows the elasticity of health expenditure to GDP.

In Figure 14.3 the increase of health expenditure is divided into a public (PHE) and a private health expenditure component (PRHE). The public health expenditure quota includes the expenditure of public health insurance funds and the spending of the state, the provinces and the local communities. The private health expenditure quota includes the expenditure of the private insurance companies and the out-of-pocket expenses of the patients. No reliable data about private health expenditure exists at the moment, although Basys estimates that 70 per cent of private health expenditure is made up of out-of-pocket expenditure and only 30 per cent is paid by the private insurance companies.[6] The ratio of private and public health care expenditure remained quite stable over the considered period. However, there is a shift in the ratio between 1970 and 1975 in favour of public health

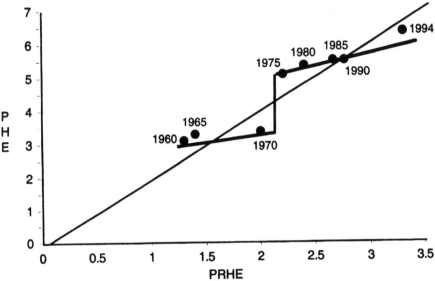

Figure 14.3 Health expenditure – public and private health care expenditure, as a percentage of GDP, 1960–94

expenditure. Within the two periods 1960–75 and 1975–95 the role of public sector decreased slightly.

The share of the main sources of financing have remained quite stable over the last 15 years. In 1992, of total health expenditure:

- 24 per cent was financed by the state;
- 54 per cent by the social insurance funds;
- 14 per cent by consumers in out-of-pocket payments; and
- 8 per cent by the private insurance companies.

Table 14.2, overleaf, shows the annual per capita growth of total health expenditure at current and constant 1990 prices and the same for important health expenditure categories for the period 1982–94.

The data shows that health expenditure increase is to a large extent a price phenomenon. This is especially true for the hospital sector, but to some extent also for expenditure on ambulatory care. Only the prices for pharmaceutical goods remained quite stable over the whole period.

614   *Health Care and Cost Containment in the European Union*

Table 14.2 Percentage growth of health expenditure categories per year – at current and constant prices, 1982–94

Period	(1)	(2)	(3)	(4)	(5)	(6)	(7)	(8)
82/83	6.0	1.5	8.4	1.8	7.6	3.4	6.3	2.9
83/84	5.3	0.0	4.9	-2.9	10.1	5.7	4.1	0.1
84/85	7.6	1.8	6.2	0.2	7.0	3.1	8.1	4.3
85/86	7.8	3.2	6.4	-0.5	6.6	0.7	3.8	1.9
86/87	5.3	0.4	7.1	-1.7	6.9	4.2	5.1	3.0
87/88	5.3	1.6	6.0	1.4	5.4	3.3	8.5	5.2
88/89	8.2	2.7	10.9	5.4	7.15	5.4	4.8	1.7
89/90	5.1	-0.8	7.1	-1.2	0.2	-1.0	3.9	0.6
90/91	7.5	1.7	5.7	0.3	14.1	9.7	5.3	2.4
91/92	9.4	1.3	7.3	-0.1	9.0	-0.3	6.9	3.3
92/93	8.2	2.0	10.8	3.9	9.4	5.4	7.9	5.7
93/94	9.8	2.0	17.9	10.5	6.7	0.1	5.7	4.3

Notes:
(1) Total expenditure on health, per capita, current prices.
(2) Total expenditure on health, per capita, constant prices (1990).
(3) Expenditure on in-patient care, per capita, current prices.
(4) Expenditure on in-patient care, per capita, constant prices (1990).
(5) Expenditure on ambulatory care, per capita, current prices.
(6) Expenditure on ambulatory care, per capita, constant prices (1990).
(7) Expenditure on pharmaceutical goods, per capita, current prices.
(8) Expenditure on pharmaceutical goods, per capita, constant prices (1990).
Source: OECD Health Data, 1996.[5]

14.4 Cost containment strategies in selected sectors of the Austrian health care system

From a global perspective the structure of the Austrian health care system has not changed significantly in recent years. In the past, several efforts were made to contain costs in the hospital sector and to increase efficiency, but they did not fundamentally change the structure of the system. However, a major reform of the financing system of in-patient care is now under way, having started at the beginning of 1997. Therefore the description of cost containment strategies will begin with this reform.

14.4.1 Hospital care

A short description of the basic structure and the main problems of the Austrian hospital system must be presented in order to understand the current cost containment strategies. Table 14.3 shows the development of important characteristics of the hospital sector over the last 15 years.

It should be noted that the private hospital sector is dominated by not-for-profit organizations and that the role of the private sector differs widely between the provinces. In some provinces, private hospitals provide acute care, while in others only specific forms of care (long-time care) is provided by the private sector. Every public hospital may use up to 25 per cent of the available beds for private patients. These patients have to pay extra fees to the hospital: normally doctors in the hospital (including specialists) are paid on a salary basis. Doctors working in the private sector of a public hospital are paid – based on private contracts – on a fee-for-service basis.

Key deficiencies of the Austrian hospital system include the following:

- Compared with other EU-countries the density of hospital beds in Austria is high (See Table 14.3). This has led to both a high (and increasing) hospitalization rate and a high average length of stay. The

Table 14.3 Capacities and throughputs in the Austrian hospital system, 1980–94

Year	Number of beds per 1000 inhabitants	Public beds (% of all beds)	Hospital admissions per 100 inhabitants	Hospital days per 100 inhabitants	Average length of stay	Occupancy rate in hospitals in %
1980	11.2	72.2	19.5	350	17.9	84.4
1983	11.0	72.9	20.7	340	14.8	81.9
1986	10.9	70.5	22.2	330	13.7	82.4
1989	10.5	70.0	25.5	320	12.4	82.2
1992	9.7	n.a.	26.0	290	11.1	80.7
1994	9.4	n.a.	26.5	270	10.3	80.0

Source: OECD Health Data, 1996.[5]

616 *Health Care and Cost Containment in the European Union*

expenditure per bed and per case treated on the other hand, is quite low by international comparison. A 1990 Basys-Study[7] showed that : when we standardize the average cost per case in acute hospital care for Austria with the value of 1, then for selected countries we get the following values (based on purchasing power parities): Germany 1.15, Switzerland 1.7, France 1.16, Sweden 1.9, Netherlands 1.7, United States 3.3. In Austria the annual growth rate of hospital expenditure amounted to between 10 and 12 per cent in the last ten years. Attempts to cut down hospital beds in recent years were successful only to a very limited degree. This can be traced back to the institutional framework of hospital care in Austria, as already discussed in this chapter. Every central plan to cut down the hospital capacities has to be agreed by the provincial governments.

- The financing system of hospitals is characterized by the separation of investment costs and current costs. This separation induces non-optimal investment decisions of the hospital owners. Current costs are financed according to a fixed *per diem* fee by the social health insurance system (until the end of 1996). Because this fee does not cover all the current costs, the arising deficits are paid by the hospital coordination fund, the provinces, the local communities and the owners of the hospital. This method of retrospective hospital financing has led to several inefficiencies in the hospital system.[8] Table 14.4 shows the main revenue sources of public hospitals in Austria in 1994.

- No structured coordination of medical equipment and medical technology, at either macro or micro level, existed in the past.[9] The above mentioned federal-level hospital coordination fund could fulfil this task only to a very limited extent, although several plans on restructuring hospital facilities were made and some work on the evaluation of new technologies was carried out. The regional allocation of medical technology was achieved by this fund. The composition of this fund is seen as the main reason for the deficiencies described. Capital investment on a macro level was controlled by the hospital coordination fund and by the provinces. No specific technology assessment organization currently exists to evaluate medical technology on a scientific level.

Several attempts to reform the hospital financing system have been undertaken in recent years, but have met with only limited success. The conclu-

Table 14.4 Revenue sources of public hospitals in 1994

Revenue source	ATS billion
Health insurance funds	37.1
Per-day reimbursements	26.7
Transfers via KRAZAF	10.3
Private insurance funds	4.1
Federal government	3.9
Subsidies to teaching hospitals	0.9
Transfers via KRAZAF	3.0
Provincial and local governments	30.0
Transfers via KRAZAF	2.9
Pension payments	4.1
Transfers to cover deficits	22.9
Other	6.5
Total revenues	81.6

Source: OECD, 1997.[10]

sion of coalition negotiations following the 1995 general election led to a restructuring of hospital financing in Austria in the course of the pruned 1996/97 budget – and this could yet be of some significance to cost containment strategies. The reform took effect from the beginning of 1997, and the agreement will last for the next four years. The reform concentrates on the public hospital sector, and its essential elements are outlined below.

The current system of hospital financing through per-day reimbursements is to be replaced by a financing system based on DRGs (Diagnosis Related Groups). The basic framework for this case-mix-based financing was created with the introduction of compulsory documentation of all hospital cases in 1989. The classification of the hospital cases was based on ICD-9 (International Classification of Diseases). Beginning with 1991, the cost of the given hospital treatment was gathered in 20 selected hospitals. Based on this information homogeneous groups of patients were indentified. In the next step, a regression tree algorithm was used to derive cost-

618 *Health Care and Cost Containment in the European Union*

homogeneous groups. The median values of the observed cases were used to fix the points per case in order to correct for outliers.

In addition to the DRG-based financing mode, additional dimensions are used to determine the sum which the hospital gets for a specific case:

- short length of stay (including, day-care, ambulatory surgery);

- long length of stay for specific cases (is allowed for in a degressive way);

- patient-days in intensive-care units (based on the intensity of care);

- patient-days of remobilization;

- long-term care (financed outside the DRG-system);

The details of these financing mechanisms are fixed by the provinces.

Besides these dimensions, additional factors are used to distribute the money to the individual hospitals. These additional factors account for special features of the hospitals. Such factors are: the quality of care, the role of research and medical education, the type of hospital, the mix of medical personnel, and technical equipment. The weight of these factors is fixed by the provinces. Currently, it is unclear whether these additional factors should only be used for a transitional period.

The DRG-based financing mode has been used in the province of Vorarlberg since 1994 on a test basis. This test has shown that the financing model functions in principle. The separation of financing investment costs from running costs, which characterized the hospital financing system in the past, will also characterize the financing mechanism in the future.

At the level of every province a hospital committee (*Länderkommission*) is established. Members of this committee are appointed by the government of the province, by the local government, by the owners of hospitals, by the social insurance system and by the central state. Delegates from the provincial government form the majority of members in these hospital committees. The main task of the hospital committee is to steer the hospital system at province level. This includes the distribution of financial resources to the individual hospitals according to the DRG-system and the additional factors mentioned above, control of the quality of hospital services and control of the coding of DRG-points by the hospitals. As an important part of the reform, a compulsory hospital plan and a large-scale

Health Expenditure and Cost Control in Austria 619

technical equipment plan will be agreed between the federal government and the provinces. This plan will include a substantial restructuring of hospital capacities (closing of hospitals), while the number of beds will not change dramatically. The political process of establishing these plans is underway. This process is very complex, because it involves harmonization between the state and provinces. At the federal level, a committee for restructuring the hospital system is being introduced as a substitute for the existing hospital cooperation fund. This committee will have a majority of delegates from the Austrian federal government.[11] The main tasks of this committee will be:

- the restructuring and development of the health care system;

- a comprehensive plan of hospital out-patient services including the services of doctors outside the hospital;

- the development of a case-based hospital financing system and its application to other sectors of the health care system;

- the development of the hospital plan to a comprehensive health care plan; this comprehensive health plan should include all health care services, not only in-patient capacities; and

- setting up a system of quality control of hospital services.

Budgets for individual hospitals are allocated in two stages, first at provincial level and then at the level of individual hospitals. In the first stage, the allocations from the hospital coordination fund (financed by the federal government from general taxes) and the social insurance systems, are fixed. The distribution of hospital coordination fund resources to the provinces was, in the past, based upon several criteria (i.e. hospital days, educational services, high quality medicine, a hospital's deficit), but overall the number of inhabitants was the dominant factor. The contribution from the federal state has now been fixed at the 1994 level for the years 1997 to 2000. Previously, the amount of financial resources allocated directly from the social health insurance funds to the hospitals was based on a per diem fee and was therefore related to the number of days of hospitalization. Under the new system this money is given as a block transfer to the hospital committee of the province and is independent of the health care services provided by their hospitals. The amount of resources allocated to each province

620 *Health Care and Cost Containment in the European Union*

in 1997 was the same as that directly allocated by the social health insurance funds in 1994. Any subsequent increases (to the year 2000) are dependent on the social health insurance funds' revenues during this period. As a result, this part of the budget is prospectively fixed at state level. But this does not mean budgets for individual hospitals are fixed. Another source of hospital expenditure is financed by the provinces and local communities. It is not yet clear whether this will also be fixed prospectively; leading to a fixed prospective global budget for a province's hospital sector.

In the second stage, the financial resources will be distributed to individual hospitals according to the criteria mentioned above. Currently, the form of the distribution of financial resources within hospitals (i.e. to the departments of the hospital) is not fixed in detail, but medical heads of the departments are likely to be given limited budget responsibility.

The cost containment effect of the hospital financing reform is based on several premises. In particular, that it is necessary that an overall budget for the hospitals in a province to be tightly fixed. There is currently no fixing of prospective budgets for hospital expenditure in Austria. Ex-ante budgets only exist for single institutions financing parts of the hospital bill. They also exist for the transfers from the state and for the payments of the social insurance funds. No prospective budgets are given for the provinces and the local communities.

14.4.2 Ambulatory care

Health care outside hospitals is supplied by local doctors. Ambulatory care is mostly provided in single practices. The following section will concentrate on ambulatory care financed by the social health insurance funds. The conditions of market entry and remuneration of medical services are determined within a model of group bargaining between the regional chamber of doctors and the social insurance funds. Market entry for doctors is limited by contract agreed by this bargaining group. Table 14.5 shows the development of the number of doctors holding a contract with the social insurance funds between 1980 and 1994. Although the number of doctors is high in Austria, this bargaining model has been useful in containing costs in the ambulatory sector in the past. About 75 per cent of general practitioners and about 40 per cent of specialists have contracts with the social insurance system, but the latter percentage differs widely between the different special-

Health Expenditure and Cost Control in Austria 621

Table 14.5 Number of doctors contracted by the social insurance system

	1980	1994	Change 1980/94
Total	7,414	7,869	6.1%
General practicioners	4,234	4,317	1.9%
Specialists	3,180	3,552	11.6%

Source: Hauptverband der Sozialversicherungsträger, 1981, 1995.[12]

ists. To a limited degree, patients of the social insurance system can also consult doctors who do not hold contracts with the social insurance system.

An important part of this collective agreement is the agreement on doctors' incomes. In principle, the general law on social health insurance provides for remuneration based on fees-for-services. In reality, however, various systems of remuneration exist, depending on the health insurance fund:

- remuneration on a fee-for-service basis, without expenditure limits;

- remuneration on a fee-for-service basis, with global expenditure limits for all doctors (not used at present);

- remuneration on a fee-for-service basis, with expense limits per doctor and per case treated;

- capitation payments per patient and time period (not used at present);

- capitation payments per patient and time period in combination with remuneration on a fee-for-service basis in special cases with expense limits per doctor and per case treated.

It is the last method of paying doctors which dominates in the Austrian health care system. The health insurance funds, which are organized on a territorial basis and which cover 80 per cent of the Austrian population, finance the services of doctors in this way. The impact of this system on the development of health care costs outside hospitals is not quite clear. On the one hand, the different forms of capitation payments and expenditure limits have helped to contain the development of the costs in the ambulatory sector. Figure 14.4 shows the development of the cases treated and the costs per case in the period 1980–94. The cases per (insured) person remained quite stable until 1988 but have grown since that time. The costs per case increased over the whole period at different rates of growth. On the other hand, the current method of paying office-based doctors is considered the main reason for the high rate of hospitalization in Austria. This is because few incentives exist to keep patients out of hospital. No financing mechanism exists to interest the doctor in his patients' hospital costs. These weak incentives were reduced by the reform of financing the hospitals. The social insurance funds have to pay the cost of treatments outside hospitals. On the other hand the funds give block transfers to hospitals, which are independent of the marginal costs of treating different numbers of patients. Therefore the incentives for the social insurance funds to keep patients out of hospital by evolving new forms of cooperation between doctors (group

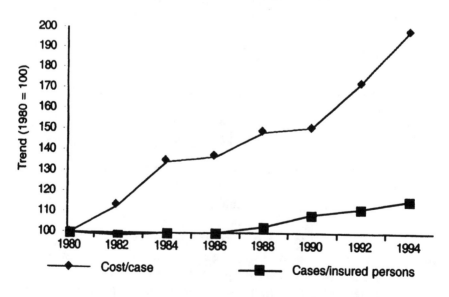

Figure 14.4 Out-patient cases treated and cost per out-patient case – (members of the social health insurance fund), 1980–94

Source: Hauptverband der Sozialversicherungsträger, Jahrbuch der Sozialversicherung, Vienna, several years.[12]

practice, fundholder-model, HMO-models) outside hospitals is reduced. Furthermore, incentives to control the total costs of the health care system independent of the level of the health care service will be reduced. Reforms to institutionalize the general practitioner as a 'gate-keeper' for the whole health care sector are therefore blocked by the hospital financing reform, because the representatives of the social insurance funds argue that these reforms would increase their expenditure for ambulatory care without reducing their expenditure for in-patient care. This is especially problematic, because the Austrian health care system is very accessible to the patient, while the referral system does not work very well.

In the recent past, several attempts have been made to control the costs in the ambulatory sector of the Austrian health care system. Methods of bureaucratic control of doctors are favoured over methods which offer positive incentives for the doctor (i.e. fundholder-models, HMO-models). No global ex-ante budgets exist for ambulatory expenditure within the health insurance funds. In 1996, guidelines for the consideration of economic principles in the treatment of patients were produced by the social insurance system and enforced. The basis of these guidelines is that the treatment of patients has to be sufficient, but should not go beyond the necessities of treatment. Doctors should especially take care that:

- in the case of equivalent medical procedures the least costly procedure is chosen;

- the potential of preventive methods is used; and

- decisions to refer patients to hospital should be made by taking into account the alternative forms of care (out-patient hospital department, home care).

Through adherence to these principles the work of doctors is controlled by the social insurance funds on the basis of comparisons with average prescribing and treatment patterns, and random tests.

A cost-sharing scheme (amount ATS 50 = ECU 3.50) was introduced for every permit (*Krankenschein*) to visit a doctor within the social insurance system at the beginning of 1997. This scheme is only valid for the first contact with the doctor. No additional money has to be paid for referrals to specialists. One aim of this cost-sharing scheme was to give incentives to use the general practitioner as a gate-keeper. There is some evidence that the

624 *Health Care and Cost Containment in the European Union*

system is working in this way, on the other hand the administrative costs of the cost-sharing scheme are very high and the abolition of the scheme is likely.

In Austria the potential for substituting in-patient care with ambulatory care without lowering the quality of care is estimated as being quite high. A study on the province of Salzburg concluded that 42 per cent of all hospital cases in 1990 could have been treated outside the hospital. These figures were based on the restructuring of health care provision. The study also concluded that, even with the existing structure of health services, 21 per cent of all hospital cases could have been treated outside the hospital.[13]

The high degree of misallocation of hospital resources in the past can be traced back to several factors: to the mechanism of financing of in-patient and out-patient care, to the definition of disease in the health insurance system, to the regulation of the cooperation of office-based doctors and to the non-existence of services outside hospital (i.e. long-term care, ambulatory services). These factors have been addressed in recent legislation. In the last few years concepts for 'Integrated Health and Social Administrative Districts' have been worked out and have been implemented in the different provinces. The DRG-based hospital financing system will create incentives for a more efficient structure of long-term care and ambulatory services.

14.4.3 The role of co-payments/cost-sharing in the Austrian health care system

The illustration of the role of cost-sharing in the Austrian health care system is a difficult task, because different forms of cost-sharing and co-payment are used for different procedures and by different insurance funds. In 1992, 24 per cent of total health care expenditure was financed by the state (state, provinces, and the local communities); 54 per cent by the social insurance system, 8 per cent by the private insurance system and 14 per cent by direct financing from the patient. This financing structure had been quite stable over the previous 15 years.

A co-payment of ATS 42 is charged for every prescription of drugs covered by the social health insurance system. People on welfare programmes (a kind of minimal living standard) and those with incomes below a certain level are exempted from this co-payment. All non-prescription drugs must be paid for by the patient. The co-payment has not changed dramatically in

Health Expenditure and Cost Control in Austria 625

the recent past. The drug policy of the social health insurance funds is based on a positive list. The prices of pharmaceuticals are regulated by the social health insurance funds. Table 14.6 gives some additional information about the role of the co-payment for drugs.

Table 14.6 The role of co-payment for drugs in the health insurance funds, 1980–94

Year	Expenditure of the social insurance system on pharmaceuticals (ATS 1,000s)	Revenues from user charges (ATS 1,000s)	% of revenues from user charges to expenditure on pharmaceuticals
1980	5,572	911	16.3
1983	6,171	1,097	17.7
1986	7,479	1,308	17.4
1989	9,187	1,630	17.7
1992	10,827	1,887	17.4
1994	14,367	2,397	16.6

Source: Hauptverband der Sozialversicherungsträger, Jahrbuch der Sozialversicherung, Vienna, several years.[12]

People insured under special health insurance funds (farmers, public workers, employers) have to pay 20 per cent of the fees for health services including hospital services. About 20 per cent of the Austrian population is covered under these insurance funds. This has not changed over the last few years. For therapeutic appliances, depending on the insurance agency in question, the insured person must pay between 10 and 20 per cent of the fee. Patients also pay a considerable share of the cost for dental treatment, particularly for high-quality and expensive individual technical items such as crowns and bridgework, which are not covered by the social insurance system. Since 1988, patients admitted to hospitals have to pay a small index-linked daily charge for a maximum of 28 days for standard-class accommodation, depending on the province of the hospital (between ATS 50 and ATS

626 Health Care and Cost Containment in the European Union

60 in 1997; ECU 3.50 to ECU 4.50). Supplementary insurance for covering co-payments is possible on a private basis. Exceptions exist for those on low-incomes. No substantial change has taken place recently in cost-sharing policies. A cost-sharing scheme for spa services was introduced in 1996. Scientific studies, which evaluate the effect of cost-sharing, are not available at the moment. However, there is a political consensus that cost-sharing should be used as a instrument of financing and not as a method of reducing demand.

14.4.4 cost containment strategies for pharmaceuticals

Unlike other components of medical spending, drug prices are under full control of the central government; and the market for pharmaceuticals is heavily regulated.[10] Drugs must be classified as either requiring a prescription or not requiring one. Eighty-five per cent of the drugs need registration, compared with, for example, 34 per cent in the UK, 45 per cent in Germany and 50 per cent in Switzerland.[10] The drugs must then be put on the register for approved drugs for reimbursement by the social insurance funds. Table 14.7 shows the number of registered drugs in Austria and the registered drugs on the positive list of the health insurance funds. The number of registered drugs increased sharply in recent years, while the percentage of drugs reimbursed by the health insurance funds decreased slightly.

In addition to regulations related to market entry, regulation of pharmaceutical prices occurs at all levels of the distribution chain.[14] On average only 40 per cent of the pharmacy retail price (= 100 per cent) per package goes to the manufacturer. With this, the costs of research, production, distribution must be covered. For their services, wholesalers were granted a 20 per cent mark up on the ex-factory price until 1994. In 1995, highly degressive mark up regulations for both wholesalers and pharmacies entered into force, which led to a decline in the average wholesale mark up to 16.9 per cent.[14] If a drug is paid for by the patient, pharmacies receive on average 35.01 per cent of the retail price. However, if the costs of drugs are born by the health insurance funds, the actual average gross margin drops to 19 per cent. Also this margin was reduced slightly by the reforms which took place in 1995 and 1996.

From the institutional feature of the Austrian pharmaceutical market we can conclude that the main instruments for cost containment in this sector

Health Expenditure and Cost Control in Austria 627

Table 14.7 Number of drugs on the Austrian market and on the positive list of health insurance funds, 1981–95

Year	(1) Number of registered drugs	(2) Registered drugs on the positive list of the health insurance funds	(3) (2) as % of (1)
1981	6,383	3,007	47
1982	6,292	2,916	46
1983	6,042	2,848	47
1984	5,966	2,825	47
1985	5,840	2,763	47
1986	5,832	2,734	47
1987	4,867	2,572	53
1988	5,023	2,591	52
1989	5,217	2,621	50
1990	5,476	2,595	47
1991	5,942	2,644	44
1992	6,635	2,761	41
1993	7,568	2,896	38
1994	8,773	2,766	31
1995	9,671	2,761	28

Source: Pharmig, 1996.[14]

are: the positive lists of the health insurance funds, the fixing of mark-ups for the manufacturers and pharmacies, and the different rebates which are given to the health insurance funds. Besides this, within the agreements established by the health insurance funds and doctors, there are various rules relating to the 'economic prescription' of drugs. However, there is no global prospective budget for pharmaceuticals.

628　*Health Care and Cost Containment in the European Union*

14.4.5 The reorganization of long-term care in Austria

Throughout the OECD countries, populations are ageing. Growth of the oldest population group, those aged 80 and above, is particularly rapid. As a result of this change in the demographic structure, chronic diseases are increasingly important, creating demand for both long-term care and acute care services. Therefore, reform of long-term care also has to be an integral part of health care reform from the perspective of cost containment. In the past in Austria, long-term care for the elderly was not ordered systematically and universally within the different funds of the social insurance system. The increasing need for assistance against these risks and the supply of long-term care services was covered in several ways:

- by additional transfers from the social pension system for 'helpless people'. In 1993 232,000 people received such a transfer;[15]

- by an extension of the definition of illness for hospital patients without adequate legal basis, because specific long-term care institutions were lacking;

- by increasing efforts of states and local communities within the decentralized welfare programmes (*'Sozialhilfe'*);

- by increasing the role of families.

However, several problems accompanied these methods of coping with the long-term care risk. The welfare programmes, which had figured as the lowest net against social risks, were now confronted with a normal risk of life and became overburdened. In addition to this, the means-tested welfare programme stigmatizes the recipient. Moreover, the long-term care services provided and the transfers received were different depending on the insurance fund rather than the level of care needed. Within families there existed a growing asymmetric burden for women. Finally, the extension of the definition of illness led to a misallocation of acute hospital resources. In 1993 a fundamental reform of long-term care took place. This reform included coverage of the financial risks of long-term care and an agreement between the state and the provinces to supply long-term care facilities. The basic principles of this reform are the following:

- The reform distinguishes between covering the financial risks of long-term care and the supply of long-term services. This seems positive,

Health Expenditure and Cost Control in Austria 629

Table 14.8 Financing of long-term care in Austria

Groups of intensity of care	Amount of the transfer (in ATS per month)	Percentage of the recipients of transfers in the intensity groups	Intensity of care (hours of care per month reported)	Financial burden*	Cost covering ratio**
1	2,635	10	127	3	79
2	3,688	52	139	10	65
3	5,690	20	214	20	59
4	8,.535	9	268	22	52
5	11,591	7	392	20	50
6	15,806	2	374	n.a.	50
7	21,071	1	417	n.a.	24

Notes
* % of the overall income recipients of long-term care transfers used to cover the monetary costs of long-term care.

** % of recipients of long-term care transfers which are not able to cover the monetary costs of long-term care out of the transfer

Source: Badelt *et al.*, 1997.[16]

because it offers degrees of freedom in the institutional alternatives of organizing long-term services.

- The transfers paid for long-term care are based on a system of universal coverage. The transfer does not depend on the income or the assets of the recipient, but is a simple cash transfer based only on the criteria of need for help. The need for help is based on the assessment of a doctor. Seven categories of need for long-term care were constructed depending on the amount of help needed. The transfer varies between ATS 2,635 per month in category one and ATS 21,074 per month in category seven (permanent need for care) (see Table 14.8, column 1).

- The transfers are neutral in respect of the institution of long-term care and allows for undistorted competition between the different institutional forms of care.

630 *Health Care and Cost Containment in the European Union*

- There exists no direct system of cost-sharing. However, the fact that the transfer is not based on existing costs leads to a substantial amount of cost-sharing in practice.

- The transfers are financed out of the general budget.

- The transfers are based on individual claims. Therefore no global budget constraint exists for these transfers. However, for 1996 and 1997 there has been no increase in the transfers granted as compared to those of 1995.

It is to early to give a full assessment of the long-term care reform of 1993. But several important points can already be made. Nearly all experts agree that the reform was a necessary and substantial step in the development of the Austrian welfare state. Badelt[17] estimated that, in a broader sense, 500,000 people currently need some form of care. This figure will increase sharply in the near future (600,000 by 2010 and 800,000 by 2030).[17] In 1995 about 300,000 people received a transfer for long-term care. Fifty-two per cent of the recipients received transfers of the intensity group two (see Table 14.8, column 2). Of these people, 90 per cent lived at home and 10 per cent in public or private care institutions or homes for the elderly. Handicapped people living at home get assistance from mobile institutions of care. The existence of such institutions varies widely between the provinces. But on the whole, the long-term care transfers have increased the possibilities of choice between different forms of care for handicapped people. The transfers cover only a part of the monetary costs of long-term care. The extent to which transfers cover the costs of care increases with the intensity of care needed (see also the last two columns in Table 14.8). Studies show strong consensus on the assessment of long-term care needs, although sometimes the heavy reliance on medical criteria is criticized.[17] The introduction of the transfers partly led to a (substantial) increase of the fees for institutional care. For two reasons the main task in the field of long-term care will be the improvement of the quantity and quality of services. First, the possibility of choice between different institutional forms has to be increased, and second, differences in the regional distribution of services, which are not related to need, have to be selected. Improvement of the quantity and quality of long-term care is also necessary for any substantial relief of the acute care institutions.

14.5 Summary

The institutional framework of the Austrian health care system is not an ideal basis for an efficient policy of cost containment. Authority over planning and spending is split between several institutions and no overall cost containment policies were possible in the past. Rather, cost containment policies were concentrated on individual components of the health care sector. The development of health expenditure was modest between 1980 and 1990, but since 1990 its average growth rate of health expenditure has been high and this has led to a substantial increase in health expenditure as a percentage of GDP. Cost containment strategies in the past have been modest and failed to cut back in the hospital sector. Policies were to some extent successful in the out-patient care sector, but only by shifting patients and costs to the hospital sector. cost containment policies have been related more to prices than to outputs/volume. It was possible to contain prices, however the resources used in the health care sector remained high by international standards. In 1996 a major reform of the hospital sector was established to reduce hospitalization and to contain hospital costs. The reform took effect in 1997 and includes the introduction of a DRG-based financing system, the strengthening of the federal state in allocating hospital resources at a macro-level, and the strengthening of the provinces in financing the hospital system. However, several further steps of reform are necessary to contain costs and increase efficiency. Areas of the health care sector still requiring reform are the following (see also OECD, 1997):[10]

- The basic problem of the Austrian health care system is the disintegration of political responsibilities and the divided nature of the financing system. This disintegration/divide is dysfunctional to a high degree. It does not promote efficiency but sometimes leads to efficiency-diminishing zero-sum games between political institutions (state, provinces, local communities, health insurance funds). It appears that Austria has to decide between two options: to extend the role and the financial obligations of the health insurance funds (especially in the hospital sector) or to concentrate health policy and financing at the level of the provinces. Health care resources need to be managed by a single institution, thereby improving decisions relating to allocative and technical efficiency.[10]

- On the demand side, a more systematic discussion of cost-sharing

632   *Health Care and Cost Containment in the European Union*

schemes is necessary. Currently, increases in user charges are mainly due to the exclusion of services from reimbursement by social insurance funds. However, no truly systematic discussion regarding which services should be paid for by the social insurance funds has taken place.

- The 1996 reform of the hospital sector was an important step in increasing the efficiency of the health care system and in containing costs. It strengthened the role of the provinces in health care policy. But the gap between the in-patient and out-patient sectors of health care was not reduced. Therefore an important next step of reform should include the following initiatives: the planning of in-patient and out-patient capacities should be integrated; the role of the provinces as purchasers of in-patient and out-patient care should be strengthened; incentives for more rational decision-making with respect to hospital investment are necessary; and the budget constraints on the provinces need to be tightened by reducing fiscal transfers.

- The role of the GP as a 'gate-keeper' must be strengthened in order to decrease the current burden on hospitals. For this to be achieved several initiatives are required. The barriers to group practice must be further deregulated – group practice has been illegal until recently – and the ambulatory sector needs to be developed accordingly. GPs must be offered incentives to increase the range of services they provide, including home visits and weekend services – currently doctors in the out-patient sector are neither permitted to follow their patients to hospital, nor to use hospital facilities. In this vein, GP-hospital cooperation must be improved, and a gradual shift from hospital to primary health care ought to be undertaken.

- Future expenditure trends are difficult to predict given the extent of the new policy measures introduced in recent years. Nonetheless it is likely that there will be an increase in private expenditure for spa services and for several medical goods (i.e. eye-glasses, dental care). In addition, within the public sector, a shift of expenditure from the central state and health insurance funds to the provinces and the local communities is probable.

References

1 Beirat für Wirtschafts- und Sozialfragen. *Neue Wege im Gesundheitswesen – Kurzfassung.* Wien: Beirat für Wirtschafts- und Sozialfragen, 1996.

2 Bundesministerin für Gesundheit, Sport und Konsumentenschutz. *Gesundheitsbericht an den Nationalrat 1994.* Wien: Bundesministerium für Gesundheit, Sport und Konsumentenschutz, 1994.

3 OECD. *The Reform of Health Care Systems – A Review of Seventeen OECD countries.* Paris: OECD, 1994.

4 Österreichisches Bundesinstitut für Gesundheitswesen. *Österreichischer Krankenanstaltenplan.* Wien: Österreichisches Bundesinstitut für Gesundheitswesen, 1994.

5 OECD. *OECD Health Data 1996.* Paris: OECD, 1996.

6 Basys. *Gesundheitssysteme im Internationalen Vergleich.* Ausgabe 1994, Basys, Augsburg, 1995.

7 Basys. *Wirtschaftlichkeit und Leistungsniveau Deutscher Krankenhäuser im Internationalen Vergleich.* Augsburg: Basys, 1993.

8 Theurl E. *Überleben die Krankenhäuser?* Thaur: Kulturverlag, 1991.

9 VAMED. *Österreichisches Krankenhauswesen bis 2010.* Wien: VAMED, 1988.

10 OECD. *OECD Economic Surveys, 1996-1997, Austria.* Paris: OECD, 1997.

11 Pfeiffer KP. The possible effects of a new hospital financing system in Austria. In: Schwartz FW *et al.* (eds). *Fixing Health Budgets: Experience from Europe and North America.* London: Wiley, 1996.

12 Hauptverband der Sozialversicherungsträger. *Jahrbuch der Sozialversicherung.* Wien: Hauptverband der Sozialversicherungsträger, several years.

13 Amt der Salzburger Landesregierung. *Substitutionspotentiale Stationärer Medizinischer Leistungen im Land Salzburg.* Salzburg: Amt der Salzburger Landesregierung, 1995.

14 Pharmig. *Drugs – Help and Heal, Facts and Figures 1996/97.* Wien: Pharmig, 1996.

15 Theurl E. Zur Ökonomik alter Menschen unter besonderer Berücksichtigung des Pflegefallrisikos. In: Universität Innsbruck (ed.). *Das Altern aus der Sicht der Wissenschaften.* Innsbruck. 1996.

16 Badelt Chr. *et al. Analyse der Auswirkungen des Pflegevorsorgesystems.* Wien: Bundesministerium für Arbeit, Gesundheit und Soziales, 1997.

17 Badelt Chr. *et al. Kosten der Pflegesicherung.* Wien: Böhlau-Verlag, 1996.

15 Health care reform and cost containment in Portugal

JOÃO PEREIRA, ANTÓNIO CORREIA DE CAMPOS,
FRANCISCO RAMOS, JORGE SIMÕES AND VASCO REIS

15.1 Introduction

A recent study identifies Portugal as one of five EU countries where, during the 1980s and 1990s, major health care reforms aiming to contain costs and increase efficiency were either proposed or undertaken.[1] During the same period, however, health care expenditure has been rising relatively fast. For example, according to the OECD, between 1980 and 1995 Portugal had the second highest rate of annual growth of total health expenditure (expressed as a percentage of GDP) among EU countries.[2]

This chapter focuses on both these issues – health reform and cost containment in Portugal. In view of the comments above, one would expect that a case study of Portugal could shed light on the factors which contribute to the relative success or failure of policy initiatives. Yet, for a number of reasons – chief among them the slow pace of reform and the lack of sound evidence on the impact of cost containment policies – we are only able to provide an impressionistic analysis.

Debate on reform of the health care system in Portugal has gone on since the late 1980s. There has been considerable legislative activity and some radical proposals have been put forward. In general, these proposals envisage organizational changes aimed at promoting a greater role for the private sector, individual responsibility and entrepreneurial management of Portugal's National Health Service (NHS). However, relatively few of the proposed measures have been put in place. There has not been a major reform as such; merely the slow enactment of varied policy measures which have left the system only slightly different from that of the early 1980s.

The sluggishness of the reform process is one reason for the lack of objective evidence on the impact of cost containment measures. However, it

635

is not the only one. The tradition of policy evaluation is not strong in Portugal and many analysts are closely associated with particular policy initiatives, meaning that evaluations are seldom impartial. Furthermore, for some years the low level of health care financing was identified by some observers as a critical issue, so that cost containment was not seen as a priority. Indeed, not long ago it was common to hear politicians arguing in favour of increasing the level of health expenditure to the average of the European Union (EU). Though this view has now largely been abandoned, most commentators remain uncritical about the effectiveness of health care interventions. A general belief that 'more health care is good' continues to prevail, reflecting the strength of the medical profession in shaping the reform debate. Whatever the causes, the fact remains that evidence on the impact of cost containment policies is slight, and there is an urgent need to proceed to more careful evaluation before new policies are either proposed or abandoned.

Very few measures during the 1990s that are aimed at containing costs can be identified. Perhaps the most important are the increases in patient co-payments in 1992 – though these have not been raised since – and two implicit measures: price rises below the rate of inflation for NHS contracted services and increased waiting lists for specialist care. Generally, however, most measures are scarcely motivated by cost containment concerns.

The chapter is structured in two broad sections. Section 15.2 describes the Portuguese health system and the policy reforms which have been proposed in the 1990s. The description of the system is made in terms of the departure of the existing situation from the classical NHS model which, from the mid-1970s to the mid-1980s, was widely viewed as an ideal to be attained. Reforms of the early 1990s are shown to have been, in practice, far less radical than is generally supposed. In section 15.3 an assessment of policy initiatives and developments that are related to cost containment is provided. A number of broad areas are analysed, among them NHS expenditure, the hospital and ambulatory-care sectors, payment of providers, cost-sharing and pharmaceutical expenditure. The chapter concludes with a summary assessment.

15.2 The Portuguese health care system

15.2.1 The mixed nature of the Portuguese NHS

The Portuguese health care system has often been described as conforming to the classical National Health Service model.[3] This model is characterized by universal coverage of the population, generality of benefits, national tax financing and national ownership or control of factors of production.[4] In 1979, a National Health Service with these characteristics was indeed created, together with a political commitment that it become the preponderant mode of health care financing and provision. Yet the available evidence suggests that the system has certain features which render the usual characterization somewhat incomplete.

Consider first the issue of *universal coverage*. Throughout the existence of the NHS there have co-existed a number of occupational insurance schemes – overwhelmingly non-voluntary and in the public sector of the economy – which were originally intended to be integrated in the NHS. Evidence from various sources shows that around a quarter of the population have access to the double-cover provided by these funds.[5] The delivery and payment of care in the insurance funds is similar to that in other countries: users are free to purchase care wherever they wish; most use the private sector or contracted services for ambulatory care and the NHS for non-elective surgical interventions; and the funds pay contracted services on a fee-per-item basis and reimburse patients or co-finance the use of privately provided care. Financing of the insurance schemes is also similar to that in other countries in that employees contribute a small proportion of their income, but with an important qualification: a significant proportion of expenditures are part-financed by state taxation. This is because contributions are generally insufficient to cover expenditure. For the funds operating in the public sector (e.g. ADSE which provides for public servants) the deficits are covered by taxation; whereas for others (e.g. SAMS for bank workers) the schemes simply do not pay for higher level services provided to their members by the NHS. In effect, this means that the funds are subsidised by other sectors of the economy with greater proportions of lower paid workers. The ADSE fund has the added implication of providing incentives for NHS workers not to use the NHS.

With regard to the NHS providing a *generality of benefits,* the evidence

638 *Health Care and Cost Containment in the European Union*

indicates that in key areas the NHS may not be providing the sufficiently wide range of services it promises. Table 15.1 shows that the NHS is predominant in the provision of hospital stays, GP and mother and child care, but takes a minor role in specialist and dental consultations as well as diagnostic services, where it commonly reimburses private providers. At the very least this evidence indicates the important role of private provision in the delivery of health care in Portugal. The evidence is in part explained by the perennial under-utilization of NHS equipment, either because of shortages in the supply of human resources or laxity in administrative controls over providers who work simultaneously for the NHS and the private sector, and the unequal spread of human and material resources throughout the territory.[6]

Table 15.1 Health care utilization by sector in Portugal, 1987

Type of care	NHS (%)	Private (%)
All consultations	67.0	33.0
GP consultations	76.5	23.5
Dental consultations	15.5	84.5
Specialist consultations	47.8	52.2
Family planning consultations	61.7	38.3
Ante-natal consultations	61.9	38.1
Child delivery	87.6	12.4
X-rays	47.5	52.4
Laboratory tests	29.5	70.5
Hospital stays	72.8	27.2

Source: Pereira (1995),[7] calculated from National Health Survey.

The Portuguese health care system is also seen to depart from the classical NHS model when one considers sources of finance. Table 15.2 shows the percentage of total and public health expenditure in GDP for Portugal, along with the EU average weighted by size of population, and a comparison of equivalent data for the countries with the lowest and highest shares. The proportion of Portuguese national income spent on health is not, nowadays, significantly different from the EU average. However, what is distinct, and

Health Care Reform and Cost Containment in Portugal 639

ever more so, is the high share of private expenditure, accounting for 36 and 39 per cent of total expenditure in 1980 and 1995 respectively. In countries with a tax-financed NHS this share tends to be between 10 and 20 per cent. In part, this reflects the strength of the insurance funds but it is also due to the existence of widespread co-payments in the NHS. Flat-rate payments exist for consultations and diagnostic tests, and patients pay a relatively large proportion of the cost of drugs.

Consider finally the question of ownership and control of the factors of production. Doctors and nurses in the NHS are paid on a salaried basis. However, they are generally not required to exercise their duties on a full-time basis and many tend to work for the NHS in the morning and in private practice in the afternoon, on a fee-per-item of service or contractual basis. Autonomous market or NHS provision is negligible. The incentives generated by these circumstances go some way to explaining the utilization and expenditure patterns previously described. Due to laxity in regulation, doctors are motivated to supply minimum standards of care in NHS work-settings in order to augment the potential market share of private practice.

Table 15.2 Expenditure on health as a per cent of GDP, 1980 and 1995

	Total expenditure		Public expenditure		Private as % of total	
	1980	1995	1980	1995	1980	1995
Portugal	5.8	8.2	3.7	5.0	36.2	39.0
EU weighted average	6.9	8.5	5.5	6.7	20.2	21.5
Lowest share	3.6	5.8	3.0	4.4	7.4	7.1
Highest share	9.4	10.4	8.7	8.2	36.2	39.0

Source: OECD Health Data 97.[2]

The NHS owns a sizeable majority of physical resources involved in the delivery of care, though as we have seen, provision in a private setting is far from negligible. Eighty per cent of hospital beds are in the public sector and there is a comprehensive network of health centres in primary care. The 1979 NHS legislation decreed that private practice should complement pub-

640 *Health Care and Cost Containment in the European Union*

lic provision, in the sense of operating in areas where the latter was deficient, but all available evidence points to the contrary. In the hospital sector, for example, private provision is heavily concentrated in those regions where NHS supply is more extensive, while a comparative analysis of case-mix showed that it tends to produce routine, low-cost treatments where there is no obvious shortage of supply in the public sector.[6] It is in ambulatory care, however, where financing is open-ended, that we find the most striking departure from the NHS model. The provision of medical acts arising from NHS GP visits is dominated by the private sector. Besides the private supply of pharmaceuticals, a large and rising proportion of diagnostic tests and treatments are contracted to the private sector, rather than being carried out in NHS hospitals.

In summary, although Portugal is commonly believed to have a system of the NHS type, the incentives built in to this structure are such that it has always tended to operate in a fashion not dissimilar to countries where there is collective provision of a basic level of care complemented by private individual purchase. Figure 15.1 provides a schematic view of the public–private mix in the financing and delivery of care in Portugal, bringing together the description provided above. The figure also serves as a useful backdrop to the discussion in section 15.3.

15.2.2 Reform in the 1990s

Given the various ambiguities of the health care system it was natural that in the 1990s, in the context of the international wave of reforms, policy-makers in Portugal should seek to introduce changes to the existing structure. However, contrary to the common portrayal in the international literature, there has been no major reform of the system. Instead, many of the more important changes have been of a normative nature, with new laws essentially legitimizing the situation which had evolved, while the more radical aspects of proposed reforms are still to be implemented.

A law of 1990 set the basis for future health service development.[8] The key principles of this law were:[9]

(a) that the NHS was no longer to be seen as the main form of provision, but as one of several entities (both public and private) involved in delivering care to the population;

Health Care Reform and Cost Containment in Portugal 641

Figure 15.1 Financing and delivery of care in Portugal: Public-private mix

| | FINANCING | |
	PUBLIC	PRIVATE
DELIVERY / PRIVATE	**A** • Hospitals (budgets set at central level) • Health centres (budgets set at central level and channelled through Regional Health Administrations – RHAs) • Other public facilities	**B** • Hospital care paid by occupational and private insurance schemes (prices set by government) • Patient co-payments in public facilities
DELIVERY / PUBLIC	**C** • Contracted services in NHS and public sector insurance schemes (e.g. most diagnostic tests and some hospital care) • Private medical practices, clinics and laboratories reimbursed by public sector insurance schemes (e.g. ADSE for public servants) • Drugs and therapeutic procedures (part-financed by state taxation) • Private medical care tax-deductible (all expenditures)	**D** • Private medical practices, clinics and laboratories (direct payments and reimbursement) • Health care units belonging to non-public occupational insurance schemes and insurance companies • Drugs and therapeutic procedures (part-financed by patients) • Contracted services (patient co-payments)

(b) that the State should promote the development of the private sector and provide incentives for the expansion of private health insurance;

(c) that care provided under the NHS should be 'approximately free' rather than free at the point of contact; and

(d) that management of NHS facilities could be contracted-out to the private sector.

642 *Health Care and Cost Containment in the European Union*

A law of January 1993 regulated some of these broad principles, specifically with regard to the organization of the NHS.[10] Among the more important changes were:

(a) the number of Regional Health Administrations (RHAs) was to be reduced from 18 to 5 and these were given greater autonomy and powers to coordinate the activity of hospitals;

(b) within regions, health centres were to be grouped with hospitals to form 'health units' in an effort to assure continuity of care;

(c) full-time salaried doctors were allowed to engage in private practice;

(d) various forms of private management of NHS facilities and of private health care provision according to NHS guidelines;

(e) NHS co-payments were to be established taking into account patients' ability to pay; and

(f) an 'alternative health insurance' scheme was to be created, whereby private insurance companies would receive from the government part-payment of the premium of people who opted-out of the NHS.

Very little progress has been made in implementing these changes. Administrative changes at the level of the regions have had a minor impact. For example, following the publication of the 1993 law a new directive was published which stated that hospitals were to continue to answer directly to the central level, rather than to the Regional Administrations. The creation of 'health units' has also had little visible impact with many areas of the country continuing very much as before.

Perhaps the most controversial provision in the 1993 law was the incentive for patients to move from public coverage to private insurers who would cover all their defined health needs throughout their lifetimes. In return, insurance companies would receive a subsidy from the government for each insured person (less than the average per capita cost of the NHS according to some commentators, though the actual amounts were never publicly revealed). Partly because of the lack of interest by private insurers and partly because of a change in the ministerial team, this provision never got off the ground.

Following the replacement of the Social Democratic government in late 1995 by a Socialist administration, there has been a change of emphasis in

Health Care Reform and Cost Containment in Portugal 643

health reform. For instance, in a recently published document, the Ministry of Health states that its first principle will be to 'invest in the potential of the NHS'.[11] Further to this, the government has specified other intentions, among them the development of managed competition between public and private providers, the reduction of price inflation in the health sector to levels in the general economy, and the granting of greater autonomy to hospitals and health centres.[12]

The new government also set up a Commission to produce a report on reform of the health system. Its results are due to be published in late 1997, but a preliminary report leaves the impression that the Commission will suggest changes that go beyond the spheres of management and delivery of care.[13] It is likely that new modes of raising revenues for the health service will be proposed; such as an earmarked health tax or a replacement of general tax-financing by a system based on social insurance. Should such measures be proposed they will doubtless prove controversial.

15.3 Policy measures and cost containment

The following section provides an examination of developments and policy measures which have been enacted in recent years and an assessment of their impact in terms of cost containment.

15.3.1 NHS and overall expenditure on health care

NHS services are overwhelmingly financed by general taxes from the State Budget. In 1995, around 90 per cent of expenditure was financed from this source. Expenditure is essentially controlled by the application of an annual global budget, separated into current and capital expenditure. Preparatory work for the budget is carried out by the Financial Management Department of the Ministry of Health (IGIF) detailing the financial resources needed to support programmed activities. A historical basis is generally adopted, involving an estimate of total expenditure for the current year which is adjusted by the expected increase in the level of consumption, salary levels and the rate of inflation. However, the actual amounts made available are also determined by government macro-economic strategies.

644 *Health Care and Cost Containment in the European Union*

Allocation of individual budgets to hospitals is carried out directly at the central level. This is also made on a historical basis. At the beginning of the 1990s it was envisaged that a prospective DRG system would be developed but it has since been largely abandoned. There are now plans to devolve hospital financing to Regional Health Administrations (RHAs), though no clear guidelines as to how have been outlined. A regional allocation of the NHS budget is currently made to RHAs which serves to finance primary care services managed by them. There are no separate budgets for pharmaceuticals and diagnostic tests, with financing for these being open-ended.

Though the procedure of setting global budgets has been shown in the past to contribute successfully to cost containment,[14,15] it should be noted that there are regular overshoots in budget limits which make the procedure somewhat fragile. In 1995 for instance, there was a supplementary mid-year budget of ESP 76 billion, roughly 9 per cent of the initial figure. This is common practice. Between 1990 and 1995, additional budgets were always approved: 14.9 per cent in 1990; 8.5 per cent in 1991; 6.3 per cent in 1992; 5.9 per cent in 1993; 1.9 per cent in 1994; and 9.0 per cent in 1995.[16] Despite these corrective budgets, in the same period the NHS always showed a financial deficit of between 0.1 per cent and 8.3 per cent.

Table 15.3 shows the evolution of NHS expenditure throughout the 1990s. In each year there was a real increase in expenditure ranging from 15.5 per cent in 1991 to 0.8 per cent in 1993. It is expected that figures for 1996 will show a significant rise in expenditure. Comparing the distribution of expenditure by sector shows a rise in hospital expenditure up to 1993, followed by a fall from then onwards. This is in part due to the growth of the drug bill which accounted for 16.9 per cent in 1992 and 18 per cent in 1995. It is also noticeable that the share of salary expenditure decreased from 51.7 per cent in 1990 to 45.3 per cent in 1995.[16]

Capital expenditure is centrally controlled by the Ministry of Health. An annual plan is prepared and approved by Parliament, and financed by the State Budget. Table 15.4 shows that throughout the 1990s capital expenditure – mainly the construction of new hospitals and health centres – has grown substantially. Since 1994 there is also a specific programme for investments in health care services co-financed by EU funds. This is expected to allow for further significant increases in the amount of financial resources devoted to new health facilities, although the latest figures for 1995 show a real decline.

Health Care Reform and Cost Containment in Portugal   645

Table 15.3 NHS current expenditure, 1990/95, constant prices (1991), ESP billion

Year	Current expenditure	Annual growth rate	% by sector		
			Hospitals	Primary health care	Other services
1990	393,640		47.7	46.6	5.7
1991	454,649	15.5%	49.7	44.7	5.6
1992	482,628	6.2%	49.8	45.6	4.6
1993	486,688	0.8%	51.1	44.9	4.0
1994	510,383	4.9%	50.1	45.8	4.1
1995	547,372	7.2%	49.0	46.4	4.6

Growth rate 1990–95: 39%

Source: Ministry of Health, DEPS.

Table 15.4 NHS capital expenditure, 1990/95, constant prices (1991), ESP billion

Year	Capital expenditure	Annual growth rate
1990	12,251	
1991	14,320	16.9%
1992	19,601	36.9%
1993	21,653	10.5%
1994	29,829	37.8%
1995	24,909	-16.5%

Growth rate 1990–95: 103%

Source: Ministry of Health, DEPS.

The growth in private expenditure has accompanied the relatively high increases in public expenditure. Of the 2.4 point increase in the share of health expenditure in GDP, 1.1 points are attributed to private expenditure.[2] In general, very little is known about the structure of private expenditure. However, drawing on data from two household budget surveys, Pereira *et al.*[17] showed that between 1980 and 1990 the largest real (constant prices) increases in out-of-pocket expenditure were for therapeutic appliances,

646 *Health Care and Cost Containment in the European Union*

diagnostic procedures other than X-rays and lab tests, nursing and paramedical services, doctors' fees and private insurance premiums. All of these rose by more than 190 per cent in real terms.

The increases in private expenditure are partly explained by generous tax deductions which came into force following the 1989 income tax reform. At the beginning of the 1980s there were limits on the amount of out-of-pocket health expenditure which could be deducted (50 per cent at most) and certain expenses were ineligible (e.g. pharmaceutical expenses). Following the reform no such limits prevailed and households were allowed to recoup an amount equal to their marginal tax rate (e.g. 40 per cent for the richest households). It is reasonable to suggest that this policy also provided an incentive to health care providers to increase prices beyond the underlying rate of inflation.

In summary, though the information base is not ideal, all evidence points to expenditure on health care having increased significantly in recent years. This is the result of a general understanding in political circles, only challenged very recently, that Portugal needed to make an effort to increase resources devoted to health care.

15.3.2 Hospitals

The NHS dominates the provision of hospital services in Portugal. In recent years, around 80 per cent of beds and 85 per cent of in-patient stays have been in state-owned hospitals.[13.] Unlike many other European countries, Portugal has throughout the 1990s continued a programme of hospital construction. Nevertheless, bed capacity in the public sector in 1995 was roughly the same as in 1980 (see Table 15.5). Hospital utilization, as measured by patients discharged, increased by 66 per cent in the same period. Similarly, out-patient and emergency consultations also increased by large amounts: 117 per cent and 32 per cent respectively. For all of these measures of activity, the more pronounced increases have been in district hospitals. Out-patient consultations, for example, were three times their 1980 value in 1995.

In general, throughout the same period, levels of efficiency in Portuguese hospitals appear to have improved. There has been a marked decline in average length of stay in public hospitals, from 17.1 to 9.6 days and 11.6 to 7.0 days in central and district hospitals respectively. The aver-

Table 15.5 Hospital activity (public, general and acute hospitals), 1980–95

| | | 1980 | | | 1990 | | | 1995 | |
	CH	DH	Total	CH	DH	Total	CH	DH	Total
Discharges*	2,248	2,086	4,334	3,190 *42%*	3,007 *44%*	6,197 *43%*	3,470 *54%*	3,725 *79%*	7,195 *66%*
No. of beds**	12,488	9,151	21,639	12,084 *-3%*	8,976 *-2%*	21,060 *-3%*	11,607 *-7%*	9,847 *8%*	21,454 *-1%*
Average length of stay	17.1	11.6	14.5	10.9 *-36%*	8.0 *-31%*	9.5 *-34%*	9.6 *-44%*	7.0 *-40%*	8.3 *-43%*
Occupancy rate (%)	83.8	71.9	78.1	69.2 *-17%*	73.0 *2%*	71.0 *-9%*	78.7 *-6%*	72.5 *1%*	75.9 *-3%*
Out-patient consultations*	1,771	645	2,416	2,783 *57%*	1,261 *96%*	4,044 *67%*	3,200 *81%*	2,036 *216%*	5,236 *117%*
Accident and emergency consultations	1,534	1,899	3,433	1,731 *13%*	2,671 *41%*	4,403 *28%*	1,918 *25%*	2,618 *38%*	4,536 *32%*

Notes: CH and DH refer to central and district hospitals, respectively.
Percentages in italic represent the change in the value directly above in relation to the 1980 value.
* Discharges and out-patient and accident and emergency consultations are expressed in 1000s.
** Does not include psychiatric hospitals.
Sources: DGH, Estatísticas Hospitalares, 1976/1980;
DEPS, Elementos Estatísticos, Saúde 90 e Saúde 95.

648 *Health Care and Cost Containment in the European Union*

age occupancy rate has remained more or less stagnant, having declined considerably in the 1970s.

Despite improvement in activity indicators, waiting lists in public hospitals are a growing problem. A recent study, covering eight areas of elective or non-emergency surgical interventions in Portuguese hospitals, showed that in 1992 there were a total of 92,000 potential in-patients waiting for an average of 223 days for a surgical intervention.[18] The number of patients on waiting lists amounted to almost 15 per cent of total hospital discharges in a single year.

Hospital budgets are distributed largely on a historical basis. Though a DRG patient classification system has been in place since the mid-1980s, an intention to move progressively to DRG-based financing has not materialized. At most, the system was used to determine 10 per cent of budgets in the early 1990s. Since then, even this small step has been abandoned, and DRG's are used essentially as a pricing system for non-NHS payers (e.g. the insurance companies). It is possible that the payment structure will be revitalized in the future, given that there are plans to provide greater autonomy to hospitals, possibly in the form of trusts as in the UK.

In contrast to most other European countries, the location of heavy medical equipment tends to be independent from the hospitals. The process has been led by the private sector with hospitals reimbursing private clinics for the use of equipment. In effect, 63 per cent of digital angiography capacity is in the hands of private clinics. For computerized tomography, lithotriptors and MRIs, the percentages are even higher, at 69, 75 and 86 per cent respectively.[19]

In order to control cost increases in the high-tech diagnostic sector, legislation in 1988 gave the Ministry of Health control over new purchases of heavy medical equipment, both in the public and private sector (see Table 15.6). The effects of this legislation were never thoroughly evaluated. However, there is no evidence of control either in the dissemination of modern technology or in the corresponding costs. In 1995 new legislation was passed which removed some equipment (e.g. CT scans and MRI) from the list subject to dissemination control, while for other equipment more generous population ratios were approved (Table 15.6).

The application in public hospitals since the mid-1980s of utilization review and other management techniques, with the objective of determining the clinical adequacy of admissions and length of stay, has led to reinforcement of health care alternatives. Day hospitals, particularly in the area of

Health Care Reform and Cost Containment in Portugal   649

Table 15.6 Legislation on approval of installation of heavy medical equipment. Population ratios 1988 and 1995

Equipment	Legislation	
	1988	1995
Computerized tomography	1 / 250,000 inhab.	No set ratio
MRI	1 / 3 million inhab.	No set ratio
Lithotriptors	1 / 3 million inhab.	No set ratio
Oncological radiotherapy	1 / 1 million inhab.	1 / 250,000 inhab.
PET	1 / 3 million inhab.	1 / 1 million inhab.
Digital angiography	1 / 500,000 inhab.	1 / 250,000 inhab.
Haemodialysis posts	45 / 1 million inhab.	No set ratio

Note: The population ratios are guidelines for the approval of installation of heavy medical equipment.

Sources: Decreto-Lei 445/88, Decreto-Lei 95/95 and Resolução 61/95.

oncology, and ambulatory surgery have been created in some institutions. Generally, however, there are no incentives in the system for alternatives to hospital care. It is estimated that patients in day hospitals account for around 3 per cent of all hospital in-patients, and ambulatory surgery for around 5 per cent of all surgery carried out under the NHS.

The 1990s has seen the enactment of legislation regarding the reduction of state control of health care delivery and management services. This practice was already in place with regard to the contracting out of certain tasks such as laundry and catering services. In 1996 the Fernando da Fonseca Hospital – a newly constructed institution on the outskirts of Lisbon – became the first public hospital to be managed by a private entity (a consortium led by an insurance company). The hospital is obliged to provide hospital care to all residents in a pre-defined geographical area in return for a fixed payment (i.e. independent of the level of delivery). This experiment has not yet been evaluated.

15.3.3 Ambulatory care

In ambulatory care, the number of consultations in NHS health centres increased by 32 per cent between 1985 and 1994. There are now 2.6 con-

650 *Health Care and Cost Containment in the European Union*

sultations per inhabitant compared to just 2 in 1985. During the same period there has been a sharp decline in home visits, probably due to the absence of direct financial incentives.

Reasons for the modest increase in NHS primary health care utilization are related both to supply and demand. Throughout the period, the number of new general practitioners and public health doctors has been declining relative to the number of young doctors admitted to hospital speciality training. This trend is the result of an explicit medical manpower policy which has generated more vacancies in the hospitals with the argument that new district hospitals, partially built with EU financial support, would imply a need for more doctors. On the demand side, many patients prefer to use the private sector or emergency care services in hospitals. In health centres it is extremely difficult to book a doctor visit for the same day, and given that laboratory and X-ray diagnostic units are separated from health centres, much time is needed to get a complete set of diagnostic tests. In the emergency departments on the contrary, the full range of ambulatory services can be obtained in a few hours. This deviation from regular health care system utilization involves the utilization of highly expensive emergency services to treat minor health complaints, leading to duplication of services and a considerable misuse of resources.

Since the creation of the NHS, the provision of ambulatory care has been largely immune to innovative reform proposals that may help to rationalize demand for care. Recently, however, there are signs of change. For example, under the so-called Alfa project created in 1996 by the Lisbon RHA, groups of GPs have seen their remuneration complemented by overtime payments and other incentives in return for an assurance of providing permanent care and adequate referral and follow-up of patients on their lists. It is likely that this experience will evolve towards a fundholding system as in the UK. It offers the promise of controlling the excessive use of hospital emergency departments in the cities and therefore of reducing costs. However, the experience has not yet been evaluated.

15.3.4 Providers

The payment of health care providers in Portugal suffers from a number of flaws which make cost containment policies generally ineffective. In the NHS, individual providers are paid on a salary basis and hospitals are financed through retrospective global budgets, independently of performance. However, in the private sector, providers are paid on a fee-for-service basis. This financing mix tends to jeopardize cost containment incentives. In the public sector, expenditure above budget levels is regularly covered with no penalty for managers. In the private sector budget caps do not exist. The only negative incentive for private providers is the chronic delay in the NHS paying its debts.

The duration of payment delay by the NHS depends not on the nature of care and its relative priority, but on provider bargaining power. In 1988, pharmaceutical outlets negotiated a system of reimbursement with a maximum two months' delay. A similar short delay is in place for end-stage renal dialysis. Therapists, radiologists and pathologists are much less powerful and they usually wait four to seven months to be paid. This traditional arrears system has acted as a deterrent to the creation of new private laboratories. It has also been instrumental in the trend towards horizontal concentration in the health care industry, with renal dialysis multinational providers purchasing many small-scale clinical pathology laboratories in recent years.

The accumulation of managerial functions in NHS hospitals with ownership and operation of private laboratories by senior doctors has continued to be tolerated. The 1993 legislation set a three-year period for these professionals to opt for the public or private sector. New legislation has since been enacted, delaying the option period for an additional year and no real signs of clarification are foreseen.

The payment system for hospitals provides no incentives for increasing efficiency (e.g. by reducing staff numbers or by concentrating activity in areas of comparative advantage). Overtime payments for doctors is a major problem in already over-doctored hospitals (36 per cent of all medical salary costs in the Lisbon Region hospitals are now for overtime).

A Commission recently set up by the Ministry of Health has identified public management rigidities as a serious source of inefficiency in hospitals and proposed introducing more flexibility into their structure. These proposals have been strongly opposed by doctors' unions and associations, with the argument that medical career prospects must be protected in order to maintain quality of care.

Another area of innovation has been the plans to introduce practice guidelines. Portuguese doctors have become receptive to the principle, but the idea that these may be obligatory or related to economic objectives is

652 *Health Care and Cost Containment in the European Union*

anathema to them. All initiatives to date have strictly to do with quality assurance. The President of the Medical Association regularly states that guidelines should not be used as a means to cost containment.

15.3.5 Pharmaceuticals

A continued source of concern in terms of cost containment has been pharmaceutical expenditure. As Table 15.7 shows, throughout the 1990s expenditure has increased in real terms in every year. Expenditure on drugs prescribed under the NHS grew by 45 per cent between 1990 and 1995 whereas total market expenditure increased by 41 per cent. The largest rise has been in patient co-payments which grew by 52 per cent in the same period. This rise means that the share of total NHS drug costs supported directly by patients grew from 31 per cent in 1990 to 33 per cent in 1995.

Table 15.7 Pharmaceutical expenditure, 1990–95, constant prices, ESP billion

Year	Total expenditure		NHS expenditure		NHS patient charges	
	Value	Annual growth rate	Value	Annual growth rate	Value	Annual growth rate
1990	174,427		99,601		31,285	
1991	193,005	10.7%	111,292	11.7%	34,534	10.4%
1992	209,080	8.3%	117,386	5.5%	37,654	9.0%
1993	222,702	6.5%	127,095	8.3%	42,691	13.4%
1994	226,933	1.9%	130,807	2.9%	43,222	1.2%
1995	245,629	8.2%	144,027	10.1%	47,493	9.9%
Growth rate 1990–95:	41%		45%		52%	

Source: Calculated from INFARMED *Informação Estatística*, 1994, 1995.

Despite concern over the increase in the NHS drug bill, very few policies have been put in place which effectively control it. In fact, the contrary is the case as various policy initiatives may be seen to actually be contributing to an escalation of costs. For example, in 1989 the full cost to the patient of

Health Care Reform and Cost Containment in Portugal   653

drugs (either OTC or cost-sharing component in NHS prescriptions) became deductible in income tax. The system allows for families to deduct an amount equivalent to marginal tax rates.

In 1995 a policy was enacted whereby private sector prescriptions could also be subject to cost-sharing by the NHS – previously this was only available for prescriptions provided in NHS services. The policy was motivated by a desire to end the practice whereby patients consulting private doctors took their prescriptions to an NHS health centre to have them repeated on an NHS prescription, and also to contribute to the separation of financing and provision in the health care system. However, there was an inevitable rise in the drug bill, as shown by Table 15.7.

A further example concerns the reimbursement system. From 1994 onwards it became increasingly accepted that it would be changed to one based on a reference price system. The Social Democratic government commissioned a study designing its implementation, and the Socialist opposition appeared to be in favour of such a move. However, in late 1996, the Socialist government (which had assumed power in 1995), following intense lobbying by the pharmaceutical industry, appeared to have temporarily abandoned the introduction of a reference price system. Similarly, the expansion of generic prescribing, which was part of the Socialist programme, is hardly at the forefront of current government objectives. Generic prescribing is virtually non-existent in Portugal: in 1995 it accounted for only 0.1 per cent of total market share.

As an alternative to the radical changes which had been foreseen, the government and the pharmaceutical industry have recently agreed a voluntary budget cap for 1997 as a means of controlling costs. This budget cap takes a peculiar form, whereby the pharmaceutical industry will pay back to the NHS 64.3 per cent of the excess over 1996 expenditure. However, there is a further proviso which states that this repayment will only apply to expenditure between 4 and 11 per cent above 1996 levels. Expenditure outside these limits is not liable to be returned. Additionally, another agreement between the State and the industry allows for an 8 per cent increase in the prices of drugs that retail below 1000 PTE. The price of other drugs will not be increased in 1997. In 1996 there had been no increase in prices and in 1995 they had risen by 1 per cent. In 1998 and 1999 there will be price increases amounting to 75 per cent and 80 per cent of the previous year's rate of inflation.

654   *Health Care and Cost Containment in the European Union*

15.3.6 Cost-sharing

Portugal's NHS has a fairly extensive co-payment system. Since 1992, users have been charged for diagnostic services and therapeutic procedures in ambulatory care; for hospital and health centre emergency services; and for out-patient visits to hospitals and primary care consultations in health centres. In all these cases patients pay flat fees and by law, the charges cannot exceed one third of the cost to the NHS. In practice, prices are fixed at a level around 10 per cent of the estimated production costs. The actual current levels of co-payment – set in 1992 – are shown in Table 15.8.

Table 15.8 Cost-sharing for NHS services, ESP

Item	Patient charge
Primary care visit	300
Hospital out-patient visit	
Central hospital	600
District hospital	400
Emergency visit	
Health centre	400
Hospital	1,000
Home visit	600
In-patient care	none
Diagnostic tests and therapeutic procedures	variable

Notes: Co-payments for diagnostic tests and therapeutic procedures range from ESP 150 for a simple lab test to ESP 10,000 for MRI.

There are also widespread exemptions for these charges. Exempted patient groups include people with *low family incomes* (e.g. those receiving specified supplementary income benefits and the unemployed); people with *exceptional need for health care consumption* (e.g. the handicapped and those with specified chronic conditions); and *special patient groups* (e.g. pregnant women, children, drug addicts on recovery programmes, chronic

Health Care Reform and Cost Containment in Portugal 655

mental patients, etc.).

The system is time-consuming for patients and costly to administer, as fees have to be paid at a special office before the consultation and, if laboratory tests or X-rays are prescribed, further fees have to be paid before these complementary services are received. In practice, there are many instances where services forego charging because of the bureaucracy involved. This helps to explain why the financial impact of co-payments is rather limited. In 1995, revenue raised through co-payments accounted for little over 1 per cent of the running costs of hospitals and health centres.[17]

Scarcely any studies have been carried out that measure the impact of cost-sharing on the demand for care. However, those that are available indicate that it is negligible. For example, Andrade *et al.*[20] examined the effect of co-payments in central hospitals and concluded that the only discernible effect was for emergency care utilization. Between 1991 and 1992 there was a reduction of 11.8 per cent in the number of visits. However, the fall in demand was short-lived for in 1993 utilization increased by 11.6 per cent, thus returning to the 1991 level. With regard to all types of diagnostic procedures, the same study indicates that the effect on demand was insignificant, even in the short term.

It should be noted that exemptions do not apply to drugs, where the cost-sharing mechanism is distinct. The level of co-payment varies in accordance with the 'therapeutic value' of the drug in question. Category A drugs – defined as substances vital for survival or used to treat specific chronic diseases (e.g. insulin, anticoagulants) – are entirely supported by the State. These drugs accounted for 9.4 per cent of total NHS consumption in 1994. Category B drugs – essential drugs needed in the treatment of serious illnesses which sometimes require prolonged therapy (e.g. antibiotics) require a 30 per cent co-payment by patients. They accounted for 63.1 per cent of NHS consumption in 1994. Category C drugs – non-priority medicines with confirmed therapeutic value (e.g. anti-inflammatory drugs) – require a 60 per cent co-payment and accounted for 27.5 per cent of NHS consumption in 1994. Cost-sharing of drugs included in categories B and C is decreased by 15 per cent for pensioners receiving pensions below the national minimum wage. Around 27 per cent of drug expenditure is not subsidized at all. As the previous section showed, despite the increased importance of patient cost-sharing in the drug market, pharmaceutical expenditure has continued to grow above the rate of price inflation.

656 *Health Care and Cost Containment in the European Union*

15.3.7 Private health care

The intention set out in the 1993 law to allow the development of an alternative health insurance system, partially financed by State tax rebates to those opting out of the NHS, has never been implemented due to lack of interest from insurance companies. Meanwhile, topping-up health insurance which up to 1993 had been developing smoothly, appears to have reached a plateau with the number of insured people, either through private or group insurance, having declined in 1994 and 1995. In 1995, according to figures from the insurance industry, there were 800,000 individuals (in a population of 10 million) covered by private insurance. Most of these are covered indirectly by virtue of employment or purchase of financial products. Only 115,000 had individual insurance.[21] The insurance industry often argues that its operation in the health sector is subject to low profitability. Recently an insurance company introduced a topping-up system with full control of providers, through a complex and sophisticated information system (a product known as Medis). This model is still in a state of development but there are already signs of doctors' resistance to this regulation.

Private health care has also maintained its essential topping-up nature. Recent attempts to build and equip new private hospitals have been a resolute financial failure. The private sector only prospers in Portugal where there are gaps and omissions by the public sector. Cumulative practice is an essential tool to transfer publicly financed clients complaining from lack of comfort and waiting lists in public hospitals towards private and elective practice.

15.3.8 Equity in financing

Given the increasing importance of out-of-pocket health spending, there have been concerns over the degree of inequity in the financing of the Portuguese health care system. A recent study has shown that, by international standards, the level of regressivity of direct expenditure in Portugal is rather high.[22] Analysing the period from 1980 to 1990 it was concluded that pharmaceutical expenditure was the main contributory factor to high levels of regressivity. There were minimal variations from one period to the next, suggesting that policy and behavioural changes had a negligible impact on the existing income distribution of out-of-pocket payments. Other sources of finance were shown to be progressive, though in the case of social and private insurance this is simply due to the phenomenon of the selective coverage of households that are better-off. The progressivity of the taxation system, which accounts for the greater part of health care financing in Portugal, results mainly from direct taxes (e.g. personal income tax), since indirect taxes (e.g. VAT) are roughly proportional.

The same study also computed levels of progressivity for overall health care financing, and concluded that over the 1980s, health care financing became unequivocally more favourable to richer households. In 1980, the financing system was marginally progressive, but became regressive by 1990. Comparison with international results suggests that a fundamental change took place throughout the 1980s. The burden of health care finance appears to have shifted to middle income groups, with the principal beneficiaries being households situated in the richest quintile. This was the result of two main factors: reduced progression in the tax system (following the introduction of VAT in 1986 and a major income tax reform in 1989) and an increase in the revenues raised directly from consumers. It should be noted that the estimates take no account of tax deductions which, during the 1980s, became more generous, thereby allowing richer households to recoup increased shares of private health care expenditure.

Table 15.9 Health care financing share and progressivity, 1980–90

| | % Share of total finance | | Kakwani index* | |
	1980	1990	1980	1990
Direct taxes	23.2%	20.7%	0.227	0.127
Indirect taxes	42.8%	34.5%	0.019	-0.002
Total taxes	66.0%	55.2%	0.092	0.047
Social insurance	5.2%	6.0%	0.245	0.244
Private insurance	0.6%	1.4%	0.175	0.152
Direct payments	28.2%	37.4%	-0.196	-0.186
Total payments	100.0%	100.0%	0.019	-0.027

* The Kakwani index is a measure of the degree of progressivity. It shows positive (negative) values when a financing source is progressive (regressive).

Source: Pereira (1996).[22]

658 *Health Care and Cost Containment in the European Union*

15.4 Conclusions

A recent study by WHO [23] has defined health reform as 'a progressive, dynamic and sustained process that results in systematic structural change'. By this measure, the changes which have taken place in Portugal in the 1990s cannot be considered as constituting a major reform. The most visible progress has been in legislating a set of principles which legitimized the situation that had evolved since the creation of the NHS in 1979.

The Portuguese NHS has confirmed its mix of positive and negative features. The most positive one, universal access with continuously improved care coverage, has been hampered in the last five years by a decline in overall quality of care, increasing costs, persisting inefficiencies, and more apparent social inequality.

The perceived shortage of public funds for the health care sector at the beginning of the 1990s, led to an increased availability of resources, but these were poorly planned and poorly distributed. All governments have been forced, until now, to find additional financial revenues to fill the financial gaps generated by a system that has lost control over increasing costs and persistent inefficiencies sustained by entrenched pressure groups. The country is in a curious situation where everyone complains about lack of money for health care, though every agent is spending without consideration for limits.

There appears to be some consensus among experts and politicians from different parties on a number of key issues: the need to separate health care provision from financing and regulation; the reimbursement of hospitals through performance indicators (DRGs or other patient classification systems); the regionalization of NHS health services; the distribution of funds to the regions through allocation formulae based on health needs; and the development of a stronger government regulatory capacity.

However, when it comes to practice, health care providers (doctors, nurses, the pharmaceutical industry, pharmaceutical outlets) all resist even the most minor changes. Increasing competition in delivery is seen as a threat to the present status quo that permits providers to enhance their income potential by accumulating activity in both the public and private sectors. All governments, including the present one, have been excessively careful in carrying out reform proposals. However, it is likely that the need to comply with the Maastricht criteria for joining the EU Monetary Union may serve as an accelerating factor towards reform. The margin of manoeuvre for the government has become increasingly reduced, and the bell of cost containment and health reform will soon be ringing.

Even so, it is difficult to predict how overall funding for the system will evolve in the future. A group of independent experts, who recently addressed the issue,[24] came to the conclusion that the health care service in Portugal is not under-funded. Further injection of funds, without widespread efficiency-promoting measures, would simply lead to higher levels of waste. A majority of the group also argued that taxation should continue to be the main form of finance and that out-of-pocket payments are already excessive. Two other important analyses, however, suggest that radical changes are required. Lucena et al.[25] propose the introduction of competition in financing, through the creation of public or private agencies (perhaps on a regional basis) that would establish contracts with providers on a competitive basis. The proposal would also allow for opting-out by patients, who would receive a fiscal credit to pay for alternative cover. Finally, the preliminary report of the government Commission set up to consider reform of the health care sector,[13] suggests that alternative forms of raising revenues (e.g. an earmarked health tax or social insurance) may be required. The Commission is due to produce its final report in 1998. The debate on how to finance the health care provided to Portuguese citizens is likely to continue for much longer.

References

1   Abel-Smith B, Figueras J, Holland W, McKee M, Mossialos E. *Choices for Health Policy: An Agenda for the European Union.* Aldershot: Dartmouth, 1995.

2   OECD. *OECD Health Data – A Software Package for the Cross-national Comparison of Health Systems.* Paris: CREDES/OECD, 1997.

3   WHO. *Health Services in Europe. Volume 2: Country Reviews and Statistics.* Copenhagen: WHO Regional Office for Europe, 1981.

4   OECD. *Financing and Delivering Health Care: A Comparative Analysis of OECD Countries.* Paris: OECD, 1987.

5   Pereira J, Pinto CG. *Regressivity in an NHS-type System: The Financing of Portuguese Health Care.* Documento de Trabalho 2/90. Lisbon: Associação Portuguesa de Economia da Saúde, 1990.

6   Campos AC (ed.). *A Combinação Público-Privada em Saúde: Privilégios, Estigmas e Ineficiências.* Lisbon: Escola Nacional de Saúde Pública, 1987.

7   Pereira J. *Equity, Health and Health Care: An Economic Analysis with reference to*

660   *Health Care and Cost Containment in the European Union*

Portugal. D.Phil. Thesis, University of York, January 1995.

8   Portugal. *Lei de Bases da Saúde.* Lei No. 48/90, Diário da República, I Série, No. 195, 24 August 1990:3452–59.

9   Reis V. As questões que se põem aos sistemas de saúde. *Gestão Hospitalar* 1995:21–30.

10   Portugal. *Estatuto do Serviço Nacional de Saúde.* Decreto-Lei No. 11/93, Diário da República, I Série-A, No. 12, 15 January 1993:129–34.

11   Portugal. *Saúde em Portugal. Uma estratégia para o virar do século. Orientações para 1997.* Ministério da Saúde, 1997.

12   Notícias Médicas. Reforma profunda, mas gradual, do SNS Entrevista da Ministra da Saúde. *Notícias Médicas* 27 November 1995.

13   CRES. *Opções para um Debate Nacional.* Porto: Conselho de Reflexão sobre a Saúde, 1997.

14   Campos AC. *O Controlo dos Gastos em Saúde. Racionamento ou Distribuição.* Cadernos de Saúde No. 7. Lisbon: Escola Nacional de Saúde Pública, 1987.

15   Mantas A, Ramos F, Roque e M. *Gastos Públicos com a Saúde 1974–1984.* Lisbon: Ministério da Saúde, DGFSS, 1984.

16   IGIF. *Elementos Económico-Financeiros. Agosto.* 1996.

17   Pereira J, Costa C, Rodrigues C, Ramos F, Vasconcelos H, Ibrahimo M. *Despesas com a Saúde em Portugal.* Apresentação no Forum Saúde. Lisbon: Apifarma, 1993.

18   Alves D, Cardoso L, Meneses-Correia J. PERLE. Uma medida para um problema. *Gestão Hospitalar* 1996 Ano X, No. 32, May.

19   CESO. *Avaliação Intercalar da Intervenção Operacional da Saúde: Relatório Final.* Lisbon: CESO, 1997.

20   Andrade A, Branco C. Sepúlveda R. Taxas moderadoras: sucessos e fracassos, 4 anos depois, ENSP/UNL, Curso de Administração Hospitalar, Trabalho de Economia da Saúde, mimeografia, 1996.

21   Instituto de Seguros de Portugal (ISP). Unpublished data. Instituto de Seguros de Portugal, Departamento de Estatística, 1997.

22   Pereira J. Who paid for health care in Portugal, 1980–1990? In: Vaz A, Pinto CG, Ramos F, Pereira J (eds). *As Reformas dos Sistemas de Saúde.* Lisbon: Associação Portuguesa de Economia da Saúde, 1996.

23   WHO. *European Health Care Reforms: Analysis of Current Strategies.* Copenhagen: WHO Regional Office for Europe, 1996.

24   APES. *Financiamento da Saúde em Portugal.* Lisbon: Associação Portuguesa de Economia da Saúde, 1997.

25   Lucena D, Gouveia M, Barros PP. *Financiamento do Sistema de Saúde em Portugal.* Lisbon: Ministério da Saúde, 1995.

16 Cost containment in Finnish health care

UNTO HÄKKINEN

16.1 Introduction

In its institutional structure, financing and goals, the Finnish health care system closely resembles the systems both of other Nordic countries and Great Britain, in that it covers the whole population and services are mainly produced by the public sector and financed through general taxation. In Finland, it is the municipalities (local governments) which have responsibility for providing health services. In addition, the National Health Insurance (NHI) finances the use of specific private health services and outpatient medicines.

The 1990s has seen radical changes to the Finnish economy and health care system. An extraordinary economic recession began in 1991. The unemployment rate increased from 3 to 18 per cent between 1990 and 1993 and was still fairly high in 1996 (16 per cent). Over the same three year period, GDP per capita (at 1985 constant prices) decreased by 15 per cent. Although there was some economic growth in the subsequent two years, GDP per capita in 1995 was still below that of the late 1980s (see Figure 16.1, overleaf).

The most important reform in Finnish health care this decade occurred at the beginning of 1993 as part of a reform of the total state subsidy system. An essential element of the reform was the revision of the grounds for determining state subsidies to municipalities for health services. Under the old system, state subsidies to municipalities or federations of municipalities (producers) were earmarked and related to real costs. In the reformed system, state subsidies for running costs in health services provided by municipalities are non-earmarked lump-sum grants, which are calculated prospectively by using a specific capitation formula. The aim of the reform was to reduce central government control and to increase local freedom in the provision of services. This makes it possible for municipalities

Figure 16.1. Health care expenditure per capita and GDP per capita in Finland at constant 1985 prices, 1985–95

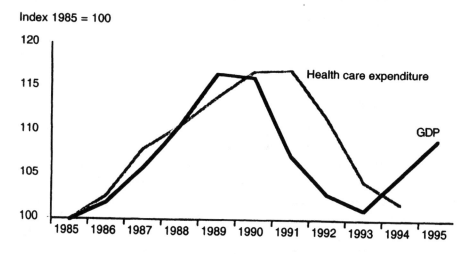

Note: 1995 estimated data.
Sources: Kansaneläkelaitos, 1996.[1]
National accounts, various years.[2]
Price index of public services, municipal health care, various years.[3]

to adopt the more active role of purchaser, instead of the previous provider/producer role. On the other hand, the reform does not alter the municipalities' responsibility for providing health and social services. Particularly in specialist hospital care, the reform has meant that the system now shifted from a somewhat public integrated model to a public contract model.

The changes in the Finnish economy and the health care system are also reflected in the usual indicators. The proportion of GDP spent on health services increased from 8.0 per cent to 9.3 per cent during the years 1990–92. The increase was mainly due to decreases in GDP itself (Figure 16.1), although in the first year of recession (1991) there was a one per cent increase in the volume of health care (measured by health expenditure at constant prices). Between 1991 and 1994 the volume of health care per capita decreased by 15 per cent. After that GDP rose again, thereby decreasing the proportion of GDP spent on health services to 7.7 per cent in 1995.

In addition to relative changes in volume, the GDP share depends on changes in the relative price levels of health care. The health sector is extremely labour-intensive and few possibilities exist to substitute labour with machines. On the other hand, the price of labour tends to increase more rapidly than the prices of other inputs. Thus, there is a general tendency for health care prices to increase more rapidly than average prices in the economy as a whole, which also tends to increase its GDP share. In Finland the relative price level of health care since 1985 has increased 17 per cent faster than the GDP price index, although the relative price level of health care personnel has remained relatively constant in the long-run (Figure 16.2). However, between 1988 and 1992 the relative development of wages of health sector personnel also affected the growth of the health sector's GDP share. After that, the relative wage level of the health sector decreased. In spring 1995 the wages of nurses were increased after their strike. This will

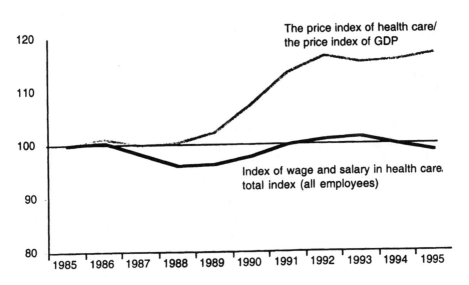

Figure 16.2 The relative price and wage level in health care compared to the average level in the economy, 1985–95 (1985 = 100)

Sources: National accounts, various years.[2]
Price index of public services, municipal health care, various years.[3]
Index of wage and salary earnings, various years.[4]

664 *Health Care and Cost Containment in the European Union*

Table 16.1 Financing of health care in Finland (%), 1990–94

	1990	1991	1992	1993	1994
National government	37.2	36.9	35.1	30.7	29.2
- income tax	14.1	11.2	7.6	5.3	5.6
- indirect tax (e.g. hypothecated taxes)	22.1	18.1	15.0	11.0	11.4
- net borrowing (debt financing)	1.0	7.6	12.5	14.4	12.2
Municipalities	35.8	35.7	33.3	34.1	33.0
Sickness insurance	10.8	11.3	11.1	12.2	13.0
Total public	83.8	83.9	79.5	77.0	75.2
Households	12.6	12.6	16.6	19.1	20.8
Other private (relief funds, employers, private insurance)	3.6	3.5	3.9	3.9	4.0

Sources: Kansaneläkelaitos, 1996.[1]
The accounts of central government, various years.[5]

increase the GDP share in future.

Justified by the poor state of the Finnish economy, the share paid by households in financing health care rose from 13 to 21 per cent between the years 1990 and 1994 (Table 16.1). This increase stemmed partly from the abolition of a tax deduction for medical expenses from income taxes, and partly from increased user fees and co-payments for health care services.

Changes have also been made to the structure of services. The share of expenditure devoted to in-patient care has decreased while the share of specialist and primary out-patient care has increased (Table 16.2). These changes are mainly due to the closure of psychiatric beds. Contrary to the trend of earlier decades, in the 1990s the share of medicines has increased; such that in 1994 about 13 per cent of health care expenditure is devoted to drugs in outpatient care (Appendices 16.1 and 16.2).

The content of this chapter was developed along the guidelines prepared for the cost-containment project coordinated by LSE Health. First the

Cost Containment in Finnish Health Care   665

Table 16.2 Health care expenditure in Finland, 1990–94

	Volume index (1990 = 100)				Share of total expenditure (%)	
	1991	1992	1993	1994	1990	1994
In-patient care	99.9	94.7	86.6	82.4	44.7	41.5
of which:						
- specialist care (including psychiatric care)	97.1	89.7	83.4	76.2	26.6	22.8
- health centres (primary hospital care)	100.7	96.4	82.4	82.4	13.1	12.1
- other hospital in-patient care (mentally retarded, military hospitals, rehabilitation)	112.8	116.5	114.7	115.7	5.0	6.6
Out-patient care (excluding dental care) of which:	102.8	98.2	93.7	92.9	28.1	29.5
- health centres	102.4	98.1	95.3	94.6	13.3	14.1
- occupational care and students health care	97.5	91.4	84.0	89.1	3.0	3.1
- out-patient departments of specialist hospitals	107.1	106.6	99.7	100.3	7.5	8.4
- private out-patient care	101.1	89.0	84.8	77.1	4.3	3.9
Dental care (including prosthesis)	92.4	89.8	87.1	86.3	5.8	5.9
Medicines and pharmaceutical products	110.3	116.4	121.3	127.8	9.4	12.8
Other running expenditure	100.0	99.5	91.4	93.1	7.4	7.8
Total running expenditure	101.7	98.3	92.8	91.8	95.4	97.5
Public investments	91.3	75.3	62.6	55.9	4.6	2.5
Total health care expenditure	101.3	97.3	91.4	89.6	100.0	100.0

Sources: Kansaneläkelaitos, 1996.[1]

Price index of public services, municipal health care, various years.[3]

Other price indices of health services, of which part are based on author's own calculations.

666 *Health Care and Cost Containment in the European Union*

budgeting system of Finnish health care is described. Secondly, several issues of cost-containment are considered. In particular, the chapter focuses on health care reforms and the effects of these in the 1990s.

16.2 Overall budgets for health care

Finnish health care consists of two main systems with different financial mechanisms: municipal health care services and private health services covered by National Health Insurance. Among municipally provided services there is no single fixed budget for health services. Instead the allocation of resources is defined in budgets, which are decided at the three levels of central government, municipalities and producers (i.e. hospital districts). Currently, the most important economic decisions are made by 455 municipal councils, which every year decide the amount to be devoted to health care (Figure 16.3). Via municipal budgets, the resources are allocated between primary and specialist care. The amount of resources spent on municipal health services in different parts of the country is also primarily defined by these budgets. Regional equality is attempted with state subsidies, which are divided between the municipalities according to certain 'need' criteria. In principle, in each of the three levels the budgets are fixed annually, but it is not unusual for municipality budgets for health services and hospital districts budgets for specialized care to be exceeded and adjusted during the year.

There is no official budget for financing the National Health Insurance. The level of employers' and insured persons' (population) contributions are decided annually by the central government. Thus the amount spent on NHI payments is not fixed. The allocation of NHI resources to different types of care, as well as their regional distribution, is based on demand for the services as well as the reimbursement system.

16.2.1 Municipally provided services

The municipalities are responsible for providing health services for their residents. In order to provide health services, the municipalities (especially the small ones) often cooperate to create a large enough catchment popula-

Cost Containment in Finnish Health Care 667

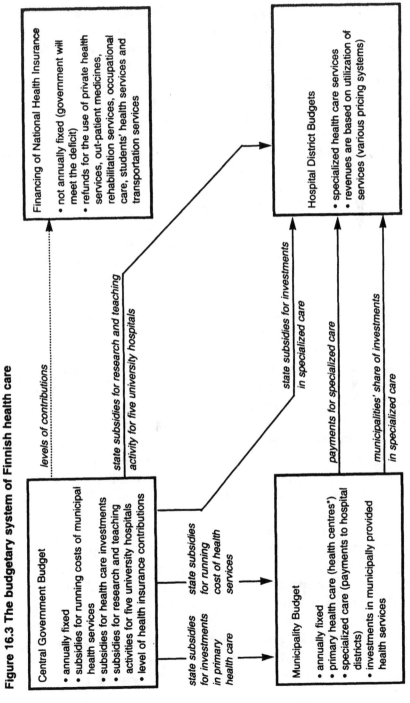

Figure 16.3 The budgetary system of Finnish health care

* About 34 per cent of health centres are federations of municipalities which have their own budgets. The remainder are owned by a single municipality and are included in its budget.

668   *Health Care and Cost Containment in the European Union*

tion. Municipally provided health services are financed by municipal taxes, state subsidies and user charges (Figure 16.4). Municipal tax revenues are not only used for health care but also for other services such as education and social services.

Primary health care is provided mainly by the public health centres, which anyone can contact for ambulatory medical services. Preventive care of communicable and non-communicable diseases, ambulatory, medical and dental care, an increasing number of out-patient specialized services and various public health programmes (e.g. maternity and school care and care for the elderly) are provided by the health centres. They are also responsible for occupational health services (e.g. for farmers). Moreover, there are specific services for particular patient groups, e.g. diabetes and hypertension clinics.

Public specialized care is provided by 21 hospital districts with their own hospitals. There are over 50 acute care hospitals and over 250 health centres, most of which also have an in-patient department. Health centre hospitals mostly provide care for elderly patients requiring long-term treatment. Some health centre hospitals also have specialized departments.

Since the state subsidy reform of 1993 there has been no overall fixed budget for public health care. Before the reform, about 70 per cent of total health expenditure was in practice tied to central government's annual prospectively fixed budget. In the old system, Cabinet annually approved a national five-year plan for public health services (provided by municipalities or municipal federations), which limited increases in manpower and levels of investments. The Ministry of Social Affairs and Health allocated these quotas to provinces and Provincial Boards, which distributed them to producers (municipal health centres and municipal hospitals). If municipalities provided services which were not in the plan, they had to do so without state subsidy.

Under the reformed system, state (central government) subsidies for health care (to municipalities) are fixed annually at an amount decided prospectively by Parliament. State subsidies for health service running costs of municipalities are calculated according to certain criteria. During the years 1993–96 these criteria included population, age structure, morbidity, population density, land area and the financial capacity of the municipality. In addition, the archipelago municipalities had a somewhat higher subsidy. The relevance of these criteria has been recently studied.[6] Based partly on the study, new criteria have been adopted since the beginning of 1997. The

Cost Containment in Finnish Health Care 669

Figure 16.4 The finance and production of municipal health services in Finland

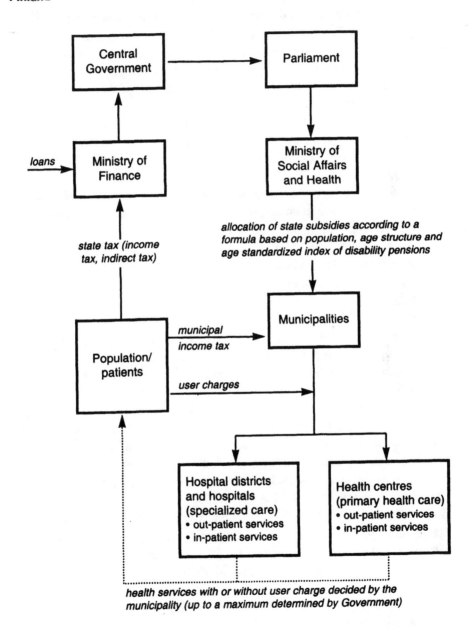

670 *Health Care and Cost Containment in the European Union*

new criteria include population, age structure and an age-standardized index of invalidity pensions for those aged under 55 years.

State subsidies are paid automatically to municipalities, who are not required to apply for them. Along with state subsidy reform, the municipalities were given a more active role in arranging services and could decide more freely on administration, personnel and user charges. They also won the right to purchase services freely from the provider of their choice and to contract out services to the private sector.

Parliament decides the total amount of subsidies for health and social services. At the same time as the implementation of the state subsidy reform, the national plan was changed from a five-year to a four-year plan and its role became less significant. The main contents of the four-year plan are general guidelines on activities in social and health care and information on the amount of state financing for running costs and capital investments.

At municipal level, the budgets for public health services are fixed annually at an amount decided by the Municipal Council. Municipal Councils are elected every four years by their inhabitants. The Councils then elect members to their Municipal Governments, which are accountable to the Councils. The Councils also elect members to the various municipality boards (e.g. the Health Boards), which may consist both of members of the Municipal Councils and other persons. The decisions concerning the planning and organization of health care are made jointly by the Health Boards, the Municipal Councils and the Municipal Governments, although variations in these arrangements exist. The leading personnel of municipal health centres are often included in the planning and organization of health services. Recently, the general trend has been towards delegating power from Municipal Councils to the Health Boards and leading officials.[7]

Although the annual budgets decided by the Municipal Councils are fixed, it is not unusual for budgets to be exceeded. When this happens the Municipal Council must decide on a supplementary budget in order to finance the deficit of the original budget. Municipalities' payments to specialist care are based more on the type and amount of different services, which are not easy to plan in advance. On the other hand, the producers of health services (hospitals and hospital districts) usually claim that the municipality budgets for specialist care are unrealistically low.

A hospital district is responsible for providing hospital services and coordinating the public specialized hospital care within its area. Each municipality located in the district area must be a member of the hospital district. Typically, the administrative organization of a hospital district is a council (whose members are appointed by each municipality), a board appointed by the council, and an executive management.

In summary, it can be concluded that the most important effect of state subsidy reform on cost containment at macro level is that the general government no longer has the chance to contain total health care expenditure directly. At the same time, the amount of state subsidies has been decreased, meaning that municipalities also have, in addition to increased freedom in the provision of services, more economic responsibility for providing services. Thus, cost containment of health care is now an acute question at municipal level. According to a recent study, the variation of health expenditure per capita between municipalities has decreased somewhat since the state subsidy reform, although the differences are still substantial.[8]

The state subsidy reform was also a radical solution internationally, since nowhere else had the pooling of financial risks been assigned to such a small unit. The median population of municipalities is 5,000. Of the 455 municipalities about 20 per cent have less than 2,000 residents and 75 per cent have less than 10,000 residents. It has been calculated that the size of a municipality must be at least between 10,000 and 15,000 in order to guarantee that the financial risk of specialist hospital care remains at a reasonable level.[9] According to the simulation for smaller municipalities, the random variation of annual costs of specialist care will annually influence the level of municipal tax rates.

16.2.2 Services covered by National Health Insurance (NHI)

The statutory National Health Insurance Scheme (NHI) is administered by the Social Insurance Institute, which is governed by Parliament. This scheme is used to finance medicines and private and occupational health care services (see Figure 16.5 overleaf).

Supplementing the network of public health services is the obligation of employers to arrange preventive occupational services for their employees to the extent prescribed by law. In addition to statutory occupational health care, employers may provide voluntary curative health care for employees and their family members. The employer is then compensated by the Social Insurance Institute for the costs of the occupational and other health care services it arranges. The compensation paid by the National

Figure 16.5 Finance and production of health services covered by National Health Insurance

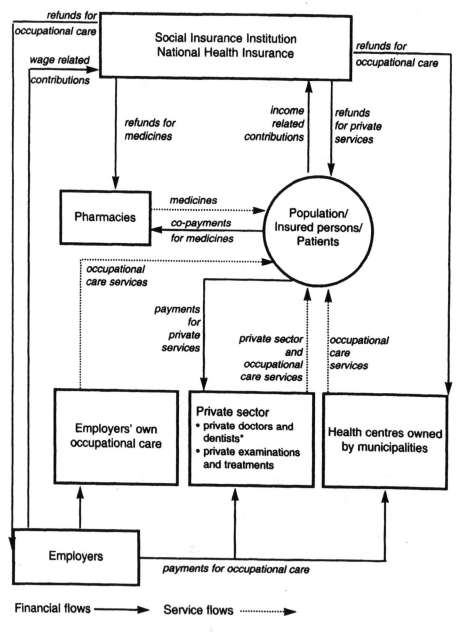

Financial flows ⟶   Service flows ┄┄▶

* only adults born after 1956 are covered

Cost Containment in Finnish Health Care   673

Sickness Insurance is 50 per cent of "all necessary and reasonable expenses". Employers can arrange occupational health care in different ways. They may produce it themselves (in their own health centre), buy services from the private sector or arrange services from a health centre owned by a municipality.

It is possible for the Social Insurance Institution to monitor the content of occupational health care services rendered. At the beginning of 1995 the reimbursement system was reformed. The aim was to emphasize preventive activities and contain costs. Maximum sums (per employee) for both compulsory and voluntary curative refunds were defined, refunds for specialist services were limited, and refunds for family member utilization were abolished.

In addition to the occupational care discussed above, the NHI also covers its members (i.e. the Finnish population) for sickness allowances, maternity allowances, special care allowances, student health services, rehabilitation services and medical expenses (drugs prescribed by doctors, private sector examinations and treatments performed or prescribed by doctors, dental care for young adults and transportation services).

Usually the NHI pays a certain percentage in excess of a fixed sum (minimum per purchase, or the so-called basic tariff). Thus the NHI covers only part of expenses, and cost-sharing is greater in those private services covered by the NHI than in municipally provided public services. In special cases (registered individuals suffering from specified conditions), nearly all medicine costs (75 or 100 per cent in excess of a fixed minimum) are refunded.

The health care payments of the NHI are financed mostly by compulsory contributions from insured persons (the population) and employers. A small part is financed from the yield of assets and a state contribution. In addition, part of the turnover tax and VAT revenues are credited to the NHI fund. With respect to the contributions from insured persons and employers, the NHI is financed on a pay-as-you-go basis. The assets of the NHI fund must, at the end of the year, equal a specified percentage (8 per cent) of total annual NHI expenditure. The government will meet any deficit.

The reimbursement system is defined by law, but government and the Ministry of Social Affairs and Health can to some extent affect the level of reimbursements. For example, the Ministry defines the principles of basic tariffs for private doctor payments and the government decides the list of specific conditions for special medicine refunds.

674   *Health Care and Cost Containment in the European Union*

16.3 Cost-containment measures

16.3.1 Changes in co-payments

During the years 1990–95 user-charges in health care were increased by about 20 percentage points more than average consumer prices (Table 16.3). The increase has been greatest in public services (hospital in-patient charges, hospital out-patient charges and health centre charges), in which, even after price increases, cost sharing is smaller than in private services (see Table 16.4).

16.3.1.1 Municipally provided services Until 1992 the cost of out-patient activities (e.g. consultations with physicians) in public health centres and psychiatric out-patient care was covered almost completely by general tax

Table 16.3 Consumer price index in health care and in all consumer goods (1990 = 100), 1991–95

	1991	1992	1993	1994	1995
Hospital in-patient day charge (specialist care including psychiatric care)	106.6	143.8	156.3	156.3	156.3
Hospital out-patient charge (specialist care)	108.8	150.0	166.7	166.7	166.7
Health centre visits charge	108.0	117.9	182.2	227.5	227.5
Private physicians' charge	113.7	125.4	127.9	128.5	128.4
Private examination and treatment charge	116.2	122.8	118.2	116.0	118.1
Medicines	107.8	117.9	129.4	136.8	143.8
of which:					
– prescribed	108.4	122..0	142..0	150.6	159.8
– over the counter	107.1	112.7	114.2	123.8	131.7
Eye-glasses	101.5	106.0	104.5	111.0	103.2
All health care charges at average	108.6	120.5	127.4	131.2	132.6
All consumer charges at average	104.3	107.4	109.7	110.9	112.0

Source: Consumer price index.[10]

Cost Containment in Finnish Health Care   675

revenues. Within municipally provided services there were user-charges for in-patient care, out-patient specialist care, dental care for adults and physiotherapy.

As part of the state subsidy reform of 1993, municipalities nowadays have the right to decide whether or not to charge for services, and to set the

Table 16.4 User-charges and cost-sharing (after the refund) share of financing different health services, 1990–94

	1990	1991	1992	1993	1994
Hospital in-patient care	6.9	6.6	7.6	9.2	10.3
Out-patient care (excluding dental care)	12.1	12.2	12.7	14.7	17.8
Health centres [a]	1.4	1.7	1.9	5.1	9.3
Occupational care and students health care services [b]	1.1	1.1	1.3	4.1	4.6
Hospital out-patient care [a] (out-patient care of specialist hospitals)	5.3	4.8	6.3	8.7	10.0
Private services (visits to a doctor and examinations and treatments)	63.6	65.8	67.3	66.9	65.9
Private doctors [b]	61.4	63.9	64.5	64.4	64.0
Private treatments [b]	65.4	67.5	69.8	69.3	67.8
Dental care (including prosthesis)	53.2	52.0	52.8	55.1	55.6
Total medicines	50.6	50.3	52.8	53.9	52.6
Prescribed medicines [b]	37.2	36.3	39.8	41.6	41.2
Totally	15.6	15.7	16.6	19.1	20.8
Including tax expenditure [c]	12.6	12.6	16.6	19.1	20.8

[a] Municipally provided services.
[b] Services covered by the National Health Insurance.
[c] Since 1992 the right to deduct medical expenses from taxation has been abolished.

Sources: Calculated from data published in: Kansaneläkelaitos, 1996.[1]

676 *Health Care and Cost Containment in the European Union*

level of these charges (up to maximum limits decided by the government). However, according to law, the following services (provided by municipalities) are still without user-charges: preventive health care, maternity and school care, psychiatric ambulatory care, immunization (in most cases), the examination and treatment of some communicable diseases specified by law (sexually transmitted diseases, tuberculosis, hepatitis and some others), treatment of patients suffering from respiratory arrest, transportation from one health care unit to another when ordered by a medical doctor, hospital treatment of under 18 year olds lasting for more than 7 days, and dental care for those under 19 years old.

If a municipality decides to levy fees on consultations with health centre physicians, it can choose between two alternative methods. The first option is either an annual payment (maximum FIM 100) which then covers all consultations during the year (i.e. the following 12 months) or a charge per consultation (maximum FIM 50) for those who do not want to pay this annual payment. The second option is to charge a maximum of FIM 50 per consultation for all patients for the first three consultations in a calendar year, with further consultations being free. There must be no charges for physician's consultations with children under 15 years.

For public specialized care (including psychiatric care) provided in hospitals, there is no annual payment system. The upper limits are FIM 100 for a specialist out-patient visit and FIM 125 per day for all short-term in-patient care. These upper limits are practically in use all over the country. In 1990 the user-charges for in-patient care increased from FIM 80 to FIM 125 per day and for out-patient visits from FIM 60 to FIM 100.

The charges for long-term in-patients are based on ability to pay and increase with the income of the patient. However, charges may not exceed 80 per cent of a patient's monthly income.

16.3.1.2 NHI scheme In principle, in 1995, the National Health Insurance (NHI) refunded the following: 50 per cent of all medicine costs in excess of a fixed minimum sum per purchase (FIM 50) or, in special cases, nearly all medicine costs (registered individuals suffering from certain specified conditions qualify for refunds of 75 or 100 per cent in excess of a fixed minimum of FIM 25); 60 per cent of the basic tariff established for private physicians' and dentists' services (90 per cent of dentist charges arising from oral or dental examination or preventive treatment); 75 per cent of examination and treatment (i.e. private laboratory, radiotherapy and physiotherapy services) charges between a fixed minimum (FIM 70) and the basic tariff for these services per prescription; all transportation costs in excess of a fixed minimum (FIM 50) per single journey. As for overnight stays, the NHI will pay all costs up to FIM 120 a day. All non-covered medicine costs in excess of FIM 3,158 a year will be paid.

As a practical example, the NHI covered 36 per cent of private doctors' patient fees in 1994, since the actual fees were higher than the basic tariffs. During the years 1991–94, actual cost-sharing, both in fees of private doctors' and private examinations and treatments, were rather stable (Table 16.4).

The refund by the NHI to employers is 50 per cent of mandatory occupational health care costs. Until 1992 these health care services were free of charge for employees. In 1993 an annual payment (FIM 100) covering all visits during a year was introduced. This fee was abolished in 1995.

The Finnish drug reimbursement system was revised in several ways between 1992 and 1994 in order to curtail the growth in NHI expenditure (Table 16.5). As a consequence, the patients' total contributions (after refunds) to the costs of prescribed medicines (covered by the NHI) rose

Table 16.5 Changes in drug reimbursement, 1990–94

	1990	1991	1992	1993	1994
Patient's share per purchase, FIM	35	35	45	45	50
Limit for additional refund, FIM*	2833	3051	2500	3100	3100
Basic refund, after patient's share per purchase	50%	50%	40%	40%	50%
Special refund category 100%	100%	100%	100%	100 %	100 % -25 FIM
Lower special refund category	90%	90%	80%	80%	75% -25 FIM

* After this all expenditure is refunded.

Source: National Agency of Medicines and Social Insurance Institution, 1995.[11]

678 *Health Care and Cost Containment in the European Union*

from 37 per cent to 42 per cent during the years 1990–93 (Table 16.4). In 1994 the revisions to the reimbursement system both increased and decreased cost-sharing depending on the refund category. The total effect of the changes was that patients' contributions to prescribed medicines decreased slightly (0.4 percentage points).

The increase in patient cost-sharing has not, however, contained the growth of total expenditure on drugs (see Table 16.2). Two main factors have influenced this growth: an increase in the number of users and the growing use of new, relatively expensive drugs in the treatment of many common diseases such as hypertension (ACE inhibitors and calcium channel blockers), depression (selective serotonin re-uptake inhibitors), psychoses (clozapine and risperdoni), diabetes (insulin pens and other devices) and asthma (salmeterol).[12,13] Since the price index of drugs does not take into account these structural changes, the increases in the volume index of drugs (almost 30 per cent during the years 1990–94) is a product of the two factors. In 1994 an additional factor influencing the expenditure of medicines was the value added tax, introduced on 1 June 1994, which increased the prices of drugs by between 3 and 5 per cent.

16.3.1.3 Medical aids and prostheses Medical aids and prostheses are generally free of charge by law. The main responsibility for providing and financing aids and prostheses lies with the municipal health services i.e. they are supplied either by health centres or hospitals. Also, other authorities such as the municipal social services authorities, the Social Insurance Institute, private insurance companies and others provide or finance medical aids to their clients if the relevant legislation obliges them to do so.

Totally excluded services from reimbursement are over-the-counter drugs, eyeglasses, private examinations and treatments not prescribed by doctors (for example surgery for purely cosmetic reasons) and alternative medicine services (such as osteopathy and chiropractice). In addition there are no public subsidies for dental care for adults born before 1956. An exemption for this is that veterans of the Second World war and individuals suffering from certain chronic disease are reimbursed for dental treatment.

All residents in Finland are guaranteed a minimum of social security. In cases where individuals (or families) are not able to support themselves, social assistance is provided. This also covers user-charges in health care. Between 1990 and 1994 the number of individuals receiving social assistance as a percentage of the total population increased from 5.9 per cent to

10.7 per cent. Thus, also the health expenses covered by social assistance have increased, although no exact data is available.

It is very hard to evaluate whether the above-described increase in cost-sharing has had effects on total health expenditure, because the increase occurred at the same time as the supply of services decreased (i.e. cuts in public health expenditure, closure of in-patient departments, decrease of personnel working in hospitals and health centres). Although there is no clear evidence, it can be assumed that the decline in health expenditure during these years was associated more with a decrease in supply than with demand-side factors. However, the increase in cost-sharing has some distributional consequences, which will be considered in detail in section 16.4.

16.3.2 Control of capital expenditure

The state subsidy reform did not cause many changes to the system of financing capital investments. The state subsidy varies from 25 per cent to 50 per cent of capital investments, depending on the per capita income of the municipality. The state subsidy decision mechanism for capital investments in municipal health services depends on the size of the investment. To get a subsidy, municipalities must submit plans to Provincial Boards, which are state authorities. Medium-size (FIM 2–25 million) investments may be approved by the Provincial Boards, but major capital investments (over FIM 25 million) require approval by the Government. The Ministry of Social Affairs and Health allocates state funding for medium-size capital investments to Provincial Boards.

Municipalities can make capital investments in health care without using a state subsidy, although this seldom happens. In addition, municipalities are allowed to borrow money from private markets to finance investments (or for other purposes).

In the 1980s, public investment's share of health care expenditure was 4–5 per cent (see Appendix 16.2). Because of the bad economic situation in the country, as well as an over-supply of hospital beds, public investment in health care decreased significantly in the 1990s. At 1990 constant prices, capital expenditure decreased by over 40 per cent during 1990–94 (Table 16.2). In 1994 its share of total expenditure was below 3 per cent. Most capital expenditure has been devoted to specialized hospitals.

During recent years the Finnish Slot Machine Association has become

680 *Health Care and Cost Containment in the European Union*

an important financier of capital investments.* However, the capital expenditure of the Association is not included in health care expenditure statistics. According to a crude estimation, the Association financed about one-third of all capital investments in health care in 1993. However, the Association does not finance any public health services, for example municipal health services.

16.3.3 Hospitals

During the 1950s and the 1960s, development of the hospital system took priority in Finnish health policy. A programme for building central hospitals, drafted in the late 1940s and early 1950s, was carried out. In addition to these, several district, local and mental hospitals were built. Thus, since 1970, Finland has had one of the highest number of hospital beds per capita of all the developed industrial countries.[14] Since the middle of the 1960s, in officially stated goals, primary and out-patient care have been emphasized. However, it was mainly the economic pressure of the 1990s which has effected the change in the balance of care. This change has been implemented mainly by closing psychiatric and somatic specialists beds. Between 1990 and 1995, the total number of hospital beds decreased by 10,000 (Table 16.6). In addition, there have been administrative changes: specialist somatic and psychiatric beds have been moved to primary care beds (i.e. beds not classified according to medical specialty).

According to crude measures, the productivity of somatic hospital care has increased in the 1990s, i.e. with decreased expenditure more services (admissions as well as many specific procedures) have been produced (see Figure 16.6). At the same time, the average length of stay has decreased. According to a DEA study (data envelop analysis) using hospital level data, the differences between hospitals in terms of productivity have been reduced. During the years 1991–94 the average inefficiency in Finnish somatic care hospitals decreased from 14 per cent to 10 per cent.[15]

There is no guarantee to patients that they will be treated within a pre-

---

* The Finnish Slot Machine Association operates slot machines, amusement machines and casino games. Its revenues are distributed to support the work of voluntary health and welfare organizations, for example service housing for the elderly and disabled, assistance for individuals and families in difficulty, and youth work.

Table 16.6 Number of hospital beds by type of care in Finland, 1990–95

Beds per 1,000 persons	1990	1991	1992	1993	1994	1995
Primary care*	3.8	4.1	4.0	4.4	4.3	4.3
Specialist somatic care	5.1	5.0	5.0	4.3	4.3	3.6
Psychiatric care	2.5	2.2	2.0	1.5	1.5	1.3
Total	11.4	11.3	11.0	10.2	10.1	9.2

*Beds not classified according to specialty.
Source: STAKES, 1996.[16]

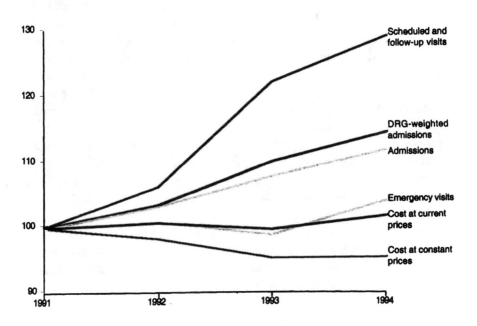

Figure 16.6 Cost and output of somatic hospital care (index 1991 = 100) based on data from a sample of acute hospitals (covering about 85 per cent of all specialized admissions), 1991–94 [15]

682 *Health Care and Cost Containment in the European Union*

determined time, although a system implemented in other Nordic countries has also recently been considered in Finland.[17] In practice there exists great differences in waiting times between hospital districts, but the reasons for these have not been carefully evaluated. For example, the median waiting time for cataract operations varied between hospital districts from 70 to 250 days in 1993.[18] Experiments with a waiting-time guarantee for elective procedures started in 1996 in three hospital districts.

The state subsidy reform of 1993 changed the financing of running costs of specialist hospital care. Before 1993, hospitals received about half of their revenues from the state via the Provincial Boards. The other half of hospital revenue came from municipalities. Since 1993 hospital revenues have depended on how many and what kind of services municipalities purchase from them.

Hospital districts determine the prices for their services without nationally set guidelines and services are defined and prices calculated in very different ways – with the possibilities for municipalities to compare prices being very limited. The pricing of hospital services is in a continuous process of change – the central trends being a move away from average (per bed-day) prices to more detailed pricing which includes service-package prices for in-patient care.[19] A service package includes certain services (the diagnoses or type of treatment, for example, childbirth or cholecystectomy). Two hospital districts have moved into a DRG-based pricing scheme at the beginning of 1997. The prices for out-patient care also vary. Normally, the price is set per visit and often according to the range and level of treatments.

The possibility for price competition in specialized hospital care is also limited, because a hospital district is a local monopoly in its area, and membership of every municipality in a hospital district is statutory. Thus there are no incentives for municipalities to try to buy services from other hospital districts, because this would make the economic situation of its own hospital district poorer. Most districts have the right to bill municipalities retrospectively on those occasions when hospital revenues are not sufficient to cover all expenditure.*

The small size of many municipalities means that they are unable to take advantage of the possibilities for cost savings offered by the revised hospital financial system. Most municipalities are economically weak compared to hospital districts, and it is unlikely that they have sufficient power

---

* In 1995, 5 out of 21 hospital districts voluntarily gave up this right.

Cost Containment in Finnish Health Care 683

to make hospitals compete with each other. In addition, it can be assumed that the asymmetry of information between providers (hospitals and hospital districts) and buyers (municipalities) is greater in small municipalities.

The central idea of the Hospital Act of 1991 was to introduce an administrative unit (hospital district) to coordinate and integrate specialized care within an area in order to avoid the duplication of services. However, in at least two of the biggest hospital districts, it is widely thought that there is an over-capacity of services. In spite of much political discussion, solutions as to how to handle this over-supply have not yet been reached.

The supply of services is not only a question of health policy: municipal decision-makers have not only considered which services to provide and to what extent, but also where (i.e. in which municipality) they are to be produced. The health sector is also an important employer, and its employees generate income tax revenues for the municipalities which host their institutions and house many of their employees.

Municipalities do not negotiate a formal contract with hospitals, rather they make an agreement with some hospitals on the provision of certain specialist services. The Council (whose members are appointed by each municipality) of a hospital district decides its annual budget. If the budget is exceeded, the municipalities must pay the deficit, usually funded by means of higher prices for services. In case of a budgetary surplus, prices can be lowered.

Most hospitals in Finland are owned by municipalities or federations of municipalities (hospital districts). The role of the private sector is minimal, constituting only around about 5 per cent of beds. In 1992 the number of private hospitals providing specialized care was 20. Usually they provide services for one specialty. In 1992, private hospitals accounted for 4.2 per cent of discharges for conservative (non-surgical) and 1.7 per cent for operative (surgical) specialties.[20] However, for some individual procedures, private hospitals have a marked significance and their role has even increased in recent years. In 1994 they performed 10.6 per cent of all procedures on heart and thoracic vessels, 6.2 per cent of procedures of the musculoskeletal system, and 5.4 per cent of eye, 6.1 per cent of breast and 4.5 per cent of skin operations.[16] The high private hospital share in orthopaedic procedures is largely due to two specialized institutions owned by non-profit foundations which provide services to the public sector. Similarly a considerable part of private hospital cardiovascular procedures, which mainly consist of coronary by-pass operations, were purchased by municipalities due to an insuf-

684 *Health Care and Cost Containment in the European Union*

ficient supply of these procedures in municipal hospitals.[21]

In principle, the state subsidy reform gives municipalities more freedom to buy hospital services from the private sector. But the fact that investments in private hospitals are not covered by state subsidies puts public hospitals in a more advantageous position.

Provincial Boards give permission to run private hospitals as well as other private services. The Board also monitors their activity. This monitoring is designed to ensure service quality and is not for prices, technology or investments.

In Finland, senior specialists working in public hospitals on a salary basis are permitted to treat private patients. These patients can choose their doctor, and their waiting times for hospital admission are believed to be shorter. The system was created in the 1950s to compensate doctors for the closure of wards for private patients in public hospitals.[21] In 1993 the proportion of these 'private' or 'pay-beds' of total admissions in all municipal hospitals was about 2 per cent. The portion is highest for specialties with many elective procedures such as ophthalmology (12.0 per cent admissions), general surgery (5.3 per cent), ear, nose and throat (5.4 per cent) and gynaecology and obstetrics (2.3 per cent).[16] Pay-bed patients pay the regular fee (FIM 125 per in-patient day) plus a supplementary fee for their doctor (maximum for a surgical procedure FIM 4,000), extra charges for each in-patient day (maximum FIM 375) and extra charges for anaesthesia procedures, X-ray and laboratory tests. These charges do not correspond to real costs, and except for bed-day charges, are paid to the attending physician as supplementary remuneration. The pay-bed charges are partly reimbursed to patients by the National Health Insurance scheme according to the same principles as the charges of private out-patient services (see above). Thus pay-bed patients do not so much increase the incomes of hospitals as the incomes of specialists.

Many hospital physicians have dual roles, working as specialists in both the public and private sectors. In 1995 about 60 per cent of hospital doctors were engaged in some kind of private practice. Most of them are specialists. If the private practice operates outside working hours the doctors must tell the hospital director. This is the most popular way to practice privately. *Permission* to practise privately is needed only if it is practised during working hours. The private sector produces about 60 per cent of out-patient services in ophthalmology and about 50 per cent in obstetrics and gynaecology.

6.3.4 Alternatives to hospital care

Most ambulatory care is provided in health centres, the out-patient departments of specialized hospitals, in private practice or by employers as part of occupational care. Between 1990 and 1994, the total number of visits to out-patient departments of somatic specialties increased by over 10 per cent (Table 16.7) while the number of other visits decreased.[22]

The municipalities are responsible for the care provided in health centres and specialist hospitals as well as social services (care of the elderly including nursing homes). Thus they have an incentive to use services more economically. On the other hand, the utilization of private and occupational services (financed partly by the NHI) can decrease the demand for public services. However, during times of economic difficulty, the demand for public-sector services has actually increased because of the lower level of cost-sharing in municipal services compared to private services.

More generally, the fact that public funds come from several different sources may result in inefficiency in the utilization of ambulatory services. The amount of public funds from sickness insurance does not affect the amount of the municipalities' state subsidy. In addition to the issue of inequality, the possibility of having other sources of funds increases the municipalities' interest in decisions which minimize their own cost but not those of the public sector or health care system as a whole.[23]

Table 16.7 Activity indicators of acute hospital care in Finland, 1990–95

	1990	1991	1992	1993	1994	1995
Admissions/1,000 inhabitants	180	181	188	192	194	193
Bed-days/1,000 inhabitants	1,292	1,268	1,160	1,086	1,109	1,088
Average length of stay (days)	7.2	7.0	6.2	5.7	5.7	5.6
Occupancy rate (%)	68.8	68.9	61.2	69.6	71.0	82.3
Out-patient visits/1000 inhabitants*	632	596	623	688	723	n.a.

*Based on data from a sample of acute somatic hospitals.[15]

Source: STAKES, 1996.[16]

686 *Health Care and Cost Containment in the European Union*

Table 16.8 Number of working-age doctors, dentists and nurses in Finland, 1990–95

	1990	1991	1992	1993	1994	1995
Doctors	12,091	12,357	12,929	13,344	13,700	13,771
Dentists	4,486	4,562	4,614	4,602	4,664	4,696
Nurses	50,616	52,059	54,587	57,202	60,578	63,499
Practical nurses*	34,212	34,682	35,401	36,702	37,188	36,382

* Nurses with less training.

Source: STAKES, various years.[24]

16.3.5 Manpower control

In practice, the state (Ministry of Education) has control over the numbers employed in the education and training of health care personnel. During 1990–94 the annual number of new doctors increased from 440 to 540. In 1995 this figure decreased to 390, which reduced the growth in total number of doctors (Table 16.8). In the 1990s the number of new students in medical schools has decreased, but this will only affect total supply later in the decade.

In the 1990s the total number of working-age nurses has increased by about 25 per cent. This increase is mainly due to a great increase in training and posts during the years 1991–94, which was based on decisions made on nursing services in the late 1980s and in 1990. At that time the lack of nurses was an acute problem in many hospitals. In the 1990s the training of new nurses and practical nurses has not been reduced because education has been used as a short-term instrument to prevent total unemployment. However, unemployment has also increased in the health sector (including doctors) from 1.7 per cent in 1990 to 8.5 per cent in 1994, although it is clearly smaller than the average for all industries (3.4 per cent in 1990 and 18.4 per cent in 1994).

Cost Containment in Finnish Health Care   687

Table 16.9 Paying doctors in Finland

Health centres

Personal doctor (40% of doctors)

- basic salary (60%)
- capitation (20%)
- fee-for-service (15%)
- local allowances (5%)

Other doctors (60% of doctors)

- basic salary and fee for services for work outside normal office time

---

Hospitals

- basic salary based on post and length of career
- additional remuneration for being on call
- fee-for-service for pay bed (private) patients

Private Sector

- fee-for-service

16.3.6 Changing the way doctors are paid

Most physicians working in the public sector draw monthly salaries, with little allowance for variations in performance (see Table 16.9). However, it should be noted that publicly employed physicians are also allowed to work in private practice. In these cases they are reimbursed on a fee-for-service basis by patients, who in turn are party reimbursed by the NHI.

Within health centres the personal physician principle is promoted by a new payment system. A list of about 2000 citizens is assigned to each physician. Personal doctors have no defined working hours, but patients have the right to see their physician within three days. A physician's total salary is a combination of basic salary (60 per cent), capitation (20 per cent), fees-for-services (15 per cent) and local allowances (5 per cent). By 1996, about 40 per cent of the population had been assigned a personal doctor.

According to studies the personal doctor system has improved the access to general practitioners and waiting times have fallen.[25] In addition, the personal doctor was found to have an impact on the total utilization of doctor services in a study using data from 1991 to 1994.[26] After controlling for relevant factors (morbidity, age, sex), physician contacts are estimated to be 20–30 per cent higher among individuals who have a personal doctor assigned by a municipality.

688   *Health Care and Cost Containment in the European Union*

16.3.7 Practice guidelines and doctors' profiles

In Finland neither practice guidelines nor doctor profiles are used for cost containment.

16.3.8 Administrative costs

In Finland it is very difficult to evaluate the development of administrative costs because of the lack of data. Health expenditure statistics include only those costs of the central administration devoted to health care and administrative costs of the National Health Insurance (NHI). The share of these costs has been about 2 per cent of total health expenditure (Appendix 16.2). The share of administration costs in 1994 was about 10 per cent of the NHI's total expenditure on health care (administration plus reimbursements). Between 1990 and 1994 the share decreased by about 2 percentage points.[1]

The state subsidy reform gave greater responsibility and decision-making power to municipalities, and decreased the administrative duties and work in central government and the Provincial Boards. Thus it can be assumed that the health care administrative costs of central government have also decreased. At least the content of work has changed: the direct administration has changed to information guidance, developmental work and research. Using the available data it is impossible to evaluate whether the decentralization of the health care system has increased administration costs for municipalities and federations of municipalities.

16.3.9 Local innovations

The new state subsidy system in 1993 created strong incentives for local innovations. The most important local efforts are devoted to integrating the administration and production of health services with social services (e.g. care of the elderly).

16.3.10 Control of drugs

Pharmaceutical products in Finland may only be sold with the permission of the National Agency For Medicines,* and retail prices of medicines distributed by pharmacies are regulated. In addition, the number and location of pharmacies for private (profit-making) licences are tightly controlled by the National Agency for Medicines. The Finnish drug reimbursement system is based on a positive list of products that can be prescribed. Before the implementation of the European Economic Area Agreement, the price of a drug was one of the factors determining whether a sales licence would be issued for it. The situation changed in January 1994. Since then, one of the criteria for licensing a medicine as a reimbursable drug has been that its wholesale price is reasonable. This is determined by considering issues such as the cost of treatment, the benefits of pharmacological treatment from the point of view of both the patient and total spending on health and social care, the cost of alternative treatment options (such as comparable drugs), the price of medicine elsewhere within the European Economic Area, the manufacturing and R&D costs of the drug, and the funds available for reimbursement.[27] The *reasonableness* of a drug's price is determined by the National Board for Drug Reimbursement. Other matters regarding reimbursement are handled by the Social Insurance Institution. The retail price is derived from the wholesale price by means of a formula defined by the Government.

The main outcome of the change in the price regulating system in 1994 is the relatively steep increase in the price of many over-the-counter drugs (such as acetylsalicylic acid and paracetamol preparations), even though, in absolute terms, they are still rather inexpensive.[12]

16.3.11 Control of dental care

The share of dental expenditure of total health care expenditure has been between 5 and 6 per cent (Appendix 16.2). As stated before, dental services are included both within services provided by municipalities (free to those aged 0–18, subsidized for those aged 19–40) and services covered by the

---

* Since 1995, in some cases the European Commission (at European Union level) can make the decision following a recommendation by the European Agency for the Evaluation of Medicinal Products.

690 *Health Care and Cost Containment in the European Union*

NHI (aged 19–40). The cuts in municipal health expenditure have somewhat decreased the supply of health centres' dental care services. In 1994, about 36 per cent of dental expenditure was financed by municipalities (including the state subsidy), 8 per cent by the NHI and 56 per cent by households. The fact that dental care for adults born before 1956 is not subsidized has contained the cost of private dental care.

16.3.12 Patient choice and referral

It is not unusual, particularly in big health centres, for patients to have no opportunity to choose the doctor who will treat them. Patients get a queue number at the reception and are treated by the doctor who happens to be free when it is their turn. In small health centres patients have a better chance of getting treatment from the same doctor on different occasions. In private physician centres, by contrast, patients may fix an appointment with the general practitioner or specialist of their own choice.

In general, patients cannot choose the hospital where they are to be treated, as the health centre informs them where they have to go. However, as far as possible, the hospital must allow patients to choose the physician responsible for their care.

For specialized (non-emergency) hospital care, the patient is expected to have a referral from a health centre physician. However these physicians cannot be considered gate-keepers, since a considerable proportion of referrals originate from the private sector (e.g. private physicians or those working in occupational care). In addition, many hospital physicians have dual roles, working as specialists in both the public and private sectors.

16.3.13 Private insurance

Private (profit-making) sickness insurance is relatively insignificant in Finland, accounting for about 2 per cent of health care financing. Private insurance is funded mainly by individuals' contributions. It is mainly taken out for children and youngsters because of queues in services in public health centres. The popularity of private insurance has been stable in recent years. In 1987 and 1995 about one-third of children under 15 years were subsidized by private insurance plans if they used private doctors' services.

Cost Containment in Finnish Health Care 691

For adults the figure was under 10 per cent in both years. Moreover, insurance premiums are not tax-deductible.

16.3.14 Quality assurance

A national policy for quality in health care was adopted in 1994 and renewed in 1995.[28] Under this policy all health care organizations and units were required to formulate a written policy on quality during 1996 and then work towards creating quality systems. Stricter measures to support this development, such as legislation, have not been considered necessary. The service producers (hospitals, health centres etc.) are responsible for the development of both policy development and enforcement.

Quality indicators have been developed for both primary and secondary care. This is done jointly by several organizations, and national registers are utilized as a basis for the system of indicators.

Accreditation systems in health care are not widely used, nor is there any pressure to start doing so. For certain specific procedures, such as organ transplantation, the Ministry may appoint the unit(s) to be used. Certification systems exist for health professionals, and for medical laboratories and voluntary certification has been available since the 1970s. Organizational certifications of quality systems are becoming increasingly popular.

The impact of cost-containment measures on quality has not been studied comprehensively. We have data on the deteriorating quality of psychiatric care that coincides with major cuts, as well as on increasing accessibility problems within primary care during the early 1990s. The cuts in maternity services do not seem to have had an impact on the quality of care or outcomes, as the cuts have usually been planned carefully and targeted to low-risk groups.

16.3.15 New technology

The Finnish Office for Health Care Technology Assessment (FinOHTA) was set up on 1 January 1995 within the National Research and Development Centre for Welfare and Health (STAKES). The task of FinOHTA in its assessment activities is to concentrate on those technologies

692 *Health Care and Cost Containment in the European Union*

that are important for the health of the citizens or for the national economy. FinOHTA's main focus is on established technology, but efforts have also been made to monitor new and emerging technologies such as telemedicine and information technology in health care.

FinOHTA has no legal authority to influence the dissemination and use of different technologies, but like other assessment agencies, FinOHTA disseminates information of good national and international assessment studies in order to have an impact on the decision-making in health care.

The National Agency for Medicines controls the conformity of medical devices marketed in Finland and supervises their use. The new device regulations came into force at the beginning of 1995.

16.3.16 Development of information systems

Statistical and other information systems for Finnish health care are very developed compared to many other countries. In the 1990s the aim has been to coordinate the different information systems at the national level. An example of this coordination is a new municipal database for social and health statistics, to be used by municipal officers and planners, which was built in 1994. This database includes some 2,700 variables on each municipality. The following topics are included: general background (e.g. land area, population density, education, unemployment, occupational structure), municipal economy, population statistics, families and housing, morbidity and mortality, social risks and challenges, social and health expenditure, the work force employed in health and social services, and utilization of these services.

16.4 Equity issues

The equity aspect of Finnish health care in the late 1980s has been evaluated by means of three dimensions: vertical equity in finance, i.e. payments for health care ought to be positively related to ability to pay; horizontal equity in utilization, i.e. those with equal need should be treated equally; and equality in health. These dimensions are emphasized in the official documents of Finnish health policy.[29] The dimensions are also used in international comparisons.[30]

The financing of health care in Finland was slightly progressive in 1990, i.e. higher income groups financed health care in proportion to their pre-tax income somewhat more that lower income groups.[29, 31] A consideration of the late 1980s reveals that total health care utilization in Finland seemed to be more closely related to need than to ability to pay. But there were differences between income groups in the utilization of various types of services. While out-patient care, provided by public municipalities, and drug utilization were generally utilized in line with need (measured by indicators of morbidity), the use of private out-patient services (private doctors' services and private examinations and treatments) was concentrated among the high income groups. In-patient care was used disproportionately by lower-income groups.[29] However, a recent study on the use of a specific surgical procedure (coronary bypass grafting) reveals clear socio-economic inequity favouring upper socio-economic groups.[21]

The latest trends in Finnish health care indicate that the changes in the system have had little effect on equity. Preliminary analyses of physician service utilization rates indicate that although the total number of visits has decreased, visits are divided between socio-economic groups according to need.[26] A microsimulation of distributional changes in the financing of health care between 1990 and 1994 indicates that financing in health care has become more regressive. However the decline has not been very substantial, and overall the health care system remained progressive in 1994. In international comparisons of different health care systems, Finland is still grouped along with other mainly tax-financed proportional or slightly progressive health care systems, while differing somewhat from so-called social insurance countries where financing is more regressive.[22, 30]

16.5 Conclusions

The Finnish health care system has been in real transition in the 1990s. Before this, cost containment was not an important issue in Finland, since the former planning and state subsidy system was an example of global budgeting which functioned effectively during a period of steady growth in the economy.[23] But in the 1990s cost containment also became an important issue in Finnish health care. There are at least three ways in which the

694   *Health Care and Cost Containment in the European Union*

changes in the Finnish health care differ from changes in other countries. Firstly, the implementation of the major reform (state subsidy reform) was performed at the time of economic crisis in the country. Thus the effects of the reform cannot be evaluated without taking into account the overall economic situation. Secondly, there have been major changes in health expenditure (a decrease of over 10 per cent) and its financing (increase of cost-sharing by 8 per cent). Thirdly, as a consequence of reform and cuts in state subsidies, local governments (municipalities) have, in addition to increased freedom in the provision of services, more economic responsibilities in providing these services. Although there is some evidence that productivity has increased and the system's equity maintained, it is too early to say anything definite regarding the overall effects of these changes.

References

1   Kansaneläkelaitos. *Terveyspalvelujen Kustannukset ja Rahoitus Suomessa 1960–1994.* Helsinki: Kansaneläkelaitoksen julkaisuja T:52, 1996.

2   *National Accounts.* Central Statistical Office of Finland.

3   *Price Index of Public Services.* Municipal Health Care Central Statistical Office of Finland.

4   *Index of Wage and Salary Earnings.* Central Statistical Office of Finland.

5   *The Accounts of Central Government.* Ministry of Finance (Finland).

6   Häkkinen U, Mikkola H, Nordberg M, Salonen M. *Tutkimus Kuntien Terveyspalveluiden Valtionosuuksien Perusteista.* Helsinki: Sisäasiainministeriön Kuntaosaston julkaisu 3/1996.

7   WHO. *Health Care Systems in Transition, Finland.* Copenhagen: World Health Organisation, Regional Office for Europe, 1996.

8   Häkkinen U, Asikainen K, Linna M. *Terveyspalvelujen, arve ja Kustannukset sekä Sairaaloiden Tuottavuus 1990-luvulla.* Helsinki: Stakes aiheita 45/1996.

9   Häkkinen U, Linna M, Salonen M. Korvausmenettelyn ja kuntakoon vaikutus erikoissairaanhoidon taloudelliseen riskiin. *Suomen Lääkärilehti* 1994;49:2454–58.

10   *Consumer Price Index.* Central Statistical Office of Finland.

11   National Agency of Medicines and Social Insurance Institution. *Finnish Statistics of Medicines 1994.* Helsinki, 1995.

12   Klaukka T, Wallenius K, Peura S, Voipio T. Highlights of drug consumption in 1994. In: *Finnish Statistics of Medicines 1994.* Helsinki: National Agency of Medicines and Social Insurance Institution, 1995. pp. 16–22.

13   Kalsta K, Martikainen J. Drug consumption in 1995. In: *Finnish Statistics of Medicines*

1995. Helsinki: National Agency of Medicines and Social Insurance Institution, 1996 pp 25–29.

14 OECD . *OECD Health Data.* Paris: OECD, 1995.

15 Linna M, Häkkinen U. Sairaaloiden tuottavuus 1991–1994. In: Häkkinen U, Asikainen K, Linna M. *Terveyspalvelujen tarve ja kustannukset sekä sairaaloiden tuottavuus 1990-luvulla.* Helsinki: Stakes aiheita 45/1996 pp. 38–51.

16 STAKES (National Research and Development Centre for Welfare and Health). *National Hospital Discharge Register.* Helsinki, 1996.

17 Hanning M. *I Väntan på vård. Vårdgarantier i Norden – Bakgrund, Utformning ock Effekter.* Stockholm: SPRI rapport 412, 1995.

18 Kekomäki M, Linna M, Rasilainen J, Alanko A. Jonotusajat elektiivisiin toimenpiteisiin 1992-93. *Suomen Lääkärilehti* 1995;50:1519–24.

19 Sosiaali- ja terveysministeriö: Sairaaloiden kuntalaskutus. *Sosiaali- ja Terveysministeriön Monisteita* 1995:24.

20 STAKES (National Research and Development Centre for Welfare and Health). Use of hospital in-patient services in Finland 1988–1993. *SVT Health* 1995:5.

21 Keskimäki I. *Social Equity in the Use of Hospital In-patient Care in Finland.* Jyväskylä: STAKES Research Reports 84, 1997.

22 Klavus J, Häkkinen U. Micro-level analysis of distributional changes in health care financing in Finland. Stakes, *Themes* 1997;4.

23 Häkkinen U. Health care in Finland: current issues. In: Alban A, Christiansen T. (eds). *The Nordic Lights. New Initiatives in Health Care Systems.* Odense: Odense University Press, 1995. pp.141–8.

24 *Central Register of Health Services Professionals.* STAKES (National Research and Development Centre for Welfare and Health).

25 Mäkelä M, Åström M, Bergström M, Sainio S. *Terveyskeskusten Alueellinen Väestövastuu.* Helsinki: Stakes Aiheita 2/1996.

26 Häkkinen U, Rosenqvist G, Aro S. Economic depression and the use of physician services in Finland. *Health Economics* 1996;5:421–34.

27 Rajamäki S. The pricing of drugs: deciding what is reasonable. In: *Finnish Statistics of Medicines, 1995.* Helsinki: National Agency of Medicines and Social Insurance Institution, 1996. pp 80.

28 STAKES (National Research and Development Centre for Welfare and Health). *Quality Management in Social Welfare and Health.* Helsinki, 1996.

29 Häkkinen U. *Terveyspalvelujen Käyttö, Terveydentila ja Sosioekonominen Tasa-arvo Suomessa.* Helsinki: Sosiaali- ja terveyshallitus. Tutkimuksia 20, 1992.

30 van Doorslaer E, Wagstaff A, Rutten F (eds). *Equity in the Finance and Delivery of Health Care: An International Perspective.* Oxford: Oxford University Press, 1993.

31 Klavus J, Häkkinen U. *Terveyspalvelujen Käyttö, Rahoitus ja Tulonjako.* Jyväskylä: Stakes raportteja 175, 1995.

696 *Health Care and Cost Containment in the European Union*

Appendix 16.1 Health care expenditure 1980–94, FIM million, at current prices

	1980	1981	1982	1983	1984
In-patient care	6,122	6,915	7,846	8,700	9,629
General and tuberculosis hospitals	4,149	4,651	5,416	6,057	7,135
Mental hospitals*	966	1,093	1,231	1,329	1,481
Hospitals for the mentally disabled	322	369	425	478	525
Other hospitals	685	802	774	836	488
Out-patient care	3,382	4,069	4,787	5,548	6,572
Out-patient care (excluding dental care)	2,632	3,213	3,805	4,446	5,298
Health centres (local authorities)	1,257	1,496	1,773	2,037	2,396
Occupational and student health care	344	410	470	531	635
Hospital out-patient care	607	817	972	1,129	1,383
Private out-patient care	423	490	589	749	883
Dental care	750	856	982	1,102	1,275
Medicines and pharmaceutical products	1,328	1,490	1,622	1,880	2,105
Medical equipment and appliances total	432	516	585	673	661
Eye-glasses	281	346	396	455	515
Prosthetic devices	75	76	83	97	104
Environmental health care	162	181	207	230	277
Administration	239	284	319	375	406
Public investment	609	781	970	1,158	1,207
Transportation	175	216	243	260	266
Running costs (total)	11,839	13,671	15,609	17,665	19,916
Total health care expenditure	12,448	14,452	16,580	18,823	21,124
Share of GDP	6.5	6.6	6.7	6.9	6.9

* The 1993–94 expenditure for mental hospital care has been included in the figures for general hospitals.

Source: Kansaneläkelaitos, 1996.[1]

1985	1986	1987	1988	1989	1990	1991	1992	1993	1994
11,125	12,017	12,890	14,205	16,114	18,374	19,847	19,455	18,020	17,454
8,273	8,977	9,658	10,659	12,320	14,147	15,703	15,553	15,338	14,699
1,676	1,771	1,813	1,932	1,983	2,162	1,625	1,211	-	-
599	619	651	697	780	889	984	1,000	824	753
577	649	767	917	1,030	1,175	1,536	1,692	1,857	2,002
7,747	8,622	9,829	10,776	12,188	13,945	15,415	15,325	14,825	14,921
6,300	7,035	8,093	8,843	10,033	11,555	12,856	12768	12,307	12,429
2,965	3,293	3,863	4,197	4,735	5,449	6,033	5,977	5,881	5,945
701	782	860	973	1,105	1,251	1,319	1,279	1,190	1,292
1,635	1,809	2,046	2,239	2,616	3,069	3,555	3,659	3,465	3,549
999	1,151	1,324	1,433	1,577	1,786	1,949	1,853	1,771	1,643
1,446	1,587	1,736	1,933	2,155	2,390	2,558	2,557	2,517	2,491
2,346	2,539	2,796	3,048	3,379	3,869	4,446	4,796	5,050	5,398
747	844	911	1,067	1,158	1,205	1,242	1,264	1,268	1,284
582	659	709	840	913	938	952	970	981	1,000
120	136	150	168	184	200	217	221	213	210
318	331	392	435	478	603	686	712	469	515
478	522	600	692	733	812	902	965	965	951
1,125	1,140	1,212	1,346	1,486	1,871	1,746	1415	1,180	1,069
298	317	350	355	386	416	450	434	437	507
23,058	25,192	27,767	30,578	34,436	39,223	42,987	42,952	41,033	41,030
24,183	26,333	28,979	31,923	35,921	41,093	44,733	44,367	42,213	42,099
7.3	7.4	7.5	7.3	7.4	8.0	9.1	9.3	8.8	8.3

698   *Health Care and Cost Containment in the European Union*

Appendix 16.2 Structure (%) of health care expenditure, 1980–94

	1980	1981	1982	1983	1984
In-patient care	49.2	47.8	47.3	46.2	45.6
General and tuberculosis hospitals	33.3	32.2	32.7	32.2	33.8
Mental hospitals*	7.8	7.6	7.4	7.1	7.0
Hospitals for the mentally disabled	2.6	2.6	2.6	2.5	2.5
Other hospitals	5.5	5.5	4.7	4.4	2.3
Out-patient care	27.2	28.2	28.9	29.5	31.1
Out-patient care (excluding dental care)	21.1	22.2	22.9	23.6	25.1
Health centres (local authorities)	10.1	10.4	10.7	10.8	11.3
Occupational and student health care	2.8	2.8	2.8	2.8	3.0
Hospital out-patient care	4.9	5.7	5.9	6.0	6.5
Private out-patient care	3.4	3.4	3.6	4.0	4.2
Dental care	6.0	5.9	5.9	5.9	6.0
Medicines and pharmaceutical products	10.7	10.3	9.8	10.0	10.0
Medical equipment and appliances total	3.5	3.6	3.5	3.6	3.1
Eye-glasses	2.3	2.4	2.4	2.4	2.4
Prosthetic devices	0.6	0.5	0.5	0.5	0.5
Environmental health care	1.3	1.3	1.2	1.2	1.3
Administration	1.9	2.0	1.9	2.0	1.9
Public investment	4.9	5.4	5.9	6.2	5.7
Transportation	1.4	1.5	1.5	1.4	1.3
Total health care expenditure	100.0	100.0	100.0	100.0	100.0

* The 1993–94 expenditure for mental hospital care has been included in the figures for general hospitals.

Source: Kansaneläkelaitos, 1996.[1]

1985	1986	1987	1988	1989	1990	1991	1992	1993	1994
46.0	45.6	44.5	44.5	44.9	44.7	44.4	43.9	42.7	41.5
34.2	34.1	33.3	33.4	34.3	34.4	35.1	35.1	36.3	34.9
6.9	6.7	6.3	6.1	5.5	5.3	3.6	2.7	–	–
2.5	2.4	2.2	2.2	2.2	2.2	2.2	2.3	2.0	1.8
2.4	2.5	2.6	2.9	2.9	2.9	3.4	3.8	4.4	4.8
32.0	32.7	33.9	33.8	33.9	33.9	34.5	34.5	35.1	35.4
26.1	26.7	27.9	27.7	27.9	28.1	28.7	28.8	29.2	29.5
12.3	12.5	13.3	13.1	13.2	13.3	13.5	13.5	13.9	14.1
2.9	3.0	3.0	3.0	3.1	3.0	2.9	2.9	2.8	3.1
6.8	6.9	7.1	7.0	7.3	7.5	7.9	8.2	8.2	8.4
4.1	4.4	4.6	4.5	4.4	4.3	4.4	4.2	4.2	3.9
6.0	6.0	6.0	6.1	6.0	5.8	5.7	5.8	6.0	5.9
9.7	9.6	9.6	9.5	9.4	9.4	9.9	10.8	12.0	12.8
3.1	3.2	3.1	3.3	3.2	2.9	2.8	2.8	3.0	3.0
2.4	2.5	2.4	2.6	2.5	2.3	2.1	2.2	2.3	2.4
0.5	0.5	0.5	0.5	0.5	0.5	0.5	0.5	0.5	0.5
1.3	1.3	1.4	1.4	1.3	1.5	1.5	1.6	1.1	1.2
2.0	2.0	2.1	2.2	2.0	2.0	2.0	2.2	2.3	2.3
4.7	4.3	4.2	4.2	4.1	4.6	3.9	3.2	2.8	2.5
1.2	1.2	1.2	1.1	1.1	1.0	1.0	1.0	1.0	1.2
100.0	100.0	100.0	100.0	100.0	100.0	100.0	100.0	100.0	100.0

17 Health care reforms and cost containment in Sweden

ANDERS ANELL AND PATRICK SVARVAR

17.1 Introduction

Total expenditure in Swedish health care, adjusted for changes in the definition of health care, has increased in current prices throughout the 1980s and 1990s. Measured in fixed prices, however, total expenditure has been rather constant over the last ten years. During this period several reforms have been introduced, varying in objectives, significance, implementation strategies and effects. Cost containment has been considered an important issue, particularly during the 1980s and in recent years. In this chapter, reforms introduced in the 1980s and 1990s will be reviewed; the particular aim being to outline those reforms relevant to the issue of cost containment, or rather, the operational measure of expenditure development. An important problem in this endeavour is that any single reform may have several purposes. For political reasons, it might also be the case that cost containment is rarely portrayed as the most important objective. We will therefore describe all reforms that can be linked to changes in micro-economic efficiency in general. In particular we will focus on:

- implementation of global budgets and resource allocation based on need (1980s);
- deregulation of patient fees (1991);
- transfer of responsibilities for care of the elderly at nursing homes to municipalities (1992);
- introduction of health care guarantee (1992);
- changes within primary care services (1990s);
- implementation of planned markets (1990s);
- changes within the pharmaceutical area (1990s).

702   *Health Care and Cost Containment in the European Union*

Regarding reforms of the 1980s, there is a link between the implementation of global budgets at national and county council level, and the slower rate of expansion of health care expenditure compared to the 1960s and 70s. Moreover, several reforms introduced in the early 1990s, focusing on the need to raise overall sector efficiency, have had important implications in this respect. However, general cut-back programmes and political decisions to down-scale the hospital sector have had a more direct effect on cost containment. Although substantial savings have been realised within the hospital sector in recent years, there is no downward trend in total health care expenditure. There is a clear upward trend in out-patient and pharmaceutical expenditure. With this development, and bearing the rather poor financial position of the county councils in mind, cost containment is likely to remain a high priority in the years to come.

Sections 17.2, 17.3 and 17.4 contain descriptions of the development of the Swedish health care system and the reforms introduced in the 1980s and 1990s, respectively. In section 17.5, the health expenditure pattern is assessed and discussed for the period 1980–94. The capacity development in terms of, for example, personnel and hospital beds, and consumption indicators, are also assessed for the same period. This, in order to be able to relate the developments in expenditure to the development in real resources and consumption. Data used in section 17.5 is presented in detail in the Appendix. In section 17.6 we aim to discuss overall linkages between developments regarding health care expenditure and the different reforms. Current and future developments are also discussed.

17.2 Developments in the Swedish health care system

The financing and delivery of health care services in Sweden are primarily the responsibility of the 26 county councils organized according to a monopolistic integrated system. Most facilities are owned and managed directly by the county councils. The private health care sector is small. Only 8 per cent of doctors work in private practices, and private health insurance is very limited. The councils finance their health care activities mainly through a proportional income tax levied on the population. Other sources of finance are block grants from central government and the social insurance system, together with flat-rate payments from patients at the point of ser-

Health Care Reforms and Cost Containment in Sweden 703

vice.*

The county councils were established as far back as 1862. Besides the municipalities, they formed a secondary level of local government and had certain decisive legislative powers, e.g. the power to levy taxes on their population. The establishment of county councils was the beginning of the basic structure of the health care system in Sweden today. A further important element in the establishment of the public Swedish health care system was the introduction of a national social insurance system in 1955. Under this system universal subsidies were provided for doctor consultations, drug prescriptions and, most importantly, for sickness compensation to cover for loss of income. The societal objective since then has been that all residents should not only have access to basic health services, but to high quality health services related to every need. Services excluded from reimbursement are limited; current examples are certain forms of plastic surgery and surgery for short-sightedness.

After the Second World War a considerable expansion of the hospital sector began, continuing throughout the 1960s and 1970s. The structural development was focused on transferring health care responsibilities from the state and the private sector to the county councils.[2] By the early 1970s, all public doctors had become salaried employees. This structural integration of activities created a basis for a total planning perspective for the implementation of overall health policy goals. The climate at the time meant that great faith was given to the possibilities of managing developments through formal planning models, both at national and county council level.

The integration of responsibilities, along with overall and rapid expansion, resulted in increasingly larger and more complex county councils. County councils became a large and important employer. More importantly, it became increasingly difficult to view and control activities through central planning, and as a consequence of these management problems, the county councils reorganized successively. Towards the end of the 1970s, most county councils were formally divided into several geographical districts, each with its own delegated political and administrative leadership.

---

* Dental care is financed and organized quite differently from general health care. About 40 per cent of dentists practice privately. Patient fees are considerably higher than for other health services; most dental services are in fact paid in full by patients. Children under the age of 19, however, are entitled to free public dental care.[1]

17.3 Reforms in the 1980s

By the early 1980s, the county councils accounted, in practice, for all publicly provided health care services. These conditions were reflected in the 1982 Health and Medical Care Act, which consolidated the power of county councils over health care activities. As the new act was being implemented, it gradually became evident that county council revenues would not increase with the same pace as they had during the 1960s and 1970s. These new conditions implied that cost containment became an important planning issue.[3] As a result, the districts gradually received more responsibility to allocate resources among activities within their respective areas. More importantly, they received more responsibility for keeping actual costs within specified budgets. The instrument used to implement this change was the *global budgets*, a method with clear incentives for providers to contain costs.

Global budgets and decentralised management were introduced at different times and with different strategies in the various county councils.[3] These differences reflect the decentralized nature of Swedish health care. In particular, since the introduction of the 1982 Act, considerable differences now exist among the county councils in terms of organization, resources and rules.[2] Generally speaking, global budgets were first implemented at the district level. The districts, basically on their own initiative, then carried out the changes involved and started to use the same method for the management of clinical and other departments. In some county councils, especially in those with a strong central leadership, the new principles were introduced in parallel for both districts and departments. With global budgets, the implementation of cost containment measures was decentralised to the district and departmental level. The central county council could, however, still intervene in district activities through guidelines and instructions; for instance when it came to control of capital investments and priorities among new activities. Usually, global budgets for recurrent and capital expenses were connected to both formal and informal rules on how to carry out activities.

The *1985 Dagmar reform*, introduced by the central government, further strengthened the planning and regulatory power of the county councils. The main motive of the reform was to cap central government grants allocated to the health care sector, and to give county councils a mandate to regulate the market for private practitioners; in particular part-time practition-

Health Care Reforms and Cost Containment in Sweden   705

ers. Before the reform, out-patient services by public providers and private practitioners were paid for by the National Social Insurance Board according to a fee-for-service system. The financing of private practitioners was in principle an open-ended system. As a result of the reform, the National Social Insurance Board now disburses general grants to the county councils based on the number of residents in each county, with some adjustment for differences in mortality rates and social factors. Private practitioners are still paid according to fees for different types of visits, but they have to negotiate with the county council in their geographic area for a contract in which the number of visits allowed per year is regulated.

By the mid-1980s, global budgets at the district level were an established practice in the majority of county councils. At the outset, this form of management did not entail any radical changes. For one thing, global budgets were usually based on the historical costs of producing services. The introduction of global budgets was, however, only the starting-point when it came to the decentralization of responsibility to the sub-county level. In some of the county councils that introduced global budgets at an early stage, it was decided that districts should, in the long-run, be responsible for the *total* costs of health services consumed by their residents. If districts were not in a position to provide appropriate care at their own facilities, services should be bought from other districts or county councils at transfer prices. Traditionally, the responsibility of districts had been limited to costs incurred at their own facilities.

17.3.1 Resource allocation based on need

In parallel with the development towards global budgets – at the national level as well as at county council and sub-county levels – it was discussed whether the overall resource allocation was fair. In the past, district administrations and heads of clinical and other departments had not paid much attention to their budgets. As it became more important to keep actual costs within a specified budget, it also became more important for districts and departments to scrutinize their own costs and compare them with those of other units. Usually, it was not hard to find differences that were difficult to explain and defend. Decades of a more or less incremental approach to resource allocation had created large differences in the supply and cost of services between districts as well as between counties. Resource allocation

706 *Health Care and Cost Containment in the European Union*

based on an assessment of need was put forward by a government report as a possible solution to the problem.[4]

By the end of the 1980s, adjustment of government grants to county councils, based on assessment of need, had been introduced. In addition, 14 of the 26 county councils had developed their own need-based model for resource allocation to districts.[3] The assessment of need was rough and based on data that was already available. In most counties, relative weights for different districts were calculated, using the total number and age-distribution of the population in each geographical area as the main explanatory variables. Thus, the models used were only loosely connected to the concept of need; but they still offered a measure of objectivity in the context of resource allocation. The new principles created winners and losers. The districts that lost out complained, and also pointed to deficiencies in the new models. As a consequence, resource allocation based on population characteristics was gradually implemented over several years.

There were also clear ambitions to continue to develop financial responsibilities at the departmental level. Heads of clinical departments were to be held responsible for total costs incurred by activities, including the indirect costs of services at diagnostic and auxiliary departments through the use of transfer prices. This development was parallel to the gradual delegation of responsibilities from the central county-council level to the districts. One of the main driving forces behind the development was the need for cost containment and the need to establish fair budgets for different departments.

17.3.2 The financial situation of the county councils

In 1988, the national parliament prohibited the county councils and municipalities from increasing their income tax rates starting from 1990. The government and the Ministry of Finance were not pleased with developments regarding public-sector expenditure during the 1980s. Another decision taken by the government in the late 1980s was to set up the Swedish Council on Technology Assessment in Health Care (SBU). The purpose was to contribute to a rational use of existing resources within the health care sector through expert assessment of medical technologies.

Squeezed between pressures of not increasing tax rates, demands from an increasingly older population and new medical technologies, the finan-

Health Care Reforms and Cost Containment in Sweden 707

cial position of the county councils gradually worsened during the latter half of the 1980s. This development was in spite of the continuing decreases in investment expenditure. In the late 1980s, several county councils had to borrow in order to pay in full for their operating expenditure. It was far from unusual that hospitals had to close wards down towards the end of the year in order to balance the budget. Not surprisingly, such measures created long waiting times.

17.4 Reforms in the 1990s

In the early 1990s, a more market-oriented approach was substituted for the predominant and earlier focus on planning, need and cost containment as the bases for reform. It was evident that global budgets and planning based on need did not promote overall efficiency. Studies pointed to a lack of incentives to use resources efficiently, and county councils were criticized for their long waiting times and poor consumer orientation.[5] The new government elected in 1992, led by the Conservatives, prolonged the decision to prohibit the county councils and municipalities from increasing their tax rates. The new Minister of Health also initiated two government committees, one on health care priorities and a second on health care financing and organization.

Similar to the developments during the 1980s, reforms of the 1990s have to a large extent been initiated at the county council level. Several important decisions have, however, been taken at national level, e.g. changes in the rules for setting patient fees in 1991, the 1992 care-of-the-elderly reform (ÄDEL), the 1992 national health care guarantee, the introduction of reference prices for generic drugs in 1993, the 1994 family doctor reform and the freedom to establish private, publicly-funded, practices, introduced in 1994.

17.4.1 Deregulation of fees

During the 1970s and 1980s, co-payments were determined by central government. Since 1991, county councils have been allowed to determine *their own fee structure* concerning out-patient care. Fees for in-patient care

708 *Health Care and Cost Containment in the European Union*

and prescription drugs are still decided at the national level by the Parliament. Further, Parliament determines the maximum amount any individual has to pay for health services and drugs for a period of one year; in 1996 this was SEK 1,800. Above this high-cost protection level, there are no charges. County councils and private practitioners are instead paid equivalent fees by the National Social Insurance Board. The government also decides on general exemptions from co-payments. Some patient groups with chronic illnesses (e.g. diabetics) have, since the mid-1950s, been given free drugs.

Cost containment has not been put forward by the county councils as the main reason behind the fee increases that have occurred during the 1990s. However, county councils have explicitly used fees as a tool in their ambitions to steer patients to primary care. In 1996, fees for visiting a doctor in primary care varied between SEK 60 and 140 depending on county council and form of provider. Fees for consulting a doctor at a hospital varied in the same year between SEK 100 and 260, depending on county council and whether or not the patient had a referral from a primary-care doctor

17.4.2 Care of the elderly reform (ÄDEL)

The so-called ÄDEL reform in 1992 is so far considered to be the most ambitious structural reform of the 1990s. The reform meant that the responsibility for providing long-term health care to the elderly and disabled was transferred from the 26 county councils to the 288 municipalities. The reform led to a 16 per cent reduction in total county council health care expenditure. The objectives for implementing the ÄDEL reform were to give municipalities total planning and financial responsibility for all services to the elderly and disabled, including home services, nursing homes and services at old peoples' homes. As part of the reform, it was decided that municipalities had to pay hospitals (or rather county councils) a fee per diem in case they were not ready to admit elderly patients being discharged from hospitals. Thus, clear incentives were introduced among municipalities to try to reduce the number of elderly patients waiting to be discharged from a hospital to, for example, a nursing home. This being the case, the reform also had an important indirect impact on the overall efficiency of hospital services.[6] There was a sharp increase in hospital turnover rates and

Health Care Reforms and Cost Containment in Sweden 709

a decrease in mean length of stay between 1991 and 1992.

17.4.3 Changes within primary care services

The structure of the primary health care delivery system, and conditions for private practitioners, was substantially changed by the central government during a short period of time. These changes had an adverse effect on the possibility of containing costs. Two changes of government during the 1990s would be one important explanatory factor for the turbulence. Moreover, the *Family Doctor Act* came into effect 1 January 1994, as did the *Act on freedom to establish private, publicly-funded practices*. Both these reforms had important and negative effects on the ability of county councils to control out-patient care expenditure. The Family Doctor Act forced the county councils to organize primary health care so that all residents within the county area were able to choose their family doctor. The reform resulted in a substantial increase in the number of private practitioners in some areas, but overall, privatization of primary care services was limited. Payments from the county councils were in part based on a monthly fixed fee for each individual, and in part on a fee for each type of visit. Each family doctor, at least in the private sector, was given clear incentives to try to attract additional patients, thereby improving his or her own personal income. The objective of the reform was primarily to improve accessibility and continuity in primary health care. The Act on freedom to establish private practices deprived the county councils of their regulatory power with respect to signing agreements with private practitioners in order to control their number and reimbursements.

The county councils were obliged to have implemented the family doctor reform by the end of 1995, but already by mid-1995 the Social Democrats, who came into power following the elections of 1994, had abolished this Act as well as the Act on freedom to establish private practices. Further, the new Social democratic government issued new directives for the ongoing government committee investigating the future financing and organization of health care, in favour of the traditional county council based model.

710 *Health Care and Cost Containment in the European Union*

17.4.4 Planned markets

In the early 1990s, some county councils initiated quite substantial changes with respect to their planning and control systems.[7,8,9] These changes included implementation of methods that had been discussed in the 1980s, such as resource allocation based on population characteristics and total cost liability at both district and clinical department levels. But the changes also included new models of control and a weak form of a purchaser-provider split.

In 1994, 14 out of the 26 county councils had established separate purchasing organizations. The organization and working methods among purchasers have varied substantially between, and in some cases within, the county councils. Developments have been strongly influenced by traditions of organizing health care activities within each county council.[7] Some county councils have introduced one large central county council purchaser, while others have chosen to establish several purchasers at the district level. The argument put forward in support of several local purchasers has been that it promotes co-operation between primary care services and social services provided by the municipalities. Initially, the restrained financial situation played a significant role for all purchasers. Price and volume negotiations and efforts to contain costs have been important issues. Other issues have been of varying importance to different purchasers; some have laid greater emphasis on the promotion of public health and collaboration with municipalities and social insurance offices, others have played greater emphasis on contracting-out and the establishment of competition among providers.

The contracts regulating the relationship between purchasing organizations and health care providers have usually been based on case-mix systems and prospective per case payments, complemented with price, volume and quality restrictions. Per case payments of in-patient hospital services have predominantly been based on diagnosis related groups (DRGs). With respect to payments to out-patient care, several county councils have developed their own classification schemes of different services, and the associated relative weights when it comes to resource use. The more detailed use of different per case payment systems, as well as the level of technical ambition, have varied substantially between county councils and hospitals.[8] *Per diem* payments have in some cases complemented per case payments, e.g. with respect to cases with an unusually long length of stay. Psychiatric, primary and geriatric care have usually been reimbursed through a combina-

Health Care Reforms and Cost Containment in Sweden   711

tion of global budgets and fees-for-services. Highly specialized, and often resource demanding, tertiary health care services have usually been reimbursed according to a fee-for-service system.

New contractual arrangements have also been arranged among those county councils that have not introduced a separation between purchasers and providers at the global level. By the end of the 1980s, it was common to introduce full-cost liability in clinical departments, meaning that transfer pricing based on per case payment schemes between clinical and ancillary departments was introduced. Furthermore, several of the nationally initiated reforms have resulted in new contractual arrangements at the county council level. For example, the ÄDEL reform introduced a contractual relationship between the county councils and the municipalities with respect to elderly patients waiting to be discharged to a nursing home or similar facility.

The patients' freedom of choice of providers was a highly important policy issue in the early 1990s, and developments have been more uniform throughout the country compared to the introduction of internal purchasing organizations and contracting. For several years now, patients in all county councils have been able to choose which family doctor or primary health centre to visit. Furthermore, in many county councils, patients have the right to choose among county hospitals with, and in some cases without, a referral. Payments to providers usually follows the choices of the patients.

Following the perceived need to strengthen the position of the individual, the Ministry of Health and Social Affairs and the Federation of County Councils agreed in 1992 to introduce a *national health care guarantee*, with the objective of reducing waiting times for certain non-acute hospital treatments.* No patient should have to wait for more than three months for these treatments. If this was still the case, the hospital had to offer treatment at another public or private hospital. Starting from 1997, the guarantee has been substituted by a new principle in which waiting times for general practitioner visits and diagnosis are regulated. Clear restrictions on the waiting times for treatment are no longer included in the guarantee.[10]

---

* These were coronary artery disease surgery, hip-joint and knee-joint replacement, cataract surgery, gallstone surgery, inguinal hernia surgery, surgery of prolapse and incontinence, and hearing aid tests.

712   *Health Care and Cost Containment in the European Union*

17.4.5 Effects due to planned markets

It is important to note that per case payment systems, increased patient choice, and the health care guarantee by no means provide incentives for cost containment. The perceived problems of the health care sector in the early 1990s were *not* focused on cost containment issues. Instead, the overall performance of the council-managed health care sector was brought up for debate. The main objective of reform was to promote productivity, and first of all to increase the volume of activity. It was only later that cost containment, or rather cost-cutting, became a more important issue. As a result, incentives of the planned market were gradually mixed with political decisions on how to cut down on expenditure.[11]

From available studies, it seems reasonably evident that there was a marked increase in productivity within the hospital sector, beginning in 1991/92. Productivity among hospitals, defined as the relation between expenditure and outputs in terms of weighted discharges and consultations, increased by 8 per cent in 1992, 6 per cent in 1993 and 2 per cent in 1994.[12] This trend can be explained first of all by a sharp increase in the volume of activity. As a result, there was a marked decrease in hospital waiting times, especially between 1991 and 1992.[13] Expenditure for in-patient care was reduced as well and, starting from 1991, overall employment in the health care sector dropped. At a lower level of aggregation, county councils differ with respect to how the increase in efficiency was accomplished. In some county councils which introduced major reforms towards planned markets (e.g. Stockholm), the development can mainly be explained by an increase in the volume of activity. In other and more traditionally managed county councils (e.g. Kronoberg), the increase in productivity can mainly be attributed to the reduction of expenditure.

It is uncertain as to what extent the overall development regarding productivity in the hospital sector in the 1990s can be attributed to national reforms (ÄDEL and the health care guarantee), county council reforms (patients' freedom of choice, purchaser–provider split and prospective per case payment systems) or other parallel changes (new health care technologies, increased unemployment and political decisions to close down activities). On the one hand, reforms can be associated with the incentives they provide to increase the volume of activity, incentives which may have a negative impact on cost containment. On the other hand, one can argue that general budget cut-backs and down-scaling in the hospital sector would have been much more difficult to achieve, had not reform components generated dynamic changes and output volume increases to the health care sector. In other words, it is quite possible that reforms associated with the objective to improve overall efficiency and increase the volume of activity, indirectly made cost containing through traditional planning activities easier to implement.

Evidence when it comes to changes in the quality and distribution of services is indirect and much more inconclusive than the available measurement of changes in the volume of services and expenditure.[14] One important reason for this is that neither quality nor equity have been regularly monitored and assessed in Swedish health care.[15] The absence of data and evidence does not of course mean that it is possible to conclude that reforms did not have any effects (positive or negative) on the quality or distribution of services. In the mid 1990s, quite a few researchers and senior doctors seemed to be of the opinion that even if negative effects could not be found at present, the new incentives introduced with planned markets involved a clear risk of negative effects in the long-run.[16,17]

17.4.6 Pharmaceuticals

Several changes have been introduced in the pharmaceutical area during the 1990s; many of which have been implemented solely for the purpose of cost containment. The trend of pharmaceutical expenditure increases (see Appendix) has been a great concern of the government since subsidies for prescription drugs are paid by the National Social Insurance Board. Patient fees, decided by the Parliament, have doubled in real terms during the 1990s. In recent years, consumers have had to pay separately for each prescription, together with an extra fee for each additional item on the prescription, and fees have been raised several times. Since 1 July 1995, fees were SEK 160 for the first item on a prescription and SEK 60 for each additional item on the prescription. Reforms have also been directed towards the pharmaceutical industry itself. In 1993, a reference price system was introduced with the intention of promoting generic drugs. According to this system, the National Social Insurance Board pays the National Corporation of Swedish Pharmacies a maximum amount that is equivalent to the lowest-priced generic plus 10 per cent. The patient can choose a more expensive drug if he or she pays the difference. The initial effect of the reference price

714 *Health Care and Cost Containment in the European Union*

system was that costs for products for which there was a reference price decreased by close to SEK 400 million in the first year.

In spite of the introduction of a reference price system and increases in patient fees, the total costs of prescribed drugs continues to increase. Gradually, it has been recognized that administrative price controls and increases in flat-rate fees do not offer a long-term solution to this development. The major explanation behind the increase in drug costs is the introduction of new and potential drugs, some of which may be working as substitutes for other treatments.[18] Thus, reforms focusing on the tail of the product-life cycle (as does the reference price system) or number of prescriptions or items on each prescription (as do flat-rate fees) may result in savings, but these are likely to be non-recurrent. Further, pharmaceutical expenditure should not be assessed in isolation.

A new drug reform, introduced in 1997, has taken this into account.[19] Part of the reform is a changed patient co-payment structure meaning that patients should pay the full drug price up to a certain limit per year (SEK 400), and a fixed percentage of the drug price in intervals above this limit. The maximum payment for individuals during a twelve-month period is SEK 1300. Costs for drugs exceeding this high-cost protection level will be fully covered by the benefit scheme. With one exception (diabetics), there will be no free drugs to the chronically ill. A more far-reaching component of the reform is that county councils, instead of the National Social Insurance Board, will be responsible for the cost of prescription drugs. This took effect in 1998. In the past, the financing of prescription drugs has been an open-ended system without cost control.

17.5 Health expenditure, 1980–94

Total health expenditure in Sweden as a share of GDP decreased rather dramatically during the period 1980–94; from 9.3 to 7.4 per cent. This trend differs from most other Western European countries, which have experienced an increase since 1980. The substantial decrease in health expenditure as a share of GDP does not, however, give a full picture of the expenditure development. One important thing to account for, is that the definition of services included in the measurement of health expenditure has changed since 1985. Figure 17.1 describes total health care expenditure in current and fixed (1980) prices (see also Tables 17.A1–17.A3 in the Appendix).

First of all, the shifts in the expenditure trend that took place in 1985 and in 1992 can for the most part be explained by changes in the definition of health care according to the national accounts. In 1985, care for the mentally handicapped was excluded. In the national accounts, this expenditure is from then on allocated to education and social services. It is difficult to estimate the effect on the accounted health expenditure, but two different estimations in the national accounts concerning 1985 indicate that the effect may be some 5–6 per cent of total health expenditure. In 1992, care for the elderly at nursing homes was transferred to the social services of the munic-

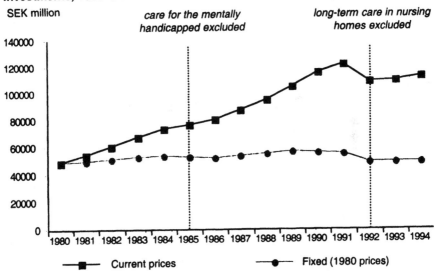

Figure 17.1 Total expenditure for health and medical care including investments, 1980–94

Source: National accounts. Price deflators from the Swedish Federation of County Councils (wage and price developments for the county councils), and from the Swedish Association of the Pharmaceutical Industry (Drug Price Index) have been used to calculate fixed expenditure.

Note: Total current expenditure includes: Private consumption (medicines, other pharmaceutical products, spectacles and other therapeutic appliances and equipment, services by doctors, etc.); general government final consumption; subsidies to doctors and dentists in private practices; subsidies to the pharmacies for drugs. The figures can be found in the Appendix, Tables 17.A1–17.A2.

ipalities (the ÄDEL reform). As a result, this cost was excluded from health care expenditure in the national accounts. According to the Ministry of Health and Social Affairs, the effect of the care-of-the-elderly reform has been estimated at SEK 20,000 million in 1991 prices, i.e. some 16 per cent of total health expenditure.[20]

As can be seen from Figure 17.1 there is an increasing trend in current expenditure for most of the 1980s, while fixed expenditure is more or less constant over the period. This gives a different picture of developments compared to the one given by the share-of-GDP measure. The difference is explained, first of all, by changes in the definition of health care, but also by changes in the total economy and in relative prices between health services

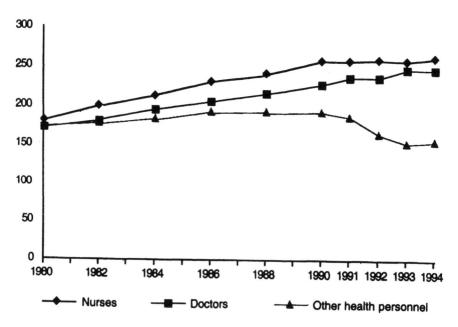

Figure 17.2 Development related to size and mix of health care personnel, 1980–94 (Index 1970 = 100)

Source: Anell & Persson, 1996, p. 15.[21]

Note: Health care personnel refers to the total number of doctors, nurses, nurse assistants, physiotherapists, etc. (excluding all administrative and technical services). Number of doctors and nurses refers to both private and public providers. The figures are reported in Appendix 17.A4.

Health Care Reforms and Cost Containment in Sweden 717

and other goods and services. As regards changes in the total economy, measured as GDP development, it can be concluded that total GDP and total health expenditure show similar development patterns over time; although total GDP has increased relatively more between 1980 and 1994 compared to total health expenditure (see Appendix, Table 17.A3). As regards changes in relative prices it has been shown that the development of the price of labour in the public health care sector has generally been relatively low compared to the private sector.[21]

Developments regarding health care personnel reveal that staff resources have increased during the 1980s, but in the 1990s developments have indeed differed between professional and non-professional groups. As can be noted in Figure 17.2 the number of doctors and nurses has more or less stabilized in recent years. When it comes to other (non-professional) types of medical personnel, however, there is a sharp drop beginning in 1991. This drop is not associated with the care-of-the-elderly reform in 1992, since personnel of nursing homes is included in Figure 17.2. As a result of the development, total employment within the Swedish health care sector has dropped.

To answer the question why current expenditure continues to increase while total employment is decreasing, it is necessary to distinguish between different activities and types of expenditure within the health care sector. Table 17.1 overleaf, gives a summary picture of current and fixed expenditure divided between in-patient care, out-patient care and pharmaceuticals. As can be seen, there has been a substantial drop in in-patient care, but on the other hand there has been an increase in out-patient care and pharmaceutical expenditure.

The changes illustrated in Table 17.1 can be explained, at least in part, by changes in medical technology; there has been a shift towards shorter periods of stay and more services performed in out-patient settings. As a result, the number of beds, bed-days and average length of stay in in-patient care has dropped substantially (see Appendix, Table 17.A5). Apparently, these shifts have been supported by new (and expensive) drugs; real pharmaceutical expenditure has in practice more than doubled during the last ten-year period (see Appendix, Table 17.A2). Several reforms have also contributed to this shift when it comes to the structure of services, and also to the marked increase in efficiency of the hospital sector that has taken place in the 1990s.

A few other development trends associated with health expenditure

718 *Health Care and Cost Containment in the European Union*

Table 17.1 Health care expenditure 1980, 1991, 1993, fixed (1991) prices

	1980		1991		1993	
	SEK million	%	SEK million	%	SEK million	%
In-patient care	59,971	68.6	65,550	62.8	45,150	47.8
Out-patient care	20,694	23.7	28,052	26.8	36,362	38.5
Pharmaceuticals	6,718	7.7	10,841	10.4	12,972	13.7
Total	87,383	100.0	104,443	100.0	94,484	100.0

Sources: The National Board of Health and Welfare (1996),[22] and estimates compiled at IHE (for 1993).

Note: Expenditure for in-patient care in 1993 does not include nursing home activities, which were transferred to the municipalities as part of the care-of-the-elderly (ÄDEL) reform. The expenditure for these services has been estimated at SEK 20,000 million. The 'Drugs' heading includes subsidies to the pharmacies for prescribed drugs and private consumption according to National accounts. Drugs for in-patient care are included in In-patient care.

may be noted. It is obvious that, especially in the 1990s, private consumption has increased substantially while general government consumption has followed a much slower rate of increase, well below the relative increase in total GDP (see Appendix, Table 17.A3). The increase in private consumption can first of all be explained by a large increase in co-payments for doctor services, and secondly by an increase in co-payments for drugs. This development is particularly significant in the 1990s, implying a relative shift in the financing of health services. While the general government consumption increase is low, subsidies for prescribed drugs and, to a lesser extent, for doctors and dentists in private practices, have increased substantially.

17.6 Discussion

There are many problems associated with the task of evaluating reform and its impact on the development of health care expenditure. To start with, it

Health Care Reforms and Cost Containment in Sweden   719

can be concluded that evaluation of reforms, or even continuous measurement of health-sector performance, has not been accorded high priority.[15] Another important problem is the abundance of parallel changes. For example, the general economic recession in Sweden has put pressure on the health sector as regards controlling expenditure, and the rapid progress in medical technology has resulted in a steady development towards shorter periods of hospitalization and more health services being provided in out-patient settings. Given these parallel changes, it is difficult to isolate the effects of individual reforms. Further, there are great variations between the county councils, since many reforms have been initiated at the county level. The variation among the 26 county councils makes it difficult to associate reforms with aggregate data on health expenditure. Ideally, evaluations should be made at lower levels of aggregation.

It is obvious that cost containment has been considered an important issue on both the national and the county political agendas, particularly during the 1980s and in recent years. Regarding developments in the 1980s, there is a link between the implementation of global budgets and the slower rate of expansion when it comes to staffing and expenditure, compared to the 1970s and 1960s. Several reforms introduced in the early 1990s, focusing on the need to raise overall sector efficiency have had important implications, but general cut-back programmes and political decisions to downscale the hospital sector have had a more direct effect on cost containment than the reforms introduced. However, one can argue that reforms towards planned markets, and more specifically the increase in productivity that followed these reforms, made implementation of cost-cutting decisions more easy.

Although substantial savings have been realized within the hospital sector in recent years, there is no downward trend in total health care expenditure. There is a clear upward trend in out-patient and pharmaceutical expenditure. With this development, and bearing the rather poor financial position of the county councils in mind, cost containment is likely to remain a high priority in the years to come. Total employment in the hospital sector is expected to drop further, and expenditure for prescribed drugs will probably be scrutinized carefully when county councils, starting from 1998, become responsible for them.

720 *Health Care and Cost Containment in the European Union*

17.6.1 Current and future developments

Regarding the future, there seems to be an agreement among the majority of the political parties to stay with the county council model. The Conservatives, being the second largest party in Sweden after the Social Democrats, are the most important exception. The Conservatives have put forward a proposal to abandon the traditional county council based model, and instead introduce a national, compulsory health care insurance system.

The transfer of financial responsibility for pharmaceuticals in out-patient care from the National Social Insurance Board to the county councils fits well with the long-term trend to decentralize responsibility to the county level. There are also, however, tendencies towards centralization. In part these tendencies can be explained by the urgent need for additional savings. In the forthcoming years, ambitions to merge several county councils (or districts within county councils) into larger units, and continuing efforts to reorganize and down-scale the hospital sector will be important activities. As in several other countries, the capacity of beds and duplication of services in nearby hospitals are discussed along with the appropriate number of hospitals with full emergency services. In recent years some small hospitals have been closed for emergency care. Some of these hospitals have been further specialized, e.g. into centres for day-care surgery or nursing homes.

In parallel to structural changes and down-scaling of in-patient hospital services, the widening gap between future health care needs and available resources, as well as the importance of priority setting, are being discussed. A final report from the government committee on priority setting was presented in early 1995.[23] The importance and final outcome of this report is, however, uncertain. First, its conclusions and policy implication have been criticized for being vague.[24,25] Second, any decision eventually taken by the Parliament is likely to be in the form of a recommendation to the 26 county councils. It will thereafter be up to each individual county council to determine their own future policy. No doubt, decisions on how to set priorities will have to be made; increases in waiting times for diagnosis and treatment have been noted in recent years throughout the country.

In parallel to cost containment activities in the public sector, the small private sector, with insurance companies offering individuals complementary insurance, will probably continue to expand. Already, there has been a significant shift in the overall mix of private and public financing during the

Health Care Reforms and Cost Containment in Sweden   721

1990s, although this change can for the most part be attributed to an increase in user charges. In 1994, 83 per cent of total financing came from public sources. This was higher than the OECD average (74 per cent) but lower compared to figures in Sweden from the mid-1970s to the early 1990s, during which about 90 per cent of total health care financing came from public sources.

Between 1991 and 1995, the number of health care personnel dropped by more than 40,000 (see Appendix 17.A4); most of those lost were assistant nurses working in hospitals. Employment is expected to drop further, although not as dramatically as in recent years. This is in spite of government promises of extra grants to both county councils and municipalities. Thus, structural change, not least affecting hospitals, and priority setting between different activities, are likely to remain highly important issues on the political agenda. At the same time the importance of planned markets and freedom of choice for patients is being played down, at least for the time being.

References

1   Lindgren B. Health care in Sweden. In: Alban A, Christiansen T (eds). *The Nordic Light: New Initiatives in Health Care Systems.* Odense University Press, 1995.

2   Heidenheimer AJ, Elvander N (eds). *The Shaping of the Swedish Health System.* London: Croom Helm Ltd, 1980.

3   Anell A. *Från central planering till lokalt ansvar* (From Central Planning to Local Responsibility). Lund: Lund University Press, 1990.

4   SOU. *Hälso- och Sjukvård inför 90-talet (HS 90)* (Health Care Services in the 1990s). Stockholm: Liber, 1984:39.

5   Arvidsson G, Jönsson B. *Valfrihet och Konkurrens i Sjukvården* (Freedom of Choice and Competition in Health Care). Stockholm: SNS Förlag, 1991.

6   Anell A, Rosén P, Svarvar P. *Health Care Reforms in Sweden. Striving Towards Equity, Efficiency and Cost Containment.* IHE Working Paper 1996:8, Lund, 1996.

7   Anell A, Svarvar P. *Landstingens Förnyelse av Organisation och Styrsystem–Är Strategierna Samordnade?* (County Council Reforms–Are strategies Co-ordinated?). IHE Working Paper 1994:8, Lund, 1994.

8   Anell A, Svarvar P. Reforms in the Swedish health care sector – survey and analysis. In: Alban A, Christiansen T (eds). *The Nordic Light: New Initiatives in Health Care Systems.* Odense University Press, 1995.

722 Health Care and Cost Containment in the European Union

9 Lyttkens C-H, Borgquist L. Organizational change in the Swedish health care sector. In: Alban A, Christiansen T (eds). *The Nordic Light: New Initiatives in Health Care Systems*. Odense University Press, 1995.

10 The Federation of County Councils. *Förbundsstyrelsens Beslut A 96:74* (Decision A 96:74 by the Federation of County Councils). Stockholm, 1996.

11 Anell A. The monopolistic integrated model and health care reform: the Swedish experience. *Health Policy* 1996;37:19-33.

12 The Federation of County Councils. *Landstingens Ekonomi: April 95*. (Financial Statements of the County Councils: April 1995). Stockholm, 1995.

13 Hanning M. Maximum waiting-time guarantee – an attempt to reduce waiting lists in Sweden. *Health Policy* 1996;36:17-35.

14 Svensson H, Nordling S. Effekter av nya styrformer i sjukvården–en litteraturöversikt. In: The National Board of Health and Welfare, *Den Planerade Marknaden–Om nya Styrformer i Hälso- och Sjukvården* (Effects of Health Care Reforms – A Survey of the Literature). Stockholm, 1995.

15 Lindgren B. Health care organisation and finance in Sweden – current issues and developments. In: Alban A, Christiansen T (eds). *The Nordic Light: New Initiatives in Health Care Systems*. Odense University Press, 1995.

16 Forsberg E, Calltorp J. *Nya Styrformer och Förändrat Medicinskt Handlande: Attityd- och Beteendeförändringar efter två år med Stockholmsmodellen.* (Health Care Reforms and Changes in Medical Activities). The Social Medicine Unit, R&D-report no. 6. Huddinge, 1994.

17 Diderichsen F. Market reforms in health care and sustainability of the welfare state: lessons from Sweden. *Health Policy* 1995;32:141-53.

18 Gerdtham U, Johannesson M, Jönsson B. Drug expenditures and new drug introductions. The Swedish experience. *PharmacoEconomics* 1993;4(3):215-25.

19 SOU. *Reform på Recept* (Reform of Prescriptions). Report by HSU 2000. Stockholm: Fritzes, 1995:122.

20 Government Bill (1990/91:150) *Kompletteringsproposition för Budgetåret 1991/92 mm* (Complementing Government Bill for 1991/92). Stockholm: Allmänna Förlaget.

21 Anell A, Persson M. *Personalresurser i Svensk sjukvård: Utvecklingslinjer och Internationell Jämförelse* (Personnel in Swedish Health Care: Development and International Comparison) IHE Working paper 1996:9. Lund, 1996.

22 The National Board of Health and Welfare. *Vad Kostar Sjukdomarna? Sjukvårdskostnader och Produktionsbortfall Fördelat på Sjukdomsgrupper 1980 och 1991* (Cost of Illnesses in Sweden 1980 and 1991). Stockholm: The National Board of Health and Welfare, 1996.

23 SOU. *Vårdens Svåra Val: Slutbetänkande av Prioriteringsutredningen* (Difficult Choices in Health Care: Final Report from the Committee on Setting Priorities). Stockholm: Allmänna Förlaget, 1995:5.

24 Lyttkens C-H. Prioritering i etik och praktik: en hälsoekonomisk analys av Prioriteringsutredningen (A health economics perspective on priority setting according to the government Committee). *Ekonomisk Debatt* 1994;22(6):595-606.

Health Care Reforms and Cost Containment in Sweden   723

25 Williams A. Prioriteringsutredningen förvirrar. Tydligare definitioner och bättre fakta krävs (The report from the Committee on setting priorities leads to confusion. Need for clear definitions and facts). *Läkartidningen* 1996;93(39)3376–81.

26 OECD. *OECD Health Data 1996.* Paris: OECD, 1996.

724 *Health Care and Cost Containment in the European Union*

Appendix: Health expenditure, personnel, hospital indicators, 1980–94

Table 17.A1 Health expenditure, current prices (SEK million)

Year	1980	1982	1984
Private final consumption	3,716	5,144	6,272
– Medicines	912	1,231	1,447
– Other pharmaceutical products	493	601	727
– Spectacles and other therapeutic appliances & equipment	672	894	1,008
– Services by doctors and other health professionals	1,639	2,418	3,090
General government final consumption	38,270	46,564	56,688
Subsidies to the pharmacies for prescribed medicines	2,326	2,919	3,490
Subsidies to doctors and dentists in private practice	1,844	1,990	2,330
Total current expenditure for health and medical care	46,156	56,617	68,780
– Pharmaceutical expenditure*	3,619	4,526	5,359
Investments	3,355	4,377	5,432
Total current expenditure + investments	49,511	60,994	74,212
GDP (purchasers value)	531,054	636,015	797,333
Health expenditure as share of GDP	9.3%	9.6%	9.3%

* Pharmacy drug sales (retail prices, VAT excluded).

Source: National accounts (various years) and the National Corporation of Swedish Pharmacies: Svensk läkemedelsstatistik 95 (drug consumption).

1986	1988	1990	1991	1992	1993	1994
7,894	9,697	11,488	13,841	15,746	17,601	18,895
1,772	2,300	2,704	3,067	3,658	4,298	4,554
889	929	1,043	1,136	1,116	1,158	1,212
1,240	1,552	1,818	1,958	1,860	1,972	1,714
3,993	4,916	5,923	7,680	9,112	10,173	11,415
60,619	71,163	88,553	90,594	74,845	73,820	73,157
4,199	4,449	6,862	7,774	8,764	9,517	11,034
2,780	3,599	4,432	4,996	4,956	4,634	5,085
75,492	88,908	111,335	117,205	104,311	105,572	108,383
6,333	8,194	10,051	11,313	12,910	14,079	15,658
5,544	6,107	5,167	5,075	4,631	4,400	4,600
81,036	95,015	116,502	122,280	108,942	109,972	112,983
947,263	1,114,502	1,359,879	1,447,327	1,441,723	1,446,212	1,524,767
8.6%	8.5%	8.6%	8.4%	7.6%	7.6%	7.4%

726 *Health Care and Cost Containment in the European Union*

Table 17.A2 Health expenditure, at constant 1980 prices (SEK million), 1980–94

Year	1980	1982	1984
Private final consumption	3,716	4,341	4,636
– Medicines	912	1,031	1,112
– Other pharmaceutical products	493	503	559
– Spectacles and other therapeutic appliances & equipment	672	758	729
– Services by doctors and other health professionals	1,639	2,049	2,236
General government final consumption	38,270	39,461	41,019
Subsidies to the pharmacies for prescribed medicines	2,326	2,445	2,683
Subsidies to doctors and dentists in private practice	1,844	1,686	1,686
Total current expenditure for health and medical care	46,156	47,933	50,024
– Drug expenditure	3,619	3,790	4,119
Investments	3,355	3,709	3,931
Total current expenditure + investments	49,511	51,643	53,954

Price deflators from the Swedish Federation of County Councils (wage and price trends in the county councils), and from the Swedish Association of the Pharmaceutical Industry (drug price index) have been used to calculate fixed expenditure.

1986	1988	1990	1991	1992	1993	1994
5,230	5,879	5,977	6,815	7,596	8,501	8,877
1,258	1,549	1,711	1,882	2,232	2,658	2,790
631	626	660	697	681	716	743
792	889	847	861	794	832	698
2,550	2,816	2,759	3,376	3,889	4,294	4,646
38,709	40,758	41,245	39,822	31,944	31,161	29,775
2,980	2,996	4,343	4,769	5,347	5,886	6,761
1,775	2,061	2,064	2,196	2,115	1,956	2,070
48,695	51,694	53,629	53,602	47,002	47,503	47,482
4,495	5,518	6,361	6,940	7,876	8,706	9,594
3,540	3,498	2,407	2,231	1,977	1,857	1,872
52,235	55,192	56,036	55,833	48,979	49,361	49,354

728   *Health Care and Cost Containment in the European Union*

Table 17.A3 Health expenditure, 1980 current prices index, 1980–94

Year	1980	1982	1984
Private final consumption	100	138	169
- Medicines	100	135	159
- Other pharmaceutical products	100	122	147
- Spectacles and other therapeutic appliances & equipment	100	133	150
- Services by doctors and other health professionals	100	148	189
General government final consumption	100	122	148
Subsidies to the pharmacies for prescribed medicines	100	125	150
Subsidies to doctors and dentists in private practice	100	108	126
Total current expenditure for health and medical care	100	123	149
- Drug expenditure	100	125	148
Investments	100	130	162
Total current expenditure + investments	100	123	150
GDP (purchasers value)	100	120	150
Health expenditure as share of GDP	100	103	100

1986	1988	1990	1991	1992	1993	1994
212	261	309	372	424	474	514
194	252	296	336	401	471	499
180	188	212	230	226	235	246
185	231	271	291	277	293	255
244	300	361	469	556	621	696
158	186	231	237	196	193	191
181	191	295	334	377	409	474
151	195	240	271	269	251	276
164	193	241	254	226	229	235
175	220	270	303	346	378	420
165	182	154	151	138	131	137
164	192	235	247	220	222	228
178	210	256	273	271	272	287
92	91	92	91	81	82	79

730   *Health Care and Cost Containment in the European Union*

Table 17.A4 Number of health care personnel*, 1980–94

Year	1980	1982	1984
Number of doctors	18,000	19,000	20,600
Number of nurses	62,478	69,181	73,743
Number of other health care personnel	178,727	181,273	188,069
Total	259,205	269,454	282,412

* Refers to the total number of doctors, nurses, nurse assistants, physiotherapists etc., including personnel at nursing homes for long-term care of the elderly, but excluding all administrative and technical services. The number of doctors and nurses refers to both private and public providers.

Sources: Landstingsförbundet, Kommunförbundet, SHSTF, Riksförsäkringsverket, Företagsläkarföreningen.

Table 17.A5 Hospital capacity and consumption indicators, 1980–94

Year	1980	1982	1984
Number of in-patient beds*	125,863	124,799	124,161
Number of acute in-patient beds**	42,285	40,677	39,566
Acute care: Average length of stay	8.5	8.2	7.8
Acute: occupancy rate–Used beds (%)	72.1	73.7	75.3
Hospital turnover rate–number of cases treated per bed and year***	12.9	14.0	14.2

*   Includes all health care beds within the definition of health care.
** Includes acute and non-acute hospital services at medical and surgical departments. Does not include hospital psychiatric and geriatric services.
*** Excludes psychiatric care.

Source: OECD Health Data 1996.[26]

1986	1988	1990	1991	1992	1993	1994
21,700	22,800	24,000	24,500	25,000	25,600	26,100
79,823	83,171	89,196	89,134	89,487	89,333	92,831
195,846	196,027	196,203	189,636	167,491	156,163	157,842
297,369	301,998	309,399	303,270	281,978	271,096	276,773

1986	1988	1990	1991	1992	1993	1994
118,714	112,094	106,484	102,152	66,045	61,258	57,159
37,773	36,323	35,403	33,943	31,737	29,659	27,871
7.3	6.9	6.5	6.2	5.8	5.5	5.3
74.2	75.3	72.2	73.0	74.8	76.2	77.4
14.8	16.2	17.1	18.4	29.0	32.0	37.0

18 Cost containment and health care reforms in the British NHS

GIOVANNI FATTORE

18.1 Introduction

In the United Kingdom, health services are primarily provided by the National Health Service (NHS), a state-owned and publicly-funded institution. Facilitated by the success of central government leadership in the hospital sector during the Second World War, the NHS was established in 1948 to make health services available to everyone free of charge and on the basis of need. Consequently, in the United Kingdom the responsibility for balancing the costs and revenues of running the NHS rests with the political system, and cost containment is an issue directly involving the funding and management of the NHS. In this chapter the nature and effectiveness of cost containment measures undertaken in the British NHS are investigated.

The next three sections present the essential features of the NHS, examine how its budget is set and briefly look at the historical trend in health care expenditure. In the two sections thereafter, the main measures undertaken to keep non-cash-limited expenditure under control are investigated. Various initiatives carried out on hospital and community care are then reviewed, and two sections concerning the relation between cost containment and the 1989 reforms follow. The chapter ends with a brief description of the private market for health services and medical insurance, a brief summary of the White Paper released in December 1997, and some concluding remarks.

18.2 The British NHS

In England, overall responsibility for the NHS rests with the Secretary of State for Health who heads the Department of Health (DoH). For many years the structure of the NHS was relatively stable, with only one impor-

734 *Health Care and Cost Containment in the European Union*

tant revision in 1974. In April 1996, however, the NHS structure and organization was substantially changed as Regional Health Authorities, the intermediate tier of the NHS, were abolished, and the traditional separation between hospital and community care and family services (mainly primary and family services) was overcome by merging District Health Authorities (DHAs) and Family Health Service Authorities (FHSAs) under the new Health Authorities (HAs). Consequently, since April 1996 the basic structure of the NHS comprises the DoH, the NHS Executive, which is the 'internal' agency of the DoH responsible for the management of the NHS, 100 health authorities in charge of purchasing care for UK citizens and about 430 NHS Trusts who are responsible for providing what purchasers require.

The basic principles of the NHS apply to the entire country. However, in Scotland, Wales and Northern Ireland the NHS is administered by the corresponding Secretaries of State and the organization and structure of the systems are little different.

The budget for the NHS is determined centrally through an annual process known as the Public Expenditure Survey (PES) and is then allocated within the NHS. Until 1995, resources were distributed from central government to FHSAs, DHAs and GP fundholders via the regions. However, since 1996/97, a single budget is now allocated to health authorities by the NHS Executive.

In the late 1980s major reforms reshaped the British welfare state. In few years legislation radically changed the funding and organization of education, health services, social services and housing programmes. Le Grand wrote in 1991 that 'if these reforms are carried through to their conclusion, the welfare state in the 1990s will be a very different animal from the welfare state of the previous 45 years'.[1] This has proven to be the case for health services.

Conceived between 1988 and 1989, incorporated in the NHS and Community Care Act of 1990, and introduced in 1991, the reforms of the NHS were based on three main principles.[2] First, the comprehensiveness, universality and equity of the NHS were preserved. Funding arrangements, criteria for entitlement to the NHS, criteria of access and the extent of coverage provided were not affected by the reforms.

Second, the responsibilities for purchasing and providing services were to be separated in order to create the conditions for competition between hospitals and other service providers. Large hospitals first, and almost all provider organizations later, were to become self-governing NHS trusts.

Cost Containment and Health Care Reforms in the British NHS 735

That meant opting out of health authority control and being freed from the main rules governing their activities. At the same time, each DHA became a purchaser and was allowed to shop around for services from both the private and public sectors. On the basis of set formulae, funds are distributed to purchasers who, in turn, give funds to providers according to contractual arrangements.

Finally, large GP practices were also allowed to become purchasers of some services for their patients. These practices receive a budget to cover the cost of prescribing and to buy a defined range of services including out-patient specialist visits, diagnostic tests, and some in-patient and day-care treatments.

18.3 Setting the limits for the NHS

The budgeting process is important in understanding cost containment in the NHS. While overspending the public budget for health care is quite common in Southern European countries, in the United Kingdom what is planned at central level generally corresponds to what is actually spent. There are several reasons why central control of public expenditure in general, and of public health care expenditure in particular, has been successful in the UK. Among these reasons, the role played by the budgeting process, better known as the Public Expenditure Survey (PES), or simply, the Survey, is crucial.

The PES has a long history and has been shaped by the encounter of two opposing forces: the search for providing a stable financial regime for public services in a long-term perspective (planning function), and the need to impose a fiscal discipline to spending departments (control function). The PES was created in the early 1960s and had two central features. First, the cabinet decided the total amount for public expenditure and, within that total, departments bid for funds. Second, the limits to spending were set out in real terms in the next four years.[3]

In the first half of the 1970s high inflation and recession made the PES inadequate, mainly because forecasting in such a situation was both difficult and politically expensive. As a consequence, public expenditure was not under control, and in 1976 the system was revised in order to strengthen the control function. This revision mainly consisted of introducing cash limits,

736   *Health Care and Cost Containment in the European Union*

that is, figures of actual spending that a department cannot overshoot. However, by imposing limits in terms of cash, rather than in real terms, budget decisions were made insensitive to the prices of goods and wages. Consequently, provision of public services was made dependent on inflation, meaning that unexpected inflation would mean a lower volume of services. During the 1980s the system was modified again, the aim being to make the control function stronger. It was then substantially revised in 1992.

The budgeting process is a yearly cycle, starting well before the beginning of the financial year. For the 1993 budget, the cycle began in March 1992, 13 months in advance (Table 18.1). It started with the Treasury issuing guidelines that departments had to follow in preparing their programmes and financial requests. In the light of these guidelines and the assumptions regarding economic development, departments submitted their bids to the Treasury. However, the process did not start from scratch because baseline figures for bids were included in the Survey of the previous year. In fact, the PES process planned expenditure for three years ahead (five in the 1970s). After discussions between the Treasury and the spending departments, bids were coordinated in a report which formed the basis for the Cabinet meeting at the end of July. In this meeting the level of total public expenditure

Table 18.1 The Public Expenditure Survey planning timetable, prior to 1993

Month	Event
March	Treasury issues guidelines
April	Baselines agreed
June	Bids submitted by departments
July	Cabinet decides overall Survey totals
September	Bilateral negotiations start
October	Star Chamber determines difficult cases and Cabinet decides on departmental totals
December	Departments submit estimates to Parliament and NHS budget is determined
March	Budget

Sources: Glennerster, 1992;[3] Liekerman, 1988.[4]

Cost Containment and Health Care Reforms in the British NHS 737

for the next three years was decided. In September a series of negotiations between spending departments and the Treasury took place to ensure that, if the total of all bids was higher than the total for public expenditure, they were to be reduced to maintain the total. As these negotiations sometimes failed to reach an agreement, pending cases were then passed to the 'Star Chamber', a special Cabinet committee of non-spending ministers or ministers who have already agreed their totals. Following these negotiations the Cabinet decided on departmental totals so as to outline the spending limits for the next financial year. It was at this stage that NHS finance officers would know how much they were likely to get. The budget finally came in March, and included proposals to change the taxes according to spending decisions.

In 1992 the PES system was substantially modified:

(a) taxation and spending decisions were unified;

(b) more stringent totals for the aggregate of public expenditure for each of the three Survey years were imposed;

(c) the Budget was moved back to December; and

(d) the Star Chamber was abolished and a new, larger and more powerful committee was created to oversee the entire Survey process: the Expenditure Committee of the Cabinet (EDX).

A full discussion of these changes is beyond the objectives of the chapter (for a detailed discussion see Thain and Wright, 1995[5]). However, it is worth mentioning that the control function was strengthened while, at the same time, decisions on the allocation of public spending were made more collectively (the establishment of EDX). Also, the 1992 revision made an important move towards more integration between taxation and spending decisions.

From the NHS perspective, a central feature of the PES is that it establishes cash limits to public funding. In particular, hospital and community expenditure, accounting for about 75 per cent of NHS expenditure, is subject to this constraint (although family services are demand-led). This means that for these services, 'volume' of care is dependent on the difference between the inflation estimates incorporated in the Budget and actual inflation. Therefore, if there is unexpected inflation, or if its value is explicitly underestimated by the Cabinet, it is likely that the level of services will be cut. Obviously, the contrary applies when predicted inflation exceeds

738   *Health Care and Cost Containment in the European Union*

actual inflation.

The role of inflation predictions is made even more important by the fact that 70 per cent of NHS expenditure is formed by labour costs. Not only does the success of trade unions in getting higher wages reduce the total amount of services made available, but the bargaining process itself is affected by the predictions reported in the Survey. Clearly, cash planning limits the scope of service planning. On the other hand, however, the advantage of cash planning from a control perspective is clear: accountability is much easier when it can be based on unquestioned numbers.

In health policy studies there is a natural tendency to investigate what lies within the health care system. The PES, however, is an important example of a political and administrative process that, from outside the health care system, determines the scope and nature of cost-containment measures undertaken within the NHS. The PES has been successful in controlling public expenditure and in putting financial resource allocation into political hands. Consequently, it has also provided the framework to keep NHS expenditure under control.

18.4 Trends in public expenditure

NHS expenditure in the UK has been under control in the sense that actual expenditure has been the result of planning and has been explicitly authorized at the political level. In this section, control over health expenditure is investigated from a different perspective, that is by comparing NHS expenditure with that of other countries.

As a proportion of the production of national wealth, as measured by the Gross Domestic Product (GDP), public health care expenditure grew from 4.1 per cent to 5.9 per cent between 1973 and 1993 (Table 18.2). The increase in the proportion of GDP publicly spent on health care in the UK (1.8 per cent) is quite similar both to those of the four largest European countries (1.8 per cent) and of the 15 EU Member States (1.7 per cent). Similarly to other European countries, the UK government has appreciably increased its commitment to funding health services. Nevertheless, three points are worth noting. First, during the 1980s the proportion of GDP publicly spent decreased; it was only after the launch of the 1989 reforms that expenditure was allowed to increase more rapidly. Meanwhile from 1983 to

Cost Containment and Health Care Reforms in the British NHS 739

Table 18.2 Health care expenditure trends in the United Kingdom, the larger four European Countries and the 15 European Union Member States, 1973–93

	1973	1983	1988	1993
Public health care expenditure as % of GDP				
United Kingdom	4.1	5.2	4.9	5.9
France, Germany, Italy and UK	4.8	5.8	5.9	6.6
15 EU Member States	4.3	5.6	5.6	6.0
Per capita public expenditure in PPPs (US$)				
United Kingdom	173	533	705	987
France, Germany, Italy and UK	209	646	888	1,180
15 EU Member States	172	572	778	1,066
Public health care expenditure as % of total expenditure				
United Kingdom	87.6	87.4	84.0	84.5
France, Germany, Italy and UK	75.9	79.4	78.4	76.0
15 EU Member States	81.8	79.3	77.6	76.7

Source: OECD Health Data, 1996.[6]

1988, the percentage of GDP spent on public health care went from 5.1 per cent to 4.9 per cent, and in the following five years it increased by 20 per cent (Table 18.2). Second, despite similarities in the trend, the UK started from a lower public expenditure in the early 1970s: public health care expenditure in the UK was lower than in the other large European countries (especially Germany and France) and the average of the 15 countries presently forming the EU. Last, the percentage of total health care expenditure publicly funded slipped from 87.6 per cent in 1973 to 84.5 per cent in 1993. Although the decrease is not very large, it indicates an increasing trend of private health care expenditure in the UK.

Looking at global expenditure data, the pattern shown in the 1973–93 period by the UK seems similar to those of the rest of the European Union: an appreciable expansion of public expenditure, backed by an even more rapid growth of private expenditure. Although the UK had a lower public

740 *Health Care and Cost Containment in the European Union*

health care expenditure 20 years ago, its long-term trend is similar to that of the rest of Europe. Nevertheless, in the last five years the growth rate of public expenditure has accelerated. Whether this acceleration is attributable to the 1989 reforms is still unclear. However, there are elements that suggest that this might be the case.

The pay bill has always been the single largest component of the NHS budget. Salaries and wages amounted to £18 billion in 1994 and accounted for about 69 per cent of revenue expenditure of Health Authorities and NHS Trusts.[7] This percentage was significantly higher during the 1980s (around 75 per cent). In fact, after the reforms the pace of growth of personnel expenditure was lower than that of the overall NHS revenue expenditure: during the period 1992–94 the former increased by 18 per cent, the latter by 23 per cent. The lower growth of personnel expenditure is due to three main factors. First, the reforms have modified the accounting system introducing new expenditure items (i.e. capital charges). Consequently, the lower expenditure rate for personnel is partly a matter of changes in accounting procedures and exaggerates a real change in the composition of NHS expenditure. Second, the number of employed staff decreased from 795,000 to 762,000, mainly because of a 10 per cent reduction in nursing and midwifery staff.[8] Third, in the period 1992–94 the NHS enjoyed a very low labour inflation rate: pay rises were 1.5 per cent in 1993 and 3 per cent in 1994.

18.5 Cost-sharing and exemptions

Out-of-pocket payments for some services provided by the NHS have long been a focus of political concern. Currently, NHS patients are charged for drugs, dental care and ophthalmic services.

For forty years, free testing of sight and the supply of spectacles were provided to the general population by the NHS, albeit with substantial cost-sharing. Since April 1989, access to these services has been restricted to children and full-time students, low-income individuals, registered blind and people suffering from specific eye diseases. These individuals, accounting for about 40 per cent of the UK population, are effectively provided with a voucher which can be spent in the private market and whose value varies annually and from one category of spectacles or lens to another.[7] Individuals who do not qualify for these exemptions are required to pay the full cost of

Cost Containment and Health Care Reforms in the British NHS   741

services.

Dental care has always been part of the benefits package provided by the NHS. However, co-payment for dental services has been significant since 1952, ranging from 20 per cent (during the 1950s and the 1960s) to almost 40 per cent (late 1980s) of total NHS dental costs. Until April 1988, patients were required to pay a flat rate per course of treatment. Since then, cost-sharing has been determined as a percentage of treatment cost up to a maximum amount per course of treatment (80 per cent of treatment cost, up to a ceiling of £325 in 1997).

In 1952, patient charges for pharmaceuticals were also introduced. Since then, with the exception of the 1965–68 period, a flat-rate charge has been paid to the pharmacist by the (non-exempt) patients when medicines are dispensed. The charge is set centrally in accordance with the government's financial targets for the funding of the NHS. Revenue raised from these charges does not accrue as government revenue, but is treated as a non-governmental source of NHS funds, and hence substitutes for government expenditure on the NHS.[9] From 1952 to 1956 the flat rate was applied to the prescription form, so that there was an incentive to increase the number of items per prescription. Since 1956 a charge has been made on each prescription item.

Particular population groups are exempt from paying prescription charges. Women over 60, men over 65, children under 16, or under 19 and still in full-time education, are automatically exempt. They are just required to sign the back of the prescription form before presenting it to the pharmacist. Other exempt population groups are: low-income individuals, expectant mothers, mothers who have had a child in the last 12 months, war/service pensioners (for prescriptions related to their accepted disablement), and people suffering from specified conditions such as diabetes, myasthenia and epilepsy. Procedures for getting exemption status vary in complexity. For example, those who receive means-tested state benefits receive exemption certificates automatically, but some other groups require the claiming person to go through an administrative procedure.

Since 1968, exemption from charges can also be purchased as a prepayment certificate, a seasonal ticket covering all prescriptions for a period of 6 months (4 months from 1980) or a year. In addition to specific population groups being exempt, contraceptive drugs and a few specific medical appliances are completely free for all UK residents.

From 1971 to 1979 the charge remained at a constant level of 20 pence.

742　*Health Care and Cost Containment in the European Union*

Since then, it has been increased sharply, and by April 1997 stood at £5.65. In real terms, the NHS charge is now almost eight times as high as at the start of 1979 (Table 18.3). However, the exemption regulation is such that more than 50 per cent of the population is exempt from paying and 87 per cent of total pharmaceutical expenditure is on non-chargeable prescriptions.

Table 18.3 Number of prescriptions dispensed by pharmacists and appliance contractors, charges and total cost of NHS prescriptions in England, 1979–86

Year	Number of prescriptions	Charge per item (1979 prices)		Total cost of NHS prescriptions (1979 prices)	
	million	£		£ billion	
1979	304.6	0.45	(0.45)	739	(739)
1980	303.3	0.70	(0.72)	898	(917)
1981	299.9	1.00	(1.03)	1,026	(1,057)
1982	311.3	1.30	(1.32)	1,281	(1,297)
1983	315.3	1.40	(1.37)	1,308	(1,277)
1984	320.5	1.60	(1.53)	1,409	(1,349)
1985	318.7	2.00	(1.84)	1,518	(1,397)
1986	322.6	2.20	(1.95)	1,643	(1,454)
1987	335.3	2.40	(2.03)	1,831	(1,548)
1988	346.5	2.60	(2.10)	2,046	(1,649)
1989	351.9	2.80	(2.21)	2,198	(1,732)
1990	360.5	3.05	(2.39)	2,402	(1,882)
1991	370.7	3.40	(2.72)	2,689	(2,152)
1992	386.7	3.75	(3.02)	2,995	(2,410)
1993	405.1	4.25	(3.35)	3,283	(2,585)
1994	414.1	4.75	(3.60)	3,404	(2,578)
1995	430.6	5.25	(3.88)	3,680	(2,719)
1996		5.50			

Notes: Values in parenthesis are expressed in 1979 prices and deflated by the implicit GDP deflator, at factor costs.

Source: Chew 1995,[7] Annual Abstract of Statistics (various years)[10] and Health and Personal Social Services Statistics in England and Wales, 1996.[8]

Cost Containment and Health Care Reforms in the British NHS 743

18.6 The impact of cost-sharing on utilization

There are five published studies on patient charges and the utilization of medicines in the British NHS (Table 18.4). All of them are time-series regressions, based on observational or self-reported data. The two most extensive studies are those by O'Brien[11] which covers the period from 1969 to 1986, and Hughes and McGuire with data from 1969 to 1992.[14]

Table 18.4 UK studies on patient charges and the utilization of NHS prescription medicines

Author(s)	Years	Place	Results
Lavers (1989)[12]	1971–82 monthly	England and Wales	Charge-volume elasticity between -0.15 and -0.2
Ryan and Birch (1991)[9]	1979–85 monthly	England	Per capita charge-volume elasticity: -0.11 in the short run -0.09 in the long run;
O'Brien (1989)[11]	1969–86 monthly	England	Charge-volume elasticity: -0.33 (1969–86) -0.23 (1969–77) -0.64(1977–86) Cross-price elasticity (OTC products): +0.22 (1969–86) +0.17(1969–77)
Smith and Watson (1990)[13]	1979–84 household data (UK Family Expenditure Survey)	United Kingdom	Charge-volume elasticity: -0.5 (1979–84)
Hughes and McGuire (1995)[14]	1969–82 annual data	England?	Charge-volume elasticity: -0.32–0.37 (1969–82) -0.125 (1969) -0.22 (1980) -0.68 (1985) -0.94 (1991)

744 *Health Care and Cost Containment in the European Union*

Based on monthly English data, O'Brien investigated the relationship between cost-sharing and utilization by means of a two-stage time series regression model. The dependent variables of the two models were the number of items dispensed with and without charge. Independent variables included: charge, income, substitute products, age, population structure, claims for sickness and invalidity benefits, and some dummy variables to take into account seasonal effects and change of legislation. The main finding was that increases in the real value of the prescription charge are associated with a reduction in the consumption of chargeable drugs. The charge-volume elasticity for the entire period (1969–86) was -0.33: that is, a 10 per cent increase in the real charge (the nominal charge adjusted for inflation) resulted in a 3.3 per cent decrease in utilization. According to sub-period estimates, the charge-volume elasticity is not stable over time and was greater for the 1977–86 period. Two other results of this study are worth mentioning: the lack of association between consumption of chargeable drugs and personal disposable income, and the value of +0.22 for over-the-counter (OTC) price elasticity, meaning that a 10 per cent increase in OTC prices results in a 2.2 per cent increase in consumption of prescribed drugs among people subject to co-payment.

Hughes and McGuire[14] re-assessed these results, introducing two major changes in the econometric model: annual data rather than monthly data, since charges are generally modified only once at the beginning of the fiscal year, and the adoption of a cointegration procedure to test and take account of stationarity of data. Despite these differences, the study found a charge-volume elasticity of -0.37 in the long run and -0.32 in the short run – values that are very similar to O'Brien's estimate.

Aggregated data covering shorter periods of time were analysed in two other studies. Using a three equation model and data from England and Wales for the period 1971–82, Lavers estimated that a 10 per cent increase in charges results in a reduction of consumption ranging between 1.5 per cent and 2 per cent.[12] Results of the second study show a lower elasticity. Both short-term and long-term per capita charge-volume elasticities are estimated at approximately -0.1.[9] Finally, the only study based on household data (the UK Family Expenditure Survey) estimated a much higher elasticity (-0.5) for the period 1979–84.[13]

From a qualitative perspective, the results of these empirical studies are clear-cut, namely, higher charges are associated with a decrease in the consumption of drugs. Similar results come from observational, quasi-experi-

Cost Containment and Health Care Reforms in the British NHS 745

mental and experimental studies performed in North America.[15,16] The British studies are also relatively clear-cut in suggesting that the demand for drugs is relatively inelastic, which implies that charge increases do not greatly affect drug consumption. Given the above-mentioned study, the best estimate of charge-volume elasticity may be around -0.3, meaning that a charge increase from £5.00 to £5.50 lowers the number of prescription items among patients subject to co-payment by 3 per cent.

The sole stated objective of using cost-sharing in the NHS is that it generates additional funds. If all prescriptions dispensed by the NHS were subject to co-payment, additional revenues would probably exceed £1 billion per year. However, the actual revenue is about £380 million, that is, approximately 13 per cent of the total cost of pharmaceutical services in England. The effectiveness of cost-sharing as a cost containment device is thus very limited. The high number of exempted people confines co-payment to a relatively small number of prescriptions. In fact, 33 million people, generating 87 per cent of total pharmaceutical expenditure, are not subject to any form of co-payment on pharmaceuticals.

The evidence reported here suggests that co-payment also moderates consumption and thus, generates additional savings to the drug bill. However, similarly to that discussed above, the fact that only a modest percentage of patients and prescribing decisions are made sensitive to price, limits its impact on the overall consumption of pharmaceuticals.

Although measuring the financial impact of co-payment on pharmaceuticals is very relevant from the health policy perspective, it should be noted that very little is known on how and why consumption of drugs is reduced by higher charges. O'Brien suggests three possible reasons behind this relationship:[11]

1. higher charges deter the marginal patient from getting his/her prescription dispensed at a chemist (i. e. reduce compliance);

2. they induce a reduction in the number of prescriptions written by GPs; and

3. they deter the marginal patient from consulting his/her GP.

Unfortunately, there is a lack of evidence to test these hypotheses. From a health policy perspective, the first possible explanation should raise some concern. If charge increases reduced compliance, it would imply that charges undermine the doctor–patient relationship and, consequently, they

746 *Health Care and Cost Containment in the European Union*

may be associated with a decrease in health status. On the contrary, the second possible explanation is relatively more reassuring: patient charges would make GPs more sensitive to the prices of pharmaceuticals and thus promote cost-effective prescribing. The third possible explanation is more ambiguous. On the one hand, opting for OTC treatments instead of visiting the doctor may be an efficient way to face minor illnesses. On the other, if people in need of care are deterred from seeing their doctor because of financial disincentives, charges on pharmaceuticals may represent a pernicious barrier to primary care.

Whatever the reason behind the charge–volume relationship, the relevant health policy question is the association between charges and outcome. That is, whether charging patients for prescriptions affects health status. There is very limited evidence from the United States that this may be the case,[17] and there are no empirical studies investigating this aspect in the UK or in other publicly-dominated health care systems. Therefore, this question remains unanswered and the need for empirical evidence is urgent, especially if European governments will keep on relying on user charges on pharmaceuticals and other services as a mechanism of rationing.

18.7 Other cost containment measures in the pharmaceutical sector

Levying patient charges was not the only measure undertaken by the British government to contain public pharmaceutical expenditure. At least three other sets of policies have played a relevant role in the last decade: the Pharmaceutical Price Regulation Scheme (PPRS), the delisting of products from NHS coverage, and the introduction of drug budgets.

In the UK, the government regulates the profitability of pharmaceutical companies, rather than prices of their products. Since 1957, profits generated by products sold to the NHS have been subject to negotiation between companies and the DoH through the PPRS. The new agreement for the period 1993–98 established that the return on capital deriving from sales to the NHS cannot exceed a ceiling that ranges from between 17 and 21 per cent, depending on the company's investments in research and its contribution to the UK economy. The new agreement also included direct regulation of prices of already marketed branded products for four years: a 2.5 per cent reduction in the first year followed by a three-year freeze.

Although some products have always been unavailable under the NHS, it was only in 1985 that the Government produced a negative list of 600 products. The list was extended in 1993. At present products as such as analgesics for mild to moderate pain, antiacids, benzodiazepines, remedies for coughs and colds, vitamins and appetite suppressants cannot be prescribed by GPs on NHS forms and are sold at full price. The aim of the negative list is to shift to the consumer the full cost of the drugs and, to a lesser extent, to curb consumption of drugs whose effectiveness is questionable. Accordingly, the Government assumed that delisting would have automatically reduced the NHS drug bill by the amount of the previous annual expenditure for the delisted products. However, it has been argued that this estimate was exaggerated because delisting may shift prescribing into other, probably more expensive, NHS-reimbursable drugs.[18] In fact, Reilly et al. found this 'shifting' effect from antiacids (delisted) to H2-antagonists (covered by the NHS).[19] Nevertheless, these results were not confirmed in other therapeutic areas and other empirical studies suggest that the introduction of the negative list did reduce the number of items prescribed by GPs. Using a time-series regression model O'Brien estimated that the introduction of the negative list in 1985 was associated with a reduction of 260,000 scripts a month.[11] Using a similar data-set, Ryan and Birch contended that the impact of delisting is greater: a 1.4 per cent reduction, that is a reduction of 300,000 items per month.[9]

Delisting can also be made in a different way: by declassifying drugs from the ethical status (prescription required) to the OTC (prescription not required, no limitation on dispensing) or the Pharmacy Only (prescription non required, but dispensing limited to pharmacies) status. This kind of delisting is actively used in the UK. As in the case of the negative list, it is expected to produce savings to the NHS drug bill. It should be noted, however, that enlarging the class of products for which a prescription is not required may have wider effects as it encourages more self-medication and less frequent GP visits.

Standard economic theory predicts that GPs will over-prescribe. As the cost of prescribing for both GPs and patients is almost zero, they do not have any incentive to curb prescribing when the cost-benefit balance of therapies is favourable from the patient's perspective (perhaps only marginally), but unfavourable from a societal perspective. Co-payment can alleviate this problem. However, although the co-payment may introduce an incentive on the patient side, it clearly affects solidarity and reduces the patient's financial risk protection. At least in theory, it is preferable to reduce over-pre-

748 *Health Care and Cost Containment in the European Union*

scribing with supply-side measures that respect decentralization of the decision-making process. In other words, to make GPs more sensitive to economic issues seems to be a better option than using incentives on the patients' side. This is the economic rationale of the Indicative Prescribing Scheme (IPS) and of GP fund-holding (for the latter scheme see below). The IPS (renamed Target Budgets in 1994) provides each GP practice with expected targets against which actual prescribing costs are compared. Targets are set by Health Authorities and, until 1992/93, were based primarily on each practice's historic spending. Since then, various attempts have been made to include list size and patients' characteristics (mainly age and sex) in the formula to calculate the Target Budget. Also, the Prescribing Analysis and CosT (PACT) information system supporting the scheme was significantly improved: lag-time for feedbacks has been reduced, effectiveness of communication has been improved, and prescribing data has been made available to the FHSAs and GPs in electronic format.

The Target Budget exercises no incentive for GPs. Neither doctors nor patients benefit from savings on the drug bill. Indeed, savings are not ring-fenced and thus do not automatically increase other components of the health care budget. In view of this situation it is unlikely that the scheme has introduced new structural incentives affecting GP prescribing behaviour. However, targets may have stimulated GP awareness on cost issues and, consequently, may have worked as an educational device. It is likely that psychological pressure on GPs to curb costs has modified prescribing patterns mainly in situations which do not involve a trade-off between costs and expected benefits, as in the case of generic substitution of branded (generally more expensive) products.

Several other measures, although not exclusively targeted to curb costs, are worth mentioning: dissemination of 'independent' information on drugs (NHS advisers on drugs, the publication of a series of *Effective Health Care Bulletins*), support to practices trying to establish formularies, and promotion of continuing education activities on rational prescribing. Some of these measures are discussed later.

18.8 Hospital services

As in many other European countries, NHS hospital services have changed dramatically in the last 20 years. Including psychiatric institutions, 1,970 hospitals were operating in Great Britain (England, Wales and Scotland) in 1993, almost 800 less than in 1975.[7] As shown in Figure 18.1, the declining number of hospitals has been accompanied by a reduction in the total number of beds: from 500,000 in 1975 to 285,000 in 1995. A substantial reduction in the number of beds occurred in the vast majority of the specialties, probably as a result of more intensive courses of treatment and the development of day-hospital and day-surgery. However, a relevant part of the decline in hospital capacity is attributable to the reduction in the number of psychiatric beds. In England, for example, between 1984 and 1994, the number of available psychiatric beds decreased by about 55 per cent, while the number of available beds in general and acute specialties decreased by only 25 per cent.

The decreasing number of hospitals and beds have not been followed by a reduction in NHS hospital staff who, in the same period, increased from 870,000 to 970,000 employees. In fact, the increasing trend in the use of resources for hospital care is evident when observing expenditure data. In 1995, hospital expenditure amounted to £22 billion, almost seven times the 1975 figure. In real terms, the average rate of increase has been 2.3 per cent per year in the 1975–95 period, with a substantially higher rate in the last five years (4.1 per cent). However, this component of NHS expenditure has increased at a lower rate than others, so that in 1995 it accounted for 54 per

Figure 18.1 NHS hospital services: expenditure, beds and employees, 1975–95

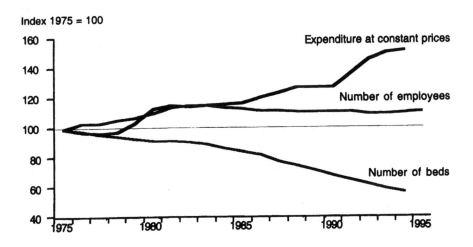

750 *Health Care and Cost Containment in the European Union*

cent of the total expenditure, 8 per cent less than in 1975.

Although the long-term trend indicates that hospital care is increasing at lower rates than those of the overall health care expenditure, latest data suggest that the situation is changing. The hospital expenditure growth rate of the last five years was higher than in the past and, as a proportion of total health care, has been stabilized above 50 per cent. It seems reasonable to assume that hospital care will continue to absorb most of health care resources.

Measuring hospital output is a very difficult task. In the US and in some European countries the Diagnosis Related Groups (DRGs) system is widely used. In the UK the main system used to measure hospital output is the Finished Consultant Episode (FCE), that is a complete period of hospital care under one consultant. Compared with DRGs, FCEs are easier to manage, but they do not differentiate according to the amount of resources expected to be needed in providing care (appendicitis and organ transplant have the same weight).

Despite these limitations and the fact that FCEs have been calculated only since 1987, it seems clear that there is an increasing trend in hospital output. The number of discharges and deaths (the traditional system to measure hospital output) increased by more than 50 per cent from 6.2 million in 1975 to 9.5 million in 1992 (Figure 18.2). This figure also reports the number of surgical and medical acute FCEs. A divergent pattern is clear. While surgical episodes have been almost constant in the last five years, medical episodes escalated from 2.3 million in 1987 to 3.2 million in 1992.

The number of out-patient attendances to clinics and accident and emergency departments shows a slightly increasing trend: from 56 million in 1975 to 63 million in 1992. Available figures on day-hospital cases indicate a rapid increase in the number of day cases: from about 1 million in 1989 to 1.5 million in 1992.

As hospital expenditure is cash limited, hospitals have never been a specific target for national cost containment measures. Specific measures were undertaken at a decentralized level, under the pressure of fixed budgets and varied from one hospital to another.

As in the rest of Europe, in the last 20 years hospitals have remained the centre of the health care system, although the rate of increase of hospital expenditure has been lower than that of the rest of the health care system. Advances in health care technology and information technology have modified and will continue to modify the nature of hospitals. Compared with 20 years ago, hospitals now use more sophisticated technologies, a larger amount of resources per unit of time and tend to focus on sicker patients. In addition, technological advancement in curative medicine directly (because it allows the treatment of 'new' patients) and indirectly (because improving survival makes it more likely that patients receive more care) increases demand for health services.

Given this scenario, whether hospital costs were contained and, if they were, at what 'price', are very challenging questions. Probably, the decreasing number of beds, mainly reflecting the reduction in the length of stay per admission, is just the result of technological change, rather than a sign that the efficiency of using existing resources has been significantly improved. However, the closure of many hospitals in recent years should have allowed the reduction of some types of costs and should have contributed to make the provision of hospital care more rational.

It is likely that the widening gap between resources to provide expensive hospital care, from one side, and resources available from the other, have put hospital administrators and health professionals under pressure. In fact, comparing hospital and community health services output, as measured

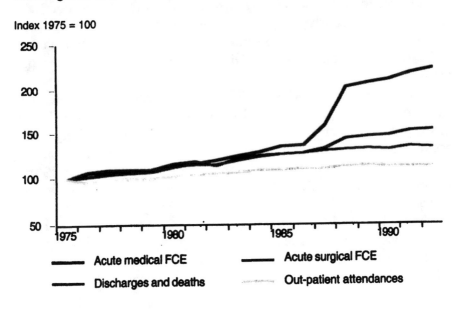

Figure 18.2 NHS hospital services: discharges and deaths, acute medical and surgical FCEs and out-patient attendances, 1975–82

752 *Health Care and Cost Containment in the European Union*

by the cost-weighted activity index, with the expenditure for these services (adjusted for changes in input unit costs) shows that this was the case for the period 1983–93. While the activity index (the output) has been increased by 28 per cent, expenditure (the input) has been increased by only 12.7 per cent.[20] These rates imply an efficiency gain over the 10-year period equal to 14 per cent (calculated as 128.5 / 112.7), a value much lower than the annual 3 per cent requested by the Government.

18.9 Technology

Technological advance is generally considered a major determinant of expenditure growth in the health care sector. It is often the case that new devices, equipment, drugs and procedures substitute less expensive technologies or represent an addition to existing practices. Moreover, even when new technologies reduce spending on individual patients, they rarely reduce spending in the health system as a whole. This is because new technologies tend to generate additional demand, either because they can benefit new patients or because they are over-utilized.

There is little research on the overall effects of introducing new technologies on health care systems. However, indirect evidence from the field of cost-effectiveness analysis suggest that new medical technologies are rarely cost-saving and they are sometimes not even cost-effective. It is therefore not surprising that the NHS is making a great effort to develop a comprehensive R&D strategy aimed at giving clear direction to research and dissemination activities.

This strategy was launched in 1991 with the creation of a Research and Development Division at the DoH. The Division is supported by the Central Research Development Committee (CRDC), a 25-member advisory body, and a regional infrastructure formed of a Director, an R&D Manager, and support staff. In order to strengthen the relationship between the NHS and the research community, in 1995 the establishment of a National Forum was also announced.

The objective of the NHS strategy on R&D is quite ambitious: to create a knowledge-based health service in which clinical, managerial and policy decisions are based on sound information about research findings and scientific development.[21] This objective is mainly pursued by R&D programmes which are prioritized at central level, are funded either nationally or regionally, and are implemented by the regional infrastructure. R&D programmes are supported by the three pillars of the NHS R&D Information Systems Strategy: the UK Cochrane Centre, the NHS Centre for Reviews and Dissemination and the NHS R&D Project Registers System.

The UK Cochrane Centre specializes in systematic reviews of randomized controlled trials and is part of the Cochrane Collaboration, an international network comprising nine centres in seven countries. The NHS Centre for Reviews and Dissemination is a 'review' facility established to support the NHS with information on the effectiveness of health care, both at clinical and organizational level. In addition to preparing and maintaining reviews, both centres make a great effort to disseminate research-based information in a user-friendly format. *Effective Health Care Bulletin* and *Effectiveness Matters*, both published by the NHS Centre for Review and Dissemination, are the best examples of this effort. Finally, the NHS R&D Project Registers System is a tool to produce information on on-going and planned research activities which aim to support effective planning (i.e. to avoid duplication of research projects) and accountability.

In order to fuel all these new activities, ministers have agreed that expenditure on R&D should be increased from the current 1 per cent towards a target of 1.5 per cent of the NHS budget.[22]

The Health Technology Assessment Programme is a pivotal feature of the NHS R&D strategy. It was established in 1993 to support the NHS with greater evidence on the cost, effectiveness and broader impact of the enormous range of interventions performed through the Service. The Programme is led by the Standing Group on Health Technology, a body whose mission is to advise on national priorities for health technology assessment and who reports to the CRDC. In performing its duties, it is supported by six advisory bodies: population screening, acute sector, primary and community care, diagnostic and imaging, pharmaceuticals and methodologies. Since Technology Assessment is demanding in terms of cost, the Standing Group follows a well-structured priorization process to commission evaluation projects, systematic reviews and dissemination activities on health technologies meant in their broader sense. As of September 1995, the NHS Health Technology Assessment Programme funded 54 projects at an estimated cost of £5.8 million.[23] The Programme is expected to spend about £20 million of NHS R&D funds between 1995 and 2000. However, the research agenda identified by the Standing Group and its advisory bodies is

Figure 18.3 The main dissemination channels aimed at improving cost and cost-effectiveness of technologies in the NHS

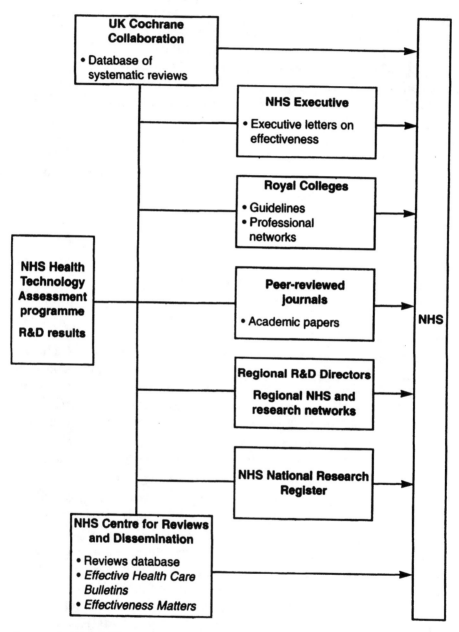

Source: DoH, 1995[23]

too expensive for the NHS to fund itself. It is therefore expected to contribute to direct research funded by other institutions such as the Medical Research Council.

Dissemination of research results is a vital issue; 'making results available to the right people in the right form is one of the key challenges for the Programme'.[23] Figure 18.3 depicts the main dissemination channels aimed at improving cost and cost-effectiveness of technologies in the NHS. In addition to the activities undertaken by the UK Cochrane Collaboration and the NHS Centre for Reviews and Dissemination, dissemination of results is promoted through an annual Executive Letter (a circular issued by the NHS Executive) listing sources of information technology effectiveness, the systematic use of research results in developing clinical guidelines, and the establishment of professional and research networks. Particular attention is also being attributed to controlling the diffusion of unevaluated technologies.

18.10 Audit and accreditation

There are at least three different types of audits that can be found in health care systems: financial, organizational and medical. Financial audit is the traditional tool to verify that public money is spent in accordance with the law and for the purposes intended by Parliament. Examination and certification of accounts are the main activities undertaken in financial audit. Two bodies are required by law to undertake the financial audit of the public sector: the National Audit Office and the Audit Commission. The former is mainly involved with central government departments, executive agencies and several kinds of public bodies, while the latter was established to manage the external auditors of local authorities. However, both of them are currently involved in auditing the NHS. Moreover, both of these bodies have evolved their audit function so as to extend the financial audit to cover effectiveness and efficiency issues. Therefore, the task of auditors is now to assess expenditure, not just for probity and regularity, but for value for money as well. The National Audit Office (NAO) has an explicit framework to undertake value for money and frequently presents to the House of Commons reports concerning the NHS. In 1995-96 these included reports on supplies in England,[24] progress the on Health of the Nation,[25] and the

756 *Health Care and Cost Containment in the European Union*

NHS Executive Initiative on Hospital Information Support Systems.[26] Similarly, the Audit Commission has issued a series of reports on key aspects of the NHS: day surgery,[27] acute hospital care,[28] prescribing in general practice[29] and GP fundholding.[30,31]

To a certain extent value for money studies are similar to organizational audits in that both review how resources are used, in order to make suggestions for improvement. The main difference, however, is that in organizational audit, the subject is treated as an organizational entity rather than a programme, piece of reform or a sector of the service. Organizational audit programmes, or accreditation programmes as they are often called, are still not very common in the UK, and only two programmes have been developed. One operates within a Regional Health Authority (South Western Region) and is directed to community hospitals, which in Britain are run by general practitioners and with no resident medical staff.[32,33] The other has been developed by an independent foundation (the King's Fund) and is mainly based on the Australian accreditation system. Both programmes are voluntary (participating hospitals are not forced to join the programme) and focus on organizational rather than clinical issues.

Although medical audit is a technique with a long history, in the UK it gained momentum only with the 1989 reforms, as these required all doctors to undertake this type of educational exercise. In fact, ring-fenced funds have been made available for this purpose, a new occupational group within the NHS emerged, i.e. the audit support staff, and tens of thousands of doctors and nurses have participated in audit meetings.

According to *Working for Patients*,[2] audit is 'the systematic, critical analysis of the quality of medical care, including the procedures used for diagnosis and treatment, the use of resources, and the resulting outcome and quality of life for the patient'. However, despite such ambitious aims, actual experience suggests that the scope of medical audit has been limited to discussion among doctors on good practices, without structurally approaching cost and quality of life issues.[34] As could be expected, medical audit has proved to be a tool in doctors' hands with reference to the most traditional component of quality of care (mainly the technical component).

All these forms of auditing represent a newly established attempt to measure performance and to facilitate improvements. Theoretically, cost considerations should be included in all types of audit because of the constraints on resources. In practice, however, clinicians tend to focus on clinical practice, neglecting the cost side of the cost-benefit equation. Thus,

Cost Containment and Health Care Reforms in the British NHS   757

while the evaluative work of both the National Audit Commission and the Audit Office are real attempts to use economic principles, at clinical level, effectiveness and ethical considerations tend to be the only relevant dimensions under investigation in most auditing exercises.

18.11 Rationing

High-profile cases have made rationing in the NHS a hot issue in the UK. Several stories attracted the attention of the national and international media.[35-37] These include the case of Child B, who had myeloid leukaemia and was denied a second transplant by her health authority, allegedly on cost considerations; the case of an 81-year-old woman who was not adequately cared for, possibly because the staff were under pressure; the case of a 73-year-old man who did not receive physiotherapy because his health authority had indicated that services should not be provided to people over 65; and the case of a man who took 10 hours to receive urgent surgery. These and other stories have made public opinion more aware that rationing is unavoidable and that rationing decisions are taken in the NHS either implicitly or explicitly.

At the same time, both the fact that rationing is controlled by the medical profession and that it is made in an implicit way have been challenged. Some health authorities have issued purchasing documents explicitly stating the exclusion of certain minor procedures. Examples of treatment excluded from purchasing or deemed to be of very low priority are: the extraction of symptomless wisdom teeth, removal of non-malignant lumps and bumps, tattoo removal, reversal of sterilization, gender identity surgery, and assisted conception techniques such as in-vitro fertilization. Concurrently, rationing is being extensively discussed in many quarters: several conferences on rationing have been organized by Royal Colleges and policy and management institutes, and various articles and books on this subject have recently been published.[37-39] Also, various attempts have been made to involve the general public in the debate on rationing.[36,40]

The debate on rationing is here to stay. It is unlikely that the NHS will go back to the times when rationing was indisputably administered by doctors according to their implicit judgements. However, *explicit* decisions to stop providing specific treatments are still very much the exception in the

758   *Health Care and Cost Containment in the European Union*

NHS[41] and are likely to remain so in the near future. There are at least two main reasons why, to a large degree, it is difficult to expand the areas where explicit rationing decisions are made. The first is related to the wide variability of effectiveness and utility among patients. Since explicit rationing tends to set up rules, the risk of denying effective and highly valued care to individual patients is great. The second reason is political: explicit rationing tends to be unpopular because it raises sensitive issues, hits specific population groups seriously, and weakens the reassuring function of the NHS.

18.12 Cost containment and the 1989 reforms: the internal market

A complete analysis and evaluation of the 1989 reforms is beyond the scope of this chapter. In this and the following section, attention is limited to how NHS expenditure is likely to be influenced by the two major components of the reforms – the creation of the internal market and the GP fundholding scheme.

The purchaser–provider split is at the heart of the NHS reforms. The first basic idea of the internal market model adopted by the British government is to create a demand-side or purchasing agency that is distinct from the supply side or providers. The model recast health authorities (and GP fundholders) as purchasers of services for people residing in their territories. These authorities are expected to assess and prioritize patients' needs and wants, and seek to use their limited resources to purchase services accordingly. Purchasers are allowed to shop around to find the 'best providers' in the market, that is the providers who present the most favourable profile in terms of prices, quality specifications, waiting times, etc.

The vast majority of secondary and community health services are now provided by publicly-owned, self-governing trusts. They are independent, non-governmental organizations directly accountable to the Secretary of State for Health. As they compete against each other to obtain contracts from health authorities and GP fundholders, NHS trusts are supposed to receive a strong incentive to control costs, to enhance quality and, more generally, to respond to purchaser expectations.

The rationale of the internal market is therefore quite straightforward: to activate the purchasing function in order to put NHS trusts (and other providers) under competitive pressure. Threatened by the risk of fewer

Cost Containment and Health Care Reforms in the British NHS 759

resources, NHS trusts are forced to be more explicit about their work, and to look for more efficiency and better quality (at least the part which is observed). Whether the internal market works as predicted is difficult to verify. It seems quite evident, however, that important changes have taken place in the NHS. These include:[42] important steps to develop the purchasing function (e.g. serious plans, priority-setting exercises, the monitoring of providers), a clear reduction of the dominance of hospital professionals in resource allocation, a better use of spare capacity in the NHS, and an enormous improvement in information flows throughout the NHS – especially with respect to the cost of clinical procedures. It is also quite clear that since 1990, the NHS has experienced an acceleration of the development of management skills and systems. Between 1989 and 1993 the numbers of senior and general managers in the NHS increased dramatically, managers from both the public and the private sectors have been hired by NHS trusts, consulting companies have intensified their work in the health care field, new management roles such as marketing manager and department administrator have been established, and relevant investments in hospital information systems have been made. Management principles, as opposed to professional or legal principles, have gained ground since the inception of the reforms.

Nevertheless, the diffusion of management techniques and skills is controversial. First, the diffusion of management ideas in the NHS was influenced by the achievement of New Public Management. This popular doctrine stresses that the public sector should be less distinct as a unit from the private sector in terms of management systems, and that the extent to which discretionary power is limited by uniform and general rules of procedures should be greatly reduced.[43] This approach is clearly consistent with the quasi-market idea behind the NHS reforms. However, it can erode the traditional public service ethos (and the trust the British citizens put in it) and can result in the loss of planning skills and strategic control of the public sector (see also below).

Second, one of the main problems associated with the NHS reforms and of direct relevance to cost containment is transaction costs. In order to work, the NHS internal market requires the provision of sophisticated administrative activities. It should be noted that these activities are managerial in nature. Consequently, even if the ultimate goal of the reforms is to provide more and better care, a clearly observable outcome of the internal market is the increase in the proportion of health care resources which are not directly spent on patient care, because they are devoted to management activities.

Not surprisingly, management costs are not very popular among the mass media and the public. The traditional view of health services as the one-to-one relationship between doctors and patients involving sophisticated knowledge and simple capital equipment, is probably one of the reasons for the mistrust of the role of management in health care organizations. Although these organizations are extremely complex, it is largely believed that their functioning depends on health professional skills only. Therefore, the role of management is clearly underestimated in the health care sector. It should be noted, however, that hostility towards resources devoted to management is probably independent of the institutional arrangement of the NHS. Since public concern is about resources not directly spent on patient care, large investments aimed at improving co-ordination, communication, monitoring and evaluation activities would probably be perceived by the general public as a waste of money even if they were undertaken in a strongly integrated NHS based on hierarchy and command/control systems.

Finally, NHS trusts and Health Authorities are making human and capital investments in order to manage the internal market. Part of these investments are highly dependent of the incentives created by the new competitive environment. If the market does not work properly (its outcome is not desirable) resources devoted to compete are socially wasted. Consequently, whether a substantial part of management activities are beneficial to social goals is dependent on the structure of incentives created by the 1991 reforms.

While there is limited evidence of the nature of these incentives and their impact on costs, there are various speculative analyses. A full account of the research on the 1989 reforms is not provided here. However, the opinions of some experts may help highlight some points. Professor Propper argues that the market introduced by the NHS reforms is underdeveloped, mainly because of poorly defined property rights.[44,45] For example, she argues that the present financial regime places a bias on current expenditure and decreases the incentives for long-term efficiency. Similarly, Dixon and Harrison suggest that the government's insistence on an annual 3 per cent increase in efficiency may have resulted in Health Authorities implementing short-term measures that actually decrease efficiency in the long term.[46]

Professor Paton is more sceptical about the potential virtues of the quasi-market.[47] He sees it as full of perverse incentives leading to higher costs without benefits: from hospital and community trusts increasingly

Cost Containment and Health Care Reforms in the British NHS   761

seeking to shift costs to each other, to marketing activities interfering with need assessment; from the DoH seeking savings by moving acute care into the community, to very high transaction costs that have to be recouped through the exploitation of workers.

The impact on costs and efficiency of additional managerial activities strictly depends on the specific incentives generated by market forces and regulatory devices. The increase in managerial costs from both the purchaser and provider sides represent an additional cost for the NHS. Whether these costs are repaid by more efficiency and effectiveness is difficult to state. While there is some evidence that providers feel a strong pressure to increase productivity, it is not clear if these productivity gains counterbalance the higher transaction costs attributable to the reform.

18.13 GP fundholding

GP fundholding is a purchasing system which overlaps with HA purchasing. In principle, a fundholding practice can be described as a 'mini-ambulatory' Health Maintenance Organization (HMO), that is, an entity that receives a fixed, pre-paid sum of money from which it must deliver or arrange for the delivery of secondary health care to a defined population.[48] Practices volunteering for the scheme are given a budget to purchase a defined list of hospital services (most out-patient clinics and elective surgery, e.g. cataract operations, hip replacements, coronary artery bypass operations), community health services (e.g. district nursing, community mental health services), direct access services (e.g. dietetics, physiotherapy), tests and investigations, drugs and appliances prescribed by the practice, and non-medical staff employed by the practice (e.g. receptionists, practice nurses).[30] For all these services, GP fundholders are free to contract with independent providers as well as with NHS providers. In the standard version of the scheme, the remaining services are still under the direct responsibility of the HAs. This includes: accident and emergency services; emergency admissions to hospitals; maternity care; residential care for people with mental illness and learning disability; cancer treatment; renal dialysis; and genito-urinary treatment. To prevent the very high costs of a few individuals absorbing a major part of the budget, and to reduce the risk of 'cream skimming', HAs also have to bear the cost of 'expensive patients',

762   *Health Care and Cost Containment in the European Union*

i.e. those whose health care costs amount to more than £6000 per year.

In the beginning, according to national guidelines, budgets were based on the use of resources by the fundholding practice in the year before the joining of the scheme. A gradual change to weighted capitation, however, is now being attempted. Components of the fundholding budget are calculated separately, although practices are responsible for the budget as a whole. A crucial feature of the scheme is that fundholders can keep any surplus, provided that is spent on facilities or on services of benefit to patients.

When the scheme started in 1991, only practices with at least 11,000 patients could become fundholders, but this lower limit has been gradually decreased to 5000 patients. A typical fundholder holds a total annual budget of about £1.7 million, or £160 for each patient on the practice list. While GP fundholders purchase more than 50 per cent of their patients' family health services (mainly pharmaceutical services), they have a limited purchasing power over hospital community services (20 per cent).[31]

In April 1995 around 40 per cent of all GP practices in England and Wales were fundholders, covering nearly half the population. However, fundholding is unevenly distributed among geographical areas and social groups. As of April 1995, the percentage of patient coverage ranged from 4 per cent (an inner London FHSA) to 84 per cent (a Southern England FHSA). Also, fundholding is less common in more deprived areas. Using 1995/96 data, a study by the Audit Commission found a statistically significant (p-value<0.0001) relationship between the percentage of FHSA population registered with fundholders and the Jarman score, a deprivation index widely used in Great Britain.[31]

Evaluating the 1989 NHS reforms poses problems, as it is very difficult to consider separately each component of such a complex 'social programme'. This is the so-called 'attributing causation' problem: it is not easy to discern between changes that are attributable to the object of the evaluation and changes that are attributable to other measures or events. Evaluation is also made difficult by the fact that social policy programmes have to be evaluated under different perspectives. These include equity and efficiency and, possibly, other issues such as freedom of choice and quality of care. And the problem is not just one of handling evaluation under several dimensions, but also of selecting these dimensions: different disciplines tend to focus on different issues and to use different methodologies.

Notwithstanding these and other difficulties,[49] and despite the lack of evaluation programmes promoted by the Department of Health, serious

Cost Containment and Health Care Reforms in the British NHS 763

attempts to evaluate the NHS reforms, and particularly the fundholding schemes do exist. The available evidence is still quite limited, at least compared with the potential implications of the programme. Nevertheless, it should not be forgotten that there is more evaluation research on the NHS now than there was before, and that in many other European countries health care reforms or other social policy programmes reforms are not evaluated at all.

Reviews of the research on fundholding can be found in Dixon and Glennerster,[50] and in Coulter[49] and Petchey,[51] whereas an update within fundholding in England and Wales is provided in a recent study by the Audit Commission.[31] This part of the chapter does not provide similar comprehensive analyses of the scheme, rather it concentrates on cost issues; that is on the costs of running the scheme and on the savings it generates.

Turning first to an examination of prescribing, various observational studies report that fundholding practices had rates of increase in prescribing costs higher than non-fundholding practices (Table 18.5 overleaf). However, a small study performed in Wales found that the cost per 1000 patients increased less among fundholders than non-fundholders.[52] Similarly, a study from the Oxford region shows that the annual increase in net cost per capita was 13.2 per cent among fundholders and 18.7 per cent* among non-fundholders.[53] Since in both studies the higher cost per patient among non-fundholders is not explained by more prescribed items, it is likely that fundholders moved to cheaper prescribing. In fact, in both studies the rate of increase in the use of generics was higher in fundholders than in non-fundholders.

A prospective study performed in Scotland provides a similar picture: fundholders increased prescribing costs less than non-fundholders,[54] mainly because they use less expensive drugs. However, the Oxford region presents different results if a longer-term perspective is taken: three years after joining the scheme, fundholders and non-fundholders have similar rates of increase in per capita prescribing costs (38.1 and 38.7, respectively) and reached similar rates of generic substitution.[55]

A much larger study was carried out in the former Mersey Regional Health Authority. Prescribing data of 100 fundholders was compared with that of 312 non-fundholders for the period 1990–94.[56] Although prescrib-

---

* It should be noted that this value refers to non-dispensing practices only. The annual increase in net cost per capita for these practices was 10.2 per cent.

764 *Health Care and Cost Containment in the European Union*

ing costs and volume rose through the study for both fundholders and non-fundholders, the former had lower rates of increase of per capita costs and volume, and higher rates of increase in generic prescriptions. Over an 18-month period, the median increase in per capita prescribing costs among fundholders was lower than among non-fundholders, by an amount that ranged from £0.68 to £1.18 according to the fundholding wave.

Table 18.5 Fundholding and drug costs

Authors	Type of study/data	Setting/size	Period
Burr et al. 1992[52]	Retrospective study with control groups.	Mid Glamorgan (Wales); 8 practices.	1990/91
Bradlow and Coulter, 1993[53]	Observational study with control groups; PACT data.	Oxford region (England); 208,398 patients.	1991/92– 1992/93
Maxwel et al. 1993[54]	Prospective controlled study; sub-set of SPA data (equivalent to PACT for Scotland); consumption measured in Defined Daily Doses (DDDs).	Grampian and Tayside regions (Scotland); 158,900 patients.	1990–92
Wilson et al. 1995[56]	Observational study with control groups: PACT data.	Former Mersey Regional Health Authority (about 2.4 million residents).	3 waves of fundholders: 1990–94
Stewart-Brown et al. 1995[55]	Updating of Bradlow, Coulter (1993). Prospective observational study with control groups: PACT data.	Oxford region (England); 208,398 patients.	1990–94
Wilson et al. 1996[57]	Multiple linear regression models on data used in Wilson et al. ,1995.[56] It tries to control for confounding.	Former Mersey Regional Health Authority (about 2.4 million residents).	3 waves of fundholders: 1990–94

Obviously, the fact that fundholders contained prescribing costs more than non-fundholders does not prove that the cause of this difference is fundholding. Since fundholding practices tend to be different from non-fundholding ones in various respects (e.g. percentage of single-handed GPs and the socio-economic environment in which they operate), it is possible that some characteristics associated with being fundholders are the true

---

Results (1 = costs, 2 = volume, 3 = use of generics)

1. Cost per 1000 patients: fundholders £14,191 to £14,533 (2.4%), non-fundholders £12,716 to £13,667 (7.5%).
2. Items per 1000 patients: fundholders 2,627 to 2,640, non-fundholders 2,390 to 2,385.
3. Analysis limited to 2 active ingredients: fundholders increase the use of generics more than non-fundholders.

---

1. Annual increase in net cost per capita: fundholders: 13.2%, non-fundholders: 18.7%.
2. Annual increase in number of items per capita: fundholders: 7.5%, non-fundholders: 6.1%.
3. Proportion of generic drugs: fundholders increase from 44.5% to 48.7%, non-fundholders from 46.5% to 46.6%.

---

1. Increase in cost per patient per year over a two year period:
   Tayside fundholders: -2.9%, Grampian fundholders: +9.8%, Grampian controls: +12.6%.
2. Increase in daily doses per patient per year over a two year period:
   Tayside fundholders: -12.3%, Grampian fundholders: -5.3%, Grampian controls: -9.3%.

---

1. Median difference of six months increase in prescribing costs per patient between non-fundholders and fundholders: first wave: £1.18, second wave: £1.68, third wave: £0.87.
2. Median difference of increase in number of items per 1000 prescriptions between non-fundholders and fundholders: first wave: 89, second wave: 100, third wave: 70.
3. Median difference in fundholders' and non-fundholders' prescribing rate of generics: first wave: 2.75%, second wave: 3.13%, third wave: 2.19%.

---

1. Increase in net cost per capita: fundholders 38.1, non-fundholders 38.7.
2. Increase in number of items per patient: fundholders 16.0%, non-fundholders 12.8%.
3. Proportion of generic drugs: fundholders increase from 44.5% to 58%, non-fundholders from 51.3% to 56%.

---

1. First and second wave fundholders associated with lower increases in prescribing costs.
2. First wave fundholders associated with lower increases in items prescribed.

determinants of the lower increase in prescribing costs. In order to ascertain if this was the case, Wilson et al. used a multiple regression model to control for confounding.[57] The results they obtained partially confirmed the influence of fundholding on prescribing costs, although, after controlling for confounding, only the first two waves of fundholders show a statistically significant (95 per cent) lower increase in prescribing costs.

Overall, the available evidence on the impact of fundholding on prescribing costs seems favourable. These results seem to support the evidence from national data regarding the sample of fundholders investigated by the Audit Commission for the period 1991–93: the cost of prescribing rose by 3–5 per cent more among non-fundholders than among fundholders.[30]

Concerning hospital and out-patient referrals, the available evidence is limited and not clear-cut. In a non-controlled study carried out in Scotland it was found that after the introduction of the scheme fundholders reduced investigation and referral rates.[58] However, in a prospective, controlled study in the Oxford region no evidence was found that budgetary pressure caused fundholders to reduce referral rates.[59,60] Nevertheless, by comparing 10 first-wave fundholding practices with six non-fundholding practices, this study found that the rate of increase in referral was higher among non-fundholders (7.5 per cent vs 26.7 per cent), particularly for general medicine, an area where there is substitution between GP and specialist services.

As fundholders are able to reinvest any savings they make, fresh resources were used by fundholding practices to develop or expand new practice-based services, such as physiotherapy and specialist outreach clinics. These services are popular among patients and thus they may be consistent with the attempt to make the NHS closer to patient expectations. However, the cost-effectiveness of these services has never been evaluated and it has been argued that they may be an inefficient way to use NHS resources.[49,51]

The NHS reforms were launched in a short period of time and they had to be based on the relatively poor management and policy information systems available at the time. In addition, the DoH gave directions to NHS purchasers not to make dramatic changes. For example, the Oxford Regional Health Authority introduced 'the 80/20 rule', under which fundholders agreed to contract at least 80 per cent of their hospital budget in the first year to the same hospitals as in the preparatory year.[59] It is therefore not surprising that fundholding budgets were set at quite generous levels and that they were almost exclusively based on previous prescribing and referral rates. Clearly, such a situation favoured the 'status quo' so that it may be premature to make generalizations on the basis of the available evidence. Also, early fundholders were not necessarily typical of their fellow practitioners because they came from well-organized practices in non-deprived areas and, probably, were determined to assure the success of the scheme.

Despite these caveats, it is, however, important to check whether the available studies provide some (even if weak) indication on the impact of the scheme on costs. Based on the available studies, it appears that fundholding has induced changes in prescribing and referral behaviour, even if the extent of this change has been smaller than originally anticipated.

Whether these changes had an overall impact on costs is more difficult to say. As a matter of fact, under fixed budgets, it is logically impossible to observe overall variations on costs attributable to decisions undertaken by GPs because the level of costs are exogenously determined by the budget. Under fixed budgets (that are not overspent) the overall costs generated by GPs are determined 'de facto' by funding decisions rather than by the GP willing to reduce costs.

Obviously, the GP fundholding scheme imposes additional costs. There are administrative costs incurred by both fundholders and providers which would not be there without the scheme. Transaction costs, which are probably a key feature of the new NHS, are likely to be much higher if the market is made of many small-scale purchasers, rather than one large health authority. The amount of these extra costs is difficult to measure. Nevertheless, some data can help understand at least the magnitude of these costs. In order to implement the scheme, in 1993–94 GP fundholding practices received £66.6 million or 3.5 per cent of the total fundholding budget. This amount was much higher than the original estimate made by the Government in 1989 (£15.6 million). Up to the end of 1994/95, fundholding practices had received a total £232 million to cover the costs of new staff, equipment and computers.

These operating costs are just a part of the transaction costs attributable to fundholding. Other costs include the substantial additional workload for GPs, and the additional burden on health authorities for setting budgets, auditing expenditure and monitoring the scheme's operation. One health authority has estimated these costs at £5,300 per practice.[51] Fundholding also imposes costs on providers who have to contract with an increasing number of small purchasers; the same study cited above reports these costs at £14,000 per practice. Clearly, the inclusion of these costs makes fund-

768   *Health Care and Cost Containment in the European Union*

holding relatively expensive. The total cost of running the scheme was estimated to be £81,638 per fundholding practice.[61]

Are the costs of this form of purchasing justified in terms of benefits? A recent Audit Commission report provides a partial evaluation of fundholding so far.[31] It compares costs in staff, equipment and computing (£232 million) with savings (allocated budget less expenditure) made by fundholders (£206 million). In making the balance, the report ignores the value of some benefits of the scheme (e.g. shorter waiting lists for some procedures, easier access to some services) and transaction costs to providers. The Audit Commission also reports that although a few fundholders have made achievements across the board, the majority have achieved only a small proportion of the benefits potentially available for their patients. Therefore, the Audit Commission seems to suggest that the answer to the above-mentioned question is 'not yet'. In fact, it is too early to make a fair judgement on fundholding. The radical nature of the programme, the lack of government interest in its evaluation (at least in the beginning), and the fact that the main benefits of the programme may be in terms of cultural and organizational changes, suggest caution in drawing conclusions from the available studies.

18.14 The private market

Approximately 85 per cent of health care needs in the UK are financed by collective and public funding. The remaining 15 per cent is funded by the private sector either directly or via Private Medical Insurance (PMI). In 1993 the sources of funding of the whole UK health care system could be estimated as follows:[7] £36.8 billion came from public sources (taxation and NHS contributions), £1.4 billion derived from co-payments on prescriptions and other services provided by the NHS, and £5.1 billion spent on non-statutory NHS services came from either PMI or from direct private payments. Most of the private expenditure in health care relates to charges on prescriptions and to expenditure on pharmaceutical products not covered by the NHS.

The private acute health care market (out-patient and in-patient services) is the second largest component of private health care expenditure. Including NHS private treatments, it was estimated at £2,192 million in

1995, some 7 per cent up on 1994 (3.5 per cent in real terms).[62] Although at a slower rate than during the 1980s, in the last years the private health care market has grown at a pace significantly in excess of the economy as a whole. The breakdown of the private acute health care market has been estimated as follows: £203 million for private patients in the NHS, £674 million for surgeons', anaesthetists' and physicians' fees, and £1,288 million for independent hospitals and clinics (Table 18.6). The NHS component of the private health care market is the most vital: NHS income from private patients is projected at £230 million, about 10 per cent of the total, up from 7.7 per cent at the launch of the reforms (1990). The reform has favoured the expansion of NHS income from private patients, although, probably, at a lower pace than expected.

There are about 1,400 beds in dedicated pay-bed NHS units. In addition, there is an average use of 1,600/1,700 beds for private patients in non-dedicated NHS wards. The capacity of the independent acute medical/surgical hospitals and clinics is much larger. In 1991, this accounted for 10,911 beds available at 216 hospitals. Sixty five per cent of these beds are supplied by profit-making organizations, while the remaining 35 per cent are run by either charitable or religious institutions.

The main funding source of the private acute health care sector is PMI. About 70 per cent of insurable private acute treatments are funded by

Table 18.6 The UK private acute health care market 1990–95, as estimated by Laing, 1996[62] (£ million)

	1990	1991	1992	1993	1994	1995
Independent hospitals and clinics (%)	884 (60.0)	971 (59.9)	1,040 (59.6)	1,112 (59.1)	1,202 (58.7)	1,288 (58.8)
Private in-patients and out-patients in NHS hospitals (%)	113 (7.7)	147 (9.1)	164 (9.4)	185 (9.8)	209 (10.2)	230 (10.5)
Surgeon, anaesthetist and physician fees (%)	477 (32.4)	504 (31.1)	542 (31.0)	584 (31.0)	636 (31.1)	674 (30.7)
Total acute in-patient and out-patient market	1,473	1,623	1,747	1,881	2,047	2,192

PMI.[62] The remaining part of private health care revenue is derived from self-paying British patients (15 per cent), non-UK patients (10 per cent) and NHS purchases (5 per cent). It is remarkable that after the launch of the internal market only such a modest part of the private provision is purchased by the NHS.

It is estimated that in 1995 the PMI market constituted 6.2 million persons covered and 3.3 million policy-holders.[62] These numbers are very similar to those of previous years. After having tripled in the period 1978–90, the number of subscribers has stabilized in the early 1990s, probably because of the economic recession. According to Laing, this situation will persist in the remainder of the 1990s.[62] The scope of private insurance will remain limited in the UK, being primarily concerned with non-life-threatening treatments required by a relatively limited portion of society seeking no waiting times and better comfort.

A few managed care initiatives have been introduced in recent years. These include the promotion of day-surgery procedures and cost containment measures. Managed care is pursued partly to contain costs and partly to enhance quality. However, it is likely that PMI will remain a luxury purchase or a senior employee benefit and thus, that very aggressive approaches to cost containment will not be used by British carriers.

Purchase of PMI depends on NHS performance, both in terms of length of waiting lists and levels of satisfaction with the NHS.[63] Although PMI can be considered a luxury purchase, a further expansion of private insurance may then depend on accessibility and perceived good quality of NHS-funded services: the better the NHS performance along these dimensions, the less scope there is for a private insurance market. It has also been suggested, on the basis of some empirical evidence, that those who are privately insured have a greater tendency than others to object to increases in public health spending[63,64] and tend not to rank public health spending as a top priority.[63] It seems plausible therefore, that poor performance (in terms of patients' criteria) induces the use of private funding sources and, consequently, alleviates the pressure to increase NHS funding. However, it also tends to weaken political support for the NHS and the popularity of its funding.

A limited private health insurance sector is compatible with an NHS type system. It is somehow unavoidable that very affluent people and very busy professionals use their income to buy more convenience, better hotel services and less waste of personal time. Provided that these patients repre-

Cost Containment and Health Care Reforms in the British NHS 771

sent a small minority, the NHS can co-exist with a public private sector. However, if the use of non-public funding is related to a perceived poor quality of (and distrust in) NHS-owned institutions, and involves the middle-class segment of the population, then the scenario may be radically different. The use of PMI may be interpreted as a signal against the NHS and its underlying values. The sustainability of adequate funding may be threatened by a vicious circle where perceived poor performance induces less funding and, in turn, inadequate funding further deteriorates provision.

Although the overall satisfaction with the NHS, as measured by the British Social Attitudes Survey, showed signs of improvement in the early 1990s, the long-term trend indicates that satisfaction with the NHS is decreasing.[65–67] Parallel to this trend, the number of PMI holders has increased. Nonetheless, the vast majority of the population still only have NHS coverage and still express strong feelings in favour of the NHS. The British system is still firmly dominated by the NHS, as is clearly shown by the fact that 85 per cent of total health care expenditure refers to the NHS. In Italy, a country where there is universal coverage and the British NHS was partly emulated, the National Health Service accounts for only 70 per cent of total health care expenditure. However, whether the NHS will continue to play this quasi-monopoly role in British health care is less certain in the future and will also depend on the adequateness of funding.

18.15 The 1997 White Paper

In May 1997 the Labour Party won a very large majority at the political election and returned to power after 19 years of Conservative governments. Six months later, the DoH released a White Paper setting out the start of 'a 10-year process' of modernization and restructuring of the NHS in England and Scotland.[68] The White Paper, *The New NHS: modern and dependable* does not suggest a radical re-structuring of the NHS. It clearly states that there will be no return to the old centralized command and control system of the 1970s and it recognizes various merits to the 1989 reform: the separation between the planning of hospital care and its provision, the important role attributed to primary care in the NHS and the decentralized responsibility for operational management.

As expected, the White Paper rejects any reference to the idea that market forces, although managed by the State, may produce incentives to promote efficiency, effectiveness and responsiveness to patients. As a consequence, it announces the abolition of the internal market which it considers divisive, unfair, and costly. However, Labour's way of modernizing the NHS appears to retain the main features of the internal market idea, introducing corrections aimed at improving fairness and at strengthening social accountability. The planning and delivery functions (in quasi-market jargon, the purchasing and providing functions) will be kept separate so to maintain one of the most innovative elements of the 1989 reform, and arrangements between purchasers and providers will be maintained, although these will now be called 'service agreements' and will be more long-term. Similarly, standard GP fundholding is to be eliminated, but budget-holding and GP-led commissioning are expected to be crucial elements of a new re-organization of primary care, envisaging the creation of Primary Care Groups (eventually Primary Care Trusts).

Despite the rhetoric, the White Paper seems to preserve the main institutional features of the NHS as it emerged in the 1990s. Although it seems likely that some measures will reduce provider competition and GP fundholding autonomy and financial accountability. Whether the quasi-market forces will survive these changes is certainly an issue. However, the White Paper may be interpreted as an evolution of the internal market, which attempts to make further steps towards ensuring a balance between local decision-making (at GP as well as Trust level) and overall social accountability.

Health Authorities are attributed a new pivotal role as they will be in charge of coordinating the commissioning function of health services, ensuring that NHS Trusts, Primary Care Groups and other organizations implement the Health Improvement Programme (the new planning procedure expected to give direction to commissioning) and to control major investment decisions. Health Improvement Programmes will assess local health needs, provide requirements for the provision of health services and define the range, location and investment required in local health services. Health Improvement Programmes will be developed under the leadership of the HAs with the participation of Primary Care Groups, NHS Trusts, Local Authorities and universities.

The establishment of Primary Care Groups is probably the most crucial part of the White Paper. The idea is to preserve the benefits of decentralized purchasing, at the same time avoiding the high transaction costs of fund-

Cost Containment and Health Care Reforms in the British NHS   773

holding and the fragmentation of the purchasing function under the internal market. Commissioning is to be attributed to groups of GPs and community nurses. Each group will have available resources for the full range of hospital and community health services, prescribing, and general practice infrastructure. These resources will allow the Group to commission and provide services. Within this cash limit, the Group is expected to give maximum choice to GPs and community nurses about how best to meet individual patient needs. Primary Care Groups are expected to serve about 100,000 patients, but their precise form will be flexible to reflect local circumstances. They will develop over time. At a minimum, they will support the health authority in commissioning care for its population, acting in an advisory capacity. However, they will be expected to progress, so that in time all Primary Care Groups assume full responsibilities, eventually becoming freestanding bodies accountable to the HA for commissioning care and with added responsibility for the provision of community health services.

NHS Trusts will retain full local responsibility for operational management. However, their strategic autonomy will be constrained by the Health Improvement Programme and a new statutory duty for NHS Trusts to work in partnership with other NHS organizations. Also, the White Paper stresses that under the internal market NHS Trusts' principal duties were financial, so that accountability to quality and effectiveness issues were often neglected. In the new NHS, the performance of NHS Trusts will be assessed 'against new broad-based measures reflecting the wider goals of improving health and health care outcomes, the quality and effectiveness of service, efficiency and access'.[68] They will sign long-term agreements (three to five years) with Primary Care Groups, typically organised around a particular care group (such as children) or disease area (such as heart disease).

The White Paper highlights the fact that the NHS requires a new national performance framework, to overcome the distortion of the Purchaser Efficiency Index, which is based on the financial bottom line and the number of 'finished consultant episodes'. The latter way of approaching performance is criticized as being too narrow because it does not reflect access, effectiveness and perceived quality. Accordingly, a new articulated framework to measure performance is launched. It will have six dimensions: health improvement, fair access, effective delivery of appropriate health care, efficiency, patient/carer experience and health outcomes of NHS care.

Commitment to improve quality, effectiveness and responsiveness to patients is also behind various other initiatives. There will be a National

774 *Health Care and Cost Containment in the European Union*

Institute of Clinical Excellence which will provide a leading role on clinical and cost-effectiveness. The Institute will also set up and disseminate guidelines from the latest scientific evidence. There will be a Commission of Health Improvement, a statutory body at arm's length from Government, in charge of guaranteeing that procedures to monitor, assure and improve quality at local level are in place, and to provide target support on request to local organizations. This body may resemble an accreditation organization, ensuring that quality programmes are adopted and providing consultative support. New evidence-based National Service frameworks will also be established to help ensure consistent access to services and adequate quality of care across the country. Finally, starting in 1998, the Government will introduce a new national survey of patient and user experience to be carried out annually, the aim being to give patients and carers a voice in shaping the NHS and to measure public satisfaction.

The White Paper announces the Government's intention to raise spending in real terms every year. However, the long-term impact of the envisaged changes on public health care expenditure is difficult to predict. It is likely that the commitment to reduce transaction costs and other administrative costs by reducing the number of purchasers and by capping management costs in Health Authorities and Primary Care Groups will produce some savings (£1 billion according to the White Paper estimate). Also, by introducing a national schedule of reference costs, the Government hopes to stimulate benchmarking exercises so to allow gains in efficiency. On the other hand, the new bodies and programmes launched by the White Paper, as well as the commitment to dramatically increase the use of information technology, are expected to require additional resources. But the critical point concerning cost containment in the long run is expected to be linked to one of the main aims of the Government plan: to harness new developments so as to ensure clinical and cost-effectiveness.

18.16 Conclusion

Until the 1990s the British NHS was the cheapest health care system among the highly industrialized European countries. In this chapter some of the measures that brought this about have been reviewed. It has also been argued that the UK Government budgeting process and the financial discipline imposed by the Treasury have played, and will probably continue to play, an important role in keeping public health care expenditure under control.

More than in other countries, in the UK the central government is the real decision-maker on public health care expenditure. It is therefore not surprising that there has always been discussion on whether the NHS is adequately funded. In the 1980s Professor Abel-Smith strongly argued that the NHS was underfunded.[69] Although in the early 1990s public health care expenditure grew rapidly and at a higher pace than the GDP or public spending as a whole, there is still a widespread perception that the NHS is underfunded. A recent report has expressed this point of view.[70] The report was produced by a team of experts set up to assess the longer-term trends and options for the provision and financing of health care services. Concerning funding, it states that even if there is no conclusive evidence that the NHS is underfunded, international comparisons, the explicit rationing of some health services and public opinion surveys, suggest that there is a gap between resources and demand. Also it forecasts that the overall impact of technological, medical and scientific advance, demographic trends, and rising consumer expectations will widen this gap.

In a provocative paper Professor Maynard has fiercely contested this argument.[71] He argued that public opinion is manipulated by health care providers to enhance expenditure (and their income) and that gross variations in clinical practice, an unwillingness to measure health care outcomes, and a reluctance to adopt more efficient practices require penalties which include spending less on both public and private health care.

In a recent series of papers published in the *British Medical Journal* a group of experts from the King's Fund Policy Institute discussed the NHS funding problem.[46,72-74] In the first article of the series (Dixon et al. 1997[72]), they reviewed all the approaches that have been used to assess whether the NHS is underfunded and concluded that there is no satisfactory answer to this question. However, underfunding may be a useful concept if it is used more specifically. Are NHS financial resources enough to cope with the functions attributed to the NHS? In this sense, determining the right level of funding is less a judgemental, and more a question of affordability.

The adequacy of funding can be assessed by investigating four main components: the level of funding, efficiency, effectiveness and demand. Deciding on the level of funding is a political question. It is thus very difficult to make predictions, although it appears unlikely that the proportion of

GDP attributed to public health care will greatly increase. Despite the fact that British citizens are more willing to pay taxes for the NHS than for other public sector spending, political parties are presently committed to not raising taxation and it appears unlikely that the NHS proportion of public spending will increase much further in the near future. On the basis of these elements, one projection is that public expenditure decisions will make NHS funding less adequate in the future.

More efficiency and effectiveness may contribute to make NHS funding more adequate because resources can be freed without reducing output (efficiency) or outcome (effectiveness). As discussed earlier, the net effect of the 1989 reforms on efficiency mainly depends on the balance between transaction costs and productivity gains generated by the purchaser-provider split. Evidence to calculate this balance is still very limited, especially concerning primary and community care. However, for hospital care the combination of Cost-weighted Activity Index data and expenditure figures adjusted for health sector inflation, suggests that there is an increasing efficiency trend (see section 18.8). As far as effectiveness is concerned, there is increased interest, both within the medical community and within the NHS in general. Growing attention in the medical community, and several NHS initiatives suggest that there is a growing motivation to work on this issue. Generally, more attention to the effectiveness of technologies used in health care is an unexpected by-product of the 1989 reforms.

Prospects on the demand-side are less favourable. There are four elements that may push for more resources: population ageing, morbidity, technological change, and rising expectations. Using a very simple method, Harrison et al. suggest that demographic change will have a moderate impact on demand for funds as it will require only a 10 per cent increase over a period of 20 years.[73] Similarly, they argue that morbidity is not expected to have a major impact, although it is possible that changes in mortality patterns may have an impact on morbidity and may involve a move towards more expensive cases.

The pressure of technological change and patients' expectations are difficult to measure but they are probably of great importance. Medical innovations do not generally allow cheaper treatments per case because they tend to be very expensive and because they are rarely labour-saving. This is suggested by real increases in the expenditure for pharmaceuticals and by the evidence derived from economic evaluation studies. Only a few of these studies have found that new technologies are cost-saving; more often they

Cost Containment and Health Care Reforms in the British NHS 777

suggest that technologies require additional resources. Paradoxically, adopting cost-effective technologies implies increasing costs.

Rising patient expectations are very important as well. The definition of health itself tends to be wider in more affluent societies, as it may include aesthetics and psychological welfare. It is also influenced by new technologies and by their availability in other countries. It is therefore likely that the expectations of people in the UK will rise in the future and that their satisfaction will be affected by the perception of the degree of completeness of NHS coverage. Education activities and encouraging public debate about priorities may alleviate the tension between what is expected and what is provided, because it may increase awareness of the scarcity of resources and of the benefits of rational approaches to deal with rationing. But it is unlikely that satisfaction with the NHS will be preserved if hard rationing becomes more explicit.

The unclear effect of technological change and rising expectations make uncertain the strength of demand pressure on the system. My impression is that this pressure is substantial and that implicit and explicit rationing decisions will become more common in the future. Since the UK has been successful in containing public and total health expenditure, the main point now is not how to further reduce NHS expenditure, but how to deal with the 'cost of cost containment', that is, how to improve cost-effectiveness and how to manage public support for a system where rationing mechanisms are becoming more evident.

The United Kingdom is an interesting case study and can provide a rich vein of experience for other European countries. Indeed, the NHS has been a sort of prototype that other countries have been examining carefully when they reform their own health care systems. The 1989 reforms seem to have further increased international interest in the NHS. In fact, both the internal market and the GP fundholding scheme can be considered large social experiments from which a tremendous amount of knowledge can be generated. Ironically, the evaluation of the 1989 reforms can be more interesting for other European countries than for the UK: the NHS has already been radically reformed, while in many other European Union members reforms are still under political discussion or are not yet implemented.

But caution has to be used in transferring policy and management solutions from one country to another, especially when there are large social and cultural differences. And transferring solutions from the UK should be done even more cautiously, since in many respects the UK is a peculiar country.

778   *Health Care and Cost Containment in the European Union*

For example, there is something unique in the strength of its public administration and in the bipolarism of its electoral and political system. There is some danger of the UK reforms being uncritically adopted by other European countries, especially by those of the southern part of the Union. While the health care systems in these countries do have similarities with the UK, their own social and cultural contexts are so different that successful policies in the UK risk becoming fiascos if uncritically transferred.

References

1   Le Grand J. Quasi-Market and Social Policy. *The Economic Journal* 1991;101:1256–67.

2   DoH. *Working for Patients*. London: HMSO, 1989.

3   Glennerster H. *Paying for Welfare: The 1990s*. New York: Harvester, 1992.

4   Liekerman A. *Public Expenditure: Who Really Controls it and How*. Harmondsworth: Penguin, 1988.

5   Thain C, Wright M. *The Treasury and Whitehall: The Planning and Control of Public Expenditure, 1976–1993*. Oxford: Clarendon Press, 1995.

6   OECD. *OECD Health Data 1996*. Paris: OECD, 1996.

7   Chew R. *Compendium of Health Statistics*. London: Office of Health Economics, 1995.

8   DoH. *Health and Personal Social Services Statistics for England. 1996 Edition*. London: The Stationery Office, 1996.

9   Ryan M, Birch S. Charging for health care: evidence on the utilisation of NHS prescribed drugs. *Social Science and Medicine* 1991;33(6):681–87.

10   *Annual Abstract of Statistics*. London: HMSO, various years.

11   O'Brien B. The effect of patient charges on the utilisation of prescription medicines. *Journal of Health Economics* 1989;8:109–12.

12   Lavers RJ. Prescription charges, the demand for prescription and morbility. *Applied Economics* 1989;21:1043–52.

13   Smith S, Watson S. Modelling the effect of prescription charge rises. *Fiscal Studies* 1990;1:75–91.

14   Hughes D, McGuire A. Patient charges and utilisation of NHS prescription medicines: some estimates using a cointegration procedure. *Health Economics* 1995;4:213–20.

15   Soumerai SB, Ross-Degnan D, Fortess E, Abelson J. A critical analysis of studies of state drug reimbursement policies: research in need of discipline. *The Milbank Quarterly* 1993;71(2):217–52.

16   Gerdtham U-G, Johannesson M. The impact of user charges on the consumption of drugs. *Pharmacoeconomics* 1996;9(6):478–83.

17   Brook R, Rogers WH, Keeler EB *et al*. Does free health care improve adults' health?

Cost Containment and Health Care Reforms in the British NHS 779

Results from a randomized controlled trial. *The New England Journal of Medicine* 1983; 309:1426–34.

18 Earl-Slater A. Privatizing medicines in the National Health Service. *Public Money and Management* 1996;1:39–44.

19 Reilly A, Brown D, Taylor RJ, Webster J. Effect of Limited List on drug use. *The Pharmaceutical Journal* 19 April 1986:480–482.

20 Harrison A (ed.). *Health Care UK 1995/96. An Annual Review of Health Care Policy.* London: King's Fund, 1996.

21 DoH. Research and Development. *Towards an Evidence-based Health Service.* Leeds: NHS Executive, 1995.

22 Henshall C, Drummond M. Economic appraisal in the British National Health Service: implications of recent developments. *Social Science and Medicine* 1994;38(12):1615–23.

23 DoH. *Report of the NHS Health Technology Assessment Programme 1995.* Leeds: Department of Health, 1995.

24 NAO. *National Health Service Supplies in England.* London: HMSO, 1996.

25 NAO. *Health of the Nation: A Progress Report.* London: HMSO, 1996.

26 NAO. *The NHS Executive: The Hospital Information Support Systems Initiative.* London: HMSO, 1996.

27 Audit Commission. *A Short Cut to Better Services: Day Surgery in England and Wales.* London: HMSO, 1990.

28 Audit Commission. *Lying in Wait: The Use of Medical Beds in Acute Hospitals.* London: HMSO, 1992.

29 Audit Commission. *A Prescription for Improvement: Towards More Rational Prescribing in General Practice.* London: HMSO, 1994.

30 Audit Commission. *Briefing on GP Fundholding.* London: HMSO, 1995.

31 Audit Commission. *What the Doctor Ordered: A Study of GP Fundholders in England and Wales.* London: HMSO, 1996.

32 Shaw CD, Brooks TE. Health Service Accreditation in the United Kingdom. *Quality Assurance in Health Care* 1991:3(3):133–40.

33 Scrivens E. *Accreditation: Protecting the Professional or the Consumer?* Buckingham: Open University Press, 1995.

34 Kerrison S, Packwood T, Buxton M. Monitoring medical audit. In: Robinson R, Le Grand J. *Evaluating the NHS Reforms.* London: Kings Fund Institute, 1994.

35 Maxwell RJ. Why rationing is on the agenda. In: Maxwell RJ (ed.). *Rationing Health Care.* London: Churchill Livingston: London, 1995.

36 New B. The rationing agenda in the NHS. *British Medical Journal* 1996;312:1593–601.

37 New B, Le Grand J. *Rationing in the NHS: Principles and Pragmatism.* London: King's Fund, 1996.

38 Harrison S, Hunter DJ. *Rationing Health Care.* London: Institute for Public Policy Research, 1994.

39 Maxwell RJ (ed.). *Rationing Health Care.* London: Churchill Livingston: London, 1995.

780 Health Care and Cost Containment in the European Union

40 Jacobson B, Bowling A. Involving the public: practical and ethical issues. In: Maxwell R J (ed.). *Rationing Health Care*. London: Churchill Livingston, 1995.

41 Redmayne S, Klein R. Rationing in practice: the case of in vitro fertilisation. *British Medical Journal* 1993;306:1521–24.

42 Robinson R, Le Grand J. *Evaluating the NHS Reforms*. London: Kings Fund Institute, 1994.

43 Dunleavy P, Hood C. From old public administration to new public management. *Public Money and Management* July–September 1994:9–16.

44 Propper C. Agency and incentives in the NHS internal market. *Social Science and Medicine* 1995;40(12):1683–90.

45 Propper C. Regulatory reform of the NHS internal market. *Health Economics* 1995;4:77–83.

46 Dixon J, Harrison A. A little local difficulty? *British Medical Journal* 1997;314:216–19.

47 Paton C. Present and future threats: some perverse incentives in the NHS reforms. *British Medical Journal* 1995;310:1245–48.

48 Weiner JP, Ferris DM. *GP Budget Holding in the UK: Lessons from America*. London: King's Fund Institute, 1990.

49 Coulter A. Evaluating general practice fundholding in the United Kingdom. *European Journal of Public Health* 1995;5:233–39.

50 Dixon J, Glennerster H. What do we know about fundholding in general practice? *British Medical Journal* 1995;311:727–30.

51 Petchey R. General practitioner fundholding: weighting the evidence. *The Lancet* 1995;346:1139–42.

52 Burr AJ, Walker R, Stent SJ. Impact of fundholding in general practice prescribing patterns. *Pharmaceutical Journal* 24 October 1992 (supplement).

53 Bradlow J, Coulter A. Effect of fundholding and indicative prescribing schemes on general practitioners' prescribing costs. *British Medical Journal* 1993;307:1186–89.

54 Maxwell M, Heaney D, Howie JGR, Noble S. General practice fundholding: observations on prescribing patterns and costs using the defined daily dose methods. *British Medical Journal* 1993;307:1190–94.

55 Stewart-Brown S, Surender R, Bradlow J, Coulter A, Doll H. The effects of fundholding in general practice on prescribing habits three years after the introduction of the scheme. *British Medical Journal* 1995;311:1543–47.

56 Wilson RPH, Buchan I, Walley T. Alterations in prescribing by general practitioner fundholders: an observational study. *British Medical Journal* 1995;311:1347–50.

57 Wilson RPH, Hatcher J, Barton S, Walley T. Influences of practice characteristics on prescribing in fundholding general practices: an observational study. *British Medical Journal* 1996;313:595–99.

58 Howie JGR, Heaney DJ, Maxwell M. Evaluating care of patients reporting back pain in fundholding practices. *British Medical Journal* 1994;309:705–10.

59 Coulter A, Bradlow J. Effect of NHS reforms on general practitioners' referral patterns. *British Medical Journal* 1993;306:433–37.

Cost Containment and Health Care Reforms in the British NHS   781

60 Surender R, Bradlow J, Coulter A, Doll H, Stewart Brown S. Prospective study of trends in referral patterns in fundholding and non-fundholding practices in the Oxford region, 1990–94. *British Medical Journal* 1995;311:1205–8.

61 Davies J. How much does the scheme cost? *Fundholding* 18 January 1995:22–4.

52 Laing W. *Laing's Review of Private Health Care*. London: Laing and Buisson Publications, 1996.

63 Besley T, Hall J, Preston I. *Private Health Insurance and the State of the NHS*. London: The Institute for Fiscal Studies, 1996.

64 Calnan M, Cant S, Gabe J *Going Private: Why People Pay for their Health Care*. Oxford: Oxford University Press, 1993.

65 Rentoul J. Individualism. In: Jowell R, Witherspoon S, Brook L (eds). *British Social Attitudes 7th Report*. Aldershot: Gower, 1990.

66 Taylor-Gooby, P. Attachment to welfare state. In: Jowell R, Brook L, Taylor B (eds). *British Social Attitudes 8th Report*. Aldershot: Gower, 1991.

67 Bousanquet N. Improving health. In: Jowell R, Curtice J, Brook L, Ahrendt D (eds). *British Social Attitudes. 11th Report*. Aldershot: Dartmouth, 1994.

68 DoH. *The New NHS: Modern, Dependable*. London: The Stationery Office, 1997.

69 Abel-Smith B. The first forty years. In: Carrier J, Kendall I. *Socialism and the NHS*. London: Gower Publishing, 1990.

70 Healthcare 2000. *UK Health and Healthcare Services: Challenges and Policy Options*. London: Healthcare 2000, 1995.

71 Maynard A. *Table Manners at the Health Care Feast. The Case for Spending Less and Getting More from the NHS* (LSE Health Discussion Paper No. 4). London: London School of Economics, 1996.

72 Dixon J, Harrison A, New B. Is the NHS underfunded? *British Medical Journal* 1997;314:58–61.

73 Harrison A, Dixon J, New B, Judge K. Can the NHS cope in future? *British Medical Journal* 1997;314:139–42.

74 Harrison A, Dixon J, New B, Judge K. Is the NHS sustainable? *British Medical Journal* 1997;314:296–98.

Index

Abel-Smith, B 164, 197, 199, 390, 775
Abril Martorell Report 419
accountability 248–59
accreditation 258–9, 755–7
Act on Freedom to Establish Private, Publicly-Funded Practices 709
activity-related payments 22–4
administrative costs 271–5, 570, 688
Advisory Council for Concerted Action in Health Care 90, 332
ageing 55–6
All Patients Diagnosis Related Groups (APDRGs) 22, 241
allocation of resources 436–7
Spain 436–7
Sweden 701, 705–6
alternatives to health insurance 642
alternatives to hospitals 282–4, 571, 685
ambulatory care
Austria 620–4
Germany 308–13
Portugal 649–50
analysis of data 209–10
Anatomical Therapeutic Chemical Classification 293
Andrade, A 655
Anell, A 701–31
Annemans, L 244, 251–2
assessment of technology, *see also* technology, 133-9
Association of British Neurologists 87
Association of British Pharmaceutical Industries 39
Association of General Practitioners 267
Association of Hospitals 569
Association of Municipalities 273
Association of Sickness Funds 127
Assurance-maladie 443–5, 448–58, 461, 463–7
Atkinson, AB 167
Audit Commission 570, 755–7, 762–3, 768
audits 433, 434–6, 755–7
Austria 605–33
auxiliary services 462

Average European Prices (AEP) 525
Aziende Sanitarie Locali 533

Badelt, C 630
bar code prescriptions 259
Barber, P 428
Basys-Study 616
Beech, R 132
Belgium 219–66
benchmarks 200–1
benefits 637–8
Berufsfreiheit 312
Bessis, N 365, 387
Beveridge model 303
biology 250–1, 462
biopharmaceuticals 86–7
Birch, S 29, 85, 747
Bismarck system 303, 605
Borst-Eilers, E 601
Britain 733–81
British Medical Journal 775
British Social Attitudes Survey 771
British United Provident Association (BUPA) 10, 104, 106, 487, 505
Brook, H 82
Buck, G 103–4
Budget Laws 422, 526
budgets 22–4, 65–8, 107–18
allocation 235–7
Denmark 271–5
Finland 666–73
Greece 363–5, 369–70
hospitals 275–7
Luxembourg 565–8
Netherlands 577, 588, 589–90
prospective 20–3
public 65, 106–7
shifting 62–5, 75–107
UK 735–8
Busse, R 115, 303–39

Caisse Médico-chirurgicale Mutualiste (CMCM) 555, 557
capital investment 237–9, 258
Finland 679–80

784 *Health Care and Cost Containment in the European Union*

Greece 385–8
Netherlands 594
Spain 425
care-of-the-elderly reform (ÄDEL) 707–8, 711–12, 716
carnet de santé 458, 465
Carte Sanitaire 444, 459
case-mix index (CMI) 489
cash benefits 596–7
Cash Plans 106
Catálogo de Prestaciones Sanitarias 420
Catálogo Nacional de Hospitales 416
Central Agency for Health Care Tariffs (GOTC) 22
Central Council for Health 368, 373, 379
Central Office on Health Care Prices (COTG) 24–5
Central Research Development Committee (CRDC) 752
Central Statistics Office (CSO) 478
Centre for Health Economics 501
Chamber of Physicians 609
charges 483–7
choice 288–9, 430, 690
Christiansen, T 267–301
Citoni, G 536
Clausen, J 267–301
Cleary, PD 131
Clinical Advice Reports 87
clinical biology reform 250–1
Closon, M-C 219–66
clubs 203–5
co-payments 10–13, 63–4, 75–83, 520
    Austria 624–6
    Finland 664, 674
    Portugal 642
    Spain 430–1
    UK 747, 768
    see also cost-sharing
Cochrane Centre 136, 753
Cochrane Collaboration 753, 755
Cohesian Fund 376, 386
Columbia/HCA Healthcare 10
Comas-Herrera, A. 197–218
Comhairle na n-Ospideal 492
Commission on Health Funding 472, 481–3, 506
Commission of Health Improvement 774
Commission of the Nomenclature 562
Commissione Unica per il Farmaco

(CUF) 524
Committee for the Health Sector 569
Committee on Hospital Deficits 371
Common Centre of Social Security 554
community care 230
community mental health services 283
Compensatory Fund 436
compulsory exceptional medical expenses scheme (AWBZ) 578–80, 584, 587, 590, 593–5
compulsory sickness fund scheme (ZFW) 578–80, 587, 590–1, 594
Consejo de Política Fiscal y Financiera 109, 413, 422, 436
constraints 422
consultation structure 249
Contracts and Agreements Commissions 237
contratos-programa 401, 416, 418, 421, 428
control 68–71, 118–33, 350–65, 367–79
    administrative costs 570
    drug expenditure 251–2
    Finland 679–80, 686, 689
    manpower 280, 569
    Netherlands 593–4, 597–8
    technology 133–9, 568–9
Conventions 444, 449, 456–7, 468
convergence 197–218
Copenhagen Hospital Cooperation 274, 281
Correia de Campos, A 635–60
cost containment
    Austria 606–11, 614–32
    Finland 674–92
    Italy 528–31
    macroeconomics 155–96
    Netherlands 589, 595–600
    overview 62–71, 71–143
    Portugal 643–57
    Spain 419–31
    UK 746–8, 758–61
cost-sharing 289–90, 324–8
    Austria 623–4, 624–6
    Belgium 254–7
    exemptions 740–2
    Finland 678
    France 444
    Greece 379–80, 385–8
    Luxembourg 556–8

Netherlands 591
Portugal 654–5
UK 740–6
Cost-weighted Activity Index 776
CosT(PACT) information system 748
Coulter, A 763
Council of Health Professionals 534
Council of Ministers 422
County Council Association 273
county councils 706–11, 719
Court of Justice 84
coverage 56–7
Crainich, D 219–66

Dagmar reform 704
Danish Council on Ethics 88–90
Danish County Councils 88–90
Danish Institute for Health Technology
    Assessment (DIHTA) 295
Dasgupta, R 130
data envelop analysis (DEA) study 680
day surgery 130–3
decentralization 532–3
decision-making 223
deductibles 292
Defever, M 201
deficits 370–2
Dekker Plan 581–3, 588
delisting 574, 590–1, 747
delivery systems 228–31
Delors II package 376
Delphi technique 91
demand 172–7
demography 174–5, 186–8
Denmark 87–90, 267–301
dental care 28–32, 231
    Denmark 290
    Finland 689–90
    Germany 313–15
    Greece 349–50
    Ireland 5–6–7
    Luxembourg 557, 560–2
    UK 740–1
Dental Health Action Plan 507
Department of Finance 107, 480
Department of Health (DoH)
    budget setting 107, 113
    Ireland 472, 475, 480, 487–9, 493–4,
        496–502, 505–6, 508
    technology assessment 136

UK 39, 60–1, 84, 733, 746, 752, 761–2,
    766, 771
VHI 106
Department of Social Welfare 475, 478,
    506
deregulation of fees 701, 707–8
deterministic trends 216–17
Dhoore Law 232
Di Biase, R 536
Diagnosis Related Groups (DRGs) 16–23,
    67, 69–71
    Austria 617–18, 624
    Belgium 241
    Denmark 277, 296
    direct controls 119
    Finland 682
    France 460
    Greece 392
    Ireland 489
    Italy 536
    Portugal 644, 648, 658
    Spain 417
    Sweden 710
    UK 750
direct controls 68–71, 118–33
Directors of Public Health 508
Disability Working Allowance 13
disease management guidelines (RMOs)
    124, 138
District Health Authorities (DHAs) 734,
    735
divergence 207, 208
diversity 199
Dixon, J 760, 763
doctors
    Austria 620–4
    Belgium 225
    Finland 677, 687–8
    France 456–8
    Luxembourg 556–7, 560–2, 569
    payment 24–6, 243
    Portugal 639, 642, 649–50
    Spain 429–30
    supply 26–7, 119–21
    Sweden 709
Drug Cost Subsidisation Scheme 485–6
Drug Refund Scheme 485–6, 502
drugs 291–3
    Denmark 251–2
    Finland 677–8, 689

786 Health Care and Cost Containment in the European Union

Spain 422–4
UK 740–1
see also pharmaceuticals
Drugs and Therapeutic Committee 483
Drummond, M 135
Dunning Committee 92, 99, 580, 598
Duphar Case 84

Economic and Monetary Union (EMU)
 159, 200, 343, 393, 658
economics literature 162–72
Effective Health Care Bulletins 748, 753
effectiveness 580, 776
efficiency 372–3, 580, 635, 646, 707, 776
Einheitlicher Bewertungs-Maßstab (EBM)
 308, 311
elderly 707, 708
Elderton, RJ 29
eligibility for health services 483–7
Elsinga, E 135
empirical remarks 162, 167–72
empirical results 178–90
Enemark, U 267–301
Engel Curve 163
Equipos de Atención Primaria 429
equity 295–6, 656–7, 691–3
Esping-Andersen, G 202, 212
Essential Scheme 106
ethics 88–90
European Commission 201, 342
European Economic Area 689
European Medicines Evaluation Agency
 86, 135
European Social Fund 472
European Union Cohesion Framework
 376, 386
Evaluation Commissions 249, 250
Evans, RG 140–1
Exceptional Medical Expenses Act
 (AWBZ) 581–2
Executive Letters 755
expenditure
 categories 51–3
 clubs 203–5
 macroeconomics 155–96
 trends 46–51
 upward pressures 53–61
Expenditure Committee of the Cabinet
 (EDX) 737
expensive pharmaceuticals 86–7

external factors 200–2

Family Budget Surveys 366–7, 377, 389
Family Credit 13
Family Doctor Act 709
Family Health Service Authorities
 (FHSAs) 734, 748, 762
Farmaindustria 116
Fattore, G 82, 201, 513–46, 733–81
Federal Association of Physicians 311,
 319
Federation of County Councils 711
*Federazione Nazionale degli Ordini dei
 Medici* 121
fee control 118–19
fee-for-service revenue 242
Ferrera, M 539
finance 3–13, 202–3, 232–46
 accountability 248–59
 capital investment 237–9
 clinical biology reform 250–1
 constraints 422
 Denmark 268–71
 information systems 599
 Ireland 480–1
 Portugal 656–7
 sources 3–5
 Spain 410–13; 425, 430–1, 436–7
 statutory health insurance 225–7
Finished Consultant Episode (FCE) 750
Finland 95–6, 661–99
Finnish National Research and
 Development Centre for Welfare and
 Health (STAKES) 95
Finnish Office for Health Care Technology
 Assessment (FinOHTA) 691–2
Finnish Slot Machine Association 679–80
Five Parties Agreement (FPA) 592
fixed reimbursement levels 126–30
Foreign Experts Committee 390–1, 395
Four Year Action Plan 508–9
France 91–2, 443–70
Friers, BE 44
Fuchs, VR 55
functions of hospitals 20–2
Fund for the Cross-Boundary Flow 436
fundholding 538, 623, 734, 748, 758,
 761–8
funding, *see also* finance, 258
The Future of General Practice in Ireland

494, 497

Garcia Cestona, MA 419
Garcia-Alonso, G 85
Geitona, M 359
General Board for Health Care Insurance 235–7
General Fund for Territorial Distribution 436
General Medical Services Committee 87
General Medical Services (GMS) 11, 56, 84–5, 493–4, 498–502
General Medical Services (Payments) Board 472, 486
General Practice Development Fund 497
General Practitioners (GPs) 483–5, 501
    agreements 285–8
    Ireland 509
    Italy 527
    Netherlands 575
    services 472, 493–8
    UK 735, 745, 747–8
    see also doctors
General Price Index 351
General Regional Health Organization Plans (SROS) 20
generality of benefits 637–8
generic prescriptions 292, 653, 707
Gerdtham, UG 60, 189
Germany 90, 303–39
Gesetz Verbesserung der Kassenärztlichen Bedarfsplanung 311–12
Gesetzliche Kranken-Versicherung (GKV) 7, 9, 303, 307, 313, 330
Getzen, T 202
Glennerster, H 763
global budgets 704
González, B 30, 426, 428, 430
Greece 341–400
Greek National Statistical Service 350
Grossman, M 162, 164
group practices 622–3
Guaranteed Health Care Entitlement (GHCE) 91, 98, 401, 422, 424–5
guidelines 124–5, 598–9
    Finland 688
    see also practice guidelines

Häkkinen, U 661–99
Harrison, A 55, 760

Harvey, AC 207
Health Authorities (HAs) 23, 28, 534–5, 538, 734, 740, 758, 760–1, 772–4
health benefits 558–60
Health Boards 21, 26, 33, 487–8, 506, 670
health care
    Austria 606–11
    delivery system 228–31
    Ireland 471–2, 472–80
    Luxembourg 550–1
    Netherlands 574–7
    Portugal 637–43
    spending 42–62
    Sweden 702–3
    systems 3–42
    UK 733–8
Health Care Prices Act (WTG) 24
Health Care Reform Act 129
Health Care Structure Act 115
Health Centres
    Spain 401, 429–30
    technology 649–50
Health Database 177, 186, 192, 208
Health Department 573–4
Health Directorates 370
Health Education Bureau 472
health expenditure
    Austria 611–14
    classification problems 43–5
    control 350–65
    convergence 197–218
    macroeconomics 155–96
    pressures 156–62
    Sweden 714–18
    value comparisons 45–6
Health Improvement Programmes 772
health insurance
    funds 225
    Greece 343–7
    Luxembourg 551–5
    Netherlands 578–87
    Portugal 642
    statutory 225–7
Health Insurance Access Act (WTZ) 586–7
Health Insurance Act 103, 503
Health Insurance Cost Containment Act 305
Health Insurance Council 597
Health Insurance Experiment (HIE) 81–2

788 *Health Care and Cost Containment in the European Union*

Health Insurance Funds Council 599
Health Maintenance Organizations
  (HMO) 10, 623, 761
Health and Medical Care Act 704
Health Services Executive Authority
  (HSEA) 482, 483
Health Tariff Act 592
Health Technology Assessment (HTA)
  committees 294–5
Health Technology Assessment
  Programme 753
health-status variable 175–6, 186–8
High Level Committee on Public Health
  91
history 20
  Belgium 221–3
  France 443–56
  Germany 305–8
  Ireland 471–2
  Italy 513–22
  Spain 410–13
  Sweden 714–18
Hospital Act 683
Hospital Association 566
Hospital Budget Commission 566
Hospital Co-ordination Fund (HCF) 23
Hospital Commission 296
Hospital Cost Containment Act 313
Hospital Council 26
Hospital Expenditure Stabilizing Act 320
Hospital Facilities Act (WZV) 122
Hospital Financing Act 304, 317
Hospital In-Patient Enquiry (HIPE) 489
Hospital Monitoring Agency 22
Hospital Restructuring Act 317
hospitals
  activities 20–2
  Austria 615–20
  beds 121–4, 374–7
  Belgium 260–3
  Denmark 275–82
  finance reform 248–50
  Finland 680–4
  France 459–60, 462
  Germany 315–20
  Greece 347–8, 367–77
  Ireland 487–93
  Italy 530–1, 535
  Luxembourg 557, 563–8, 571
  Netherlands 577, 589–90, 591

payment 16–24, 239–42
Portugal 639–40, 646–9
private 282
public 275–82
Spain 415–19, 425–9
UK 748–52
variables 176, 189–90
Howarth, C 303–39
Hsia, DC 70
Hughes, D 743–4
Hughes, J 471–511
Hurst, J 225, 226, 262, 344
Hutten, JB 36

impact of proposals 98–100
implementation problems 516–18
imports 293
in-patient care 595, 707, 768
income 178–86
Income Support 13
Indicative Prescribing Scheme (IPS) 748
indirect controls 68–71
individual responsibility 580
information systems 137–9, 599, 692
Initiative on Hospital Information Support
  Systems 756
innovation 596, 688
input control 119
INSALUD 403, 406, 409–12, 416, 420–1
  capital financing 425
  finance 436
  hospital financing 427–8
  policy-making 432
*Institut National d'Assurance Maladie
  Invalidité* (INAMI) 107, 224–5
  budget allocation 235
  clinical biology 250, 252
  community care 230
  consultation structure 249
  dental care 231
  fee-for-service revenue 242
  hospitals 248
  pharmaceuticals 244
  reform 219, 223, 226, 252–3, 258
Insurance Committee for Health Care
  113–14, 235, 237
insurance-based countries 211–13
Interministerial Committee on Economic
  Planning (CIPE) 133–5, 525
internal factors 198–200

internal markets 758–61
International Classification of Diseases (ICD) 617
International Labour Office 56
Interterritorial Committee 90
Investigative Medicine Committee 597
investment
  capital 237–9, 258
  Luxembourg 568–9
  Netherlands 594
  public hospitals 281–2
  Spain 425
Ireland 471–511
Irish Medical Organisation (IMO) 494, 496–7
Irish Pharmaceutical Health Care Association (IPHA) 498–9, 502
Italian Public Administration 534
Italy 513–46

Jarman score 762
Job Seekers Allowance 13
Joint Consultants Committee 87
Jönsson, B 60
Jospin government 468–9
Juppé Plan 443, 449, 463–6, 466–8

Kahan, JP 573–603
Kanavos, P 155–96, 208
Karokis, A 341–400, 377
KEMA organization 598
Kerkstra, A 36
Kesenne, J 257
Keynes, JM 200
King's Fund 756, 775
Klauber, J 129
Kleiman, E 163–4
Klein, R 203
Konzertierte Aktion im Gesundheitwesen 305
Koopman, SJ 207
Krankenschein 623
KRAZAF fund 609
Kyriopoulos, J 356, 359, 363, 387

Läanderskommission 618
Lancry, P-J 443–70
Lavers, RJ 744
Law of Hospitals 239
Le Fur, P 125

Le Grand, J 1–154
Leburton Law 222
length of stay 130–3
Ley de Presupuestos Generales del Estado 410
Ley General de Sanidad (LGS) 408, 428
Liaropoulos, L 389
limit-setting 735–8
literature 162–72
Local Health Care Units 142
Local Hospital Units (LHUs) 517, 519–22, 533, 534–5, 538–9
Lohr, KN 142
Loi de Financement de la Sécurité Sociale 467
long-term care 581–2, 595–6, 628–30
Long-Term Illness Scheme 485–6, 502
López, G 419, 426, 428, 429
Lopez I Casasnovas, G 401–41
Lopez-Bastida, J. 60, 414
LSE Health 664
Lucena, D 659
Luxembourg 547–72

Maastricht Treaty 200–1, 342, 362, 523, 658
McGuire, A 743–4
macroeconomics 155–96
Main Association of Social Insurance Funds 609
managerialism 533–5
manpower 280, 492
  Finland 686
  Luxembourg 569
  Netherlands 597
Mapelli, V 519
market initiatives 292–3
Maynard, A 775
medical aids 678–9
Medical Association 652
Medical Care Price Index (MCPI) 351–6
Medical College 562
Medical Council 225
medical equipment, see also technology, 568–9
medical guidelines 124–5
medical profession 177, 188–9
medical profiles 570
medical technology
  control 133–9

790 *Health Care and Cost Containment in the European Union*

see also technology
Medical Workforce Standing Committee 27
Medicare 70
medicijnknaak 594
Medicines Act 413
Medicines Evaluation Board 598
Meerding, WJ 55–6
mental health services 283
methodological issues 43–6, 205–8
microeconomics 164–7
migration of policies 201
Ministerial Decrees 86
Ministries of Health 21, 43, 87, 91
    Denmark 275, 277, 293
    France 449
    Germany 310, 318, 332
    Greece 344, 363–4, 368, 370, 372, 375, 390–3
    Ireland 482
    Italy 515, 518, 541
    Luxembourg 571
    Portugal 643, 644, 651
    priority setting 99
    reference price systems 127
    technology assessment 137
    VHI 102–3
Ministry of Budget and Economic Planning 531
Ministry of Defence 13
Ministry of Development 371, 382
Ministry for Economic Affairs 244, 254
Ministry of Economy 344
Ministry of Education 686
Ministry for the Family 571
Ministry of Health and Social Affairs 711, 715
Ministry of Health, Welfare and Sport 573, 586, 595
Ministry of Labour, Social Affairs and Health 607, 608
Ministry of Labour and Social Security 364
Ministry for Public Health 224, 227, 235, 238
    clinical biology 250
    hospitals 240, 248–9, 261
    pharmaceuticals 244
    technology 242
Ministry of Science, Transport and Arts 607

Ministry for Social Affairs, Belgium 223, 237, 243
Ministry of Social Affairs, Netherlands 597, 599
Ministry of Social Affairs and Health 668, 673, 679
Ministry of Social Security 547, 566
models 172–3, 207–8, 216
Morgan, M 131
Mossialos, E 1–154, 208, 212, 341–400, 547–72
MUFACE system 402, 421, 423, 430, 432–4
Multiple Sclerosis Society 87
Municipal Councils 670, 683
municipal service provision 666–71, 6746
Murillo, C 30, 430
Musgrave, RA 163
Mutualités 101, 112, 225
    budget allocation 237
    clinical biology 250–2
    dental care 231
    doctors 243
    hospitals 248–9
    INAMI reform 253
    pharmaceuticals 244
    prescriptions 259
    reform 219, 221–7, 257–8, 264–5
    technology 242
    VHI 232
Mutuelles 10, 32, 91, 444, 447
    France 455, 467, 469
    VHI 101

National Accounts
    France 445
    Greece 350, 356
    Ireland 478
National Advisory Ethics Committee 86
National Agency for Medicines 689, 692
National AIDS Council 86
National Audit Office (NAO) 755, 757
National Board for Drug Reimbursement 689
National Board of Health, Denmark 12, 137, 275, 280–2, 289
    quality assurance 295
    technology 295
National Board of Hospital Establishments (NBHE) 225, 238, 242

National Case-Mix Project 488
National Corporation of Swedish
  Pharmacies 713
National Drug Organization 383
National Drugs Formulary 500
National Health Fund 514
National Health Insurance (NHI) 110,
  661, 666, 671–3, 676–8
  Finland 687–8
National Health Service model 637
National Health Service (NHS) 27–30, 39,
  49, 84, 87, 733–8
  budget setting 107
  Cochrane Centre 136
  information systems 138
  policy migration 201
  reforms 199
  role 203
  technology assessment 136–7
  VHI 103–4
National Health System 369, 374, 389–90
National Hospital 269, 274
National Hospital Plan 568
National Institute of Clinical Excellence
  773–4
National Lottery 472
National Research and Development
  Centre for Welfare and Health
  (STAKES) 691
National Social Insurance Board 705, 708,
  713, 714, 720
necessity 580
need 701, 705–6
negative lists 84–6
Netherlands 92–5, 573–603
Netherlands Organization for Applied
  Science Research (TNO) 598
Networks of Primary Health Care 392,
  396
new products 86–7
New Public Management 759
Newhouse, JP 163–4, 167
NHS Centre for Reviews and
  Dissemination 753, 755
NHS and Community Care Act 734
NHS Executive (NHSE) 136, 756
NHS R&D Information Systems Strategy
  753
NHS R&D Project Registers System 753
NHS Trusts 103, 740, 758–60, 772–3

Niakas, D 356, 363, 387
Nolan, A 502
Nolan, B 487
non-convergence 212
Nonneman, W 228
North Western Health District, UK 132
Northern Ireland 734
numerus clausus 228, 259–60, 264, 456
nurses 283–4
nursing homes 283–4, 595–6
Nuttall, NM 29

objectives 198
O'Brien, B 85, 743–5
Office National de Sécurité Sociale
  (ONSS) 222, 223
office-based doctors 556–7
Offices for Health Assessment 426
Okma, KGH 573–603
ophthalmic services 740
opting-out 539–40
organization 202–3, 223–46, 225–7
Organization of General Practitioners in
  Denmark (PLO) 285, 287
out-of-hospital care 32–6
out-of-pocket payments 232
out-patient care 595, 707, 768
overview 1–154

Papandreou, A 391
parallel importation 293
Partido Popular (PP) 431–9
Patient Management Categories 417
patients
  choice 27–8, 288–9, 430
  cost-sharing 254–7
  Finland 690
Paton, C 760
Pay Related Social Insurance Scheme 506
Pay Related Social Insurance Treatments
  Benefits Scheme 481
payment
  doctors 24–6, 243
  hospitals 16–24, 239–42
  Netherlands 591–3
per diem charges 239–42
Pereira, J 635–60
Petchey, R 763
Pharmaceutical Price Regulation Scheme
  (PPRS) 38–9, 746

792 Health Care and Cost Containment in the European Union

pharmaceuticals 84–7
  Austria 626–7
  Belgium 244–6
  France 460–2
  Germany 320–4
  Greece 349, 381–5
  Ireland 498–502
  Italy 524–8
  Luxembourg 556, 562–3
  Netherlands 593–4
  Portugal 652–3
  reference pricing 126–30
  regulation 36–42
  Sweden 701, 713–14
  UK 746–8
  see also drugs
Pharmacy Benefit Managers (PBMs) 137
physicians, *see also* doctors, 308-13
Plan Beregovoy 455
Plan Seguin 455
planned markets 701, 710–13
policy migration 201
policy-making 362, 422–4, 431–9
  Austria 606–11
  Netherlands 588–600, 597
  Portugal 643–57
population 177, 190
Portugal 635–60
positive lists 84–6
Poulsen, PB 267–301
practice guidelines, *see also* guidelines,
  295, 598-9, 688
Prescribing Analysis 748
prescriptions 259, 291–2
pressures 156–62, 198–200
price agreements 293
prices 176–7, 190
Pricing Commission for Pharmaceutical
  Specialities 244
primary care
  Belgium 228–9
  Denmark 284–5
  Greece 348–9, 377–9
  Spain 429–30
  Sweden 701, 709
Primary Care Groups 16, 24, 113, 772–4
Primary Health Care Reform 421
Prior, D 429
priority setting 87–106
private health care

doctors 456–8
  expenditure 51–3, 365–7
  hospitals 282, 462, 531
  Italy 540–1
  Portugal 656
  Spain 407–8
  specialists 282–3
  UK 768–71
private health insurance
  Denmark 293–4
  Finland 690–1
  Germany 329–30
  Greece 388–9
  Ireland 503–5
  Netherlands 585–6
  Portugal 641
Private Medical Insurance (PMI) 768–71
Private Patients Plan (PPP) 10
*Programme de Medicalisation de
  Systemes d'Information* (PMSI) 460
proposals 296–8, 422, 432–4
propositions 208
Propper, C 760
prospective budgets 20–3
prostheses 678–9
Provincial Boards 679, 682, 684
provision 13–16, 650–2
public budgets 65, 106–7
Public Centres for Social Assistance
  (CPAS) 230
Public Expenditure Survey (PES) 734,
  735, 737–8
public health care expenditure 51–3,
  522–31
  Greece 359–61
  roles 203
  Spain 403–10, 413–15
  UK 738–40
Public Health Insurance 267, 271–5, 282,
  285, 287–8, 290
public hospitals 275–82
Public Servants Scheme 350, 363
Purchaser Efficiency Index 773
Purchasing Power Parities (PPPs) 41,
  45–7, 168–71, 173
  Greece 350
  Italy 525–6
  Luxembourg 550
  Spain 403, 406

Index 793

Quality Adjusted Life Years (QALYs) 93
quality assurance 295, 599–600, 691
quasi-markets 536–9, 772

Ramos, F 635–60
RAND Corporation 81–2
rationing 83–4, 558–60, 588, 757–8
Red Cross 403
Redmon, P 115
reference prices 126–30, 292–3
Reference Programmes 87, 295
Références Médicales Opposables
    (RMOs) 458, 462, 465–6
referral 690
reform 199, 219, 252–3
  Belgium 246–62
  clinical biology 250–1
  Greece 389–93
  hospital finance 248–50
  Italy 531–40
  Luxembourg 551–5
  Mutualités 257–8
  Portugal 640–3
  Spain 420, 422
  Sweden 704–14
  UK 734, 758–61
Regime General 443
Regional Doctors' Association (RDA) 117
regional governments 224
Regional Health Administration (RHA)
    642, 644, 650
Regional Health Authorities (RHAs) 406,
    426, 734, 763, 766
Regional Physicians' Associations 26
regular medical care 582–7
regulation 36–42, 408–10
Reichs-Versicherungs-Ordnung (RVO)
    303, 311–12
Reilly, A 747
reimbursement schemes 126–30, 291–2
Reis, V 635–60
Relative Value Scale 25–6, 29, 115
Research and Development Division 752
resources 232
responsibility 580
restrictions 64–5, 83–4
revenue 239–42
Revenue Commissioners 481
Root Mean Square Errors (RMSE) 207
Royal Belge 101

Royal College of General Practitioners 87
Royal Colleges 136, 757
Russell, LB 71
Rutten, FFM 135
Ryan, M 85, 747

Saez, M 189
Saltman, RB 537
Sandier, S 443–70
Schéma Régional d'Organisation Sanitaire
    (SROS) 459
Schulenburg, VD 118
Schwartz, FW 115, 201, 202, 213
Scotland 734, 749, 763, 766
Second Statutory Health Insurance
    Restructuring Act 75
secondary care 229–30
Secretary of State for Health 733, 758
Sécurité Sociale 454, 461, 463–4
Seehofer, H 332–3
Seguro de Assistencia Sanitaria 10, 103
Seguro de Reembolso 103
Sermet, C 125
setting, budgets 65–8, 107–118
Shaping a Healthier Future 492, 506,
    507–9
shifting of budgets 62–5, 75–107
Sickness Fund Council 99, 590, 599
Sickness Funds 7, 588
Sickness Funds Insurance (ZFW) 582–5
Simoes, J 635–60
single European market 104–6
Sissouras, A 341–400, 377
Sistema Nacional de Salud 415
Social Budgets 365, 367, 369, 378
Social Health Insurance Scheme 9
social insurance 5–9
social insurance funds 364–5, 475
Social Insurance Institute 671, 673, 678,
    689
social security 232
Social Security Medical Board 570
Societés d'assurance 101
Solà, M 429
sources of finance 232–5
Sozial-Gesetz-Buch (SGB) 303–5, 309,
    311–12, 321–2
Sozialhilfe 628
Sozialversicherung 606
Spain 90–1, 401–41

794 *Health Care and Cost Containment in the European Union*

Spanish Constitution 408, 435
Spanish Household Expenditure Survey 415
Spanish National Office of Technology Assessment 419
specialists 280–3
Specialty Costings programme 489
spending 42–62
Standing Group on Health Technology 753
Standing Medical Advisory Committee 87
Star Chamber 737
statutory health insurance 225–7
Statutory Health Insurance Restructuring Acts 332–3
Stockholm County Council 137
Strategy for Continuous Quality Development 295
structural time series models 207–8, 216
supplementary health insurance 587
supply
  doctors 26–7, 119–21
  restructuring 259–673
Supreme Council of Health Professionals 562
sustainability 410–13
Svarvar, P 701–31
Sweden 96–8, 701–31
Swedish Council on Technology Assessment in Health Care (SBU) 706
Swedish Parliamentary Priorities Commission 100

Target Budgets 748
Task Force on Health Care Information 599
tax-based countries 210–11, 212–13
taxation 5–9, 232
Taylor-Gooby, P 199–200
technology 57–61, 174, 189, 201–2, 242–3
  assessment 133–9
  Denmark 294–5
  Finland 691–2
  Greece 385, 387–8
  Ireland 505–6
  Luxembourg 568–9
  Netherlands 577, 597–8
  Portugal 648
  Spain 419
  Sweden 706

UK 752–5, 776–7
tests 206–7, 208, 217–18
theoretical issues 162–7
Theurl, E 605–33
Third Non-Life Insurance Directive 104–6
Transparency Commission 244
Treasury 137, 774
treatment restrictions 64–5, 83–4
Trident Management Consultants 498
Tyrie, A 200

UK Family Expenditure Survey 744
Unidades Ponderadas de Asistencia (UPAs) 416, 421
Unified Fund 391, 392
Union of Sickness Funds 113, 547, 550–5, 558, 566–7, 569
United Kingdom (UK) 733–81
universal coverage 637, 771
University of Dublin 501
upward pressures 53–61
utilization 743–6

Valor, J 426
Van Doorslaer, E 228
Van Het Loo, M 573–603
variables 174–7
Veil Plan 461
Veterans Affairs 70
Villalobos, J 426
visiting nurses 283–4
Voluntary Health Insurance Act 103, 503
Voluntary Health Insurance Board 103, 472, 481
Voluntary Health Insurance (VHI) 5, 9–10, 100–4
  Belgium 232
  Ireland 478, 487, 489, 503–5, 506
  Luxembourg 555
  Netherlands 587
  single European market 104–6
Voluntary Public Hospitals 21
von Otter, C 537

Wagner's Law 163
Wagstaff, A 427, 428, 429
waiting lists 280
Wales 734, 744, 749, 763
welfare convergence 199–200
Wennberg, JE 69–70

Wet op de Toegang tot Ziektekostenverzekeringen (WTZ) 586–7, 590–1
White Paper 733, 771–4
Wildavsky, A 1
Wilson, RPH 766
Working Group for Health Finance 413
Working for Patients 756
World Bank 201
World Health Organization (WHO) 201, 384

Yakobski, P 115
Yfantopoulos, J 155–96
Yule, B 82

Zammit-Lucia, J 130
Ziekenfondsraad 599
Zorgvernieuwingsfonds 596